Histology and Embryology

(Chinese and English Edition)

组织学与胚胎学（中英文版）

主　编◎郑英　傅奕

Editor-in-Chief Zheng Ying　Fu Yi

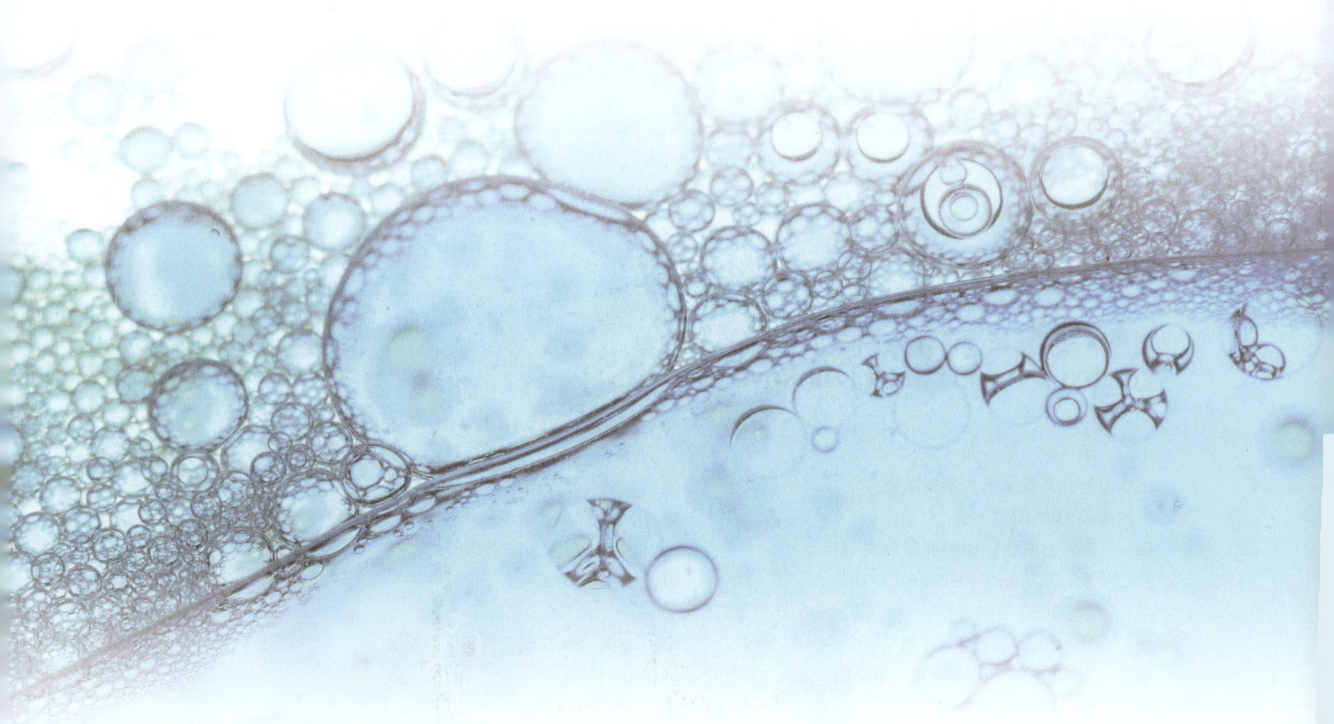

上海交通大学出版社

SHANGHAI JIAO TONG UNIVERSITY PRESS

内容提要

本书涵盖组织学和胚胎学两个部分，其中组织学包括四大基本组织、循环系统、免疫系统等共计 19 章，胚胎学包括胚胎发生总论、颜面和四肢的发生、消化系统的发生、呼吸系统的发生等共计 7 章。全书紧紧围绕医学各专业培养具有国际视野的复合型医学本科人才的目标，将英文和中文两种语言的内容结合起来，并配有中英文标注的高质量图片，便于读者学习。本书可供医学类各专业中外合作办学项目学生、国际医学生、医学类各专业本科生及研究生学习使用。

图书在版编目（CIP）数据

组织学与胚胎学：汉文、英文/郑英，傅奕主编.
上海：上海交通大学出版社，2025.7. —ISBN 978 - 7
- 313 - 32813 - 7

Ⅰ. R32
中国国家版本馆 CIP 数据核字第 20258M7L71 号

组织学与胚胎学（中英文版）
ZUZHIXUE YU PEITAIXUE（ZHONGYINGWENBAN）

主　　编：郑　英　傅　奕
出版发行：上海交通大学出版社　　　　　　　地　　址：上海市番禺路 951 号
邮政编码：200030　　　　　　　　　　　　　电　　话：021 - 64071208
印　　制：上海锦佳印刷有限公司　　　　　　经　　销：全国新华书店
开　　本：787mm×1092mm　1/16　　　　　印　　张：36.25
字　　数：1080 千字
版　　次：2025 年 7 月第 1 版　　　　　　　印　　次：2025 年 7 月第 1 次印刷
书　　号：ISBN 978 - 7 - 313 - 32813 - 7
定　　价：138.00 元

编委会

张　玲　　徐州医科大学

赵奕淳　　扬州大学

郑　英　　扬州大学

周慧萍　　扬州大学

祝　辉　　南京医科大学

Editorial Committee

Zhang Ling	Xuzhou Medical University
Zhao Yichun	Yangzhou University
Zheng Ying	Yangzhou University
Zhou Huiping	Yangzhou University
Zhu Hui	Nanjing Medical University

前　言

　　医学教育的核心在于培养兼具理论素养与实践能力的复合型人才,而教材作为知识传递的载体,需与时俱进地回应时代需求。在此背景下,我们编写了《组织学与胚胎学(中英文版)》教材,旨在为医学及相关专业学生、教师和临床工作者提供一部兼具科学性、前沿性与实用性的双语教学工具。

　　组织学与胚胎学是一门医学基础学科,由组织学和胚胎学两个部分组成,主要研究人体的正常组织结构和人体胚胎的正常发育过程。随着医学教育全球化的推进,双语教学已成为我国高等医学教育的重要模式。本教材基于组织学与胚胎学教学大纲,借鉴了国内外权威教材的组织架构,同时结合我国医学教育实际需求,删繁就简、优化编排,形成适应本土化双语教学的核心框架。教材以"结构-功能-临床"为主线,突出基础医学与临床实践的有机衔接,注重学科交叉与前沿进展的融入,旨在帮助学生掌握人体微细结构与胚胎发育规律,同时提升专业英语能力,为后续临床课程和科研工作奠定坚实基础。

　　本教材的编写有以下几个特点:①科学编排,层次清晰。教材分为组织学与胚胎学两大部分。组织学部分以四大基本组织为起点,逐步延伸至器官系统的显微结构,涵盖上皮组织、结缔组织、肌组织、神经组织,以及循环系统、免疫系统、内分泌系统、消化系统、呼吸系统、泌尿系统及生殖系统等,共计19个章节。胚胎学部分从胚胎发生总论出发,系统阐述生殖细胞的发生与成熟、三胚层分化、器官系统发育及先天畸形机制,特别强化消化系统、呼吸系统、泌尿生殖系统、心血管系统及神经系统等关键系统的器官发生内容。②双语对照,精准表达。教材采用中英文双语形式,英文内容部分精选自国际经典教材,语言规范且符合医学语境;中文部分由国内专家审校,确保术语准确性与表述流畅性,通过双语注释和示意图双重视角解析,助力学生突破语言与专业双重障碍。③图文并茂,资源立体。全书包含400余幅高清彩图,涵盖苏木精-伊红染色切片、电镜图像及三维模式图,直观展示细胞、组织的形态特征。

　　本教材由国内高校富有组织学与胚胎学教学经验的专家共同编写。编写过程中,编委们提供了大量原创切片照片,力求内容精准、视觉直观。此外,本书编写和出版过程中得到了苏州大学、南京医科大学、徐州医科大学、南方医科大学附属广东省人民医院及上海交通大学出版社等单位的大力支持。本书的出版得到了扬州大学精品本科教材建设工程项目及苏州大学的资助。在此表示衷心感谢。

　　本教材可供临床医学(MBBS)、护理学(中外合作办学)、基础医学、预防医学、医学检验技术、药学、中医学、中西医临床医学、口腔医学等专业国内外本科生及研究生使用,亦可作为高校教师、临床医师、医学类研究生的参考用书。

医学教育任重道远,教材编写亦需不断精进。尽管我们力求完美,疏漏之处仍在所难免,恳请广大师生与读者不吝指正,共同推动组织学与胚胎学教学的创新发展。

郑 英 傅 奕

2025 年 5 月

Prologue

The core of medical education is to cultivate interdisciplinary talents with both theoretical accomplishments and practical skills. As carriers of knowledge transmission, textbooks need to keep pace with times and meet the requirements of the era. Under the circumstances, we have compiled the textbook *Histology and Embryology (Chinese and English Edition)*, aiming to provide a scientific, leading and practical teaching tool for students majoring in medicine and related health sciences, teachers and clinical professionals.

Histology and Embryology is a fundamental medical discipline, in which Histology primarily studies the normal structures of tissues in human body and Embryology mainly focus on the developmental process of human embryo. With the advancement of medical education globalization, bilingual teaching has become an important model in China. This textbook is based on the syllabus, draws on the organizational structure of authoritative textbooks both domestically and internationally, and also considers the practical needs of medical education in China. It simplifies and optimizes content arrangement to form a core framework suitable for domestically bilingual teaching. It follows the "Structure-Function-Clinic" approaches, emphasizing the organic connection between the basic medicine and the clinical practice, and integrating interdisciplinary knowledge and cutting-edge advances. It aims to help students master the microstructure of human body and the embryonic development, and improve their professional English skills, laying a solid foundation for subsequent clinical courses and scientific researches.

This textbook has the following characteristics. ① It is scientifically organized with clear hierarchy. The textbook is divided into two major parts: Histology and Embryology. The Histology part starts with the four primary tissues, gradually extending to the microscopic structures of organs and systems, covering a total of 19 chapters including the epithelial tissue, connective tissue, muscular tissue, nervous tissue, and systems such as the circulatory system, immune system, endocrine system, digestive system, respiratory system, urinary system and reproductive system. The Embryology part begins with an overview of embryogenesis, systematically explaining the development and maturation of germ cells, three germ layer differentiation, organ and system development, and mechanisms of the congenital malformations, particularly emphasizing organogenesis in key systems such as the digestive system, respiratory system, urogenital system, cardiovascular system and nervous system. ② It is bilingually presented with precise expression. The English content is carefully adapted from international classic textbooks with standardized language, conforming to medical contexts. The Chinese content has been reviewed by domestic experts to ensure accuracy of terminology and fluent expression. Through bilingual annotations and schematic diagrams, it helps students overcome both language and professional barriers. ③ It is richly illustrated with comprehensive resources. The book includes over 400 high-definition images, covering HE-stained sections, electron microscope images and three-dimensional model diagrams, visually displaying the morphological features of cells and tissues.

This textbook was co-authored by experienced experts in Histology and Embryology from domestic universities. During the writing process, the authors provided a large number of original histological images, striving for accurate content and intuitive visual presentation. Moreover, we received strong supports from Soochow University, Nanjing Medical University, Xuzhou Medical University, Guangdong Provincial People's Hospital Affiliated to Southern Medical University and Shanghai Jiao Tong University Press. The publication of this textbook was funded by Yangzhou University's Quality Undergraduate Textbook Construction Project and Soochow University. We express our heartfelt thanks for all the supports.

This textbook is suitable for both domestic and international undergraduate and postgraduate students majoring in Clinical Medicine (MBBS), Nursing (Sino-Foreign Cooperative Program), Basic Medicine, Preventive Medicine, Medical Laboratory Technology, Pharmacy, Traditional Chinese Medicine, Clinical Medicine of Chinese and Western Medicine, and Stomatology. It can also serve as a reference book for university faculties, clinicians, and medical postgraduate students.

Medical education carries a heavy burden of responsibility and still has a long way to go, so the textbook compilation requires continuous improvement. Despite our efforts to achieve perfection, some flaws and omissions are inevitable. We sincerely welcome comments and suggestions from teachers, students and readers to jointly promote the innovative development of Histology and Embryology teaching.

Zheng Ying, Fu Yi
May 2025

目　　录

Chapter 1

Introduction to Histology

1 Definition of Histology

Histology is defined as the scientific study of microscopic anatomy of human tissues and their related biological functions. The study includes not only tissues, but also cells, organs and systems.

The cell is the basic structural and functional unit of life forms. There are over 200 different cell types and 60×10^{12} cells in the human body. Each type of cells shows specialized morphology due to their unique functions.

Tissues are made of cell populations and intercellular substance, which show similar morphology and functions. Intercellular substance is also known as intracellular matrix, which is produced by cells. Four fundamental tissues are recognized according to the origin in embryology, the morphology and functions of cells and intercellular substance: epithelial tissue, connective tissue, muscular tissue, and nervous tissue.

Organs, which consist of four fundamental tissues, have unique morphology and biological functions. They can be classified as solid organs or hollow organs due to the differences in anatomy. The hollow organs are the heart and blood vessels of the circulatory system, the stomach and intestines of the digestive system and so on. There are central lumen and walls with multiple layers in these organs. For example, the wall of digestive tract is divided into four layers: the mucosa, submucosa, muscularis, and serosa; the wall of blood vessels is divided into three layers: the tunica intima, tunica media, and tunica adventitia. The solid organs are the liver, pancreas, thymus, spleen, lung, kidney, etc. They consist of the capsule, parenchyma and stroma. Most capsules are made of the connective tissues; the parenchyma, which is composed of the cells with unique functions and intercellular substance, is essential to the normal specific physiological functions of organs; the stroma is composed of the connective tissue, blood vessels, nerves, lymphatic vessels, etc.

The system, which is composed of the organs with different morphology, structural continuity and similar functions, has specialized biological functions, such as the digestive system, the respiratory system, and so on.

Histology is an important basic medicine course, which is closely related to the other medicine courses including physiology, pathology, internal medicine, obstetrics and gynecology, pediatrics and so on. With the moving forward of researches of life science, histology is constantly updated and more closely related to other courses of life science. Therefore, mastering microscopic anatomy of human tissues systematically by learning theory of histology and observing tissue slides will lay a solid foundation of morphology for medical students to learn other medical courses.

2　Methods of Study

2.1　Light Microscopy

The microscopic structures of tissues are usually observed under microscope in histology. The most common length unit of light microscopy is micrometer (μm), which of electron microscopy is nanometer (nm).

2.1.1　Ordinary Light Microscopy

The most common procedure used in the study of histology and embryology is observing the microscopic structures of the organism under light microscope. The light microscope allows magnifications of $1\,000\sim1\,500$ times with a resolution of $0.2\,\mu$m. Tissue slides should be prepared and stained before observation using microscope. The preparation methods include sectioning and non-sectioning.

2.1.1.1　Sectioning

Paraffin sectioning is the most commonly used technique including several steps: sampling, fixation, dehydration, transparency, embedding, sectioning (thickness 5 – 8 μm), staining, mounting. The most common staining procedure is the combination of hematoxylin and eosin (HE). Tissue components that stained more readily with basic dyes are termed basophilic; those with a high affinity for acid dyes are termed acidophilic; those with a low affinity for both basic dyes and acid dyes are termed neutrophilic. Hematoxylin behaves like a basic dye, that is, it stains the acidophilic tissue components including cell nucleus and ribosomes of cytoplasm. Eosin is an acid dye, which can stain cytoplasm and collagenous fibers red (Figure 1 – 1). There are also some other dyes such as silver nitrate and toluidine blue. Silver stains the tissue components brownish-black with (argentaffin) or without the supplementation of reducing agents (argyrophilic) (Figure 1 – 2). The colour that toluidine blue stains the tissue components are different from the colour of the dye itself, which is termed metachromasia. Besides paraffin sectioning, frozen sectioning is also performed for the detection of unstable active substances and quick pathological diagnosis by freezing and sectioning tissues quickly with the liquid nitrogen and freezing microtomes.

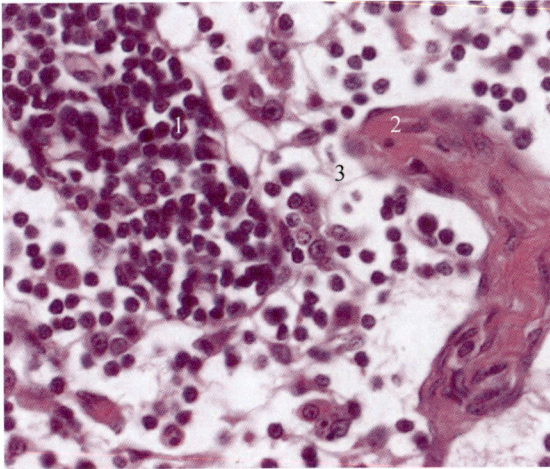

1. Basophilic; 2. Acidophilic; 3. Neutrophilic
Figure 1 – 1   Hematoxylin and eosin staining (HE, Lymph node)

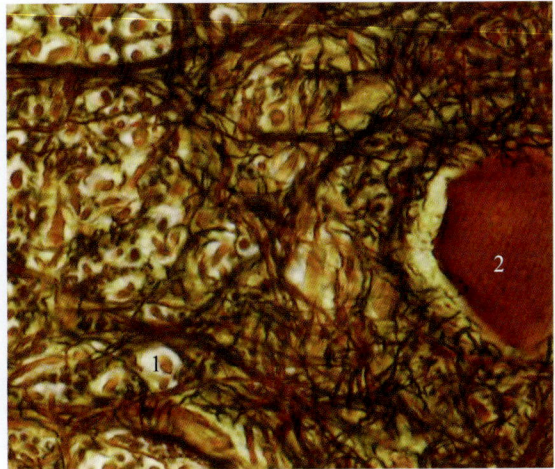

1. Nerve fiber; 2. Neuron
Figure 1 – 2   Silver nitrate staining (Spinal cord)

2.1.1.2   Non-Sectioning

In a smear preparation, liquid samples including the blood and cerebrospinal fluid can be spread over a small area of the microscope slide, dried, fixed, and then stained (Figure 1 – 3). In a stretched preparation, soft tissues including the connective tissue and mesenteries can be spread in a thin film over slides (Figure 1 – 4), dried, fixed and then stained. Cutting and grinding methods are designed for the preparation of slides of hard tissues such as bones, teeth, and so on (Figure 1 – 5).

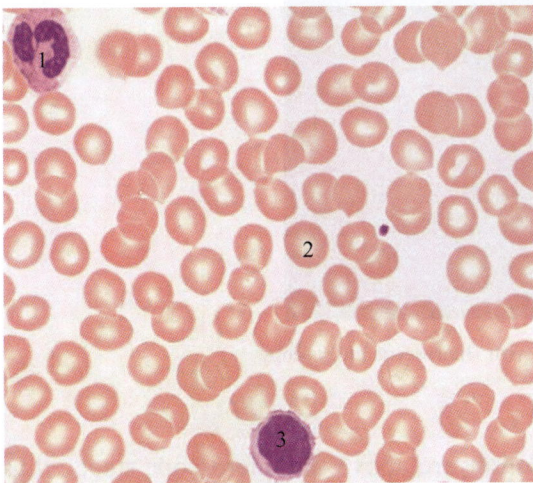

1. Neutrophil; 2. Erythrocyte; 3. Lymphocyte
Figure 1 – 3   Blood smear (Wright stain)

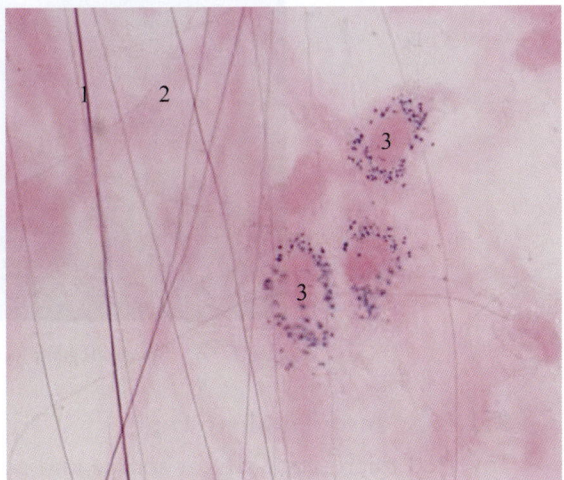

1. Elastic fiber; 2. Collagen fiber; 3. Macrophage
Figure 1 – 4   Loose connective tissue spread (Special stain)

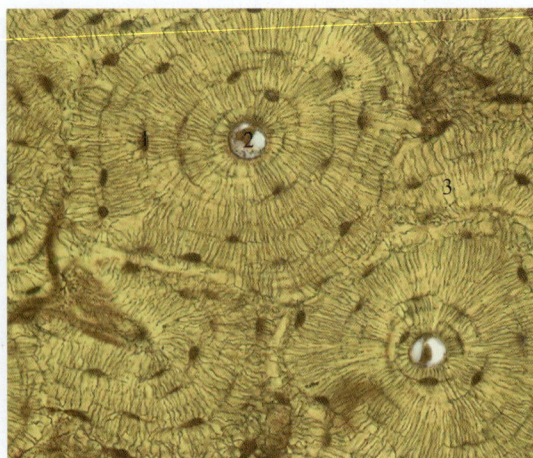

1. Osteon; 2. Central canal; 3. Interstitial lamellae

Figure 1 – 5   Long bone (Thionine staining)

2.1.2   Special light microscopy

2.1.2.1   Fluorescent microscopy

Generally, high-pressure mercury lamps and arc lamps are used as light sources to excite fluorescent molecules in biological samples to emit fluorescence. Fluorescence microscopy can be performed to identify, localize and quantitate specific substances by determining the distribution of fluorescent molecules (Figure 1 – 6).

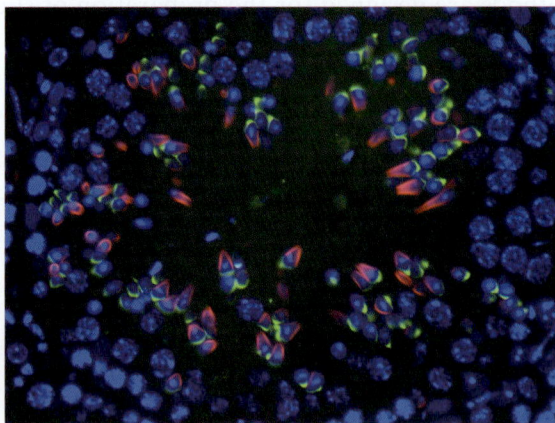

Figure 1 – 6   Spermatogenic cells with fluorescent microscopy

2.1.2.2   Inverted Microscopy

Inverted microscope's light source and condenser are above the microscope stage, thus increasing the height of the stage to place the sample. It is useful for observing cultured cells in vitro, and checking cell growth continuously.

2.1.2.3   Phase Contrast Microscopy

It is based on the principle that light changes its speed when passing through cellular and extracellular structures with different refractive indices. These changes are used by the phase contrast system to cause the structures to appear lighter or darker relative to each other, which makes this kind of microscopy a powerful tool to observe living cells. An inverted phase contrast microscope is made from the phase contrast microscope and inverted microscope, which can be used to study the biological processes of living cells including morphology, division, proliferation, movement and so on (Figure 1 − 7).

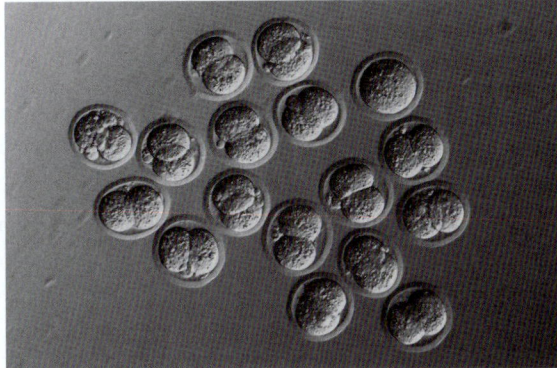

Figure 1 − 7　Appearance of two-cell embryos in phase-contrast microscopy

In addition, there are ultraviolet microscopes, confocal microscopes and so on. The ultraviolet microscope is designed to determine the distribution and quantification of nucleic acids. The confocal microscope can be used to reconstruct the three-dimensional structure of cells and perform quantitative analysis of stereology.

2.2　Electron Microscopy

Electron microscopy is a technique using the beam of electrons instead of the visible light, and the electromagnetic lens instead of the optical lens. The image can be finally projected on a fluorescent screen. Ultrastructure will be observed under the electron microscope. At present, the commonly used electron microscopes are transmission electron microscope and scanning electron microscope.

2.2.1　Transmission Electron Microscopy

The transmission electron microscope is an imaging system that permits a very high resolution (0.2 nm), which allows magnifications of up to hundreds of thousands times. To provide a good interaction between the specimen and the electrons, electron microscopy requires ultrathin sections (50 − 80 nm). The preparation procedure includes fixation with glutaraldehyde and osmic acid, dehydration, embedding in epoxy resins, sectioning and staining. The beam of electrons passes through the specimen, and the electrons either scatter or hit a fluorescent screen. An image of the specimen with its assorted parts shown in different shades according to its density appears on the screen. Dark areas of an electron micrograph are usually called electron dense, whereas light areas are called electron lucent

(Figure 1 – 8).

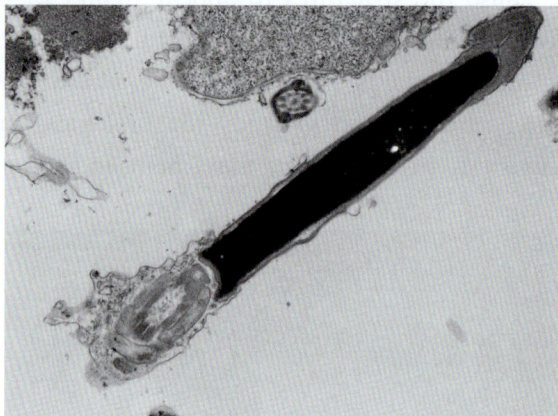

Figure 1 – 8   The ultrastructure of sperm in transmission electron microscopy

2.2.2   Scanning Electron Microscopy

This electron microscopy produces a very narrow electron beam that is moved sequentially (scanned) across the surfaces of the specimen. Then the electrons are captured by a detector that transmits them to amplifiers and other devices so that in the end the signal is projected into a cathode ray tube (a monitor), resulting in a black-and-white image. The resolution of this electron microscopy is around 2 nm, and it can be used to observe the surface morphology and 3-dimensional structure of the tissues and cells (Figure 1 – 9).

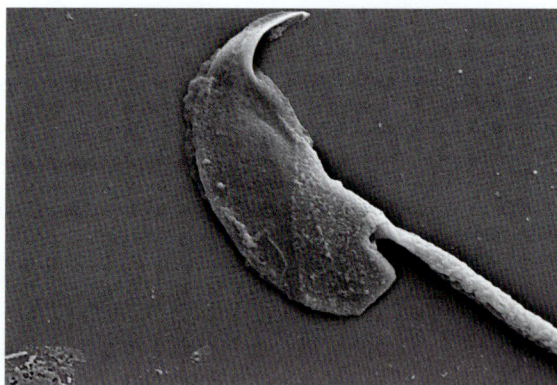

Figure 1 – 9   The morphology of sperm in scanning electron microscopy

2.3   Other Histological Techniques

2.3.1   Histochemistry and Cytochemistry

The terms histochemistry and cytochemistry are based on specific chemical reactions or on high-affinity interactions between macromolecules. These methods usually produce insoluble colored or electron-dense compounds that enable the localization of specific substances by means of light or electron microscopy. For example, the periodic acid—Schiff (PAS) reaction can detect the polysaccharides or proteoglycans in cells and tissues (Figure 1 - 10). The periodic acid oxidizes the polysaccharides to aldehydes, which combines with the Schiff's reagent (fuchsin and sodium bisulfite) to produce a purple or magenta colour.

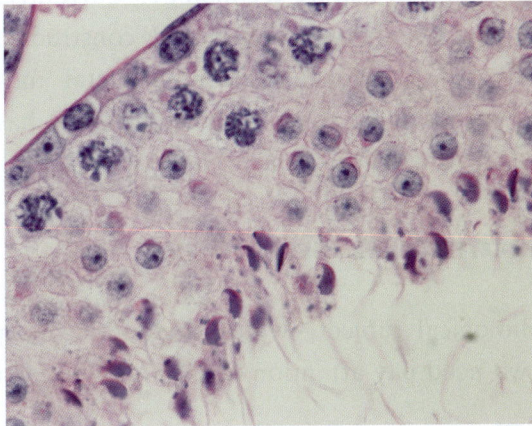

Figure 1 - 10   Periodic acid-Schiff (PAS) staining (Testis)

2.3.2   Immunochemistry and Immunocytochemistry

This technique is used for the localization and quantification of the peptides and proteins in cells and tissues, which is based on the highly specific interaction between an antigen and its antibody. To detect a specific antigen such as peptide or protein, the antibody that reacts specifically and binds to this antigen will be marked with a label, and then the antigen can be detected under microscope. The most commonly used labels are fluorescent compounds (fluorescein isothiocyanate), enzymes (horse radish peroxidase), etc.

2.3.3   In Situ Hybridization

In Situ Hybridization (ISH) is also known as the nucleic acid hybridization histochemistry for the localization of specific RNA or DNA sequences in a portion or section of tissue. The principle is RNA or DNA sequences in tissue sections or cells are hybridized with a segment of single-stranded DNA or RNA called as probe that is complementary to the target sequence. The probe must be tagged with a label, usually a radioactive isotope, digoxygenin or fluorescein, which can be identified by immunocytochemistry.

2.3.4   Cell and Tissue Culture

Cell and tissue culture is a technique that living tissues or cells are collected and cultured in vitro for experiments (Figure 1 - 11). The culture medium, temperature, concentrations of O_2 and CO_2, and pH are all critical for the long-term expansion of cells. Flasks, dishes, and plates are commonly used for in vitro culture. The proliferation,

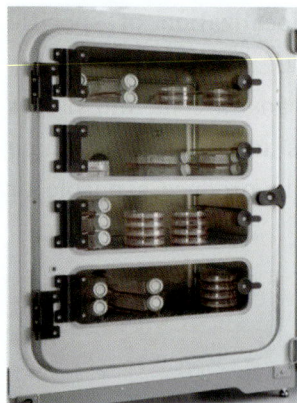

Figure 1 - 11　Cell incubator

differentiation, phagocytosis and other biological processes of cells can be observed and recorded under the inverted phase contrast microscope. This technique can be used to study the effects of various factors on living cells, which is difficult to achieve in vivo experiments. Tissue engineering is a technology that simulates the construction of body tissues or organs in vitro using cell culture technology. Currently, the tissues and organs that are being studied and constructed mainly include skin, cartilage, bone, tendon, skeletal muscle, blood vessel and cornea. The tissue-engineered skin has been used in clinical treatment for burns, venous skin ulcers, etc.

3　Learning Methods in Histology

Histology is a morphological subject, which studies the morphology and its related functions. In the study, we need pay attention to the following points.

3.1　Combination of Theory and Practice

In the study of histology, the combination of theory and practice is essential. Remembering the illustrations with the description in the books, observing the slices carefully in the classes, and understanding the relationship between histological theory with the images, which are all essential and effective ways to learn histology and embryology.

3.2　Combination of Morphology and Function

Histology is the study of the microstructure of the organism and its related functions. The unique functions of the cells and tissues are based on their specific morphology, and the specific morphology is also essential to the unique biological functions. So, it will be beneficial to study the histology when combining the morphology and functions of the organism. For example, abundant ribosomes in the cytoplasm cause increased cell protein synthesis, and HE staining will stain the cytoplasm blue because of the nucleic acid in the ribosomes. Rich mitochondria in the muscle fibers will supply energy to the skeletal muscle contraction. Macrophages are professional phagocytes because they contain more lysosomes, phagosomes, pinocytotic vesicles, etc.

3.3　Combination of Two Dimensions and Three Dimensions

When a three-dimensional volume is cut into very thin sections, the sections seem to have only two dimensions: length and width. For example, not all neurites of a neuron can be observed in one section. It is difficult to find the primary oocyte in some sections of the secondary follicle. The inner and outer layers of the muscle fibers of the intestinal tract show different under the microscope. Therefore, in the learning process, we should actively cultivate our spatial thinking ability, and strive to restore two-dimensional images to the three-dimensional structure, so as to better understand the structure of the organ.

3.4 Combination of Similarity and Difference

The comparative analysis could be performed to determine the similarity and difference in the structure and functions of the organism. The human body has many organs with different structures. However, the general structural framework of the organ can be deduced if we know it is a hollow or solid organ. Then we can deduce the structural characteristics of each part according to the unique functions of this organ. Finally, there will be a basic and flexible grasp of the organ structure.

3.5 Combination of Occurrence, Development and Evolution

The morphological structures of human organs are gradually formed in the long-term evolution from low level to high level, from simple to complex. The tissues have been in the dynamic changes of metabolism, development and differentiation.

In brief, correct learning methods can improve learning efficiency, firmly grasp knowledge, and flexible apply the basic medical theories to other disciplines.

(Zhou Huiping, Zheng Ying)

第一章　组织学绪论

第一节　组织学的定义及研究内容

组织学是研究人体的微细结构及其相关功能的科学,其研究内容包括细胞、组织、器官及系统。

细胞是机体形态结构和功能活动的基本单位。人体由 200 多种、约 60×10^{12} 个细胞组成,这些细胞由于承担的功能不同而形态各异。

组织由形态和功能相似的细胞群和细胞间质有机结合而成。细胞间质又称为细胞外基质。细胞间质由细胞所产生。根据胚胎时期的发生来源、细胞与细胞间质的形态及功能等可将组织分为上皮组织、结缔组织、肌组织、神经组织 4 种。

器官由 4 种基本组织按不同数量和不同方式组合而成,具有特定的形态和功能。根据结构的不同,人体器官可分为中空性器官和实质性器官两大类。中空性器官,如循环系统的心脏、血管,消化系统的胃、肠等。这些器官中央有管腔,管壁可分为不同层次,如消化管管壁可分为黏膜、黏膜下层、肌层和外膜四层,血管管壁可分为内膜、中膜和外膜三层。实质性器官,如肝、胰腺、胸腺、脾、肺和肾等,其结构一般包括被膜、实质和间质三部分,被膜大多由结缔组织构成;实质由各器官具有特异性功能的细胞和间质构成,是各器官完成特异性生理功能的基础;间质一般由结缔组织、血管、神经、淋巴管等构成。

系统是形态各异、结构连续、功能相关的器官按照一定的顺序组合而成,能够完成特定的生理功能,如消化系统、呼吸系统等。

组织学是重要的医学基础课程,与生理学、病理学、内科学、妇产科学、儿科学等其他医学课程有着密切的联系。随着生命科学研究的不断深入,组织学内容不断更新,与当代生命科学各学科相互渗透、相互促进,关系日益密切。因此,医学生通过对组织学理论知识的学习及组织切片的观察,系统地掌握正常人体的微细结构,可为学习其他医学学科奠定良好的形态学基础。

第二节　组织学的基本研究方法

一、光学显微镜技术

组织学主要用显微镜观察组织的微细结构,常用的光镜长度单位为微米(μm),电镜的常用长度单位为纳米(nm)。

(一) 普通光学显微镜

应用光学显微镜观察机体微细结构是组织学与胚胎学最常用的研究方法。光镜可将观察的物象放大 1000～1500 倍,分辨率可达 0.2 μm。用显微镜观察前需将观察的材料制成很薄的标本并进行染色,制作方法包括切片法和非切片法。

1. 切片法

石蜡切片术是最常用的技术,其基本程序如下:取材、固定、脱水、透明、包埋、切片(厚度 5～8 μm)、染色、封片。最常用的染色法是苏木精-伊红染色法,又称 HE 染色法。苏木精为碱性染料,主要使胞核内染色质与胞质内核糖体染成紫蓝色,组织结构与碱性染料亲和力强的现象称嗜碱性;伊红为酸性染料,可使细胞质和胶原纤维等染成粉红色,与酸性染料亲和力强的现象称嗜酸性。对碱性和酸性染料亲和力均不强的结构,称中性(图 1-1)。除 HE 染色法外,还有许多特殊染色方法。如银染法,即用硝酸银染色,使相应的组织结构呈棕黑色(图 1-2)。组织结构直接使硝酸盐还原显色称亲银性;添加还原剂使硝酸银还原显色称嗜银性。有些结构染色后所呈现的颜色与所用染料的颜色不同,如甲苯胺蓝染色肥大细胞时,其颗粒显示为紫红色,称为异染性。除石蜡切片法外,还有冷冻切片法,即应用液氮、低温制冷装置和恒冷切片机等将组织迅速冷冻并切片,常用于不稳定活性物质的研究和快速病理诊断。

2. 非切片法

血液和脑脊液等液体样本,可直接在载玻片上涂片,干燥后再进行固定和染色,称涂片法(图 1-3)。疏松结缔组织和肠系膜等软组织,可在载玻片上铺开展平,制成薄片,待干燥后进行固定和染色,称为铺片法(图 1-4)。骨和牙等坚硬组织可直接磨成薄片进行染色观察,称为磨片法(图 1-5)。

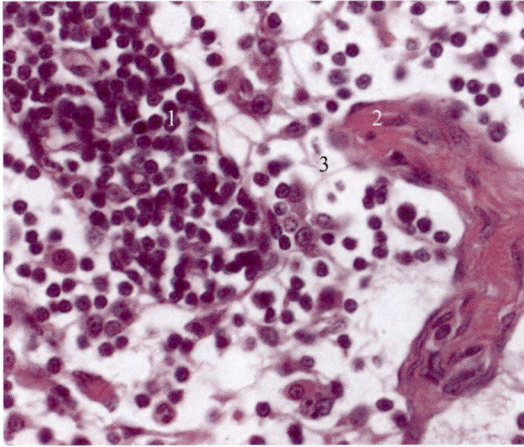

1—嗜碱性;2—嗜酸性;3—中性
图 1-1　HE 染色法(淋巴结)

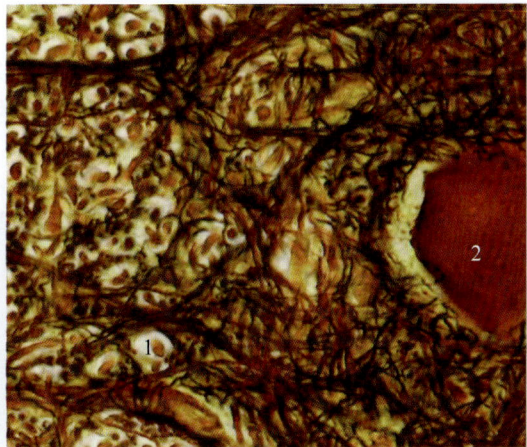

1—神经纤维;2—神经元
图 1-2　硝酸银染色法

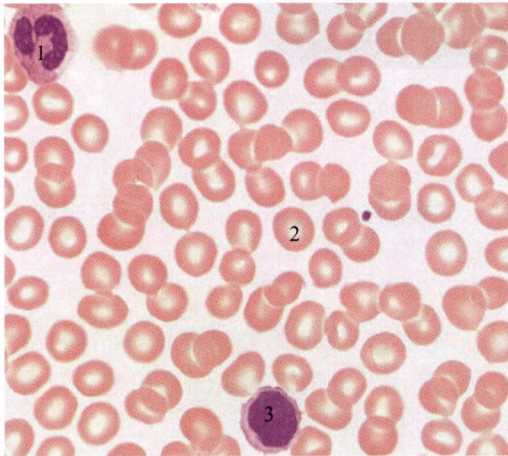

1—中性粒细胞;2—红细胞;3—淋巴细胞
图 1-3　血涂片

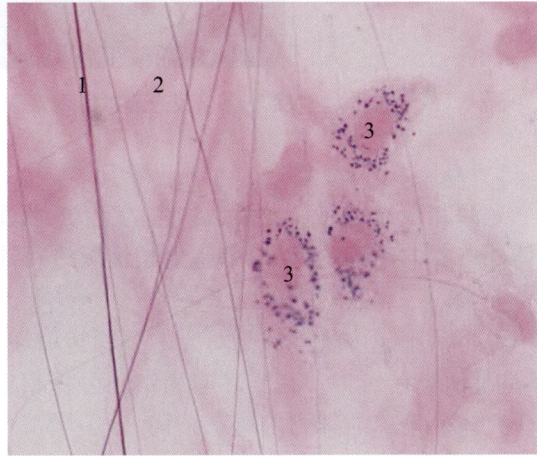

1—弹性纤维;2—胶原纤维;3—巨噬细胞
图 1-4　疏松结缔组织铺片(特殊染色)

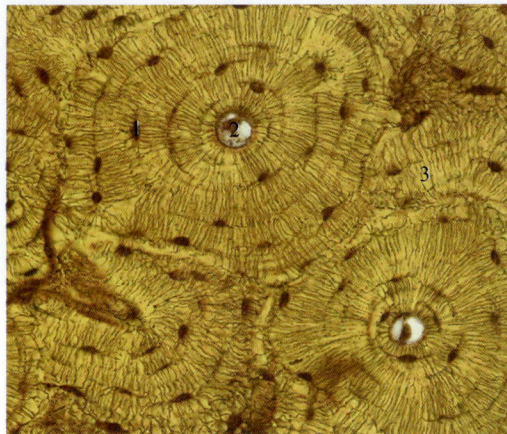

1—骨单位;2—中央管;3—间骨板
图 1-5　长骨磨片(硫堇染色)

(二)几种特殊的光学显微镜

1. 荧光显微镜

一般采用高压汞灯和弧光灯作为光源,激发生物样本中的荧光物质,产生各种荧光。利用荧光显微镜可研究荧光物质或带有荧光标记的物质在组织细胞中的分布,以达到对特定物质进行定性、定位和定量观察的目的(图1-6)。

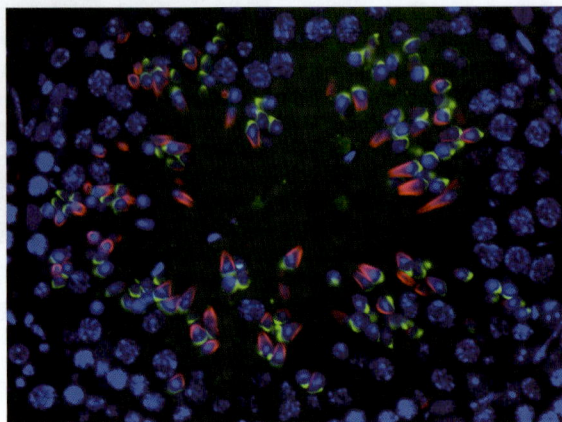

图 1-6　荧光显微镜观察睾丸中生精细胞的亚细胞结构

2. 倒置显微镜

光源和聚光器在显微镜载物台的上方,从而增大了载物台放置样本的高度。主要用于观察体外培养的活细胞,可对细胞生长情况进行连续观察。

3. 相差显微镜

可将活细胞内各种结构对光的不同折射转换为光密度差异(明暗差),使镜下结构反差明显,呈现清晰的影像。在实际应用中还可将相差显微镜和倒置显微镜制成倒置相差显微镜,用于研究体外培养活细胞的形态结构、分裂增殖及运动等过程(图1-7)。

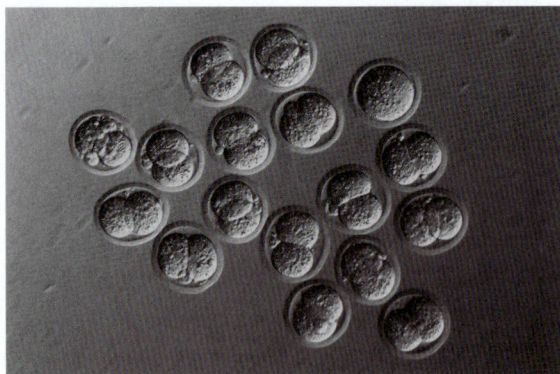

图 1-7　相差显微镜观察二细胞期胚胎

此外,还有用来研究核酸分布和定量的紫外光显微镜,以及能重建细胞三维结构、进行体视学定量分析的激光扫描共聚焦显微镜等。

二、电子显微镜技术

电子显微镜技术简称电镜技术,是以电子束代替可见光,以电磁透镜代替光学透镜,最后将物像投射到荧光屏上进行观察。在电镜下可以观察到的结构,称为超微结构。目前常用的电镜有透射电镜和扫描电镜。

1. 透射电镜

透射电镜的分辨率为 0.2 nm,放大倍数为几万到几十万倍。用透射电镜观察的样本必须制备成超薄切片(通常厚为 50~80 nm)。其制备过程主要包括戊二醛和锇酸固定、脱水、环氧树脂包埋、超薄切片机切片、电子染色等。电子束投射到样本时,可随组织构成成分的密度不同而发生相应的电子散射,如电子束投射到质量大的结构时,电子被散射的多,因此投射到荧光屏上的电子少而呈暗像,称为电子密度高;反之,则为低电子密度(图 1-8)。

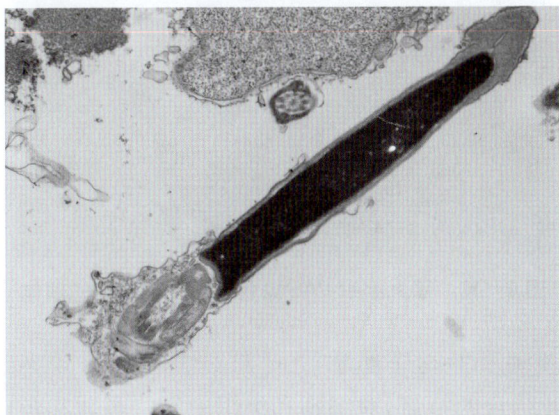

图 1-8　透射电镜观察精子的超微结构

2. 扫描电镜

扫描电镜是用极细的电子束在样本表面扫描,将产生的二次电子用特制的探测器收集,形成电信号运送到显像管,在荧光屏上显示图像。其分辨率一般为 2 nm,主要用于观察组织和细胞的表面形态和立体结构(图 1-9)。

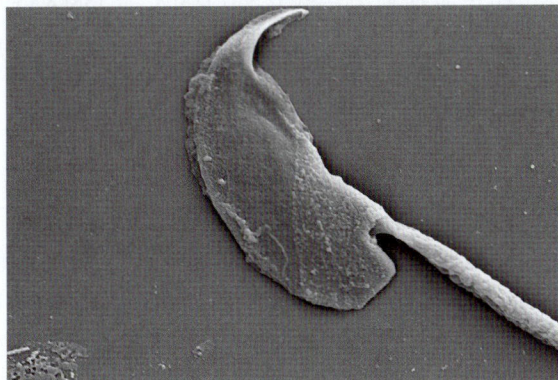

图 1-9　扫描电镜观察小鼠精子形态

三、其他组织学技术

1. 一般组织细胞化学技术

其原理是在切片上加入能与组织细胞中某种待检物质发生化学反应的试剂,其最终产物为有色沉淀物或重金属沉淀,以便用光学显微镜观察。如显示细胞、组织内的多糖或蛋白聚糖的常用方法是过碘酸希夫染色(简称 PAS 染色,图 1-10)。糖被过碘酸氧化后形成多醛,后者与品红硫酸复合物(希夫试剂)结合,形成紫红色反应产物。

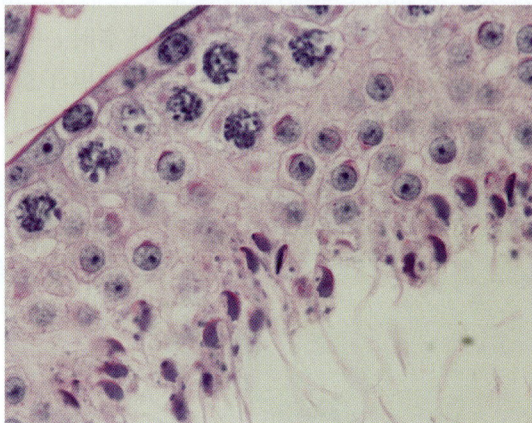

图 1-10　睾丸组织 PAS 染色显示生精细胞的顶体

2. 免疫组织化学与免疫细胞化学技术

利用抗原抗体特异性结合的特点,对细胞和组织中某些多肽和蛋白质等大分子进行定位、定量的技术。其基本原理是将组织中待测的多肽或蛋白质作为抗原,将与待测抗原相对应的抗体用显微镜下可见的标记物进行标记,通过抗体与抗原特异性结合,从而显示待测的抗原。常用标记物有荧光素(如异硫氰酸荧光素)、酶(如辣根过氧化物酶)等。

3. 原位杂交技术

原位杂交技术又称核酸分子杂交组织化学术,是检测 RNA 或 DNA 序列片段的主要方法。其基本原理是应用含有特定序列、经过标记的 DNA 或 RNA 片段作为核酸探针,与组织切片或细胞内待测核酸(RNA 或 DNA)片段进行杂交,从而获知待测核酸的有无及相对量。常用标记物有放射性核素、地高辛、荧光素等。

4. 细胞培养技术

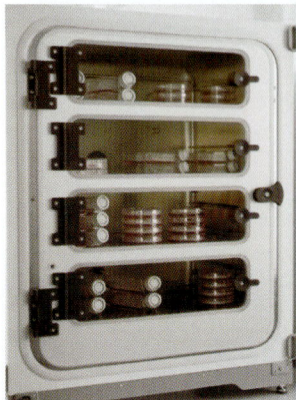

图 1-11　细胞培养箱

体外培养技术包括组织培养和细胞培养技术,是指从机体取得的活组织或活细胞在体外一定环境条件下进行培养并进行实验的技术(图 1-11)。培养液要具有适合细胞生存的必需条件,包括细胞所需的各种营养物质,一定温度,适宜的 O_2 与 CO_2 浓度、pH等条件。体外培养常用的容器有培养瓶、培养皿、培养板等。在倒置相差显微镜下可直接观察细胞的增殖、分化、吞噬等动态变化,并可用显微录像或显微摄影真实地记录活细胞的连续变化过程。

此技术可用于研究各种因素对活细胞的影响,可获得单纯体内实验难以达到的效果。组织工程是用细胞培养技术在体外模拟构建机体组织或器官的技术。目前正在研究构建的组织器官主要有皮肤、软骨、骨、肌腱、骨骼肌、血管及角膜等,其中以组织工程皮肤的研究较为成功,并已应用于临床治疗烧伤、皮肤静脉性溃疡等。

第三节　组织学的学习方法

组织学是一门形态学科,其研究的是形态及其相关功能,在学习中需要注意并做到以下几点。

1. 理论与实际相结合

形态结构的掌握,百闻不如一见。因此对于形态学科的学习,理论与实践相辅相成,密不可分。在教材描述性理论的指导下,看懂教材的插图;重视实验课,仔细观察并比较、分析、记录相关切片;利用所观察到的图像去理解记忆相关理论,均是学好组织学与胚胎学的必要而有效的手段。

2. 形态与功能相结合

组织学研究的是机体的微细结构及其相关功能,一定的形态总是为一定的功能服务;一定的功能活动,必须具备一定的形态学基础。因此,形态与功能结合,有助于知识的灵活掌握。例如,合成蛋白质功能旺盛的细胞,胞质内核糖体较丰富,核糖体含有核酸成分,故 HE 染色胞质多为嗜碱性,呈蓝紫色;肌肉收缩需要耗能,因此肌细胞内具有较多的线粒体;巨噬细胞具有吞噬功能,因此细胞内有较多的溶酶体、吞噬体、吞饮小泡等。

3. 平面与立体相结合

立体的细胞、组织或器官随着切面部位和角度的变化,所呈现的形态结构也不尽相同。例如,单一切片内并非能看到所有的神经元突起;次级卵泡的有些切面看不到初级卵母细胞;肠道纵、横切面的内外层肌纤维断面不一致等。因此,在学习过程中,应积极培养自己的空间思维能力,努力将看到的平面和局部的二维图像还原为实物的三维结构,以便更好地理解机体的结构。

4. 共性与特性相结合

组织学的学习应善于比较分析,努力掌握其共性和特性。如人体内脏器官数量很多、结构各异,但一般只要了解其为中空性或实质性器官,即可推断出该器官的大概结构框架,再结合功能的不同,推断出框架各个部分的特征性的结构,这样便可对该器官结构有一个基本而又灵活的掌握。

5. 发生、发展与进化相结合

人体各器官的形态结构是在漫长的由低级向高级、简单向复杂的进化过程中逐步形成的。这些组织结构一直处于新陈代谢、发育分化的动态变化之中。

总之,正确掌握学习方法可以提高学习效率,牢固掌握知识,并能将所学到的医学基础理论灵活运用到其他各学科中去。

（赵奕淳　郑　英）

Chapter 2

Epithelial Tissue

Epithelial tissue is one of the four basic tissues, with a wide distribution and many functions. It is composed of closely aggregated polyhedral cells with little extracellular substance. These cells have strong adhesion and form cellular sheets that cover the surface of the body and line its cavities. An important feature of epithelia is their polarity. The region of the cell contacting the connective tissue is called the basal pole and the opposite end, usually facing a space, is the apical pole. The 2 poles of epithelial cells differ in both structure and function. Epithelia lack a direct blood supply and are fed via diffusion from underlying basement membrane. These nutrients and precursors of products of the epithelial cells then diffuse across the basal lamina and are taken up through the basolateral surface of the epithelial cell, usually by an energy-dependent process. Most epithelial tissues receive a rich supply of sensory nerve endings from nerve plexuses in the basement membrane. The principal functions of epithelial tissues include covering, lining, absorption, secretion, and protecting surface.

According to their structure and function, epithelial tissues are divided into covering epithelia, glandular epithelia, germinal epithelia, sensory epithelia and so on. Among them, covering epithelia and glandular epithelia are two main groups. Covering epithelia cover exposed body surface or line internal cavities, such as those of cardiovascular, digestive, respiratory tract. Glandular epithelia secret mucus, hormones, enzymes and so forth from various glands.

1 Covering Epithelium

Covering epithelia are tissues in which the cells are organized in layers that cover the external surface or line the cavities of the body. They can be classified according to the number of cell layers and the morphologic features of the cells in the surface layer (Table 2-1). Simple epithelia contain only one layer of cells, and stratified epithelia contain more than one layer. Simple epithelia can, according to the morphology of the cells, be squamous, cuboidal and columnar. Stratified epithelia are classified by the morphology of the cells in their superficial layer: squamous, cuboidal, columnar, and transitional.

Table 2 - 1   Types and distribution of epithelium

Types	Distribution
Simple squamous epithelium	Endothelium: Lining of vessels Mesothelium: Serous lining of cavities: pericardium, pleura, peritoneum
Simple cuboidal epithelium	Covering the ovary, thyroid
Simple columnar epithelium	Lining of intestine, gallbladder, etc.
Pseudostratified cilliated columnar epithelium	Lining of trachea, bronchi, nasal cavity
Stratified squamous epithelium	Nonkeratinized (moist): Mouth, esophagus, larynx, vagina, anal canal Keratinized (dry): Epidermis
Stratified columnar epithelium	Conjunctiva
Transitional epithelium	Bladder, ureters, renal calyces

1.1   Simple Squamous Epithelium

Simple squamous epithelium is formed of a single layer of flat cells (Figure 2 - 1). When viewed from the surface, the epithelial sheet looks much like a tile floor, with a bulging nucleus placed centrally in each cell. The endothelium that lines the heart, blood and lymph vessels and the mesothelium that lines certain body cavities, such as the pleural and peritoneal cavities, and covers the viscera are examples of simple squamous epithelium.

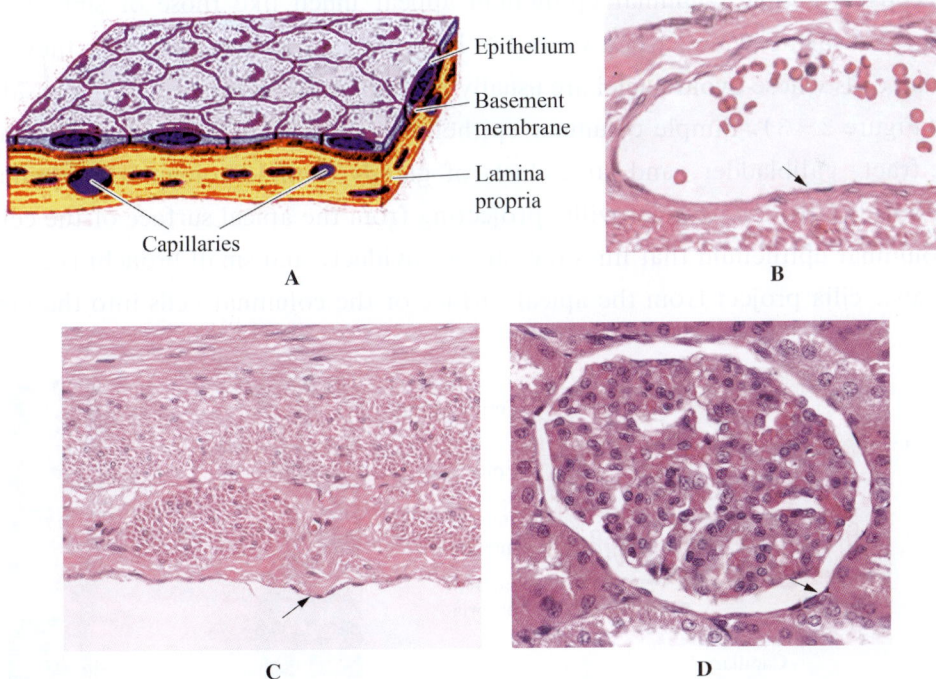

Figure 2 - 1   Simple squamous epithelium

A. Diagram of simple squamous epithelium; B. Endothelium, small vein; C. Mesothelium, vermiform appendix; D. Parietal layer of glomerular capsule (HE)

1.2　Simple Cuboidal Epithelium

Simple cuboidal epithelium is composed of a single layer of cells shaped like truncated hexagonal solids (Figure 2 - 2). When viewed in a section cut perpendicular to the surface, the cells present a square profile with a centrally placed round nucleus. Simple cuboidal epithelia make up the ducts of many glands of the body, form the covering of the ovary, and compose some kidney tubules.

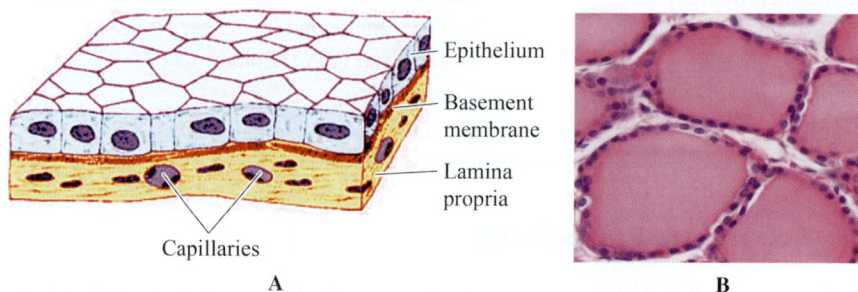

Figure 2 - 2　Simple cuboidal epithelium

A. Diagram of simple cuboidal epithelium; B. Thyroid follicular cells (HE)

1.3　Simple Columnar Epithelium

The cells of simple columnar epithelium appear much like those of simple cuboidal epithelium in a surface view; when viewed in longitudinal section, however, they are tall, rectangular cells whose ovoid nuclei are usually located at the same level in the basal half of the cell (Figure 2 - 3). Simple columnar epithelium is found in the lining of much of the digestive tract, gallbladder, and large ducts of glands. Simple columnar epithelium may exhibit a striated border, or microvilli, projecting from the apical surface of the cells. The simple columnar epithelium that lines the uterus, oviduct, and small bronchi is ciliated. In these organs, cilia project from the apical surface of the columnar cells into the lumen.

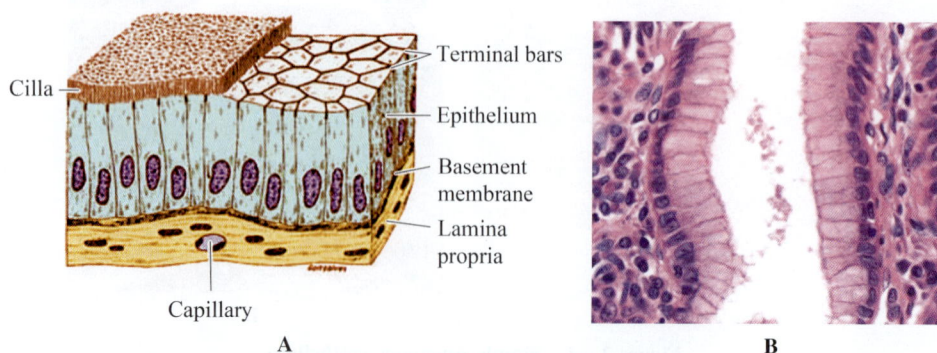

Figure 2 - 3　Simple columnar epithelium

A. Diagram of Simple columnar epithelium; B. Surface mucous cells of stomach (HE)

1.4　Pseudostratified Columnar Epithelium

As the name implies, pseudostratified columnar epithelium appears to be stratified but it is actually composed a single layer of cells (Figure 2 – 4). All cells are attached to the basement membrane, but only some cells reach the surface of the epithelium. Because the cells of this epithelium are of different heights, their nuclei are located at different levels, giving the impression of a stratified epithelium even though it is composed of a single layer of cells. A good example of this tissue is the ciliated pseudostratified columnar epithelium in the respiratory passages.

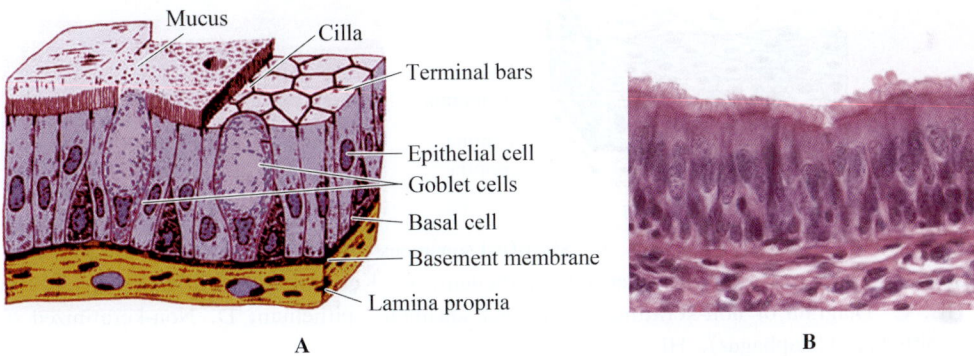

Figure 2 – 4　Pseudostratified columnar epithelium
A. Diagram of pseudostratified columnar epithelium; B. Respiratory epithelium of trachea (HE)

1.5　Stratified Squamous Epithelium

Stratified squamous epithelium is a tough, resilient multilayered epithelium that mainly protects against abrasion and dehydration. Its name derives from the shape of the outer layer of flattened cells. The cells closer to the underlying connective tissue are usually cuboidal or columnar. Basal cells are mitotically active and continuously divide into daughter cells that mature and are pushed toward the surface. The very thin surface cells of stratified squamous epithelia can be "keratinized" (filled with keratin intermediate filaments, Figure 2 – 5) or "non-keratinized" (with relatively sparse amounts of keratin, Figure 2 – 6). Stratified squamous keratinized epithelium is found mainly in the epidermis of skin, where it helps prevent dehydration from the tissue. The cells become irregular in shape and flatten as they get progressively closer to the surface, where they become thin, metabolically inactive packets of keratin lacking nuclei. Stratified squamous non-keratinized epithelium lines wet cavities (e. g., mouth, esophagus, and vagina) where water loss is not a problem. Here the fattened cells of the surface layer contain much less keratin, retaining their nuclei and metabolic function.

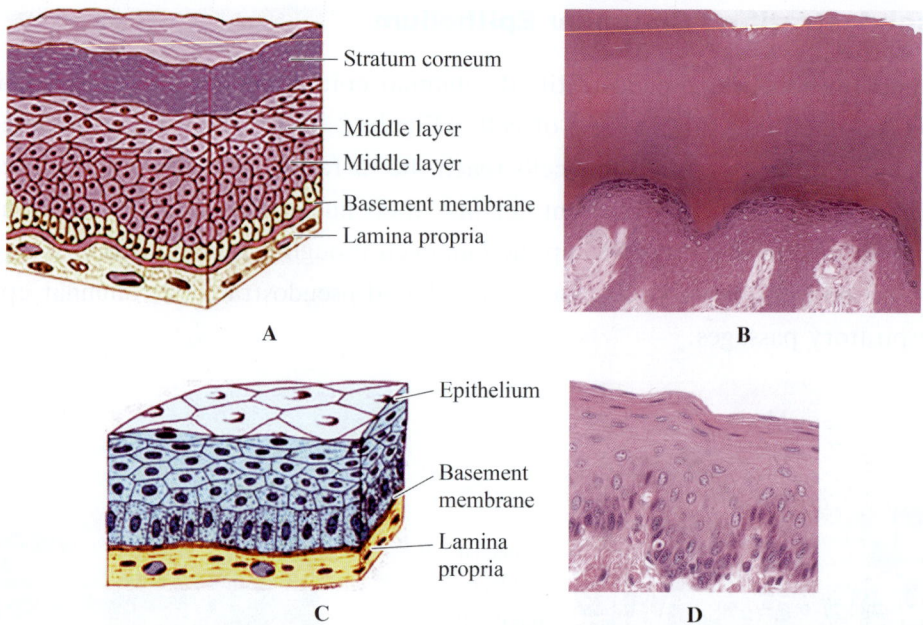

Figure 2 - 5   Stratified squamous epithelium

A. Diagram of keratinized stratified squamous epithelium; B. Keratinized stratified squamous epithelium (Skin), HE; C. Diagram of non-keratinized stratified squamous epithelium; D. Non-keratinized stratified squamous epithelium (Esophagus), HE

1.6   Stratified Columnar Epithelium

Stratified columnar epithelium is rare. It is present in the human body only in small areas (Figure 2 - 6), such as the ocular conjunctiva and the large ducts of salivary glands.

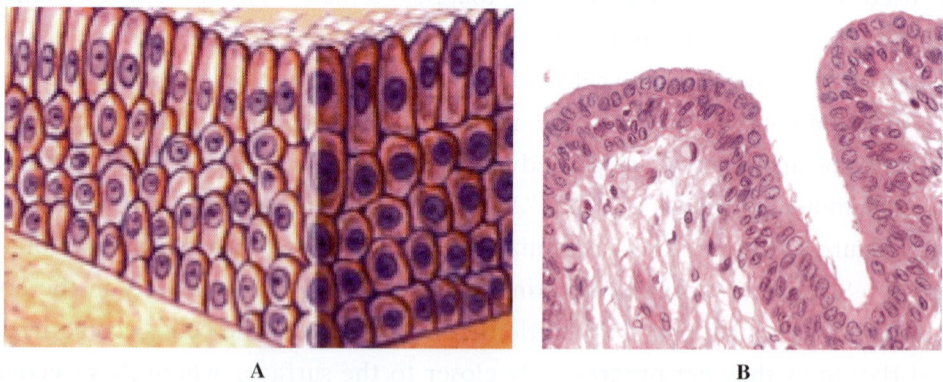

Figure 2 - 6   Stratified columnar epithelium

A. Diagram of Stratified columnar epithelium; B. Urethra (HE)

1.7   Transitional Epithelium

Transitional epithelium lines the urinary bladder, the ureter, and the upper part of the urethra, and is characterized by a surface layer of domelike cells that sometimes called umbrella cells (Figure 2 - 7). These cells are specialized to protect underlying tissues from the hypertonic and potentially cytotoxic effects of urine. The form of these cells changes according to the degree of distention of the bladder.

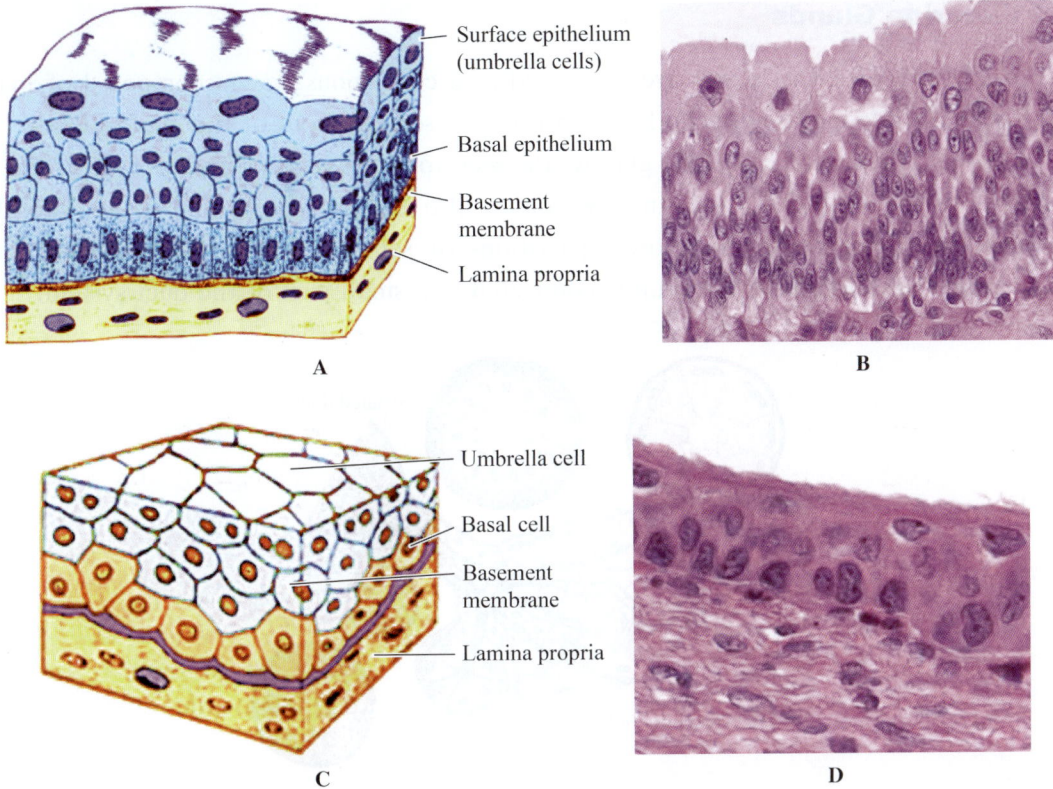

Figure 2 - 7   Transitional epithelium
A. Diagram of transitional epithelium when bladder is empty; B. Bladder (empty), HE; C. Diagram of Transitional epithelium when bladder is full; D. Bladder (full), HE

2   Glandular Epithelium and Glands

Epithelial cells that function mainly to produce and secrete various macromolecules may occur in epithelia with other major functions or comprise specialized organs called glands. The molecules to be secreted are generally stored in the cells in small membrane-bound vesicles called secretory granules. Secretory epithelial cells may synthesize, store, and release proteins, lipids, or complexes of carbohydrates and proteins. The cells of some glands have little synthetic activity and secrete mostly water and electrolytes (ions) transferred from the blood. Secretory cells are common in simple cuboidal, simple columnar, and pseudostratified epithelia of many organs.

Glands are classified into 2 major groups on the basis of the method of distribution of their secretory products. Exocrine glands secrete their products via ducts onto the external or internal epithelia surface from which they originated. Endocrine glands are ductless, having lost their connections to the originating epithelium, and thus secrete their products into the blood or lymphatic vessels for distribution.

2.1 Exocrine Glands

Epithelia of exocrine glands are organized as a continuous system composed of many small secretory portions and ducts that transport the secretion out of the gland (Figure 2 - 8). In both exocrine and endocrine glands, the secretory units are supported by a stroma of connective tissue. A layer of connective tissue also encloses the gland as its capsule, surrounds the larger ducts, and forms partitions or septa that separate the gland into lobules, each containing secretory units connected to a small part of the duct system.

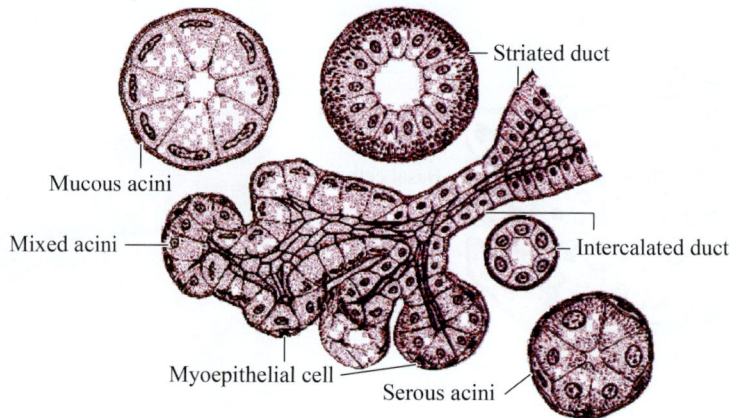

Figure 2 - 8 General structure of exocrine glands

Exocrine glands can be further categorized as either serous or mucous according to the nature of their secretory products, which give distinct staining properties to the cells (Figure 2 - 9). Serous cells synthesize proteins that are mostly non-glycosylated, such as digestive enzymes. The cells have well-developed RER and Golgi complexes and are filled apically with secretory granules in different stages of maturation. Serous cells therefore stain intensely with basophilic or acidophilic stains. Acini of the pancreas and parotid salivary glands are composed of serous cells. Mucous cells, such as goblet cells, also have RER and Golgi complexes and are filled apically with secretory granules, but these contain heavily glycosylated proteins called mucins. When mucins are released from the cell, they become hydrated and form mucus. Most of the hydrophilic mucins are washed from cells during routine histological preparations, causing the mucinogen granules to stain poorly with eosin. Sufficient oligosaccharides usually remain, however, to allow mucous cells to be stained by the periodic acid-Schif (PAS) method. Some salivary glands are mixed seromucous glands, with both serous acini and mucous tubules capped by groups of serous cells. The product of such glands is a mixture of digestive enzymes and watery mucus.

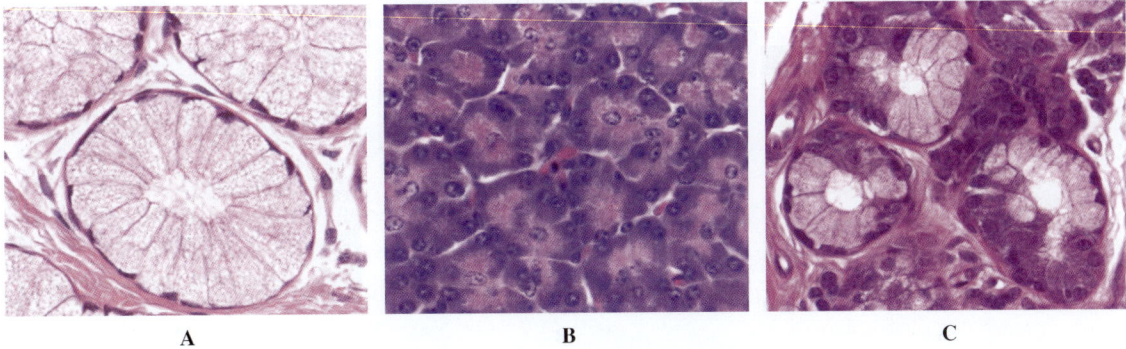

Figure 2 – 9   Serous, mucous and mixed acini
A. Mucous acini (Esophagus); B. Serous acini (Pancreas); C. Mixed acini (Trachea)

2.2   Endocrine Glands

Endocrine glands release their secretions, hormones, into blood or lymphatic vessels for distribution to target organs. The cells of endocrine glands are usually specialized for either protein or steroid synthesis, with cytoplasmic staining characteristic of RER or SER, respectively. The proteins are released by exocytosis and the lipophilic steroids by diffusion through the cell membrane for uptake by binding proteins outside the cell. Endocrine signaling involves hormone transport in the blood to target cells throughout the body, often within other endocrine glands. The receptors may also be on cells very close to the hormone-secreting cell or on the secreting cell itself, in these cases the signaling is termed paracrine or autocrine, respectively.

3   Specializations of the Cell Surface

The free surface of some epithelial cells shows specializations to increase cell surface area or to move foreign particles.

3.1   Microvilli

Microvilli are small finger-like cytoplasmic projections emanating from the free surface of the cell into the lumen (Figure 2 – 10). They range in number from a few to many. In absorptive cells, such as the lining epithelium of the small intestine and the cells of the proximal renal tubule, orderly arrays of many hundreds of microvilli are encountered. Each microvillus is $1\,\mu$m high and $0.08\,\mu$m wide. Each microvillus contains a core of actin filaments, cross-linked by villin, attached to an amorphous region at its tip and extending into the cytoplasm, where the actin filaments are embedded in the terminal web. The terminal web is a complex of actin and spectrin molecules, as well as intermediate filaments located at the cortex of the epithelial cells. Microvilli represent the striated border of the intestinal absorptive cells and the brush border of the kidney proximal tubule cells observed by light microscopy.

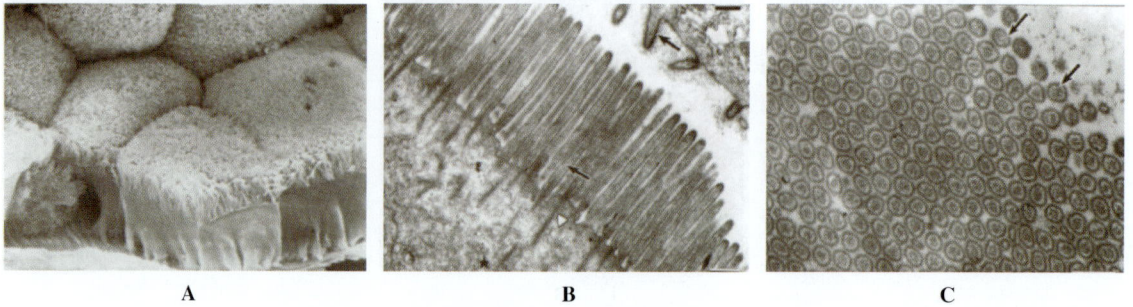

Figure 2 - 10   Microvilli
A. SEM of microvilli; B. & C. TEM of microvilli (Vertical section & horizontal section)

3.2 Cilia

Cilia are long, motile, hair-like structures emanating from the apical cell surface (Figure 2 - 11). Their core is composed of a complex arrangement of microtubules known as the axoneme. The axoneme is composed of a constant number of longitudinal microtubules arranged in a consistent $9+2$ organization. Two centrally placed microtubules are evenly surrounded by 9 doublets of microtubules. The 2 microtubules located in the center of the core are separated from each other, each displaying a circular profile in cross-section, composed of 13 protofilaments. Each of the 9 doublets is composed of 2 subunits. In cross-section, subunit A is a microtubule composed of 13 protofilaments, exhibiting a circular profile. Subunit B possesses 10 protofilaments, exhibits an incomplete circular profile in cross-section, and shares three protofilaments of subunit A.

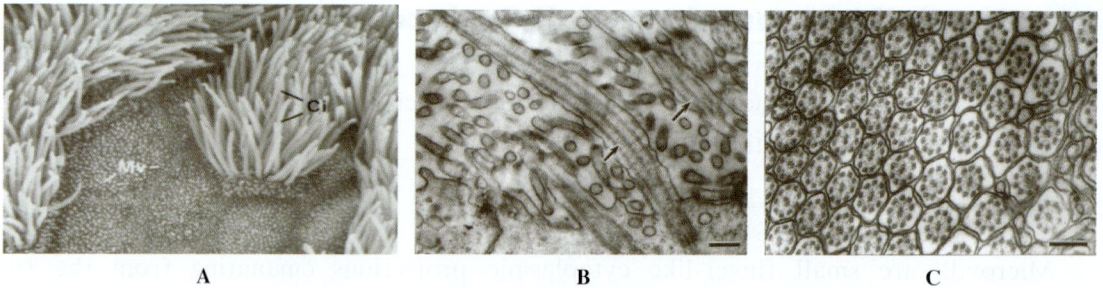

Figure 2 - 11   Cilia
A. SM of cilia; B. & C. TM of cilia (Vertical section & horizontal section)

In living organisms, cilia have a rapid back-and-forth movement. Ciliary movement is frequently coordinated to permit a current of fluid or particulate matter to be propelled in one direction over the ciliated epithelium. A ciliated cell of the trachea is estimated to have about 250 cilia.

3.3 Intercellular Junctions

Epithelial cells adhere strongly to neighboring cells and basal laminae, particularly in epithelia subject to friction or other mechanical forces. Lateral surfaces of epithelial cells exhibit several specialized intercellular junctions, which serve different functions (Figure 2-12). In some epithelia the various junctions are present in a definite order from the apex toward the base of the cell.

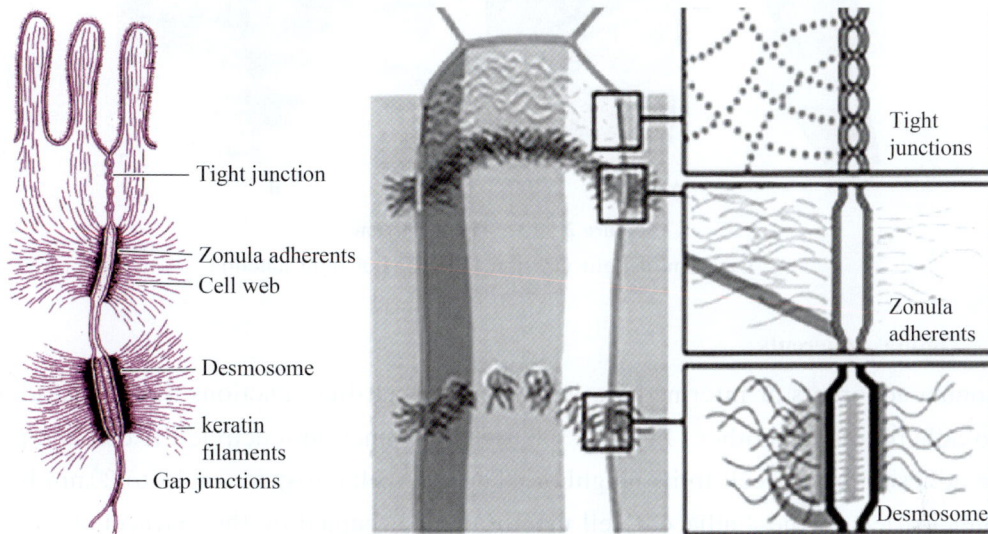

Figure 2-12   Diagram of intercellular junctions

3.3.1   Tight Junctions

Tight junctions, or zonulae occludens, are the most apical of the junctions. These junctions prevent movement of membrane proteins and function to prevent intercellular movement of water-soluble molecules. "Zonula" refers to the fact that the junction forms a band completely encircling the cell, and "occludens" refers to the membrane fusions that close off the intercellular space. In properly stained thin sections viewed in the electron microscope, the outer leaflets of adjacent membranes are seen to fuse, giving rise to a local pentalaminar appearance (Figure 2 – 13). One to several of these fusion sites may be observed, depending on the epithelium. After cryofracture, the replicas show anastomosing ridges and grooves that form a netlike structure corresponding to the fusion sites observed in conventional thin sections. The number of ridges and grooves, or fusion sites, has a high correlation with the leakiness of the epithelium. Epithelia with one or very few fusion sites (e. g., proximal renal tubule) are more permeable to water and solutes than are epithelia with numerous fusion sites (e. g., urinary bladder). Thus, the principal function of the tight junction is to form a seal that prevents the flow of materials between epithelial cells (paracellular pathway) in either direction (from apex to base or from base to apex). In this way, zonula occludens participates in the formation of functional compartments delimited by sheets of epithelial cells.

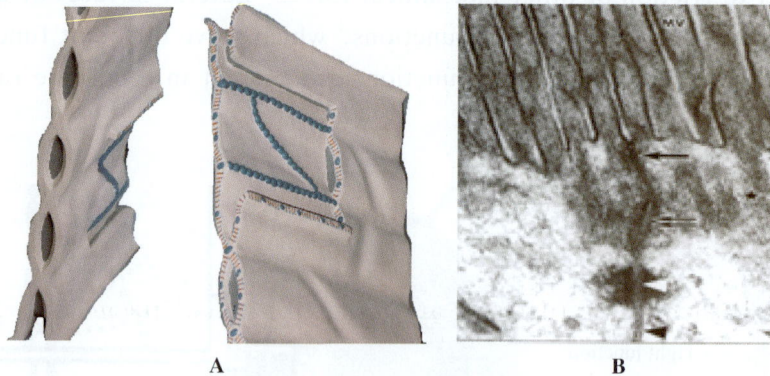

Figure 2 – 13 Tight junction
A. Diagram of tight junction; B. TEM of tight junction

3.3.2 Zonula Adherents

Zonula adherents or intermediate junction, are belt-like junctions that assist adjoining cells to adhere to one another (Figure 2 – 14). These junctions encircle the cell and provide for the adhesion of one cell to its neighbor. The intercellular space of 15 to 20 nm between the outer leaflets of the 2 adjacent cell membrane is occupied by the extracellular moieties of cadherins. These Ca^{2+}-dependent integral protein of the cell membrane are transmembrane linker proteins. Their intracytoplasmic aspect binds to a specialized region of the cell web, specifically a bundle of actin filaments that run parallel to and along the cytoplasmic aspect of the cell membrane. The actin filaments are attached to each other and to the cell membrane by vinculin and alpha-actinin. The extracellular region of the cadherins of one cell forms bonds with those of the adjoining cell participating in the formation of the zonula adherens. Then this junction not only joins the cell membranes to each other but also links the cytoskeleton of the 2 cells via the transmembrane linker proteins.

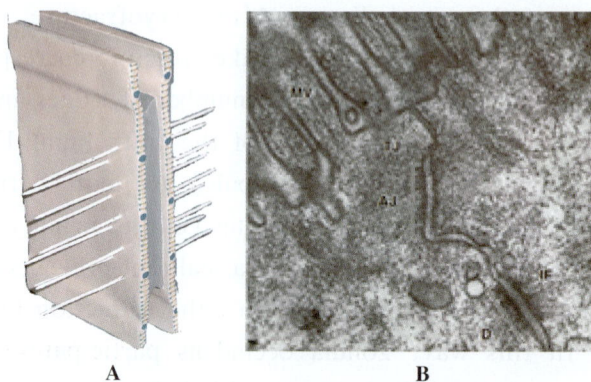

Figure 2 – 14 Zonula adherents
A. Diagram of zonula adherents; B. TM of zonula adherents

3.3.3 Desmosome

Desmosome, or macula adherens, is a complex disk-shaped structure at the surface of one cell that is matched with an identical structure at the surface of the adjacent cell (Figure 2 – 15). The cell membranes in this region are very straight and are usually somewhat farther apart (>30 nm) than the usual 20 nm. On the cytosolic side of the membrane of each cell and separated from it by a short distance is a circular plaque of material called an attachment plaque, made up of at least 12 proteins. In epithelial cells, groups of intermediate keratin filaments are inserted into the attachment plaque or make hairpin turns and return to the cytoplasm. Because intermediate filaments of the cytoskeleton are very strong, desmosomes provide a firm adhesion among the cells.

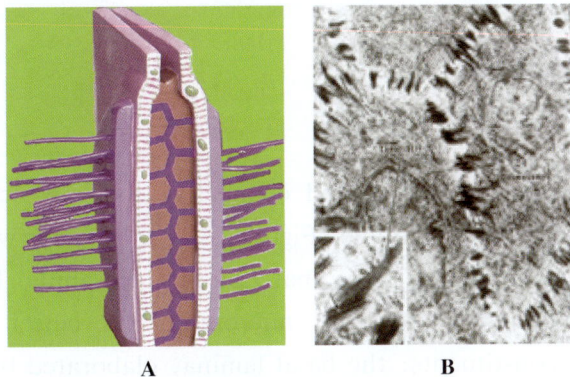

Figure 2 – 15 Desmosome
A. Diagram of desmosome; B. TEM of desmosome

3.3.4 Gap Junctions

Gap junctions, also called communicating junctions, are regions of intercellular communication. Gap junctions are widespread in epithelial tissues throughout the body as well as in cardiac muscle cells, smooth muscle cells, and neurons. The intercellular cleft at the gap junction is narrow and constant at 2 to 3 nm. Gap junctions are built by 6 closely packed transmembrane proteins (connexins) that assemble to form structures called connexons, aqueous pores through the plasma membrane extending into the intercellular space (Figure 2 – 16). When a connexon of one plasma membrane is in register with its counterpart of the adjacent plasma membrane, each connexon juts out of the plasma membrane about 1.5 nm into the intercellular space. The 2 connexons fuse, forming the functional intercellular communication channel. With a diameter of 1.5 to 2.0 nm, the hydrophilic channel permits the passage of ions, amino acids, cyclic adenosine monophosphate (cAMP), molecules smaller than 1 kD in weight, and certain hormones. However, gap junctions are regulated, so they may be opened or closed. In addition, gap junctions have different properties with diverse channel permeabilities in different cells.

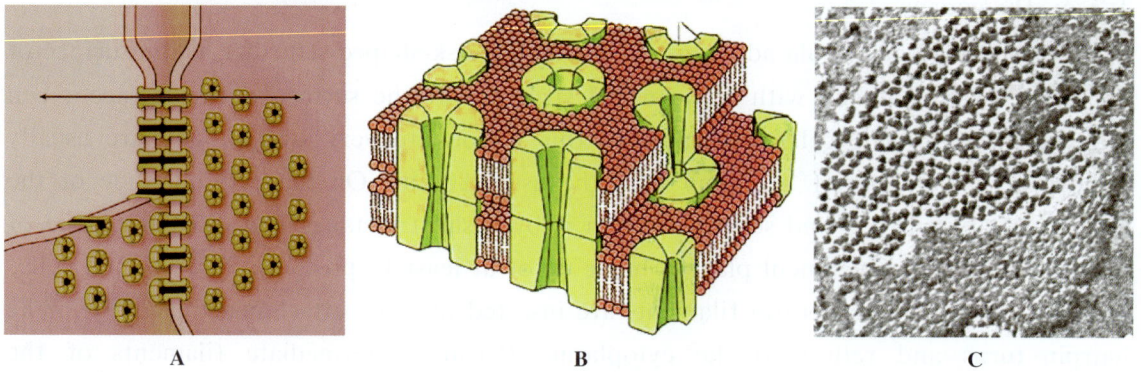

Figure 2 – 16   Gap junctions

A. & B. Diagram of gap junctions; C. TM of gap junctions

3.4   Basal Specializations

3.4.1   Basement Membrane

The interface between epithelium and connective tissue is occupied by a narrow, acellular region, the basement membrane (Figure 2 – 17), which is well stained by the PAS reaction and by other histological stains that detect glycosaminoglycans (GAGs). The basement membrane, as visible by light microscopy, is better defined by electron microscopy as having 2 constituents: the basal lamina, elaborated by epithelial cells, and the lamina reticularis, manufactured by cells of the connective tissue. The basal lamina is visible only with the electron microscope, where it appears as a dense layer, 20 – 100 nm thick, consisting of a delicate network of fine fibrils (lamina densa). In addition, basal laminae may have electron-lucent layers on one or both sides of the lamina densa, called

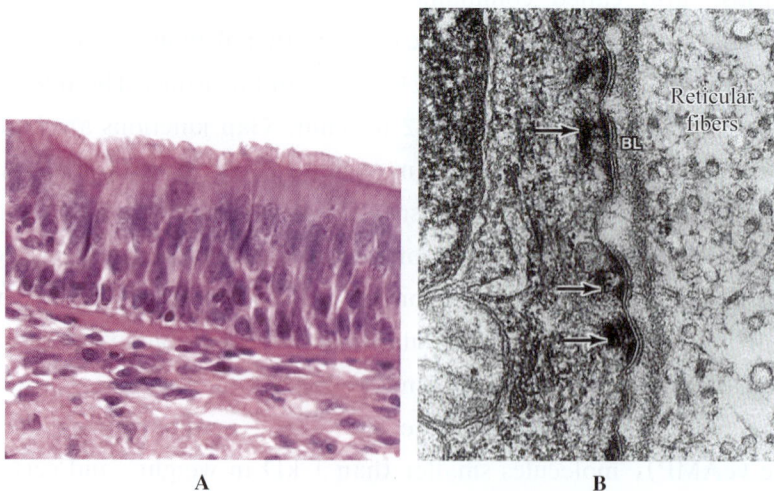

Figure 2 – 17   Basement membrane

A. LM of basement membrane, Trachea (HE); B. TEM of basement membrane laminae rarae or laminae lucidae. The main components of basal laminae are type IV collagen, the glycoproteins laminin and entactin, and proteoglycan. The basal lamina functions both as a molecular filter and as a flexible, firm support for the overlying epithelium. An additional function of the basal lamina is to direct the migration of cells along its surface. The lamina reticularis, a region of varying thickness, is manufactured by fibroblasts and is composed of type I and type III collagen. It is the interface between the basal lamina and the underlying connective tissue.

3.4.2   Plasma Membrane Enfoldings

The basal surface of some epithelia, especially those involved in ion transport, possesses multiple enfoldings of the basal plasma membranes (Figure 2 - 18). These enfolding, which increase the surface area of the plasma membrane, partition the basal cytoplasm and many mitochondria into the finger-like enfolding. The mitochondria provide the energy required for active transport of ions in establishing osmotic gradients to ensure the movement of water across the epithelium, such as those of kidney tubules.

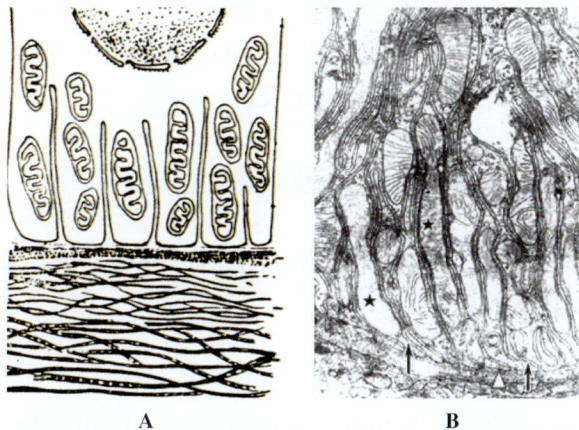

Figure 2 - 18   Plasma membrane enfoldings
A. Diagram of plasma membrane enfoldings; B. TEM of plasma membrane enfoldings

3.4.3   Hemidesmosomes

Hemidesmosomes resemble half desmosomes and serve to attach the basal cell membrane to the basal lamina. However, in desmosomes the attachment plaques contain mainly cadherins, whereas in hemidesmosomes the plaques are made of integrins, a family of transmembrane proteins that are receptor sites for the extracellular macromolecules laminin and collagen type IV.

(Yang Fan, Zheng Ying)

第二章　上皮组织

　　上皮组织是由大量形状较规则且排列紧密的细胞和少量的细胞间质组成,细胞间以间质和特殊结构相连。上皮细胞具有明显的极性,上皮细胞朝向身体表面或有腔器官腔面的一面称为游离面,另一面为基底面,一般均附着在基膜上,借此与结缔组织相连。上皮细胞的游离面和基底面在结构和功能上具有明显的差别。上皮组织内大多无血管与淋巴管,其营养由深层结缔组织的血管提供,来自血液中的营养物质通过基膜渗透到上皮细胞的间隙中。上皮内一般富有神经末梢,神经末梢终止在上皮细胞。如表皮、角膜上皮和支气管上皮等,均有丰富的游离神经末梢。上皮组织具有保护、吸收、分泌和排泄等功能。

　　根据上皮组织的分布、功能的不同,可将其分为被覆上皮、腺上皮、生殖上皮和感觉上皮等。其中被覆上皮和腺上皮是两种主要的上皮。被覆上皮覆盖于身体表面或衬贴在有腔器官的腔面。腺上皮以分泌功能为主,构成腺体的上皮。

第一节　被覆上皮

　　被覆上皮覆盖于身体表面或衬贴在有腔器官的腔面,分布广泛。被覆上皮的细胞形状规则,排列紧密、成层,位于身体的界面。

一、被覆上皮的类型和结构

　　被覆上皮根据构成细胞的层数,分为单层上皮和复层上皮;由一层细胞组成的上皮称为单层上皮,由多层细胞组成的上皮称为复层上皮。根据单层上皮的细胞形状及复层上皮表层细胞的形状可进一步将其分为扁平、立方、柱状等多种类型(表 2-1)。

表 2-1　被覆上皮的分类及主要分布

细胞层次	上皮类型	主要分布
单层上皮	单层扁平上皮	内皮:心、血管和淋巴管的腔面 间皮:胸膜、腹膜和心包膜的表面及部分器官表面 其他:肺泡和肾小囊壁层的上皮
复层上皮	单层立方上皮	肾小管和甲状腺滤泡等
	单层柱状上皮	胃、肠和子宫等
	假复层纤毛柱状上皮	呼吸道等
	复层扁平上皮	未角化:口腔、食管和阴道等 角化:皮肤的表皮等
	复层柱状上皮	眼睑结膜和男性尿道
	变移上皮	肾盏、肾盂、输尿管和膀胱等腔面

（一）单层扁平上皮

单层扁平上皮由一层很薄的扁平细胞组成。从上皮表面观，细胞呈不规则多边形，边缘呈锯齿状，相互嵌合，核扁圆，位于细胞中央。垂直切面观，细胞中央含细胞核的部分略厚，其余部分的胞质很薄，细胞核扁长（图2-1A）。

衬于心、血管和淋巴管腔面的单层扁平上皮称为内皮，表面光滑，有利于血液和淋巴液的流动（图2-1B）。衬于胸膜、腹膜和心包膜及部分器官表面的单层扁平上皮称为间皮，可减缓器官间的摩擦（图2-1C）。此外，I型肺泡上皮和肾小囊壁层的上皮也是单层扁平上皮（图2-1D）。

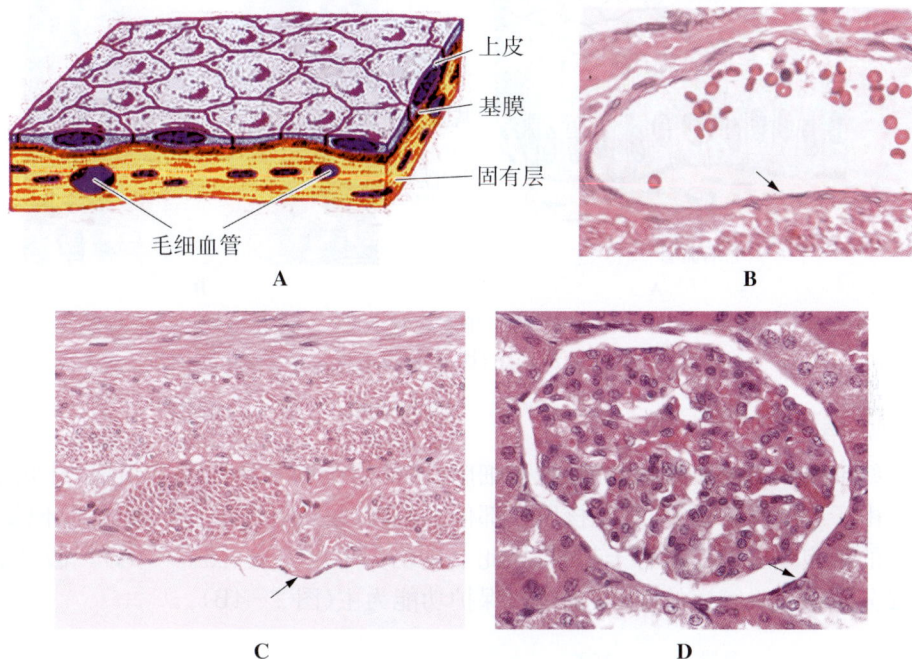

图2-1 单层扁平上皮
A.模式图；B.内皮；C.间皮；D.肾小囊壁层

（二）单层立方上皮

单层立方上皮由一层近似立方形的细胞组成。从上皮表面观，每个细胞呈六角形或多边形；垂直切面观，细胞呈立方形，核圆形，位于细胞中央（图2-2A）。这种上皮见于肾小管、甲状腺滤泡和视网膜色素上皮等处，具有分泌和吸收功能（图2-2B）。

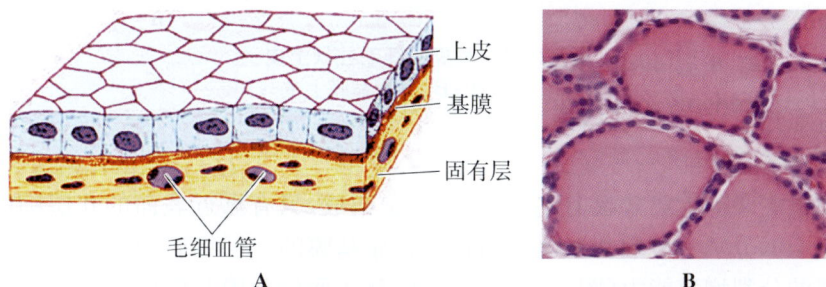

图2-2 单层立方上皮
A.模式图；B.甲状腺滤泡上皮

(三）单层柱状上皮

单层柱状上皮由一层棱柱状细胞组成。表面观,细胞呈六角形或多边形,垂直切面观,细胞呈柱状,核椭圆,靠近细胞基底部(图 2-3A)。这种上皮分布于胃、肠、胆囊和子宫等器官,有吸收或分泌功能(图 2-3B)。在小肠腔面的单层柱状上皮内散布有杯状细胞。杯状细胞形似高脚酒杯,底部狭窄,含深染的三角形细胞核,顶部膨大,充满黏原颗粒,黏蛋白分泌后与水结合形成黏液,对上皮表面有保护和润滑作用。

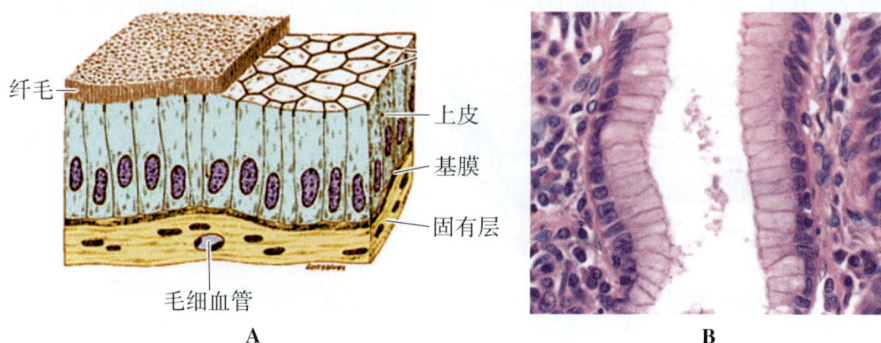

图 2-3　单层柱状上皮
A.模式图;B.胃黏膜上皮

(四）假复层纤毛柱状上皮

假复层纤毛柱状上皮由柱状细胞、梭形细胞、锥体形细胞和杯状细胞组成,柱状细胞游离面有纤毛。由于细胞高矮不等,细胞核所在部位也不同,故从上皮垂直切面观,酷似复层,但这些高矮不等的细胞基底面都附着于基膜,故此上皮仍为单层上皮(图 2-4A)。假复层纤毛柱状上皮主要分布在呼吸管道的腔面,主要以保护功能为主(图 2-4B)。

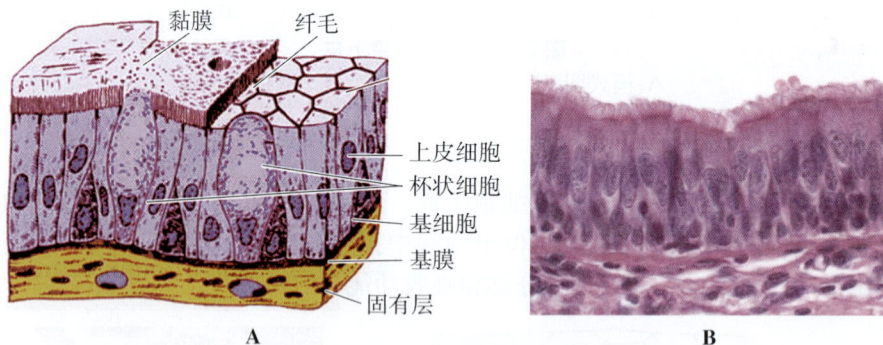

图 2-4　假复层纤毛柱状上皮
A.模式图;B.气管黏膜上皮

(五）复层扁平上皮

复层扁平上皮又称复层鳞状上皮,由多层细胞组成,只有靠近表面的几层细胞呈扁平状,中间数层由浅至深分别为梭形和多边形细胞。紧靠基膜的一层细胞为立方形或矮柱状,此层细胞具有较强的分裂增殖能力(图 2-5A)。上皮基底面借基膜与深面的结缔组织相连,其连接面呈波浪形,扩大了两者的接触面。复层扁平上皮是最厚的一种上皮。位于表皮的复层扁平上皮,浅层细胞的细胞核消失,细胞质中充满角蛋白,细胞干硬并不断脱落,称角化的复层扁平上皮,具有很强的耐摩擦和保护功能(图2-5B)。铺衬在口腔和食管等腔面的复层扁平上皮,浅层细胞有核,含角蛋白少,称未角化的复层扁平上皮(图2-5C、D)。

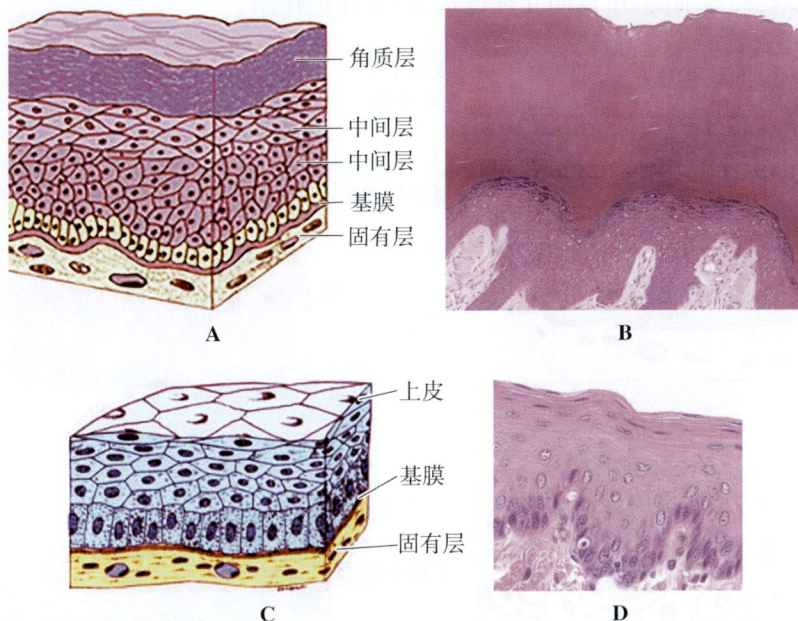

图2-5　复层扁平上皮

A.角化的复层扁平上皮模式图;B.手指掌侧皮肤(HE染色);C.未角化的复层扁平上皮模式图;D.食管上皮(HE染色)

(六) 复层柱状上皮

复层柱状上皮的表层细胞为柱状,排列整齐,中间几层细胞为多边形,基底层是矮柱状细胞。此种上皮只见于眼睑结膜和男性尿道等处,具有保护作用(图2-6)。

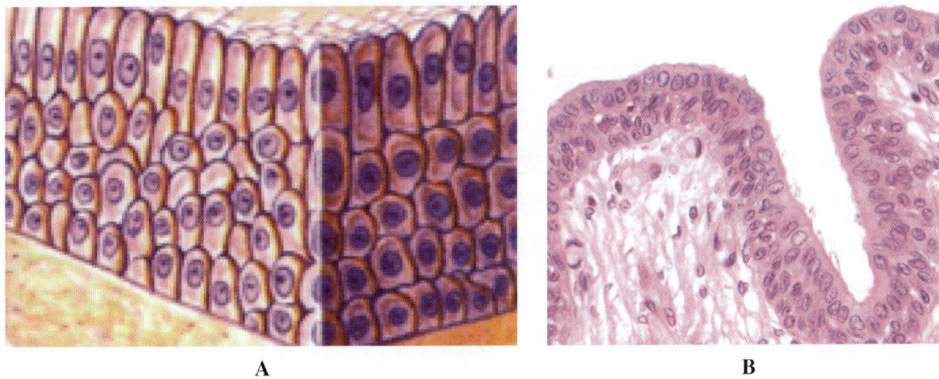

图2-6　复层柱状上皮

A.复层柱状上皮模式图;B.尿道黏膜上皮(HE染色)

(七) 变移上皮

变移上皮又称为移行上皮,上皮细胞的形态和层数可随所在器官的收缩和扩张状态不同而改变(图 2-7A)。如膀胱收缩时,上皮较厚,细胞层数较多,细胞较高(图 2-7B);反之,上皮变薄,细胞层数减少,仅 2～3 层,细胞变扁(图 2-7C、D)。上皮细胞按核位置的深浅可分为表层细胞、中间层细胞和基底层细胞。表层细胞较大,质膜较厚,胞质丰富,常有双核,可覆盖几个中间层细胞,称盖细胞,可以防止尿液侵袭,有保护作用。

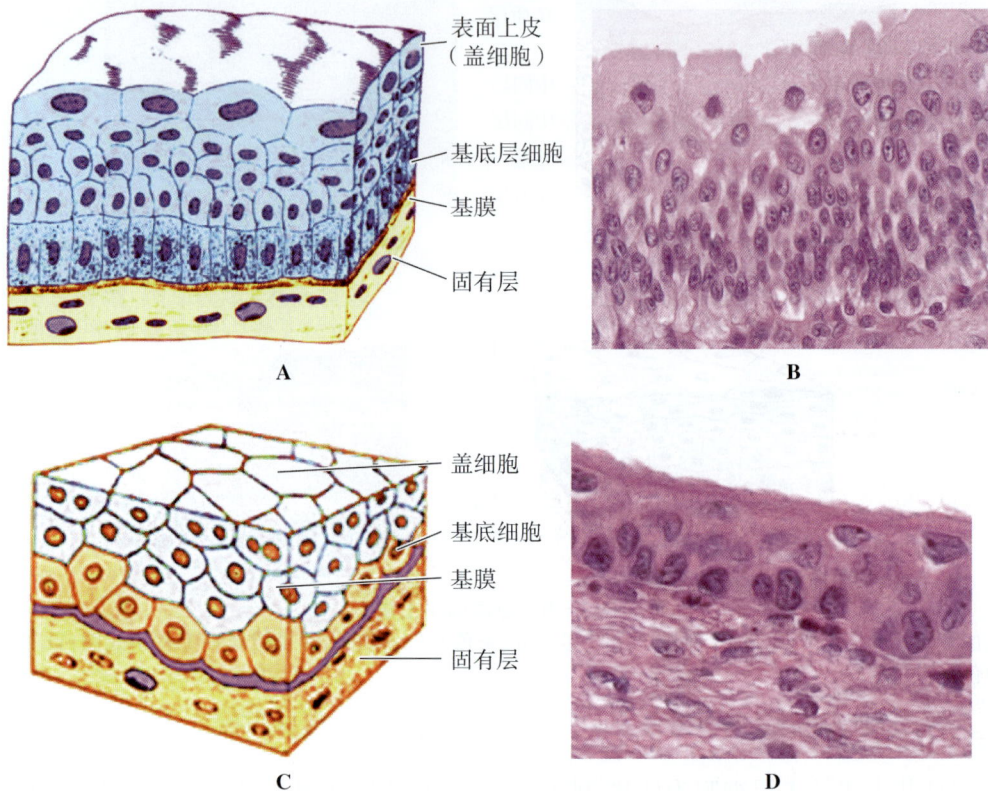

图 2-7 变移上皮
A.空虚膀胱变移上皮模式图;B.空虚膀胱上皮;C.充盈膀胱变移上皮模式图;D.充盈膀胱上皮

第二节 腺上皮和腺

由腺细胞组成,以分泌功能为主的上皮称腺上皮。以腺上皮为主要成分的器官称腺。凡是分泌物经导管排至体表或器官腔内的称外分泌腺,如汗腺、胃肠腺等;另一些腺体没有导管,分泌物(激素)释放入血液,称内分泌腺,如甲状腺、肾上腺等。本节只介绍外分泌腺的结构和分类。

(一)外分泌腺的结构

人体绝大多数外分泌腺属于多细胞腺。多细胞腺大小不等,一般由分泌部和导管两部分组成(图 2-8)。

1. 分泌部

由单层腺细胞围成腺泡,中央有腺泡腔。腺细胞的形态结构因种类、分泌物的性质和功能状态不同而有明显差异。黏液性腺泡由黏液性腺细胞组成(图 2-9A);浆液性腺泡由浆液性腺细胞组成(图 2-9B);混合性腺泡由上述两种腺泡共同组成(图 2-9C)。

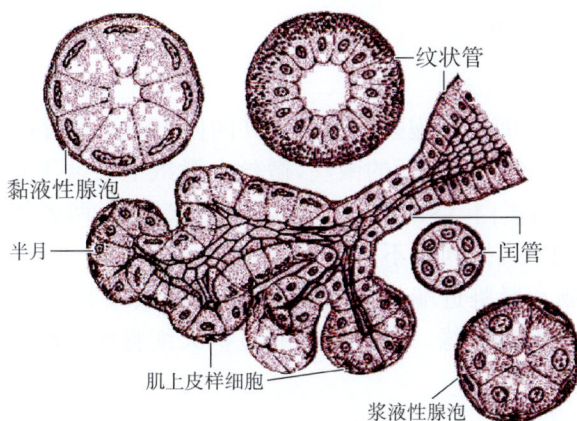

黏液性腺泡

半月

肌上皮样细胞

纹状管

闰管

浆液性腺泡

图 2-8 外分泌腺结构模式图

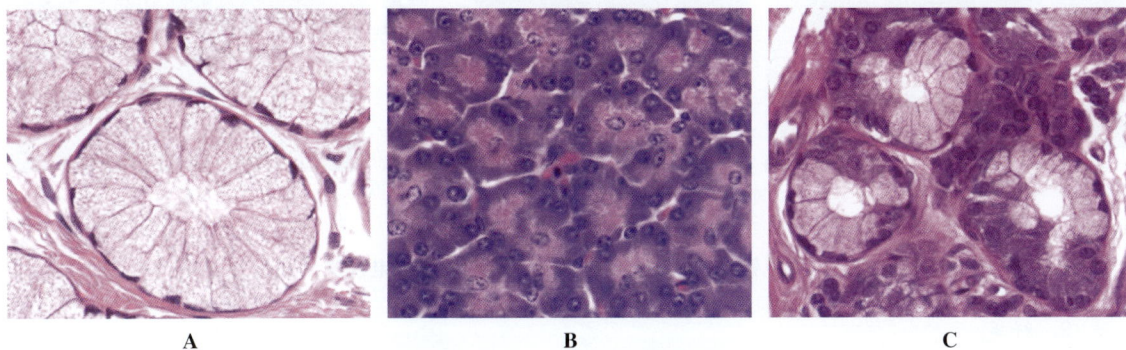

A   B   C

图 2-9 三种类型的腺泡

A. 黏液性腺泡(食管);B. 浆液性腺泡(胰腺);C. 混合性腺泡(气管)

2. 导管

导管与分泌部直接相通,由单层或复层上皮构成。导管主要功能是排出分泌物,有些腺导管还有吸收或分泌水和电解质的功能。按其导管有无分支,外分泌腺可分单腺与复腺。通常把分泌部的形态与导管是否分支两个因素结合考虑对外分泌腺进行分类、命名。

(二) 外分泌腺的分类

外分泌腺有多种分类方法。按组成腺的细胞数可分为单细胞腺(如杯状细胞)和多细胞腺;按导管是否分支可分为单腺(如汗腺和肠腺)和复腺;按分泌部的形状分为管状腺、泡状腺与管泡状腺;按腺细胞分泌物排出的方式分为局部分泌腺、顶浆分泌腺与全浆分泌腺;按腺细胞分泌物的性质分为浆液性腺、黏液性腺与混合性腺。

第三节 细胞表面的特化结构

上皮组织有极性,与其功能相适应,在上皮组织每个细胞的各个面分别形成一些具有重要生理功能的特殊结构,这些结构有的是由细胞质和细胞膜构成,有的是由细胞膜、细胞质和细胞间质共同构成。

一、上皮细胞的游离面

1. 微绒毛

微绒毛是上皮细胞游离面的细胞膜和细胞质共同伸出的细小指状突起。在电镜下微绒毛外包细胞膜,轴心的胞质中有许多纵行的微丝,微丝自微绒毛尖端下行,与细胞质顶部终末网的微丝相连,微丝内含肌动蛋白,终末网的微丝内含肌球蛋白,两者相互作用,致使微绒毛伸长或缩短。微绒毛长短不一,排列也不整齐,并可有分支(图 2-10)。在一些具备活跃吸收功能的上皮细胞,如小肠和肾脏近端小管上皮,其游离面微绒毛多而长,且排列整齐,构成光镜下细胞游离面的纹状缘和刷状缘。微绒毛可明显扩大细胞的表面积,有利于细胞对物质的吸收。

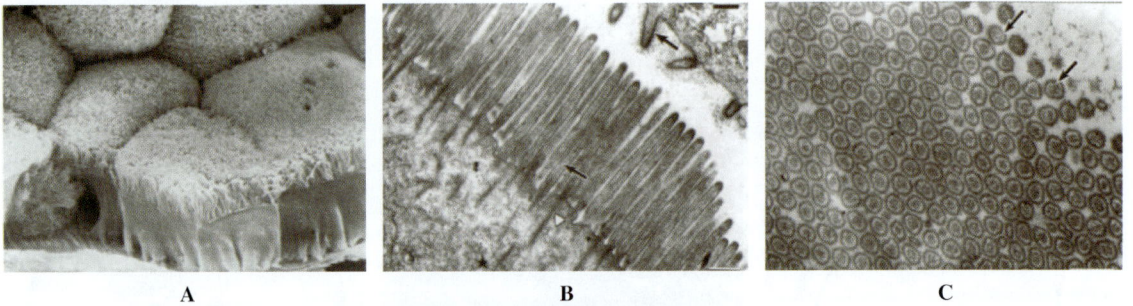

A   B   C

图 2-10 微绒毛电镜结构
A.扫描电镜结构;B.透射电镜纵切面;C.透射电镜横切面

2. 纤毛

纤毛是细胞游离缘细胞膜与细胞质伸出的能摆动的细长突起,长 $5\sim10\mu m$,宽约 $0.2\mu m$,较微绒毛粗而长。在电镜下,纤毛表面有细胞膜,内为细胞质,其中有纵向排列的微管。微管的排列有一定的规律,中央为 2 条完整的微管,周围为 9 组成对的双联微管(图 2-11)。每根纤毛的根部有一个致密颗粒,称基体,基体的结构与中心粒基本相同,有产生纤毛的功能。纤毛具有向一定方向做有节律性摆动的能力,纤毛的摆动与双联微管的相互滑动有关;许多纤毛的协同摆动像风吹麦浪一样,能把黏附在上皮表面的分泌物和颗粒状物质向一定方向推送。如呼吸道的腔面是有纤毛的上皮,通过纤毛的定向摆动,可将被吸入的尘埃和细菌等排出。

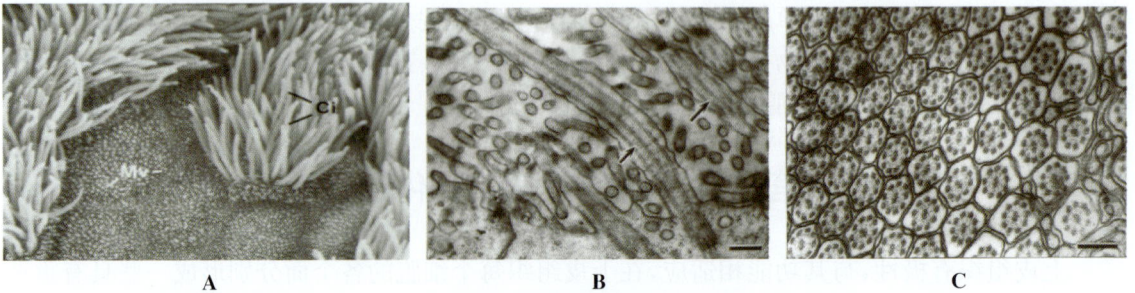

A   B   C

图 2-11 纤毛电镜结构
A.扫描电镜结构;B.透射电镜纵切面;C.透射电镜横切面

二、上皮细胞的侧面

上皮细胞之间排列紧密,间隙很小,其间含有少量糖蛋白等物质,可起着黏着作用。在相邻上皮细胞的侧面上,还分化出一些特殊结构称为细胞连接,主要包括紧密连接、黏合带、桥粒和缝隙连接(图 2-12)。除游离的细胞外,细胞连接也存在于其他组织细胞,如心肌细胞、骨细胞和神经细胞之间。

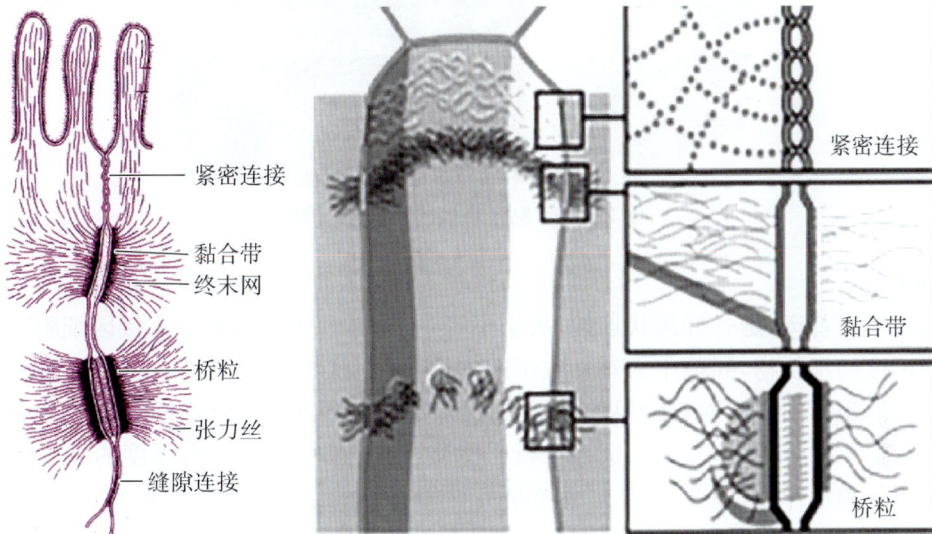

图 2-12　细胞连接模式图

1. 紧密连接

紧密连接又名闭锁小带,位于两相邻细胞侧面的顶端,为长短不等的带状。电镜下,相邻细胞膜外侧的膜蛋白颗粒相互对接,呈网格状融合,细胞间隙消失,将上皮细胞的间隙在近顶端处封闭,未融合处留有间隙(图 2-13)。紧密连接除有机械性连接作用外,更重要的是封闭了相邻细胞顶部的间隙,防止大分子物质由细胞间隙进出。

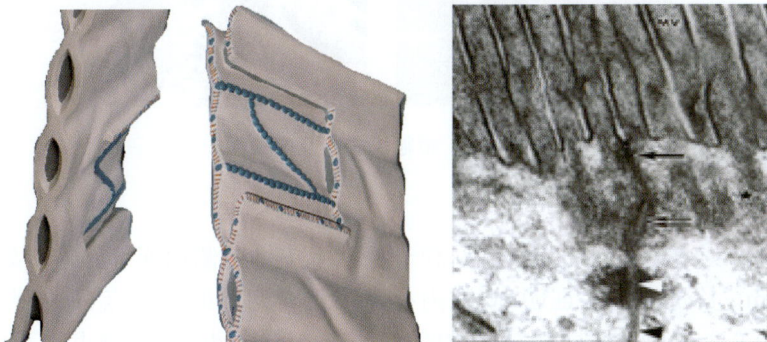

图 2-13　紧密连接模式图及电镜图

2. 黏合带

黏合带又称中间连接,位于紧密连接下方,呈连续带状,环绕上皮细胞。相邻细胞膜间隙较宽,其中充以较致密的丝状物。在细胞膜的胞质面,附着有薄层致密物质和微丝,该处的微丝参与构成细胞顶部胞质中的终末网(图2-14)。黏合带除有黏着作用外,还能使终末网绷紧,保持细胞形状和传递细胞收缩力。

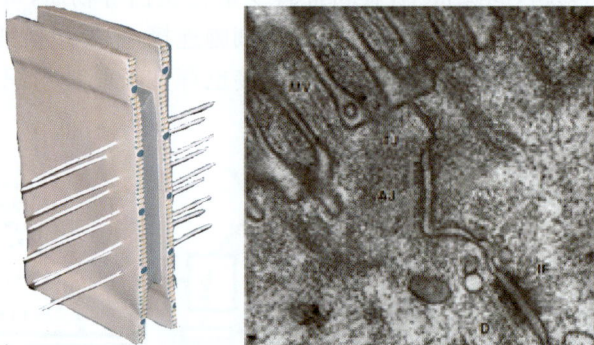

图2-14　黏合带模式图及电镜图

3. 桥粒

桥粒又称黏着斑,是一种斑状连接,大小不等,位于黏合带的深部。连接区细胞间隙较宽,其中有低密度的丝状物,间隙中央有一致密的中线,由丝状物交织而成,这些丝状物属于钙黏蛋白家族。细胞膜的胞质面有较厚的电子致密物质构成的椭圆形附着板,胞质中有许多微丝(角蛋白丝)插入附着板中,并常形成襻状折回胞质,构成有很大抗张力强度的细胞骨架,在细胞内起支持和固定作用(图2-15)。桥粒是一种很牢固的细胞连接,多见于易受机械性刺激或摩擦的部位,如皮肤的复层扁平上皮。

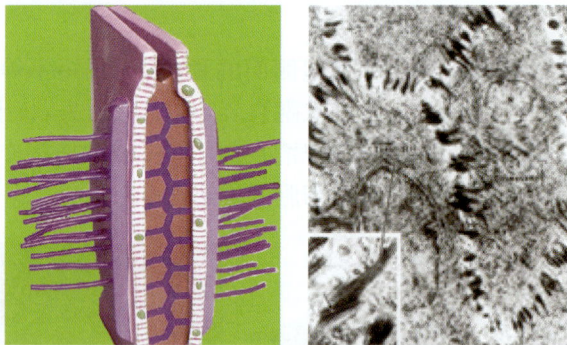

图2-15　桥粒模式图及电镜图

4. 缝隙连接

缝隙连接又称为通信连接,呈斑块状,位于柱状上皮细胞侧面深部。连接处的细胞间隙很窄,仅有2~3 nm。冷冻蚀刻法证明,间隙内有许多距离相等的连接点,连接点是相邻对应的细胞膜内镶嵌的6个亚单位蛋白颗粒围成的直径1.5 nm的小管,两侧小管互相接通,成为细胞间的交通管道(图2-16)。在钙离子和其他因素作用下,管道可以开放或闭合。一般分子量小于1500的物质,包括离子、cAMP等信使分子、氨基酸、葡萄糖、维生素等,均可以在细胞间交换,使细胞在营养代谢、增殖分化和功能等方面成为统一体。

以上四种细胞连接,只要有两个或两个以上连接同时存在,即称为连接复合体。

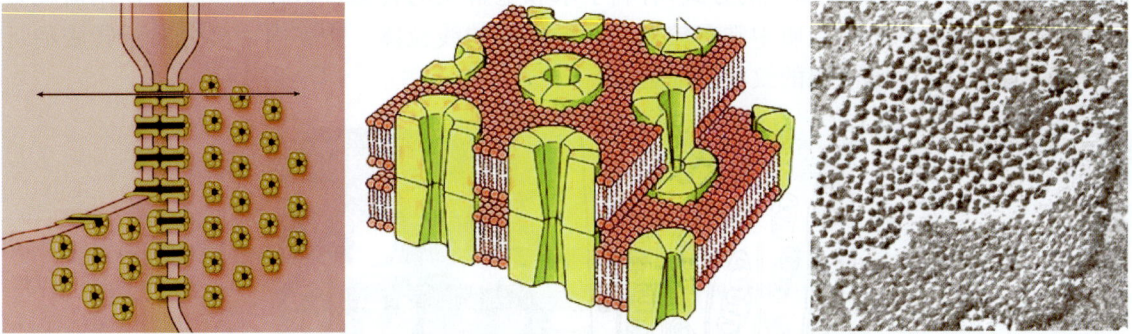

图 2-16　缝隙连接模式图及电镜图

三、上皮细胞的基底面

1. 基膜

基膜是上皮细胞基底面与深部结缔组织之间的薄层膜状结构。由于很薄，在 HE 染色切片中一般不能分辨，但假复层纤毛柱状上皮和复层扁平上皮的基膜较厚，呈粉红色（图 2-17A）。用镀银染色时可见基膜呈黑色。在电镜下，基膜由靠近上皮的基板和与结缔组织相连的网板所构成（图 2-17B）；也可由两层基板构成，如肾血管球的基膜；还有一些上皮的基膜仅由基板组成。

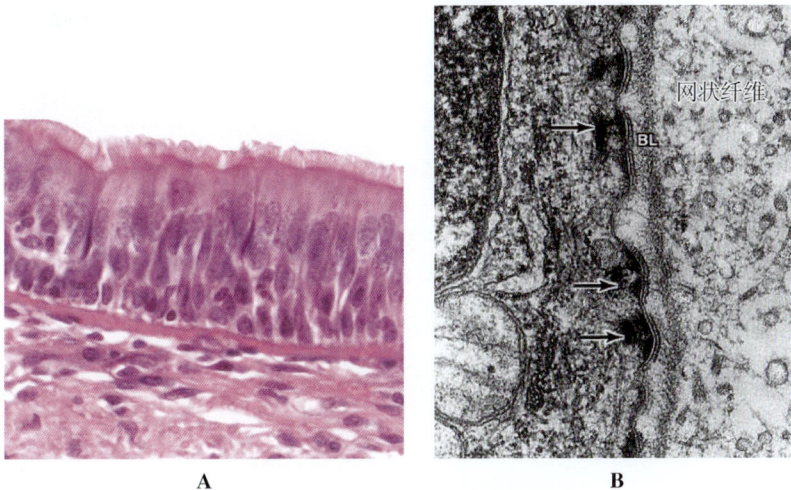

图 2-17　基膜光镜图及电镜图
A.气管，HE 染色；B.基膜电镜图

基板主要是上皮细胞的产物，构成基板的主要成分有层粘连蛋白、Ⅳ型胶原蛋白和硫酸肝素蛋白聚糖等。网板由结缔组织内成纤维细胞产生，主要由网状纤维和基质构成。

基膜除具有支持、连接和固着作用外，还可作为半透膜使上皮细胞与深部结缔组织进行物质交换。基膜还能引导上皮细胞移动，影响细胞的增殖和分化。

2. 质膜内褶

质膜内褶是上皮细胞基底面的细胞膜折入胞质所形成的许多内褶（图 2-18）。质膜内褶是一种扩大细胞基底面表面积的方式,有利于水和电解质的转运。这种物质转运作用需耗费能量,故质膜内褶附近的胞质中常有较多的纵行排列的线粒体。质膜内褶多分布于肾脏的近端小管、远端小管及唾液腺的纹状管细胞内。

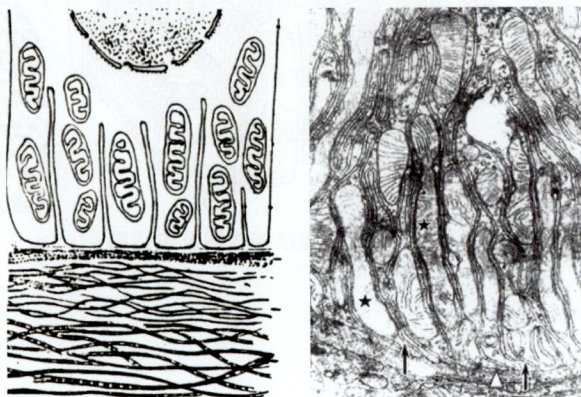

图 2-18　质膜内褶模式图及电镜图

3. 半桥粒

半桥粒位于上皮细胞基底面,为上皮基底面上形成的半个桥粒结构,将上皮细胞固着于基膜上。

（赵奕淳　郑　英）

Chapter 3

Connective Tissue

Connective tissue includes a variety of tissues with different functional properties in the human body. Connective tissue consists of two major constituents: cells and extracellular matrix. Cells in the connective tissue are relatively small in number, and the extracellular matrix is generally the dominant component, which includes ground substance, protein fibers and tissue fluid. The connective tissue shows differences when compared with the epithelial tissue: many complex extracellular components, a low number of cells, no polarity, and different types of cells in different connective tissues. Nutrients and metabolic wastes are exchanged between the tissue fluid and blood because of the enriched blood vessels in the connective tissue. The connective tissue has the functions of support, connection, defense, protection, nutrition, repair and so on.

The connective tissues originate from the mesenchyme, an embryonic tissue formed by elongated cells, the mesenchymal cells. The mesenchyme is the mesoderm during the embryonic period, which fills between the ectoderm and the endoderm, and consists of the mesenchymal cells and matrix without fibers. Mesenchymal cells are poorly differentiated, which can differentiate into multiple connective tissue cells, endothelial cells, smooth muscle cells and so on. There are still a small number of undifferentiated mesenchymal cells in the adult connective tissue.

According to the composition and organization of cellular and extracellular components, connective tissues are classified into various types. The generalized connective tissue includes the connective tissue proper, cartilage, bone, blood and lymph. The narrow connective tissue refers to the connective tissue proper. The connective tissue proper can be further divided into loose connective tissue, dense connective tissue, adipose tissue and reticular tissue based on the variations in the types and number of the cells and fibers.

1 Loose Connective Tissue

Loose connective tissue, also called areolar tissue, is characterized by a relatively large number of different cell types, abundance of ground substance and loosely arranged thin fibers. It fills spaces between organs, tissues in the organs, and cells, which are rich in blood vessels. It has many functions such as support, nutrition, defense, protection, repair, etc.

1.1 Cells

Several types of cells are found in the loose connective tissue: fibroblasts, macrophages, plasma cells, mast cells, adipose cells and undifferentiated mesenchymal cells. The number, proportion and distribution of cells can vary depending on the functional state of the loose connective tissue. In addition, granulocytes and lymphocytes in the blood can be transient inhabitants of the loose connective tissue during inflammation and immune response.

1.1.1 Fibroblasts

Fibroblasts are the most common cells in the connective tissue. They are large and flat, have abundant and irregularly branched basophilic cytoplasm. Its nucleus is large, ovoid, with a prominent nucleolus. The cytoplasm is rich in rough endoplasmic reticulum and free ribosomes, and the Golgi complex is well developed (Figure 3 - 1), indicating enhanced protein synthesis. Fibroblasts can synthesize proteins, such as collagen and elastin, that form collagen fibers, reticular fibers and elastic fibers, and the glycosaminoglycans, glycoproteins of the extracellular matrix.

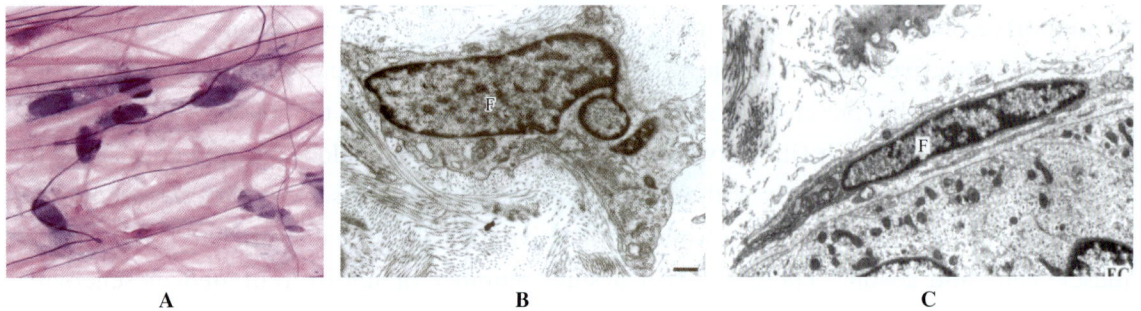

A   B   C

Figure 3 - 1 Fibroblasts & fibrocyte
A. LM of fibroblasts (CT, HE); B. EM of fibroblast; C. EM of fibrocyte

The quiescent fibroblast, or fibrocyte, is smaller than the active fibroblast and tends to be spindle-shaped. It has fewer processes; a smaller, darker nucleus; an acidophilic cytoplasm; and a small number of organelles (Figure 3 - 1). The fibrocyte reverts to the fibroblast state during wound healing and regeneration of the connective tissue. Meanwhile, the fibroblast can undergo division and proliferation.

1.1.2 Macrophages

Macrophages were characterized by their potent phagocytic ability, and also called histiocytes in the loose connective tissue. They are often scattered throughout the fibers, and will be activated into wandering macrophages with the stimulation of inflammation or foreign bodies. Macrophages have a wide spectrum of morphologic features that correspond to their state of functional activity, such as oval, round or irregular surface with protuberant pseudopodia. They often have an oval or kidney-shaped nucleus located-eccentrically, and an acidophilic cytoplasm. Under electron microscope, macrophages are characterized by an irregular surface with pleats, protrusions, and indentations, a morphologic expression of their active pinocytotic and phagocytic activities. They generally have many lysosomes, phagosomes, pinocytotic vesicles and residual bodies (Figure 3-2). There are many microfilaments and microtubules near the cell membrane.

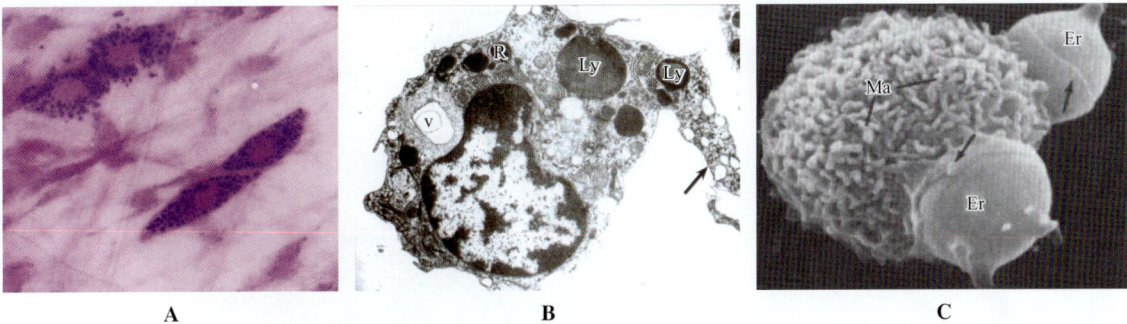

Figure 3-2   Macrophages
A. LM of macrophages (Connective tissue); B. & C. EM of macrophages

Macrophages derive from monocytes that circulate in the blood. The monocytes which derived from bone marrow precursor cells cross the wall of capillary and venules to penetrate the connective tissue, where they mature and acquire morphologic features of macrophages. Their main functions include: ①Chemotaxis and deformation: macrophages will migrate directionally in response to the concentration gradients of a chemical stimulus such as bacterial metabolites and denatured products of inflammatory tissue. ②Identification, adhesion and phagocytosis: macrophages can identify, adhere and phagocytize foreign bodies and senescent cells to become phagosomes or swallowing vesicles, and then fuse with the primary lysosomes to form the secondary lysosomes for intracellular digestion, which will produce residual bodies. ③Involved in immune response: macrophages can not only capture, process and store antigens, but also present them to lymphocytes to initiate the immune response of lymphocytes. The macrophages themselves are also immunocompetent cells. The macrophages that stimulated by lymphokines have enhanced biological functions and can directly kill tumor cells. The interferon and interleukin-1 they secrete can significantly enhance the immunocompetence of lymphocytes. ④Secretion: macrophages can produce an impressive array of bioactive substances, such as interferon, complement, interleukin-1, angiogenesis factor, etc. They are involved in the regulation of body defense and cell functions. In addition, the secretory products released by the macrophage can release hydrolytic enzymes in lysosomes to dissolve senescent cells and tissues, and produce negative oxygen ions, hydroxyl radicals and other oxidants to sterilize and kill tumor cells.

1.1.3 Plasma Cells

Plasma cells are round or ovoid cells that have a basophilic cytoplasm. The nucleus of the plasma cell is spherical and eccentrically placed, containing compact, coarse heterochromatin alternating with lighter areas of approximately equal size. Under the electron microscope, a large number of rough endoplasmic reticulum and well-developed Golgi complexes can be observed in the cytoplasm of plasma cells. The Golgi complexes and the centrioles occupy a region that appears pale in regular histologic preparations (Figure 3 – 3).

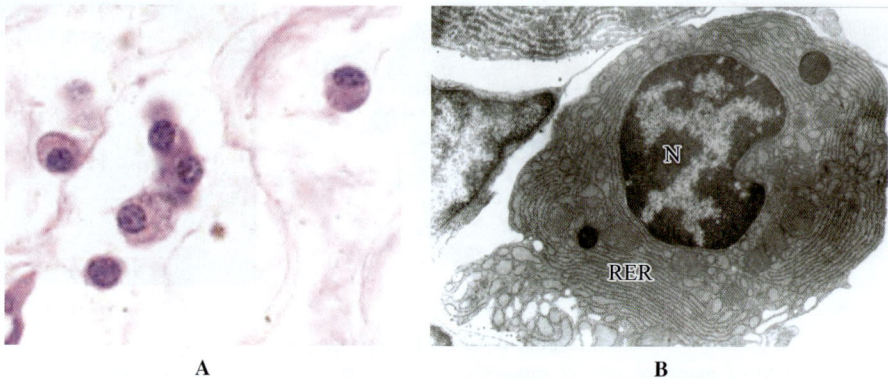

A   B

Figure 3 – 3   Plasma cells
A. LM of plasma cells (Connective tissue); B. EM of plasma cell

Plasma cells are derived from B lymphocytes with the stimulus of the antigen. There are few plasma cells in most connective tissues, and more cells in the places that susceptible to the antigen invasion including connective tissues of the respiratory tract and digestive tract and the lesions of chronic inflammation.

1.1.4   Mast Cells

Mast cells are large, round or ovoid cells with small nuclei. Their cytoplasm is filled with basophilic secretory granules (Figure 3 – 4), which have two characteristics. ①Metachromatic: the colour that mast cells stain with the dye is different from the dye's original colour. For example, the granules are stained purple with toluidine blue. ②Water-soluble: it is difficult to distinguish mast cells from other cells because the granules are dissolved in water. Under the electron microscope, there are a small number of microvilli on the surface of mast cells. Their interior is heterogeneous in appearance, with a prominent scroll-like structure that contains pre-formed mediators such as heparin, histamine, eosinophil chemotactic factor of anaphylaxis, leukotriene (slow reacting substance), prostaglandin and other bioactive substances. Mast cells are widely distributed in the human body but are particularly abundant in the dermis of the skin and in the digestive and respiratory tracts. Mast cells are involved in allergic or immediate hypersensitive reactions. The process of anaphylaxis consists of the following sequential events: the first exposure to an antigen (allergen), such as bee venom, results in production of IgE, a type of immunoglobulin (antibodies) by plasma cells. IgE then binds to the IgE receptor on them mast cell membrane. A second exposure to the same antigen results in binding of the antigen of IgE on the mast cells. This event triggers degranulation of mast cells and release of granular content, causing allergic reactions.

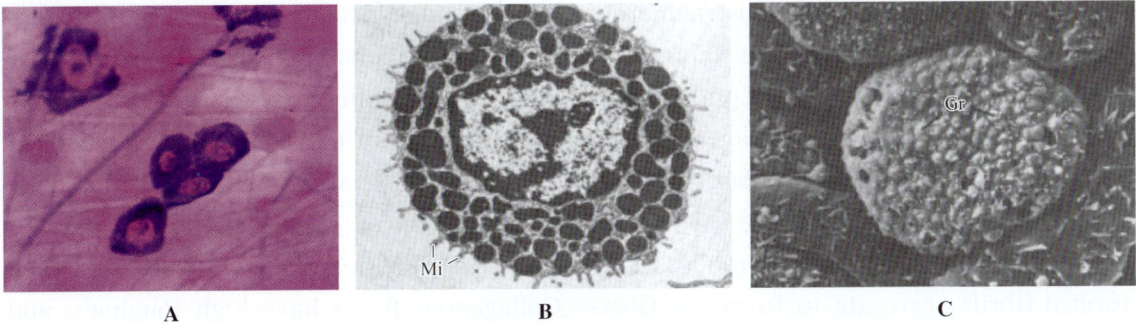

Figure 3 – 4   Mast cells
A. LM of mast cells (Connective tissue, toluidine blue staining); B. & C. EM of mast cell

1.1.5   Adipocytes

Adipocytes are large, spherical or polygonal cells. There is a large central lipid droplet in the cytoplasm of the mature adipocyte. The cytoplasm is squeezed by the lipid droplet to form a thin layer, and the nucleus is also squeezed into an oblate shape. The cytoplasm and the nucleus together are crescent-shaped and biased to one side of the cell. In HE sections, adipocytes show vacuolated cytoplasm as the lipid droplets are dissolved (Figure 3 – 5). Adipocytes can synthesize and store fat, and participate in energy metabolism.

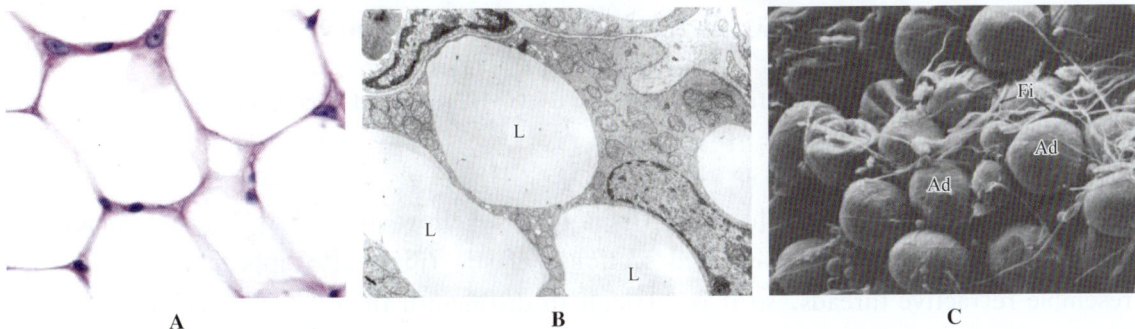

Figure 3 – 5   Adipocytes
A. LM of adipocytes (Connective tissue); B. & C. EM of adipocytes

1.1.6   Undifferentiated Mesenchymal Cells

The morphology of undifferentiated mesenchymal cells is similar to the fibroblasts, whereas they are smaller. They are often associated with the small blood vessels, especially capillaries. They maintain developmental multi-potentiality of embryonic mesenchymal cells. The cells can differentiate into fibroblasts, adipocytes, endothelial cells and smooth muscle cells during physiological regeneration, inflammation and damage repair.

1.2   Fibers

There are three types of fibers in connective tissue: collagenous fibers, reticular fibers and elastic fibers.

1.2.1 Collagenous Fiber

Collagen fibers are the most numerous in loose connective tissue. Fresh collagenous fibers appear white; they are therefore called white fibers. In HE-stained sections, collagenous fibers are stained pink, and organized in parallel to each other, forming collagenous fiber bundles. Collagenous fibers are composed of collagen fibrils. Under the electron microscope, collagenous fibrils have transverse striation with a characteristic periodicity of 64 nm (Figure 3 - 6). They are composed of collagen types Ⅰ and Ⅲ. Collagen is secreted by the fibroblasts and aggregates into the collagen fibrils, and then formed fibrils aggregate to form the fibers. Collagenous fibers have high toughness and high tensile resistance.

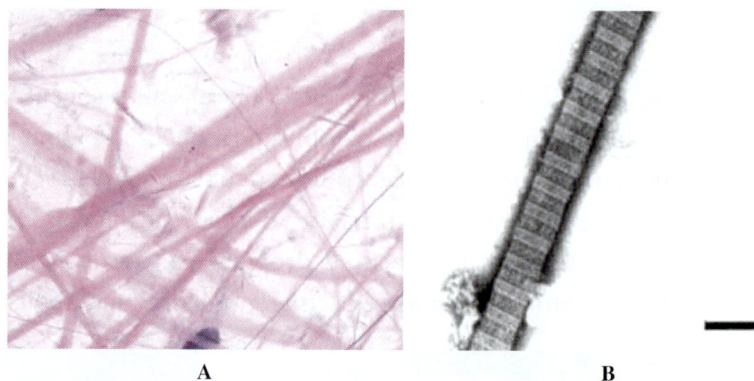

Figure 3 - 6   Collagen fibers

A. LM of collagen fibers (Connective tissue, HE); B. EM of collagen fiber

1.2.2 Elastic Fiber

Sufficient number of fresh elastic fibers have a yellow colour, so they are sometimes termed yellow fibers. In HE-stained sections, elastic fibers also appear weak pink but resemble refractive threads, so it is difficult to distinguish them from collagenous fibers. The elastic fibers can be clearly seen with some special stains, including resorcin-fuchsin, eosin, nigrosine and so on. They are thinner than collagenous fibers, and are arranged in a branching pattern to form an irregular network. Electron microscopic observations reveal that elastic fibers are composed of elastin and microfibrils. Elastin can crimp arbitrarily, and the molecules are connected by covalent bonds to form a network (Figure 3 - 7). There is a 2.5-times difference in the length of elastin with or without the effect of external force. Elastic fibers can be elongated and restored easily because they are elastic. They are intertwined with collagen fibers to make the loose connective tissue tough and elastic. Elastic fibers are derived from fibroblasts, chondrocytes and smooth muscle cells.

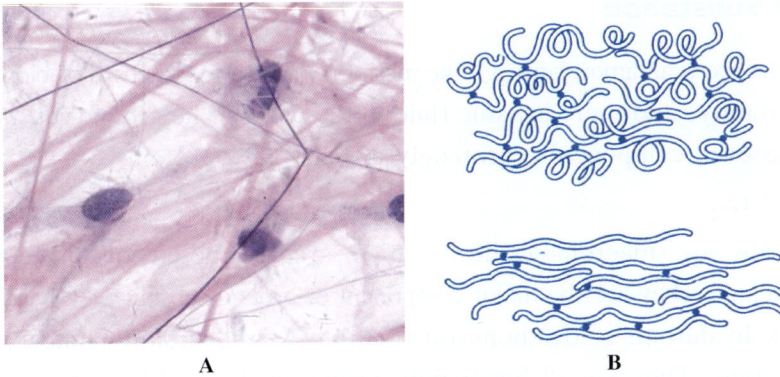

Figure 3 - 7　Elastic fibers
A. LM of elastic fibers (Connective tissue); B. Molecular structure of elastic fibers

1.2.3　Reticular Fibers

Reticular fibers are not visible in HE preparations but can be easily stained black brown by impregnation with silver salts. Because of their affinity for silver salts, these fibers are called argyrophilic (Figure 3 - 8). Reticular fibers are extremely thin, and arranged in a branching pattern to form an irregular network.

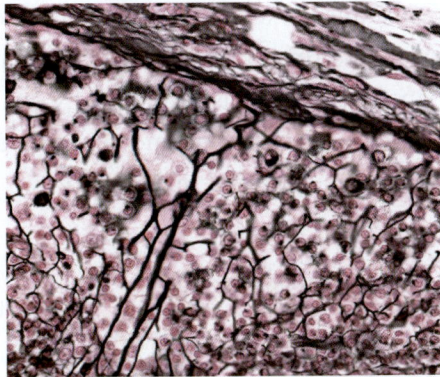

Figure 3 - 8　Reticular fibers (Lymph node, silver staining)

Reticular fibers are composed mainly of collagen type III. Under the electron microscope, reticular fibers also have transverse striation with a characteristic periodicity of 64 nm. They are widely distributed at the junction of the connective tissue and other tissues, and have the functions of connection and fixation. The small diameter and the loose disposition of reticular fibers create a flexible network in organs that are subjected to changes in form or volume, such as lymphoid tissue, lymphoid organs and hematopoietic organs.

1.3　Ground Substance

Ground substance is an amorphous gel-like substance, which is composed of biomacromolecules. It is viscous certainly, and there is tissue fluid in the pores. The ground substance is formed mainly of 2 classes of components: proteoglycans and glycoproteins.

1.3.1　Proteoglycans

Proteoglycans are macromolecules, which are composed of proteins and many glycosaminoglycans. They are the major component of ground substance. Glycosaminoglycans (GAGs) include hyaluronic acid, chondroitin sulfate A, chondroitin sulfate C, keratin sulfate and heparan sulfate. They are all linear polysaccharides formed by repeating disaccharide units. Hyaluronic acid, the predominant GAG in loose connective tissue, is a long and rigid molecule. The other GAGs bind to the core protein to form a subunit of proteoglycan, which can bind to the hyaluronic acid by means of linker proteins, and finally form molecular sieve (Figure 3 - 9). There are many anions on the chains of polysaccharides, which can bind to the cations in inorganic salts and water molecules to maintain the characteristics of water as a solvent, playing a role of ion exchangers in regulating metabolism and transportation of water and salt. Water, water-soluble nutrients, metabolites, hormones and gas molecules can pass the molecular sieve freely, which is beneficial to the substance exchange between blood and cells. Conversely, molecular sieve acts as a barrier to prevent the spread of pathogenic microorganisms and bacteria. The hyaluronidase enzyme, which is produced by snake venom, cancer cells and hemolytic streptococcus, will break down hyaluronic acid and destroy the barrier, thereby allowing the spread of toxins, cancer cells and inflammation.

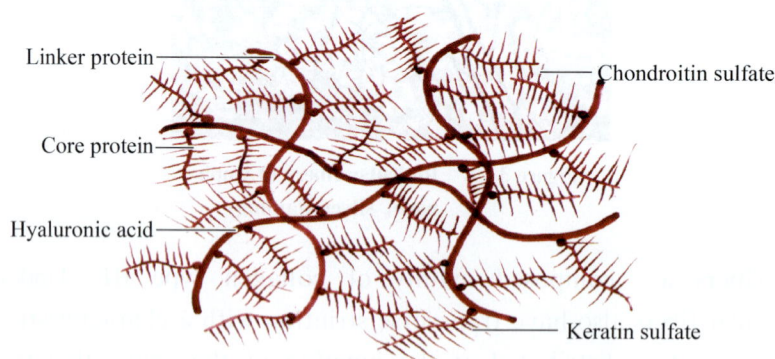

Figure 3 - 9　General structure of molecular sieve

1.3.2　Glycoproteins

Glycoproteins are another type of biomacromolecules in the ground substance, mainly including fibronectin, laminin and chondronectin. They are not only involved in the formation of the molecular sieve, but also affect cell adhesion and migration through connection and mediation. They are also involved in the regulation of cell growth and differentiation.

There is also a very small amount of tissue fluid in the ground substance. The fluid passes through the capillary walls as a result of the hydrostatic pressure of the blood (Figure 3 - 10). Normally, water passes through capillary walls to the surrounding tissues at the arterial end of a capillary, and water is drawn back into the capillary at the venous end of the capillary. In this way, blood brings to connective tissue the various nutrients required by its cells and carries metabolic waste products away to the detoxifying and excretory organs. In several pathologic conditions, the quality of tissue fluid may increase or decrease considerably, causing edema or dehydration, which both affect the normal physiological activities of cells.

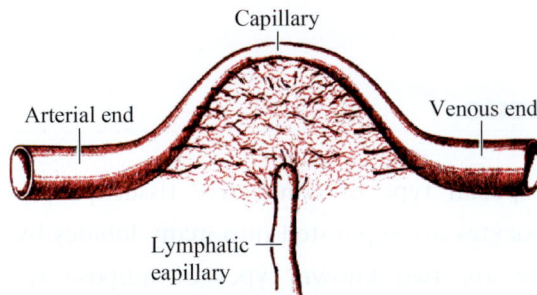

Figure 3 - 10   Formation of tissue fluid

2   Dense Connective Tissue

Dense connective tissue consists of the same components found in the loose connective tissue, but there are fewer cells and a clear predominance of collagen fibers in it (Figure 3 - 11). The collagen fibers are aligned with the linear orientation of fibroblasts in response to prolonged stresses exerted in the same direction. According to the differences of collagen fibers, dense connective tissue can be divided into dense regular connective tissue and dense irregular connective tissue. Tendon and aponeurosis are common examples of dense regular connective tissue. They have parallel, closely packed bundles of collagen separated by a small quantity of intercellular ground substance. There are fibroblasts with special morphology between the fiber bundles, which are named tenocytes. The dermis, dura mater, sclera and some endocrine glands are known as the dense irregular connective tissue, because the collagen fibers are arranged in bundles without a definite orientation and there are few cells between the fibers. The major functions of the dense connective tissue are connection, support and protection.

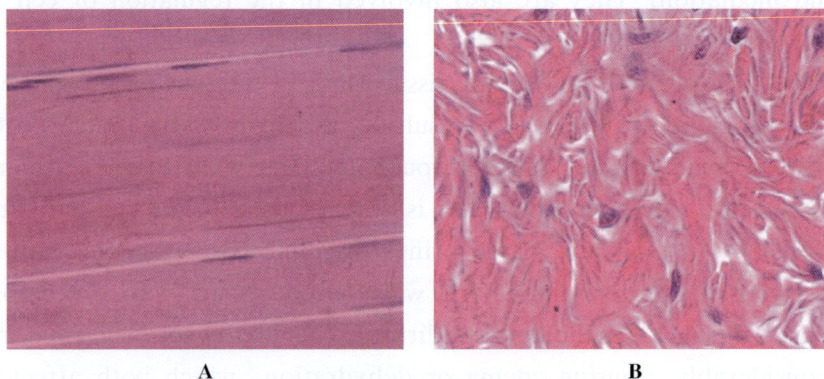

Figure 3 – 11   Dense connective tissue

A. LM of dense regular connective tissue (Tendon, HE); B. LM of dense irregular connective tissue (Small intestine, HE)

3 Adipose Tissue

Adipose tissue is a special type of connective tissue proper in which adipose cells predominate. Many adipocytes are separated into many lobules by a small amount of loose connective tissues. There are two known types of adipose tissue that have different morphological structures and functions: yellow (common, or unilocular) adipose tissue and brown (multilocular) adipose tissue (Figure 3 – 12).

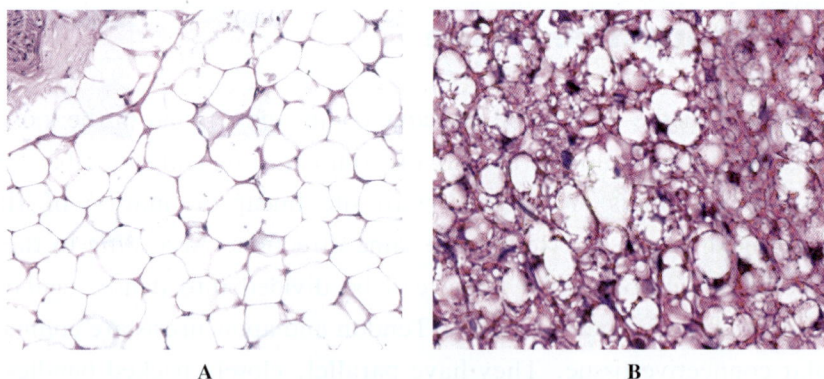

Figure 3 – 12   Adipose tissue

A. LM of yellow adipose tissue; B. LM of Brown adipose tissue

Yellow adipose tissue is composed of cells that, when completely developed, contain one large central droplet of yellow fat in their cytoplasm. Most adipose tissues in the bodies of adult are yellow adipose tissues that can storage the most energy, and have functions of maintaining body temperature, buffering, protecting, supporting and filling. They are mainly distributed in the subcutaneous tissue, omentum, mesentery, etc.

Brown adipose tissue is composed of cells with numerous lipid droplets and abundant brown mitochondria. Brown adipose tissue has a rich blood supply and many nerves. There is little brown adipose tissue in the adult, whereas more (2%~5% of the body weight) in the newborn. When this type of tissue is stimulated in the cold, stored lipids will be decomposed and oxidized, which can release a lot of heat to warm the body.

4 Reticular Tissue

Reticular tissue is composed of reticular cells, reticular fibers and ground substance. Reticular cells are star-shaped cells with abundant and irregularly branched basophilic cytoplasm. They have large nuclei with prominent nucleoli. Their cytoplasm is rich in rough endoplasmic reticulum. Reticular fibers, which are produced by reticular cells, have many branches that are located in the cell body and processes of reticular cells, forming the scaffold of reticula tissues (Figure 3 - 13). Reticular tissue provides the architectural framework that creates a special microenvironment for hematopoietic organs and lymphoid organs.

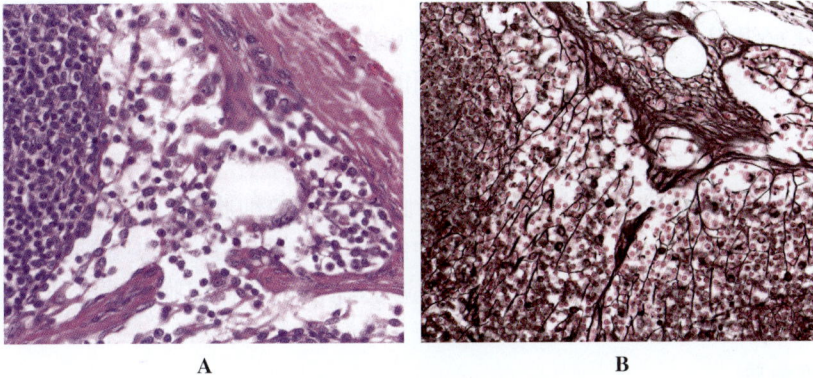

Figure 3 - 13　Reticular tissue
A. LM of Reticular tissue (Lymph node, HE); B. LM of reticular tissue (Lymph node, silver staining)

(Ge Tingting, Yang Fan)

第三章　结 缔 组 织

　　结缔组织是人体内分布最广泛、结构和功能最多样的一种组织。由细胞和大量的细胞间质构成。细胞散在于细胞间质内。细胞间质包括细丝状的纤维、无定形的基质和组织液。与上皮组织相比,结缔组织的细胞间质成分多且复杂,细胞数量少,没有极性,细胞的类型和数量随结缔组织的类型不同而有差异。结缔组织含有丰富的血管,细胞通过结缔组织内的组织液与血液进行物质交换。结缔组织具有支持、连接、防御、保护、营养和修复等功能。

所有的结缔组织都是由胚胎时期的间充质演变而来。间充质是胚胎时期填充在外胚层和内胚层之间的散在的中胚层组织,由间充质细胞和基质组成,无纤维成分。间充质细胞是一种低分化的细胞,不但能分化为多种结缔组织细胞,还能分化为内皮细胞和平滑肌细胞等。成体的结缔组织内仍保留有少量的未分化间充质细胞。

根据细胞和纤维的种类及基质的状态不同,结缔组织可分为多种类型。广义的结缔组织包括固有结缔组织、软骨组织、骨组织、血液和淋巴。狭义的结缔组织是指固有结缔组织,其基质呈胶状,细胞和纤维散在分布其中,根据细胞的类型和数量及纤维的种类和含量的不同,可分为疏松结缔组织、致密结缔组织、脂肪组织和网状组织。

第一节　疏松结缔组织

疏松结缔组织纤维细而少且分布比较疏松,细胞种类多,而基质比较丰富,呈疏松网状结构,故又称为蜂窝组织。疏松结缔组织富含血管,在体内广泛分布于器官之间和器官内部的各种组织、细胞之间,具有支持、营养、防御、保护和修复等多种功能。

一、细胞

疏松结缔组织中细胞种类较多,包括成纤维细胞、巨噬细胞、浆细胞、肥大细胞、脂肪细胞和未分化的间充质细胞等。细胞的数量和各种细胞的比例及分布,均可因疏松结缔组织的功能状态不同而有变化。此外,在炎症和免疫反应时,血液中的粒细胞和淋巴细胞也可游走入疏松结缔组织中。

1. 成纤维细胞

成纤维细胞是疏松结缔组织中的主要细胞。细胞大而扁平,多突起,胞质嗜碱性,核较大,呈卵圆形,核仁明显。电镜下,胞质内可见丰富的粗面内质网和游离的核糖体,高尔基复合体发达,表明其具有旺盛的蛋白质合成功能。成纤维细胞的功能是形成纤维和基质。成纤维细胞能合成和分泌胶原蛋白和弹性蛋白,形成胶原纤维、网状纤维和弹性纤维。同时还能分泌糖胺聚糖和糖蛋白形成基质。

处于功能静止状态的成纤维细胞称纤维细胞,其胞体较小,突起少,呈梭形,核小而着色深,胞质嗜酸性。电镜下,胞质内细胞器不发达。纤维细胞在创伤修复和结缔组织再生时,能转化为成纤维细胞(图 3-1),同时成纤维细胞也能分裂增生。

2. 巨噬细胞

巨噬细胞是体内吞噬能力最强大的细胞,在疏松结缔组织中也称为组织细胞。常沿纤维散在分布,在炎症或异物的刺激下,活化成游走的巨噬细胞。其胞体形态可随其功能状态不同而呈现多样,如卵圆形、圆形或带有伪足样突起的不规则形。其胞核较小,呈卵圆或肾形,着色较深。其胞质丰富,多呈嗜酸性。电镜下,细胞表面具有许多微皱褶及突起,胞质内含有大量的初级溶酶体、次级溶酶体、吞噬体、吞饮小泡和残余体,细胞膜附近有较多的微丝、微管等(图 3-2)。

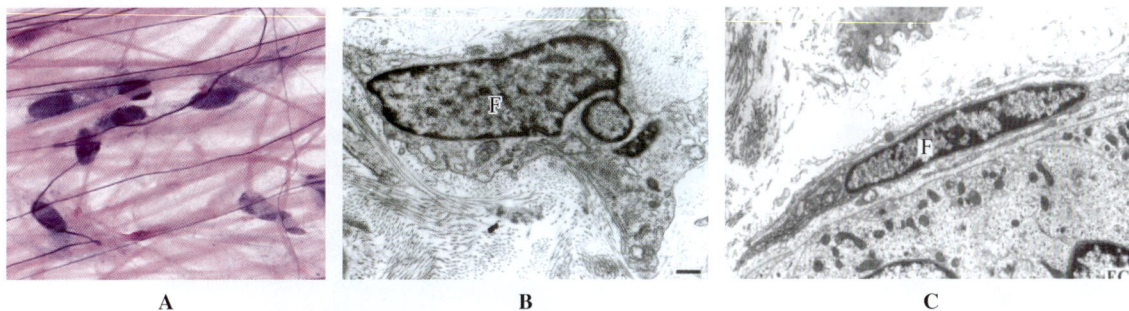

图3-1 成纤维细胞和纤维细胞
A. 成纤维细胞光镜结构(疏松结缔组织,HE染色);B. 成纤维细胞电镜结构;C. 纤维细胞电镜结构

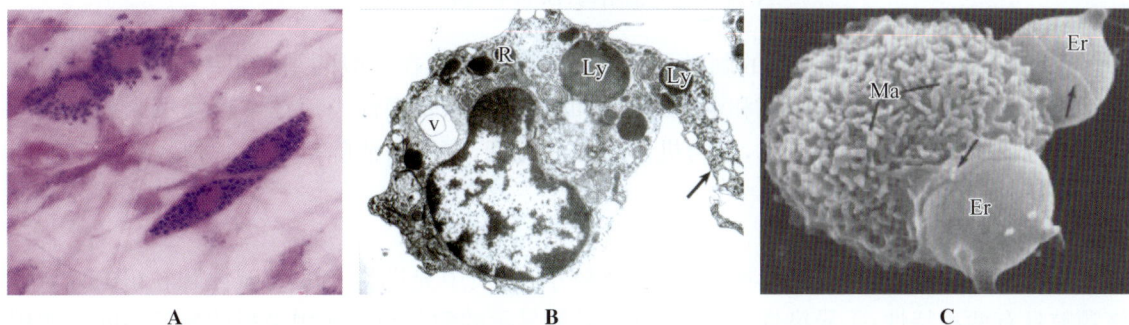

图3-2 巨噬细胞
A. 巨噬细胞光镜结构(疏松结缔组织);B、C. 巨噬细胞电镜结构

巨噬细胞是由血液中的单核细胞穿越毛细血管壁或微静脉壁,进入结缔组织分化而成的。其主要功能有:①趋化性与变形运动。当巨噬细胞受到细菌代谢产物和炎症组织的变性产物等化学性趋化因子吸引时,就能沿着这些化学物质的浓度梯度,定向地进行活跃的变形运动,向着趋化因子浓度最高的地方集聚。②识别、黏附和吞噬功能。巨噬细胞能识别外来的异物和体内衰老变性的细胞等成分,将其黏附于细胞表面,再伸出伪足,包围并吞噬入胞内,成为吞噬体或吞饮小泡,并与初级溶酶体融合成次级溶酶体,进行细胞内消化,消化分解后的残留物称残余体。③参与免疫应答。巨噬细胞不仅能捕捉、加工、处理和储存抗原,还能将抗原呈递给淋巴细胞,启动淋巴细胞的免疫应答。而其本身也是免疫活性细胞,被淋巴因子活化的巨噬细胞的各种功能大大加强,能直接杀伤肿瘤细胞,其分泌的干扰素和白细胞介素-1等能明显地增强淋巴细胞的免疫活性。④分泌功能。巨噬细胞能合成分泌数十种生物活性物质,如干扰素、补体、白细胞介素-1、血管生成因子等,参与机体防御、激活并调节相关细胞的功能。此外,巨噬细胞还能释放溶酶体中的水解酶,溶解衰老的细胞和组织,释放负氧离子、羟自由基等氧化剂杀菌和杀伤肿瘤细胞。

3. 浆细胞

浆细胞呈圆形或卵圆形,核小而圆,常偏于一侧,染色质粗大、呈块状,常位于核膜内面,排列呈车轮状。胞质丰富,嗜碱性,近核侧常有一浅染区。电镜下,胞质中可见大量呈层板状排列的粗面内质网和发达的高尔基复合体,中心粒位于核旁浅染区(图3-3)。

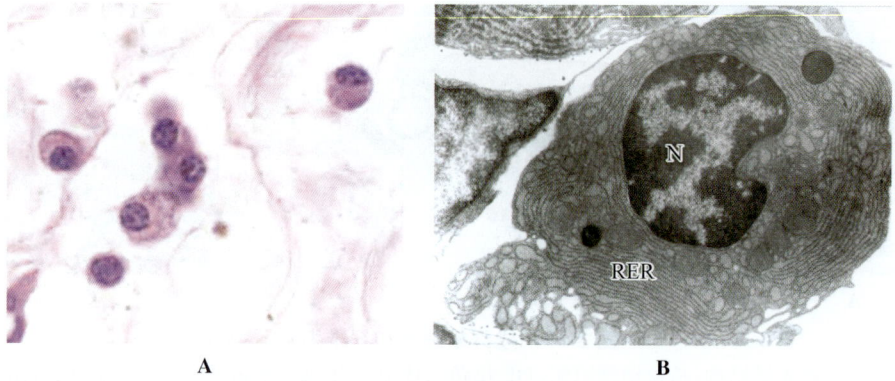

图 3-3 浆细胞
A.浆细胞光镜结构;B.浆细胞电镜结构

浆细胞是由 B 细胞在抗原的刺激下增殖分化而成的。在一般的结缔组织中较少见,但在易受抗原入侵的部位,如呼吸道和消化道黏膜的结缔组织及慢性炎症灶中较多见。浆细胞能合成与分泌免疫球蛋白,即抗体,参与机体的体液免疫,中和并清除抗原。一种浆细胞只能产生一种特异性的抗体。

4. 肥大细胞

肥大细胞胞体较大,呈圆形或卵圆形,核较小,胞质中充满粗大的嗜碱性颗粒(图 3-4),该颗粒具有两种特性:①异染性,即颗粒染色后所显示的颜色与所使用染料的颜色不同。如用甲苯胺蓝染色后颗粒呈现紫色。②水溶性,在常规 HE 染色过程中,因颗粒被水溶解而不易与其他细胞区别。电镜下,肥大细胞表面有少量的微绒毛,胞质内的颗粒均有单位膜包裹,内含有肝素、组胺、嗜酸性细胞趋化因子等,胞质内还有白三烯(慢反应物质)、前列腺素等多种生物活性物质。肥大细胞膜表面有能与免疫球蛋白 E(IgE)结合的受体,能与浆细胞产生的 IgE 抗体结合。肥大细胞广泛存在于体内,常沿小血管和淋巴管分布,在真皮、消化道和呼吸道黏膜中尤多,与这些部位的变态反应密切相关。当机体受到致敏原刺激后,浆细胞产生的 IgE 与肥大细胞膜上的受体结合,使之致敏。当该致敏原再次进入机体时,即与肥大细胞膜上 IgE 的抗原结合端结合,从而使肥大细胞的颗粒内容物释放至细胞外,引起过敏反应。

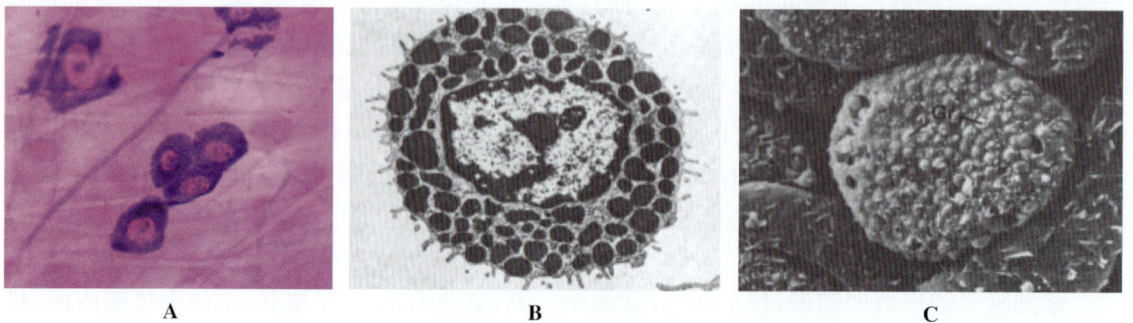

图 3-4 肥大细胞
A.肥大细胞光镜结构(疏松结缔组织,甲苯胺蓝染色);B、C.肥大细胞电镜结构

5. 脂肪细胞

胞体较大,呈圆球形或多边形。成熟的脂肪细胞胞质内有一个很大的中心脂滴,胞质被挤到周边成一薄层,胞核也被挤成扁圆形,连同核周的胞质呈新月形,偏于细胞的一侧。在 HE 染色切片中,因脂滴被溶解,故细胞呈空泡状(图 3-5)。脂肪细胞能合成和贮存脂肪,参与能量代谢。

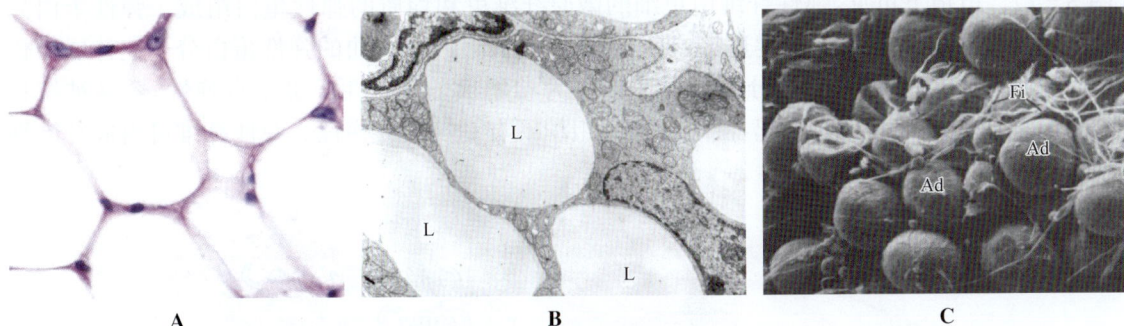

图 3-5 脂肪细胞
A.脂肪细胞光镜结构(皮下组织,HE 染色);B、C.脂肪细胞电镜结构

6. 未分化的间充质细胞

未分化的间充质细胞形态类似成纤维细胞,但胞体较小,常分布在小血管,尤其是毛细血管的周围。它保持着胚胎时期间充质细胞的一些分化潜能,在生理性再生、炎症与损伤修复时,能分化为成纤维细胞、脂肪细胞、内皮细胞和平滑肌细胞等。

二、纤维

疏松结缔组织中的纤维有胶原纤维、弹性纤维和网状纤维三种。

1. 胶原纤维

胶原纤维是疏松结缔组织中分布最广泛、含量最多的一种纤维,新鲜时呈亮白色,又名白纤维,在 HE 染色的标本中,胶原纤维被染成粉红色,成束分布,方向不定,粗细不等,长短不一,呈波浪状并交织成网。胶原纤维由胶原原纤维组成。电镜下,胶原原纤维有明暗相间的横纹,横纹周期为 64nm,其化学成分为I型和Ⅲ型胶原蛋白(图 3-6)。胶原蛋白由成纤维细胞分泌,在细胞外聚合为胶原原纤维,再聚合为胶原纤维。胶原纤维具有韧性大、抗拉力强的特性。

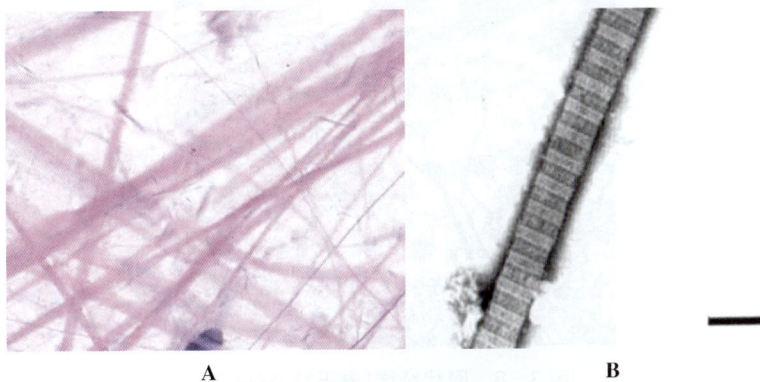

图 3-6 胶原纤维
A.胶原纤维光镜结构(疏松结缔组织,HE 染色);B.胶原纤维电镜结构

2. 弹性纤维

新鲜的弹性纤维肉眼观呈黄色,故又称为黄纤维。弹性纤维在 HE 染色的切片中呈浅红色,不易与胶原纤维区别,但折光性较强。弹性纤维可被多种染色剂如雷锁辛复红染色、地伊红染色、苯胺黑染色等清楚地显示。弹性纤维比胶原纤维细,常呈直线行走,有分支,交错成网(图3-7)。电镜下可见,弹性纤维由更细的微原纤维束和均质的弹性蛋白组成。弹性蛋白分子能任意卷曲,分子间借共价键连接成网。在外力的作用下,卷曲的弹性蛋白分子能伸展增长2.5倍;外力消除后,弹性蛋白分子能迅速恢复为卷曲状态。弹性纤维富有弹性,容易被拉长和复原,与胶原纤维交织在一起,使疏松结缔组织既有韧性又有弹性。弹性纤维可由成纤维细胞、软骨细胞和平滑肌细胞产生。

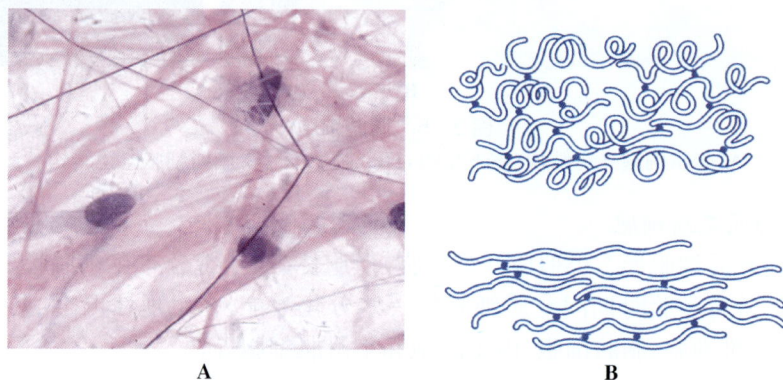

图3-7 弹性纤维
A.弹性纤维光镜结构(疏松结缔组织,HE 染色);B.弹性纤维分子结构模式

3. 网状纤维

网状纤维在 HE 染色标本中不着色,但可被银盐染成黑褐色,故又称嗜银纤维(图3-8)。网状纤维是一种很细的纤维,分支多,相互交织成网。网状纤维主要由Ⅲ型胶原蛋白构成,电镜下,也具有 64 nm 的周期性横纹。网状纤维主要分布在结缔组织与其他组织的交界处,具有连接固定功能。同时还构成淋巴组织、淋巴器官和造血器官的支架。

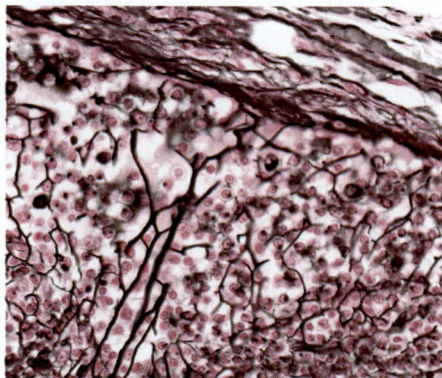

图3-8 网状纤维(淋巴结,银染)

三、基质

基质是一种由生物大分子构成的无定形胶状物,具有一定的黏性,孔隙中有组织液。构成基质的大分子物质主要是蛋白聚糖和糖蛋白。

1. 蛋白聚糖

蛋白聚糖是由蛋白质和大量的糖胺聚糖相结合而形成的大分子化合物,是基质的主要成分。糖胺聚糖包括透明质酸、硫酸软骨素 A、硫酸软骨素 C、硫酸角质素和硫酸乙酰肝素等。它们都是以含有氨基己糖的双糖为基本单位聚合而成的长链状化合物。其中透明质酸为曲折盘绕的长链大分子,是蛋白聚糖复合物的主干;其他糖胺聚糖则以蛋白质为轴心,构成蛋白聚糖亚单位,并借助连接蛋白接合到透明质酸分子上,从而形成带有许多微小孔隙的复杂大分子立体结构,即分子筛(图 3-9)。多糖链上带有密集的阴离子,它们能与无机盐中阳离子和极性的水分子结合,保持水作为溶剂的特性,在调节局部水盐代谢与运输的过程中,发挥离子交换剂的作用。小于分子筛微孔的水和溶于水的营养物质、代谢产物、激素和气体分子等可以自由通过,便于血液与细胞之间的物质交换。大于分子筛孔隙的物质,如致病的微生物等,则不能通过,使之成为限制细菌扩散的防御屏障。而蛇毒、癌细胞和溶血性链球菌等产生的透明质酸酶,能分解透明质酸,破坏屏障,从而使毒素、癌细胞和炎症扩散。

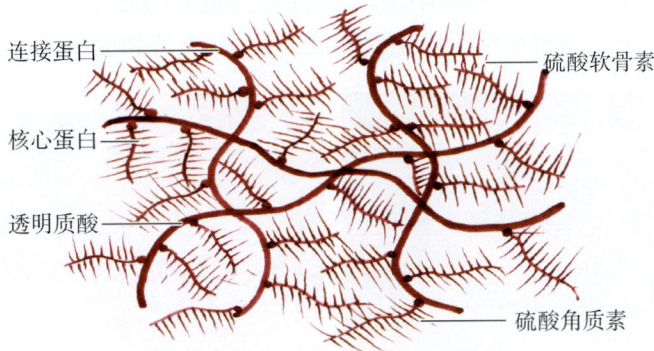

图 3-9 分子筛结构模式图

2. 糖蛋白

糖蛋白是基质中另一类生物大分子物质,主要有纤维黏连蛋白、层黏连蛋白和软骨黏连蛋白等,它们不仅参与基质分子筛的组成,而且通过它们的连接、介导等作用,影响细胞的黏着与移动,并参与调节细胞的生长与分化。

基质中还有少量的组织液。它们是从毛细血管动脉端渗入基质的液体,经毛细血管静脉端和毛细淋巴管回流入血液或淋巴,处于不断更新的动态平衡之中(图 3-10)。组织液将血液中的氧和营养物质带给各种组织细胞,同时将细胞的代谢产物与二氧化碳带回血液。在病理情况下,基质中的组织液可增加或减少,前者称为水肿,后者称为脱水,均可影响细胞的正常生理活动。

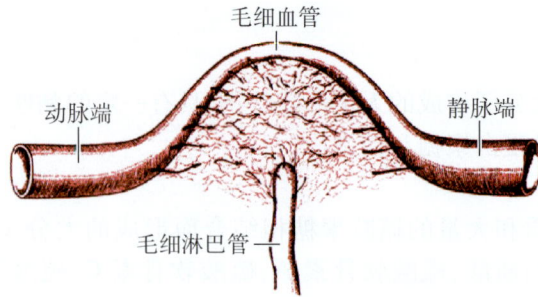

图 3-10 组织液形成示意图

第二节 致密结缔组织

致密结缔组织的组成成分和疏松结缔组织相似,但以纤维成分为主,细胞种类和数量较少,主要是成纤维细胞。致密结缔组织的纤维粗大,排列紧密,且与所承受的张力方向一致。根据纤维的性质和排列方式,可将致密结缔组织分为规则的致密结缔组织和不规则的致密结缔组织两种(图 3-11)。肌腱和腱膜为规则的致密结缔组织,由大量密集成束的胶原纤维平行排列成束,纤维束之间有形态特殊的成纤维细胞,称为腱细胞。而真皮、硬脑膜、巩膜和一些内分泌腺的被膜均为不规则的致密结缔组织,其特点为粗大的胶原纤维纵横交织,排列紧密,纤维之间细胞成分较少。致密结缔组织主要功能为连接、支持和保护。

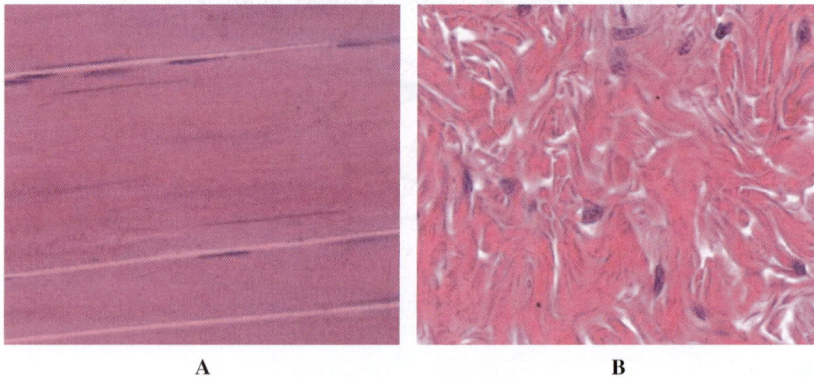

图 3-11 致密结缔组织

A.规则致密结缔组织光镜结构(肌腱,HE 染色);B.不规则致密结缔组织光镜结构(小肠,HE 染色)

第三节 脂 肪 组 织

脂肪组织是以脂肪细胞为主要成分的结缔组织。大量的脂肪细胞被少量疏松结缔组织分隔成许多小叶。按其形态结构和功能的不同,可以分为黄色脂肪组织和棕色脂肪组织两种类型(图 3-12)。

黄色脂肪组织即通常所说的脂肪组织,其脂肪细胞如前所述,细胞内只有一个大的脂滴,称为单泡脂肪细胞,成人大多数的脂肪组织均属此类,主要分布在皮下组织、网膜、系膜等处,

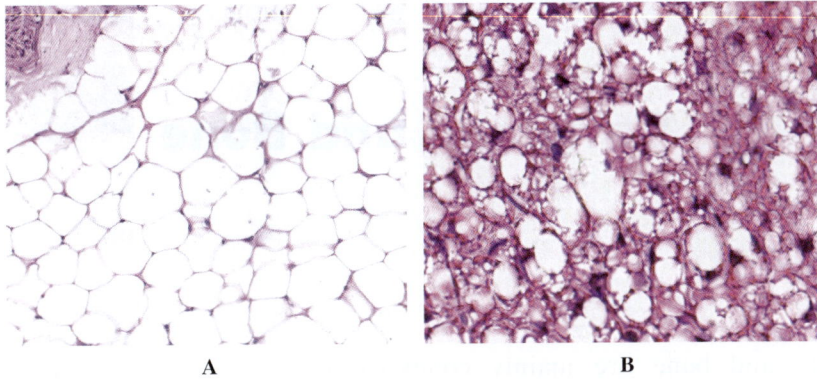

图 3-12 脂肪组织
A.黄色脂肪光镜结构;B.棕色脂肪光镜结构

是体内最大的储能库,并具有维持体温、缓冲、保护、支持和填充等作用。

棕色脂肪新鲜时呈棕色,其脂肪细胞内有丰富的小脂滴和线粒体,故称多泡脂肪细胞。该组织中还含有丰富的血管和神经。棕色脂肪组织在成人很少,新生儿含量较多,占体重的2%~5%。棕色脂肪组织在寒冷刺激下,其贮存的脂类被分解和氧化,可释放大量的热能。

第四节 网 状 组 织

网状组织由网状细胞、网状纤维和基质组成。网状细胞为星形多突的细胞,核大,着色浅,核仁明显,胞质弱嗜碱性,电镜下可见胞质内有发达的粗面内质网。相邻细胞的突起互连成网。网状纤维由网状细胞产生,分支交错,且大多陷于网状细胞的胞体和突起中,成为网状组织的支架(图 3-13)。网状组织多为造血组织和淋巴组织的基本成分,构成血细胞和淋巴细胞发育的微环境。

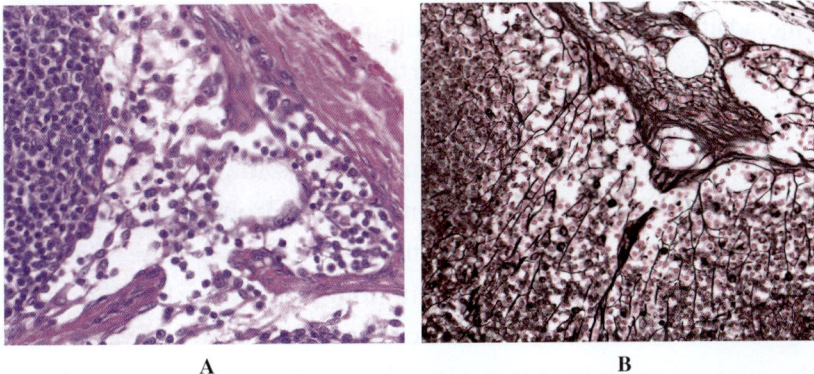

图 3-13 网状组织
A.网状组织光镜结构(淋巴结,HE 染色);B.网状组织光镜结构(淋巴结,银染)

(赵奕淳 郑 英)

Chapter 4

Cartilage and Bone

Cartilage and bone are mainly composed of cartilage tissue and bone tissue, respectively. Like all connective tissue, they are composed of a limited number of cells and a large number of intercellular substances.

1 Cartilage

Cartilage is composed of cartilage tissue and the perichondrium. The intercellular substance of cartilage tissue consists of fibers and gelatinous ground substance, making it tough and elastic. Chondrocytes are embedded in the intercellular substances. Due to the lack of blood vessels, the vessels in the perichondrium will provide nutrition for the cartilage tissues. On the basis of characteristics of the matrix, 3 types of cartilage can be distinguished: hyaline cartilage, elastic cartilage, and fibrocartilage.

1.1 Hyaline Cartilage

Hyaline cartilage is the most common and best studied of the 3 forms. Fresh hyaline cartilage is bluish-white and translucent. In the embryo, it serves mainly as the skeleton of the fetus. In the adult, it serves as the skeleton of the nose, throat, trachea, and bronchus. Additionally, articular cartilage and costal cartilage are also hyaline cartilages.

1.1.1 Matrix

The main component of the extracellular matrix is the cartilage proteoglycan except 70% of water. Cartilage proteoglycans contain chondroitin A-sulfate, chondroitin C-sulfate, and keratan sulfate, covalently linked to core protein. Up to 200 of these proteoglycans are noncovalently associated with long molecules of hyaluronic acid, forming molecular sieve which is structurally similar to that in loose connective tissue. The cartilage cells or chondrocytes are contained in cavities in the matrix, called cartilage lacunae. The cartilage matrix surrounding each chondrocyte is rich in glycosaminoglycan and poor in collagen. This peripheral zone, called the capsular, stains differently from the rest of the matrix (Figure 4-1). There are no blood vessels in the cartilage tissues, but nutrients can be delivered to the deep parts of the cartilage tissues because of the rich of water and high permeability in the matrix.

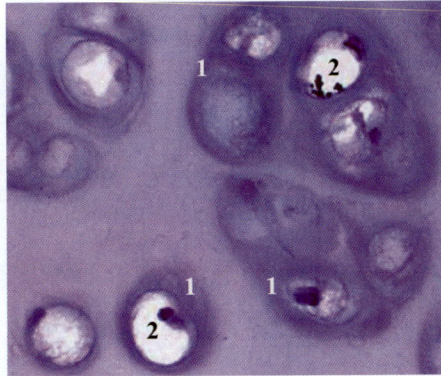

1. Cartilage capsular; 2. Cartilage lacunae
Figure 4 – 1   Hyaline cartilage (Trachea, HE)

1.1.2   Collagen Fibril

The fibers of the hyaline cartilage are collagen fibrils, which are composed of the type II collagen and embedded in the matrix. Collagen fibrils are very thin and only 10 – 20 nm in diameter. They have no periodic striations. It is difficult to observe them under the light microscope because the refractive index is the same as the one of matrix.

1.1.3   Chondrocyte

Chondrocytes occupy small cavities termed lacunae. In living tissue, the chondrocytes fill the lacunae completely, but in histological preparations, the cells and the matrix shrink, resulting in the irregular shape. Young chondrocytes have an elliptic shape, with the long axis parallel to the surface. In the deeper part of the cartilage, cells are more mature and rounder, often appearing in groups of 2 – 8 cells originating from miotic divisions of a single chondrocyte. These groups are called isogenous. Chondrocytes have a round or elliptic nucleus with a prominent nucleolus. The cytoplasm is basophilic in the most immature chondrocytes. Under the electron microscope, numerous rough endoplasmic reticulum and large Golgi apparatus are observed in the cytoplasm, as well as glycogen and lipid droplets. Chondrocytes obtain energy through glycolysis. They can synthesize and secret fibers and matrix (Figure 4 – 2).

1.1.4   Perichondrium

Except in the articular cartilage of joints, all hyaline cartilage is covered by a layer of dense connective tissue, the perichondrium. There are many dense fibers in the outer layer of perichondrium, and fewer fibers and more cells with blood vessels and nerves in the inner layer. Although fusiform cells in the inner layer of the perichondrium resemble fibroblasts, they are chondroblasts and easily differentiate into chondrocytes. Perichondrium can protect and nourish cartilage tissues, and plays an important role in the growth and repairment of the cartilage.

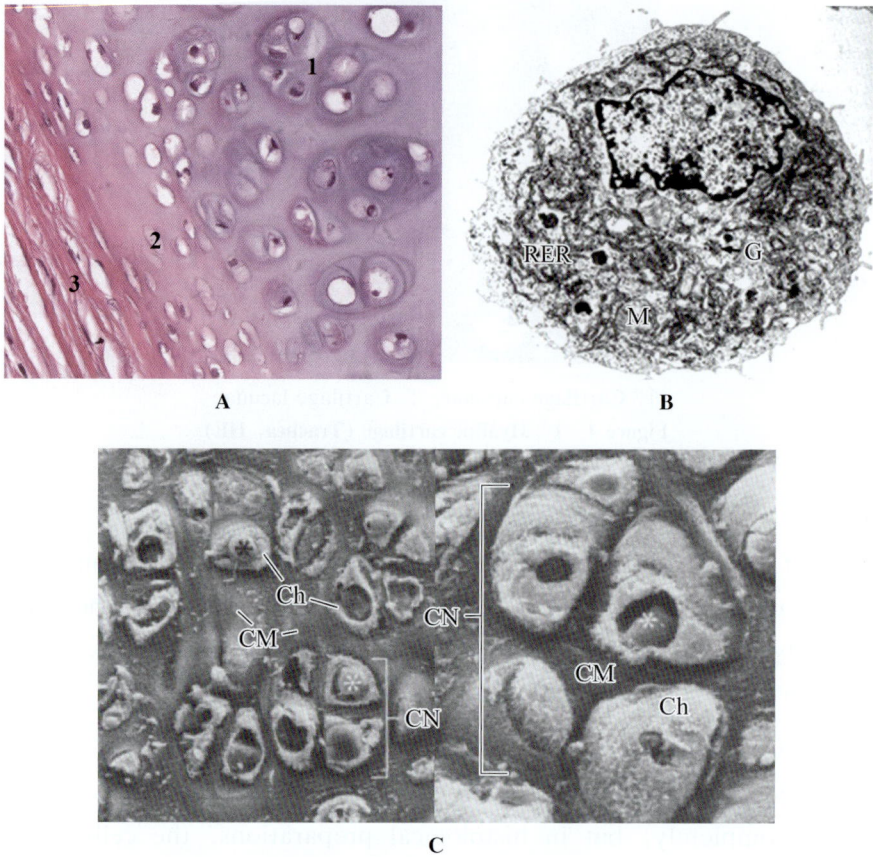

Figure 4 - 2 Hyaline cartilage
A. LM of hyaline cartilage (1. Isogenous group; 2. Immature chondrocytes; 3. Perichondrium); B. & C. EM of hyaline cartilage

1.2 Elastic Cartilage

Elastic cartilage, found in the auricle of the ear and the epiglottis, is similar to the hyaline cartilage in the structure. However, the elastic cartilage is more elastic because of an abundant network of fine elastic fibers (Figure 4 - 3).

1.3 Fibrocartilage

Fibrocartilage can be found in the symphysis pubis, intervertebral disks and articular discs. In fibrocartilage, the numerous collagen fibers either form irregular bundles between the groups of chondrocytes or are aligned in a parallel arrangement along the columns of chondrocytes, which makes it tough. Because it is rich in collagen type I, the fibrocartilage matrix is acidophilic, there is a few ground substance can be seen near the chondrocytes (Figure 4 - 4).

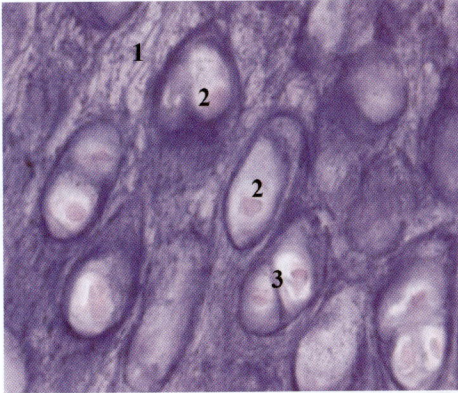

1. Elastic fiber; 2. Chondrocytes; 3. Isogenous group

Figure 4 − 3   Elastic cartilage (External ear, aldehyde fuchsine staining)

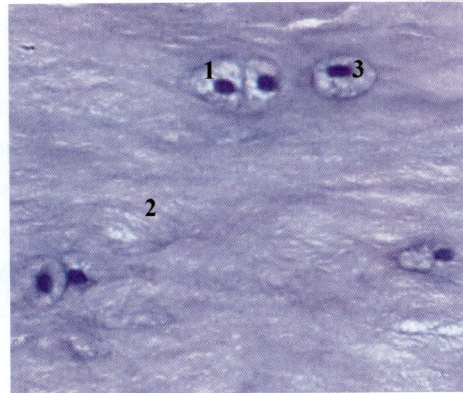

1. Isogenous group; 2. Collagen fiber; 3. Chondrocytes

Figure 4 − 4   Fibrocartilage (Intervertebral disc, HE)

2   Bone

Bone is composed of bone tissue, periosteum, and bone marrow. It has the functions of support, moving and protection in the body. Bone serves as a reservoir of calcium and phosphate to maintain their constant concentrations.

2.1 Bone Tissue

Bone tissue is one of the hardest tissues in the human body, which is composed of a large amount of intercellular calcified material, the bone matrix, and 4 cell types: osteoprogenitor cells, osteoblasts, osteocytes and osteoclasts. The osteocytes with the largest number are located within the bone, and the other three are located at the edge of the bone.

2.1.1   Bone Matrix

Bone matrix includes inorganic and organic matter.

Inorganic matter is also known as bone mineral, and represents about 65% of the dry weight of the bone tissue. Its chemical component is the hydroxyapatite crystal, an insoluble neutral salt. In electron micrographs, inorganic matters appear as fine needles that lie alongside the collagen fibrils. The association of minerals with collagen fibers is responsible for the hardness and resistance of bone tissue.

The organic matter consists of many collagen fibers and a little ground substance, accounting for about 35% of the dry weight of bone tissue. The non-calcified extracellular matrix of bone is also called osteoid. This gel-like matrix containing neutral and weakly acidic glycosaminoglycans can work as the adhesive. In addition, the ground substance also contains osteonectin and osteocalcin, which participate in the binding of collagen fibers and bone salt, adhesion of cells to bone, and regulation of bone calcification. Osteocollagenous fibers are mainly composed of type I collagen, accounting for 90% of the organic components. In the bone matrix, collagen fibers are parallel to each other and arranged in lamellae, it is therefore called lamellar bone. In adjacent lamellae, the collagen fibers are oriented in different directions. The presence of large numbers of lamellas with differing fiber orientations provides bones with great strength (Figure 4 – 5). There are blood vessels in the bone tissues, which is different from the cartilage tissues.

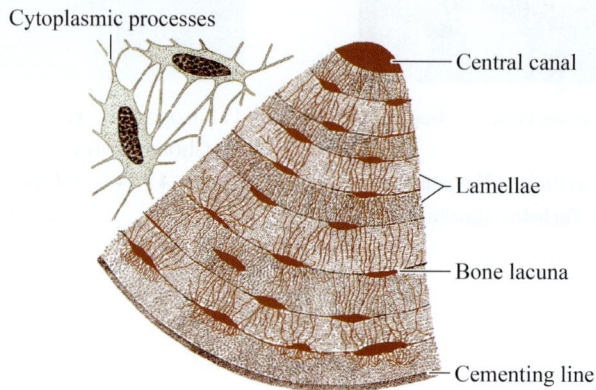

Figure 4 – 5　General structure of osteocyte and bone matrix

2.1.2　Cell

2.1.2.1　Osteoprogenitor Cell

Osteoprogenitor cells are found on the inner layer of the periosteum, the endosteum, and the surface of central lumen. They appear as small size, spindle-shaped, ovoid nuclei, and slightly basophilic cytoplasm (Figure 4 – 6). Osteoprogenitor cells are stem cells of the bone tissue. They can self-renew and differentiate into osteoblasts when the bone tissues are growing or reconstructing.

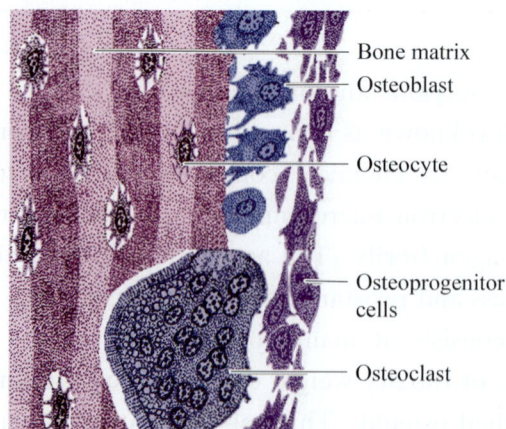

Figure 4 – 6　Diagram of osteoprogenitor cells

2.1.2.2 Osteoblast

Osteoblasts are located on the surfaces of osseous tissues. Most of them appear as columnar or oval, branched cytoplasm and single-layer arrangement. The size of their cell bodies is larger than the one of osteoprogenitor cells. They can form gap junctions with adjacent osteoblasts or osteocytes. Osteoblasts have big and round nucleus with obvious nucleoli, basophilic cytoplasm, and abundant alkaline phosphatase. Under the electron microscope, osteoblasts are found to have abundant rough endoplasmic reticulum and well-developed Golgi apparatus. Osteoblasts synthesize and secret both collagen fibers and ground substances to constitute the osteoid. Because of the secreted alkaline phosphatase, a large number of hydroxyapatite crystals are deposited, and the osteoid will become the bone matrix. In the process of osteogenesis, some osteoblasts are also gradually surrounded by the matrix and become osteocytes (Figure 4 – 7). When bones continue growing, the osteoprogenitor cells will be always dividing and differentiating into new osteoblasts to form new bones. Calcitonin can promote this process.

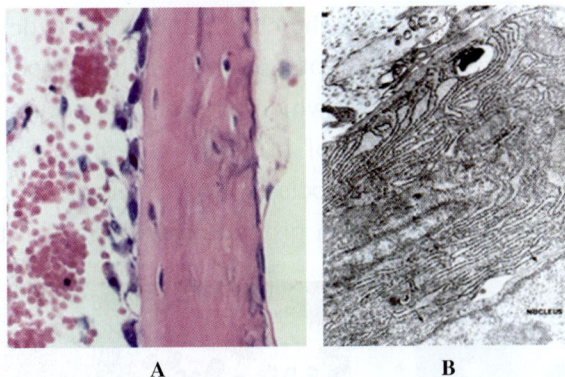

Figure 4 – 7 Osteoblast
A. LM of Osteoblast; B. EM of Osteoblast

2.1.2.3 Osteocyte

Osteocytes are scattered between or within the bone plates. Oval osteocytes have many slender protrusions, which can form gap junctions between the osteocytes. They are lying in a space called bone lacuna, situated between the lamellae of bones. The osteocytes extend cytoplasmic processes through the fine tunnels termed bone canaliculi (Figure 4 – 8). There is tissue fluid in the bone lacuna and bone canaliculi, which guarantee the nutrition supply of osteocytes and the excretion of metabolites. Under the control of parathyroid hormone and calcitonin, osteocytes can perform weak osteolysis and osteogenesis, and participate in the regulation of calcium and phosphorus balance.

2.1.2.4 Osteoclast

Osteoclasts are located in the depression of the bone resorption site. They are large, multinucleate cells with a diameter of up to 100 μm. Dilated portions of the cell body contain from 5~50 nuclei. The cytoplasm is eosinophilic, and ruffled border can be observed

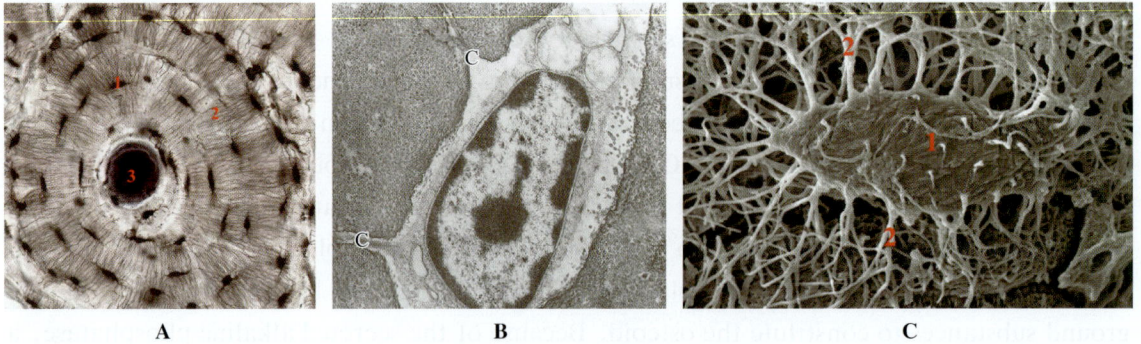

Figure 4 - 8 Osteocyte

A. LM of osteocyte (Long bone; 1. Osteocyte; 2. Cytoplasmic processes; 3. Central canal); B. TEM of osteocyte (C. Cytoplasmic processes); C. SEM of osteocyte (1. Cell body; 2. Cytoplasmic processes)

on the side close to the bones. Osteoclasts are phagocytotic cells derived from bone marrow. Under the electron microscope, it can be observed that the ruffled border is formed by many microvilli with different lengths and irregular arrangements. Surrounding the ruffled border is a cytoplasmic zone, the clear zone, that is devoid of organelles, yet rich in actin filaments. This zone is a site of adhesion of the osteoclasts to the bone matrix and creates a closed microenvironment in which enzymolysis occurs. The cytoplasm in the deep of the ruffled border contains lots of primary lysosomes, swallowing vesicles, and secondary lysosomes (Figure 4 - 9). Osteoclasts have a strong function in dissolving and absorbing bones. Parathyroid hormone can promote osteolysis of osteoclasts.

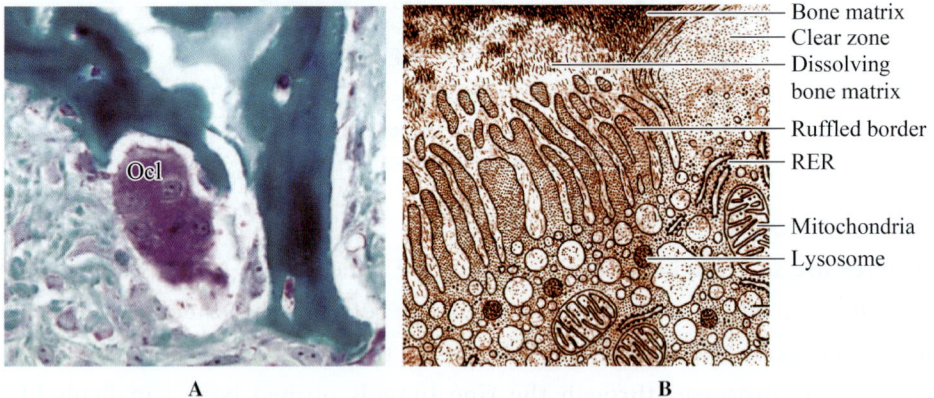

Figure 4 - 9 Osteoclast

A. LM of osteoclast (Ocl. Osteoclast); B. EM diagram of osteoclast

2.2 Long Bone

The long bones are composed of compact bones, cancellous bones, periostea, articular cartilages, bone marrows, etc.

2.2.1 Compact Bone

The compact bones are distributed in the shafts of long bones and on the surfaces of the epiphyses as well. The compact bones in the shafts of long bones are thicker, and their lamellae are arranged in a compact and orderly manner. The lamellae in the compact bones are regularly arranged in 3 patterns: circumferential lamellae, osteons and interstitial lamellae (Figure 4 – 10).

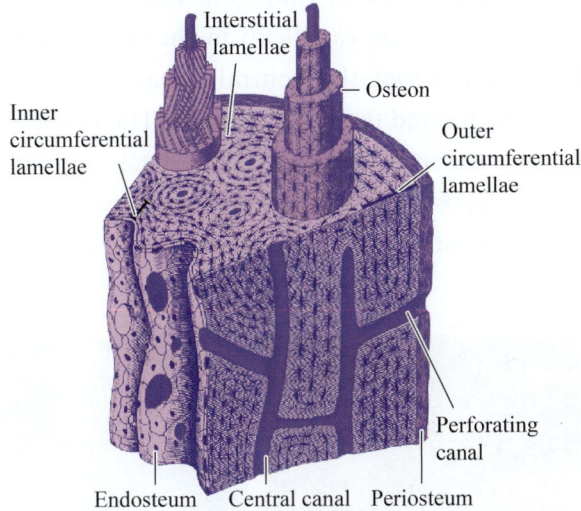

Figure 4 – 10   General structure of long bone

2.2.1.1   Circumferential Lamellae

The bone lamellae on the external surfaces and inner surfaces of long bones are called outer circumferential lamellae and inner circumferential lamellae, respectively (Figure 4 – 11). The outer circumferential lamellae are thicker and composed of 10 – 20 layers of bone lamellae. They are located beneath the periosteum, running parallel with the surfaces. The inner circumferential lamellae are only composed of several layers of bone lamellae, and located above the endostea.

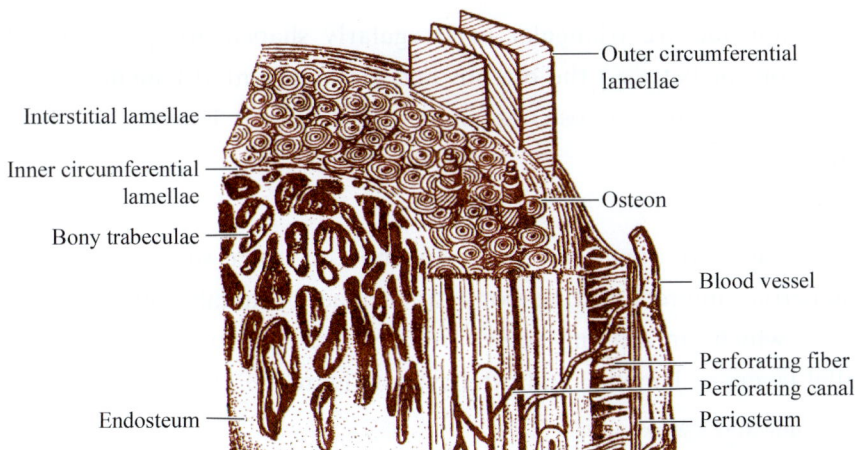

Figure 4 – 11   Diagram of circumferential lamellae

2.2.1.2 Osteon

Osteons or Haversian systems, the basic structural units of the compact bones, are located between the outer and inner circumferential lamellae. This cylindrical structure consists of 4~20 concentric bone lamellae surrounding a central canal. The central canal is connected with the perforating canal, and they both contain small blood vessels, nerves, and a little connective tissue. The bone canaliculi in the osteons connect with each other. The inside bone canaliculi start from the central canals and serve for the passage of substances between the osteocytes and the blood vessels. The outside bone canaliculi cannot connect with the adjacent osteons, and will turn back within the cementing line. Surrounding each osteon is a deposit of amorphous material called the cementing substance, or cementing line, that consists of mineralized matrix with few collagenous fibers (Figure 4-12).

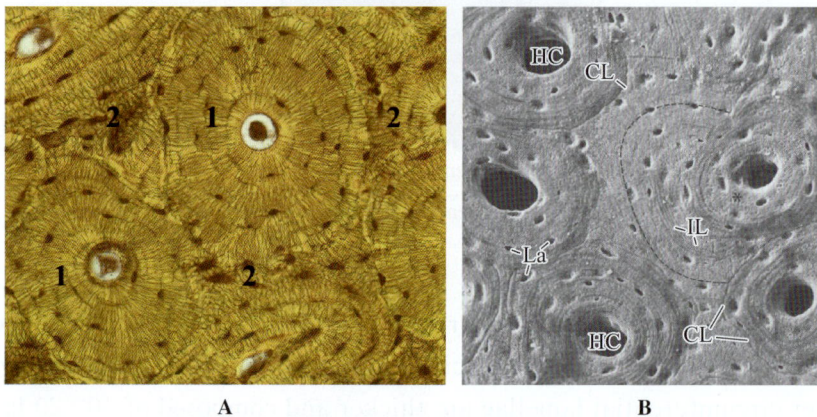

Figure 4 - 12   Osteon

A. LM of osteon (Long bone, thionine staining; 1. Osteon; 2. Interstitial lamellae); B. SEM of osteon (HC. Haversian canal; CL. Cementing line)

2.2.1.3 Interstitial Lamellae

Interstitial lamellae are triangular or irregularly shaped groups of parallel lamellae between the osteons or between the osteons and circumferential lamellae (Figure 4-13). They are remnants of previous osteons and circumferential lamellae in the growth and remodeling of bones.

2.2.2 Cancellous Bone

Cancellous bones are found in epiphyses and the inner surface of diaphysis. They consist of numerous interconnecting bony trabeculae by a labyrinth of interconnecting marrow spaces, which, in a living bone, are occupied by marrow. Trabeculae consist of several parallel layers of lamellae and osteocytes (Figure 4-14).

2.2.3 Endosteum and Periosteum

Except the articular surfaces, external and internal surfaces of bones are covered by the connective tissue called endosteum and periosteum (Figure 4-15).

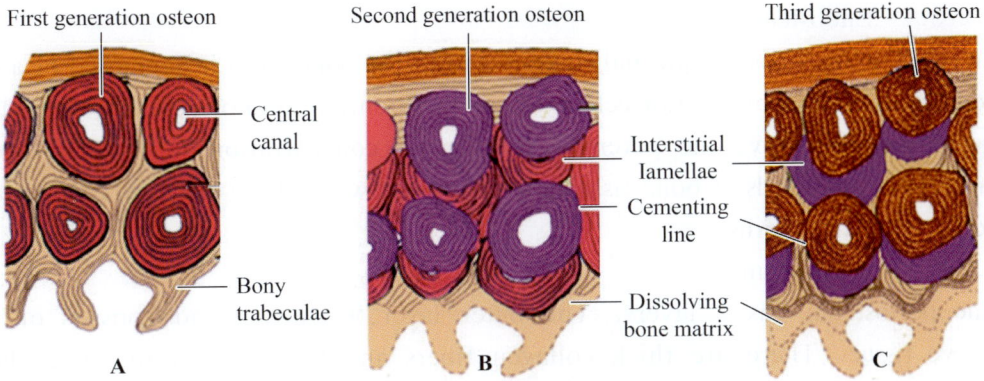

Figure 4 - 13   Remodeling of compact bone

A. The formation of first generation osteon; B. The formation of second generation osteon; C. The formation of third generation osteon

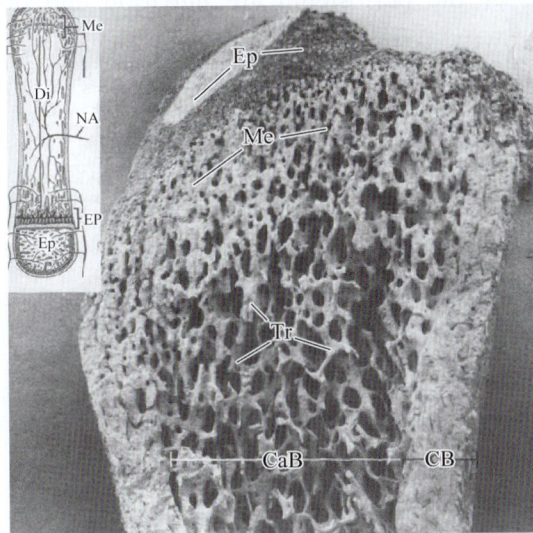

Figure 4 - 14   SEM of cancellous bone

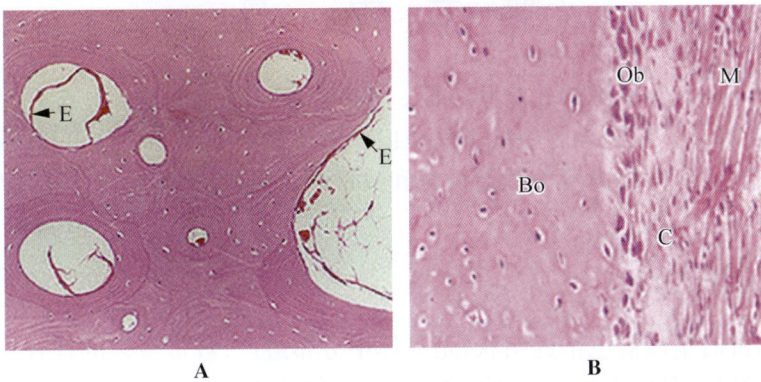

Figure 4 - 15   Periosteum

A. LM of endosteum (E. Endosteum); B. LM of periosteum (Bo. Bone matrix; Ob. Osteoblast; M. Periosteum; C. Connective tissue)

2.2.3.1　Endosteum

The endosteum lines all internal cavities within the bone, and is composed of a single layer of flattened osteoprogenitor cells that can differentiate into osteoblasts. In addition, the endosteum may have the potential to regulate concentrations of ions, because it separates the tissue fluids of bone tissue and bone marrow that have different concentrations of calcium and phosphorus.

2.2.3.2　Periosteum

The periosteum has 2 layers. The outer layer is thicker and consists of dense connective tissue. There are thick collagen fibers and few cells in the outer layers. Periosteal collagen fibers, called Sharpey's fibers, penetrate the bone matrix, binding the periosteum to bones. The inner layer is thinner and consist of loose connective tissue containing less fibers, osteoprogenitor cells, small blood vessels, nerves, etc.

The major functions of the periosteum are nutrition and protection of bones, and involved in the normal growth, remodeling, and repair of bones.

(Yuan Lu, Yang Fan)

第四章　软 骨 和 骨

软骨和骨是构成身体支架的器官,它们分别以软骨组织和骨组织为主要结构成分,均属于广义的结缔组织,由少量的细胞和大量的细胞间质组成。

第一节　软　　骨

软骨由软骨组织及其周围的软骨膜组成。软骨组织的细胞间质由纤维和呈凝胶状的基质构成,使之坚韧有弹性。软骨细胞包埋于间质内。软骨组织中无血管分布,其营养由软骨膜内的血管供应。根据细胞间质内所含纤维种类和数量的不同,可将软骨分为透明软骨、弹性软骨和纤维软骨三种。

一、透明软骨

透明软骨新鲜时呈浅蓝色半透明状,是人体中分布最广、数量最多的软骨。它是胚胎时期胎儿主要的支撑结构,是成人构成鼻、喉、气管、支气管的支架。此外,关节软骨和肋软骨也是透明软骨。

1. 透明软骨的组织结构

（1）基质：除含 70% 水分外，基质的成分主要为软骨蛋白聚糖，它以透明质酸为主干，通过连接其上的蛋白短链，与硫酸软骨素 A、C 和硫酸角质素等，形成瓶刷状大分子即分子筛，并和胶原原纤维结合形成固态结构。软骨基质内的小腔称为软骨陷窝，在软骨陷窝周围的基质内，含较多硫酸软骨素，HE 染色呈强嗜碱性，似囊状包绕软骨细胞，称为软骨囊（图 4 - 1）。软骨组织内无血管，但由于基质富含水分，通透性强，故营养物质可通过渗透进入软骨组织深部。

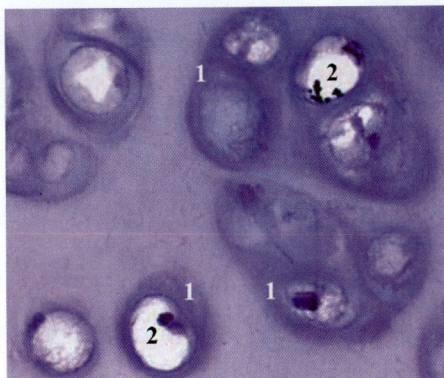

1—软骨囊；2—软骨陷窝
图 4 - 1　透明软骨（气管，HE 染色）

（2）胶原原纤维：透明软骨中的纤维是胶原原纤维，由 Ⅱ 型胶原蛋白组成，相互交织埋于基质中。胶原原纤维很细，直径为 10～20 nm，无明显的周期性横纹，其折光率与基质一致，因而在光镜下不易辨认。

（3）软骨细胞：位于软骨陷窝内。新鲜时，软骨细胞充满软骨陷窝，在石蜡切片中软骨细胞因收缩呈不规则形，使细胞和陷窝壁之间出现明显的空隙。软骨细胞的大小、形态不一，近软骨膜边缘部位的细胞小而扁圆，单个分布，为幼稚的软骨细胞；自边缘向中央，软骨细胞渐趋成熟。位于软骨中部的软骨细胞体积较大，呈圆形或椭圆形，成群分布，每群由 2～8 个细胞组成，群内细胞常呈半圆形互相紧靠，细胞间常隔有薄层的软骨囊。它们是由同一个软骨细胞分裂增生而来，故称同源细胞群。软骨细胞核圆，着色浅，核仁清楚，胞质嗜碱性。电镜下可见胞质内有丰富的粗面内质网和发达的高尔基复合体，还可见糖原和脂滴。软骨细胞主要依靠糖酵解获取能量，它具有合成和分泌纤维和基质的功能（图 4 - 2）。

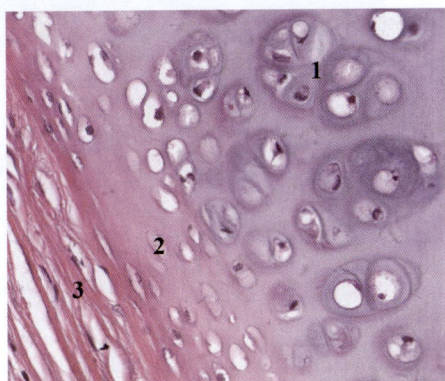

A

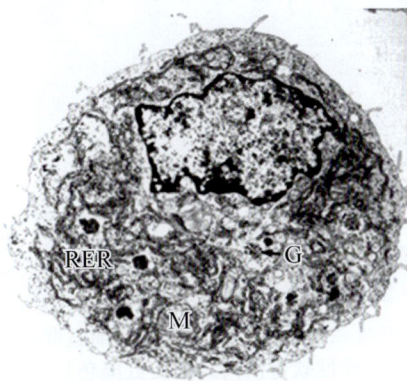

B

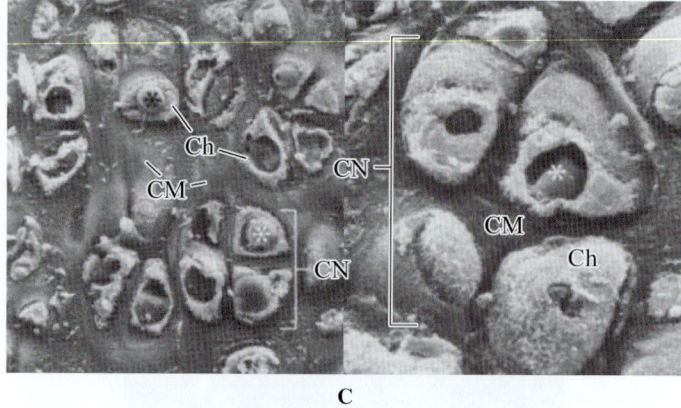

图 4-2　透明软骨

A.透明软骨光镜结构(1—同源细胞群;2—幼稚的软骨细胞;3—软骨膜);B.软骨细胞透射电镜图;C.透明软骨扫描电镜图

2. 软骨膜

　　除关节软骨外,软骨周围均裹有一层由结缔组织构成的软骨膜。软骨膜的外层纤维多,较致密;内层纤维少,细胞多,较疏松,并富含血管和神经。其紧贴软骨组织处,有一种较小的梭形细胞,即骨祖细胞,能分裂分化为软骨细胞。软骨膜能保护、营养软骨组织,并在软骨的生长与修复中起重要作用。

二、弹性软骨

　　弹性软骨分布于耳郭、会厌等处,其结构与透明软骨相似。主要区别在于其间质中含有大量的弹性纤维,相互交织成网,使其具有很大的弹性(图 4-3)。

三、纤维软骨

　　纤维软骨分布于耻骨联合、椎间盘和关节盘等处。其结构特点是间质中含有大量平行或相互交错排列的胶原纤维束,具有较强的韧性。在 HE 染色切片中,纤维软骨呈红色,基质较少,软骨细胞较小,常成行分布于纤维之间(图 4-4)。

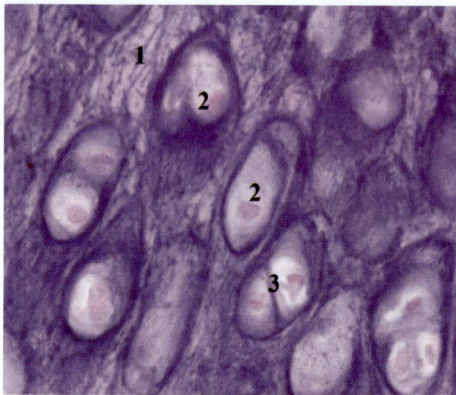

1—弹性纤维;2—软骨细胞;3—同源细胞群
图 4-3　弹性软骨(耳郭,醛复红染色)

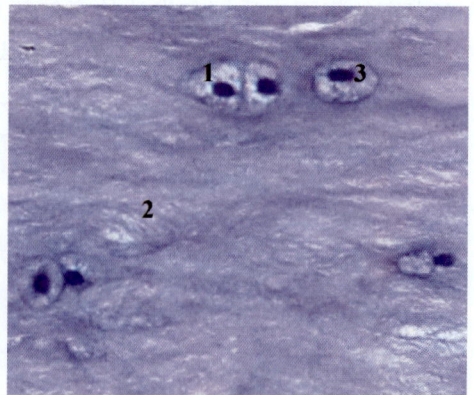

1—同源细胞群;2—胶原纤维;3—软骨细胞
图 4-4　纤维软骨(椎间盘,HE 染色)

第二节 骨

骨是由骨组织、骨膜和骨髓等构成,在机体中起支持、运动和保护作用。骨中含有大量的钙和磷,是机体钙、磷的储存库,在钙、磷的代谢调节中起重要作用。

一、骨组织的结构

骨组织是人体最坚硬的组织之一,由大量钙化的细胞外基质和细胞构成,前者又称为骨质。骨组织的细胞有骨祖细胞、成骨细胞、骨细胞、破骨细胞,其中骨细胞的数量最多,位于骨质内,其余三种细胞位于骨质的边缘。

1. 骨质

骨质由无机成分和有机成分构成。

无机成分又称骨盐,占骨组织干重的65%,其化学成分是羟基磷灰石的结晶,属不溶性中性盐。电镜下呈细针状,有规律地沿胶原原纤维的长轴排列,借助于骨粘连蛋白与之紧密结合,它是骨质坚硬的成因。

有机成分由大量的胶原纤维和少量无定形的基质组成,约占骨组织干重的35%。这种未钙化的细胞外基质又称为类骨质。基质呈凝胶状,主要是中性和弱酸性糖胺聚糖,具有黏合作用。此外,基质中还含有骨粘连蛋白和骨钙蛋白,它们参与胶原纤维和骨盐的结合、细胞和骨质的黏附,并调节骨的钙化。骨胶原纤维主要由Ⅰ型胶原蛋白构成,占有机成分的90%。在骨质中,胶原纤维规律地成层排列,且与骨盐晶体和基质紧密结合,形成薄板状结构称骨板。层层叠叠的骨板犹如多层木质胶合板。同一层骨板内的胶原纤维互相平行,相邻层骨板内的胶原纤维互成一定角度,从而有效增加了骨对多方压力的承受力(图4-5)。与软骨组织不同,骨组织内有血管穿行的管道。

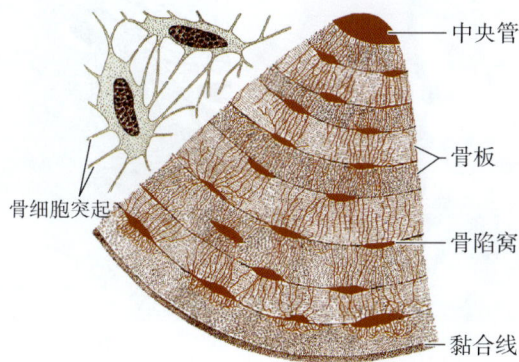

图4-5 骨细胞与骨板排列结构模式图

中央管
骨板
骨陷窝
黏合线
骨细胞突起

2. 细胞

(1)骨祖细胞:分布于骨外膜内层、骨内膜及中央管腔面,细胞胞体小,呈梭形,核卵圆,胞质少,胞质嗜碱性(图4-6)。骨祖细胞是骨组织的干细胞,当骨组织生长或改建时,能分裂分化为成骨细胞。

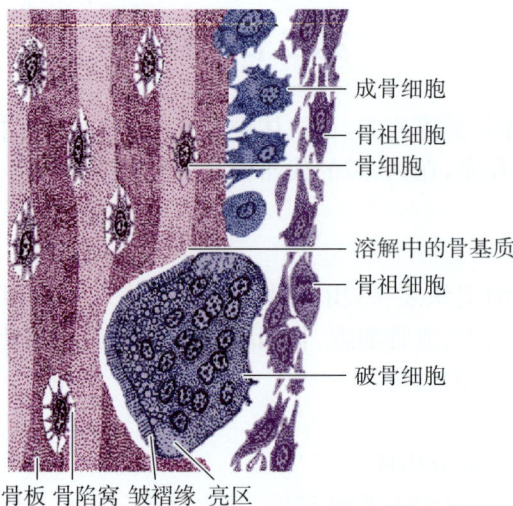

成骨细胞

骨祖细胞

骨细胞

溶解中的骨基质

骨祖细胞

破骨细胞

骨板 骨陷窝 皱褶缘 亮区

图4-6 骨祖细胞模式图

（2）成骨细胞：分布于骨组织表面，成年前较多，成年后较少。成骨细胞常呈单层排列，胞体较骨祖细胞大，呈矮柱状或椭圆形，表面伸出许多细小突起，并与邻近的成骨细胞或骨细胞的突起形成缝隙连接。成骨细胞的核较大，呈圆形，核仁明显，胞质嗜碱性，含丰富的碱性磷酸酶。电镜下可见丰富的粗面内质网和发达的高尔基复合体。成骨细胞的功能是合成和分泌骨胶纤维和基质，形成类骨质。而后，在其分泌的碱性磷酸酶的作用下，沉积大量的羟基磷灰石结晶而成为骨质。成骨细胞在成骨的过程中自身也被埋入骨质中，成为骨细胞（图4-7）。当骨质继续增长时，骨膜内层的骨祖细胞不断分裂分化为新的成骨细胞，贴附于骨质表面，继而形成新的骨质。降钙素能促进成骨细胞的成骨作用。

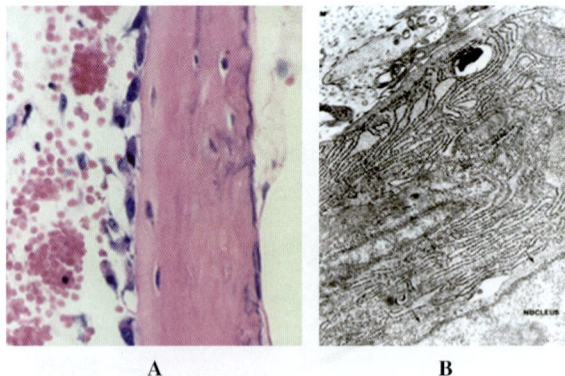

A   B

图4-7 成骨细胞

A.成骨细胞光镜结构；B.成骨细胞电镜结构

（3）骨细胞：单个散在分布于骨板间或骨板内。骨细胞为扁圆形多突起的细胞，表面伸出许多细长突起，相邻骨细胞的突起间形成缝隙连接（图4-8）。骨细胞胞体所在的腔隙称为骨陷窝，其突起所在的位置称为骨小管。相邻骨陷窝借骨小管相连通。骨陷窝和骨小管内含组织液，通过组织液循环，保证了骨细胞的营养供给与代谢产物的排泄。骨细胞能在甲状旁腺激素和降钙素的调控下,进行较弱的溶骨和成骨,参与钙、磷平衡的调节。

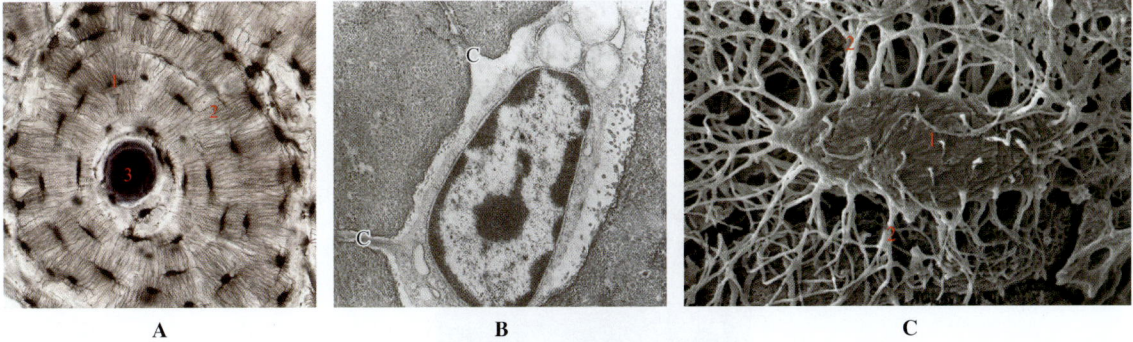

图 4-8 骨细胞

A.骨细胞光镜结构(长骨骨干,自然色,1—骨陷窝;2—骨小管;3—中央管);B.骨细胞透射电镜结构(C—骨小管);C.骨细胞扫描电镜结构(1—胞体;2—突起)

　　(4)破骨细胞:常位于骨质吸收部位的凹陷处,是一种多核的大细胞,细胞直径可达 $100\mu m$,有 5~50 个核,胞质嗜酸性,在贴近骨质的一侧可见皱褶缘(图 4-9)。一般认为破骨细胞由多个单核细胞融合而成。电镜下可见皱褶缘是由许多长短不一、排列不齐的微绒毛形成的。皱褶缘周围有一环形的细胞质区,含大量微丝,缺乏其他细胞器,称为亮区,该处的细胞膜平整且紧贴于骨质表面,犹如一道围墙,形成一个密封的酶解微环境。皱褶缘深部的胞质含大量初级溶酶体、吞饮泡和次级溶酶体。破骨细胞有极强的溶解和吸收骨质的作用。甲状旁腺素可促进破骨细胞的溶骨作用。

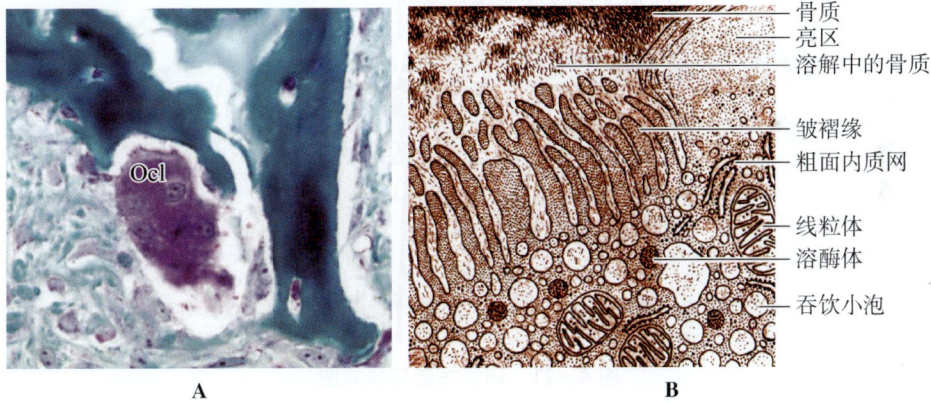

图 4-9 破骨细胞

A.破骨细胞光镜结构(Ocl—破骨细胞);B.破骨细胞电镜结构模式图

二、长骨的结构

长骨由骨密质、骨松质、骨膜、关节软骨和骨髓等构成。

1. 骨密质

骨密质分布于长骨骨干和骨骺的外侧部分,长骨骨干的骨密质较厚,其骨板排列紧密有序,按其排列的形式不同,可分为环骨板、骨单位和间骨板三种(图 4-10)。

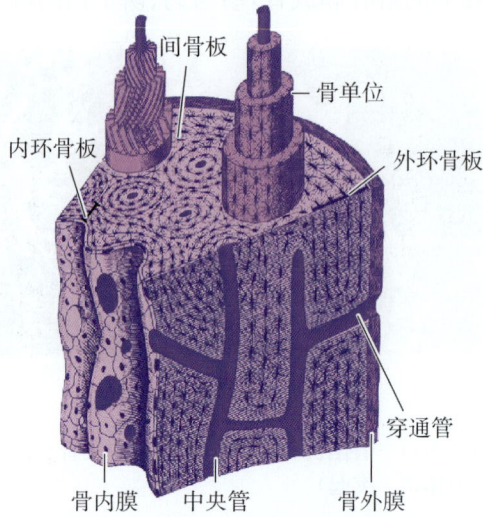

图 4 - 10　长骨骨干立体结构模式图

（1）环骨板：是环绕骨干外表面和内表面的骨板，分别称为外环骨板和内环骨板（图 4 - 11）。外环骨板较厚，10～20 层，环绕骨干外表面平行排列，最外层与骨外膜相贴。内环骨板较薄，仅由数层骨板组成，其内面衬有骨内膜。

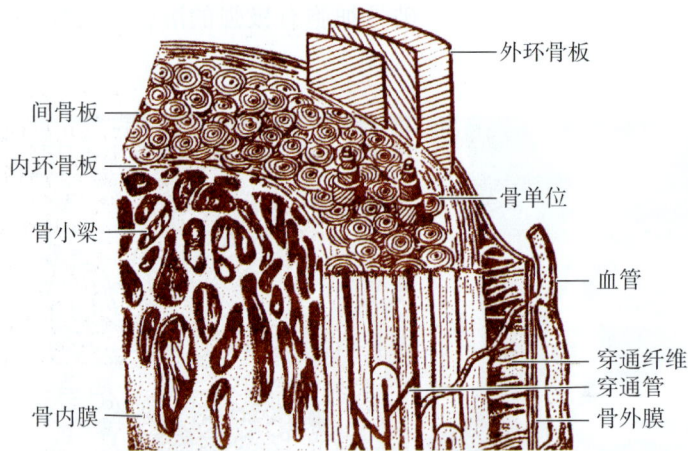

图 4 - 11　环骨板结构模式图

（2）骨单位：又称哈弗斯系统，位于内、外环骨板之间，数量最多，是长骨起支持作用的主要结构单位。骨单位呈纵行的圆筒状，以中央管为轴心，由 4～20 层同心圆排列的骨板层层环绕形成。中央管与穿通管相通，它们都含有小血管、神经和少量结缔组织。骨单位内的骨小管相互通连。最内层的骨小管开口于中央管，形成血管系统与骨细胞之间营养物质和气体交换的通道。骨单位最外层的骨小管在黏合线以内返折，与相邻骨单位的骨小管不相通。骨单位表面有一层黏合质，是含骨盐较多而胶原纤维很少的骨质，在骨磨片上呈折光较强的轮廓线，称黏合线（图 4 - 12）。

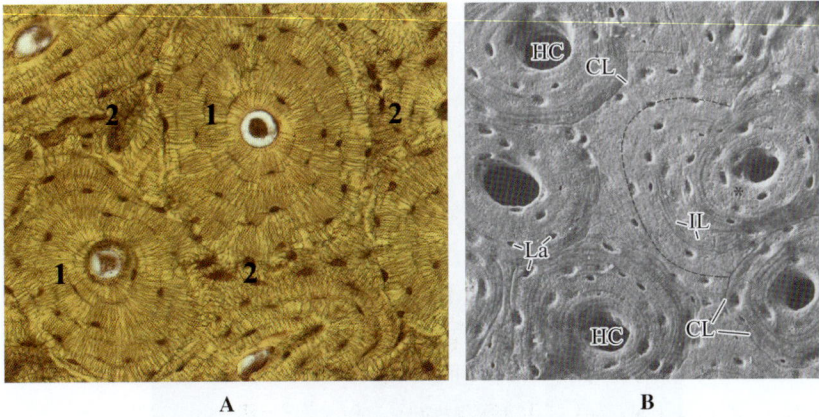

图 4-12　骨单位

A. 骨单位光镜结构(长骨骨干,硫堇染色,1—骨单位;2—间骨板);B. 骨单位扫描电镜图(HC—中央管;CL—黏合线)

（3）间骨板:是填充于骨单位之间和骨单位与环骨板之间的不规则骨板(图 4-13)。它们是骨生长和改建过程中原有的骨单位和环骨板被吸收后的残留部分,其中无血管。

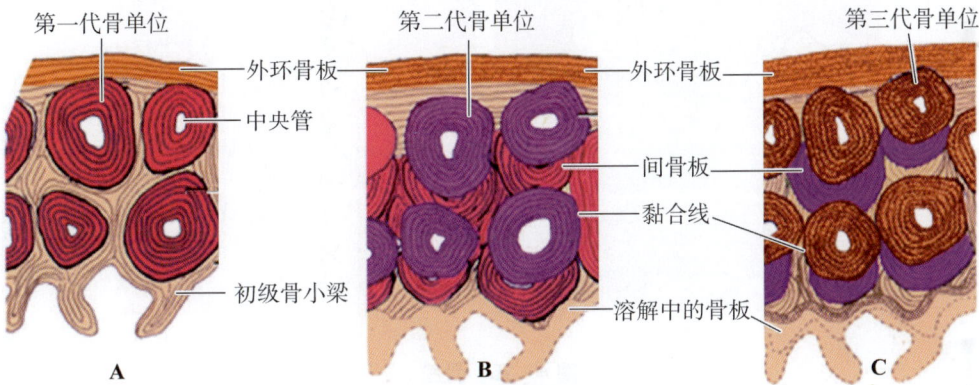

图 4-13　骨密质改建模式图

A. 第一代骨单位形成;B. 第二代骨单位形成;C. 第三代骨单位形成

2. 骨松质

分布于骨骺和骨干的内侧部分,是由大量针状或片状的骨小梁搭建成的多孔隙网状结构,孔隙中充满着红骨髓。骨小梁由数层平行排列的骨板和骨细胞构成(图 4-14)。

3. 骨膜

除关节面以外,骨的内、外表面均覆有一层结缔组织,分别称为骨内膜和骨外膜(图 4-15)。

（1）骨内膜:衬贴于骨髓腔面、骨小梁的表面、穿通管和中央管的内表面。骨内膜的骨祖细胞在骨表面排列成单层扁平形,细胞间有缝隙连接,这些细胞可分化为成骨细胞。此外,由于骨内膜分隔了骨组织和骨髓两种钙、磷浓度不同的组织液,可能具有离子屏障功能。

（2）骨外膜:分为内、外两层。外层较厚,为致密结缔组织,胶原纤维粗大而密集,细胞较少。有些纤维穿入到外环骨板,称为穿通纤维,将骨外膜固定于骨。内层较薄,为疏松结缔组织,纤维较少,含有骨祖细胞、小血管和神经等。

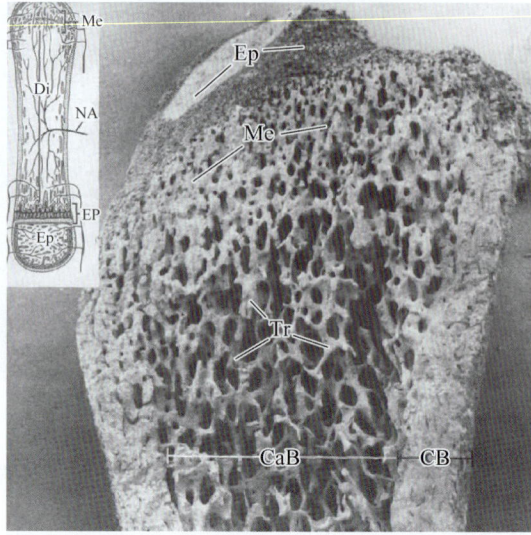

图 4-14　骨松质扫描电镜结构

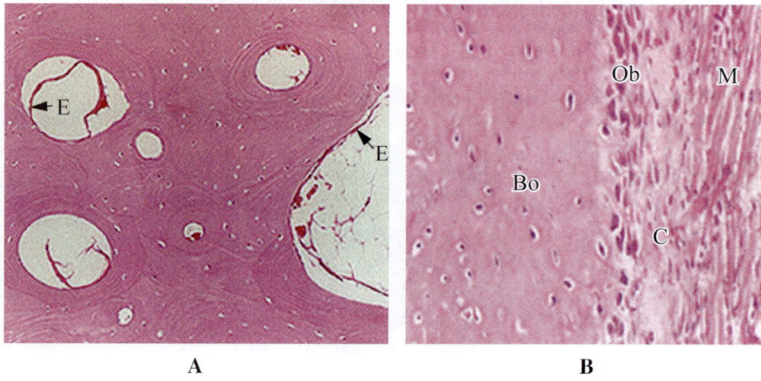

图 4-15　骨膜

A. 骨内膜光镜结构(E—骨内膜);B. 骨外膜光镜结构(Bo—骨组织;Ob—成骨细胞;M—骨外膜;C—结缔组织)

　　骨膜的主要功能是营养、保护骨组织,并参与骨的正常生长、改建和修复。

（赵奕淳　郑　英）

Chapter 5

Blood and Hematopoiesis

Blood is the liquid tissue that flows in a regular unidirectional movement within the closed circulatory system. It is about 5 L in an adult and consists of plasma and blood cells. Blood that is collected and kept from coagulating by the addition of anticoagulants (e. g. , heparin, citrate) separates, when centrifuged, into 3 layers that reflect its heterogeneity. The upper layer is yellowish plasma, the lower layer are dark red erythrocytes, and the middle thin layer are milk-white leukocytes and blood platelets.

Plasma is like the intercellular substance in connective tissue, accounting for 55% of the volume of blood. Ninety percent of the plasma is water, and others include plasma proteins (albumins, globulins, fibrinogen, etc.), sugar, lipoproteins, vitamins, enzymes, hormones, inorganic salts, and metabolites. When blood leaves the circulatory system, either in a test tube or in the extracellular matrix (ECM) surrounding blood vessels, plasma proteins react with one another to produce a clot, which includes formed elements and a yellowish liquid called serum. The stable properties of the plasma are essential to maintaining appropriate conditions for physiological activities of tissues and cells, including specific gravity $(1. 05 - 1. 06)$, pH $(7. 3 - 7. 4)$, osmolarity $(313 \text{ mmol/L},$ equivalent to $0.9\% \text{ NaCl})$, viscosity and chemical components.

Blood cells account for 45% of the volume of blood, including erythrocytes, leukocytes and platelets (Figure 5 - 1). Normally, Wright and Giemsa staining are performed to stain the blood cells on blood smears. Under normal physiological conditions, blood cells are usually uniform in morphology and number. In clinical, the detection of blood cell morphology, quantity, proportion and hemoglobin content is called hemogram. There will be significant changes in hemogram when people are sick, so detection of hemogram is critical for learning body conditions and diagnosing diseases.

Classification and normal values of blood cells are as follows:

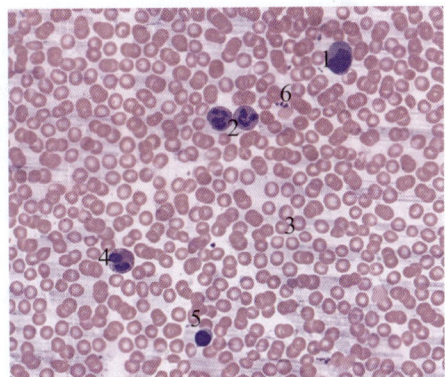

1. Monocyte; 2. Neutrophil; 3. Erythrocytes;
4. Eosinophil; 5. Lymphocyte; 6. Platelets
Figure 5 - 1　Blood cells (Wright staining)

$$\text{Blood cell}\begin{cases}\text{Erythrocyte } (3.5-5.5)\times10^{12}/L\\[4pt]\text{Leukocyte } (4-10)\times10^{9}/L\begin{cases}\text{Neutrophil } 50\%-70\%\\\text{Eosinophil } 0.5\%-3\%\\\text{Basophil } 0-1\%\\\text{Lymphocyte } 25\%-30\%\\\text{Monocyte } 3\%-8\%\end{cases}\\[4pt]\text{Platelet } (1.0-3.0)\times10^{11}/L\end{cases}$$

1 Erythrocyte

Erythrocytes are $7.5-8.5\,\mu m$ in diameter. They are biconcave disks with thin center and thick edge, so the staining shows light colour in the center and dark in the edge (Figure 5 - 2). The biconcave shape increases the surface area of erythrocytes and facilitates gas exchange.

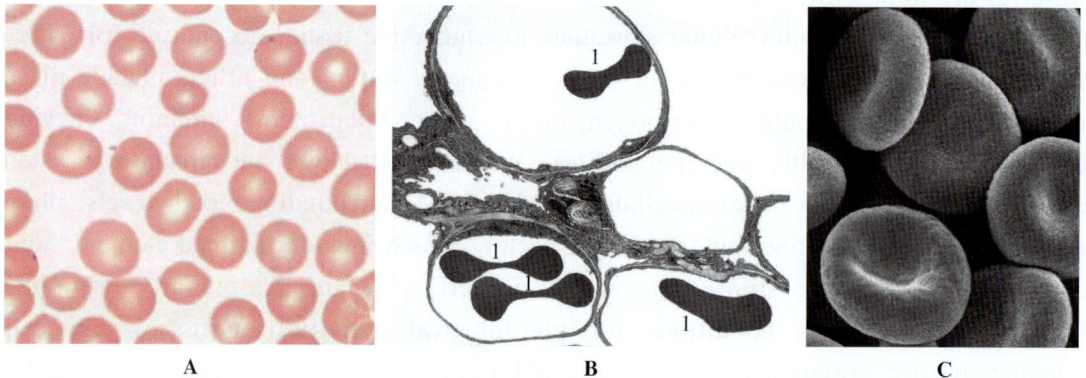

Figure 5 - 2   Erythrocytes
A. LM of erythrocytes; B. TEM of capillaries showing erythrocytes; C. SEM of erythrocytes

There are no nuclei and organelles in the mature erythrocytes. They appear red because the cytoplasm is filled with hemoglobin. Hemoglobin is a kind of protein containing iron, accounting for about 33% of the weight of erythrocytes. Hemoglobin can provide O_2 to tissues and take some produced CO_2 away by combining with O_2 or CO_2 and transporting them. When blood flows through lungs, the high partial pressure of O_2 and low partial pressure of CO_2 in the pulmonary alveolus will be observed, hemoglobin will release CO_2 and combine with O_2. When blood flows through other tissues and organs, the low partial pressure of O_2 and high partial pressure of CO_2 will be observed, hemoglobin will release O_2 for local metabolism and take away CO_2. Because CO has a greater affinity for hemoglobin than O_2, hemoglobin will combine with a large amount of CO if there is a lot in the air. CO poisoning will result in a lack of O_2 in the tissues and cells, even death.

The average concentration of erythrocytes in blood of the adult is $(4.0-5.5)\times10^{12}/L$ in men and $(3.5-5.0)\times10^{12}/L$ in women. The average concentration of hemoglobin in blood is 120 – 150 g/L in men and 110 – 140 g/L in women. The concentrations of erythrocytes and hemoglobin will change when the physiological or pathological conditions change. Normally, when the concentrations of hemoglobin are less than 100 g/L, anemia will be diagnosed. The size and morphology of erythrocytes will change in anemia.

Immature erythrocytes in blood that come from bone marrow are called reticulocytes. There are some ribosomes left in these cells. It is difficult to distinguish reticulocytes and mature erythrocytes following conventional dyeing. However, brilliant cresyl blue staining can stain the ribosomes blue in reticulocytes, which indicates the ability of synthesizing hemoglobin (Figure 5 – 3). When staying in the peripheral blood for 1 – 3 days, reticulocytes will become mature erythrocytes with the disappearance of ribosomes and no more increase of hemoglobin. Reticulocytes account for 0.5%– 1.5% of the total number of erythrocytes in adults and 3%– 6% in newborns. This value can be used to assess the hematopoiesis of bone marrow.

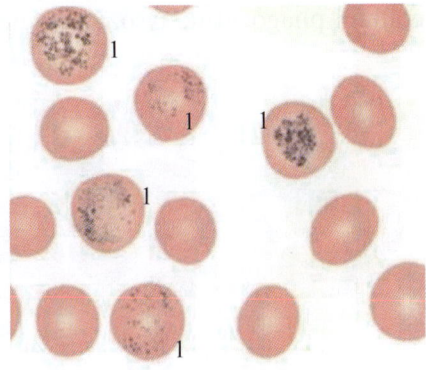

1. Reticulocytes

Figure 5 – 3 LM of erythrocytes

The life span of erythrocytes is about 120 days. Aging erythrocytes will be phagocytized by macrophages in liver and spleen.

2 Leukocyte

Spherical leukocytes are larger than erythrocytes. They can pass through the capillaries into the tissues through amoeboid movement, playing defense and immune functions. Under the light microscope, according to the special granules in the cytoplasm, leukocytes can be divided into 2 types: granulocytes and agranulocytes. With the different colour of special granules following staining, granulocytes can be divided into neutrophils, eosinophils, and basophils. Agranulocytes include lymphocytes and monocytes.

2.1 Neutrophil

Neutrophils are the most abundant type of leukocytes. Spherical neutrophils are 10 – 12 μm in diameter. They have clump-like nuclear chromatin with deep staining. The nucleus has a variety of forms, some are salami-shaped, called rod-shaped nuclei; some are lobulated, with thin filaments connecting the lobes, called lobed nuclei. The nucleus is usually divided into 2 – 5 lobes. The nuclei with 2 – 3 lobes are mostly observed in normal people. The cytoplasm of neutrophils is stained pink, and there are many fine neutral granules that distributed evenly in it. The granules include azurophilic granules and specific granules (Figure 5 – 4). Azurophilic granules constitute 20% of total granules and can be stained light purple. Azurophilic granules show bigger size and high electron density. They are lysosomes containing acid phosphatase, peroxidase and acid hydrolases. Azurophilic granules can digest and decompose swallowed foreign bodies. Specific granules account for 80% of the total number of granules in neutrophils. These granules are fine, distributed evenly, and stained light red. Specific granules exert bactericidal effect because they contain phagocytin, lysozyme, etc (Figure 5 - 5).

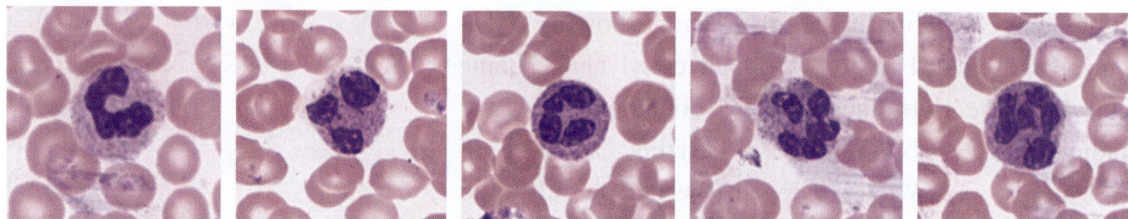

Figure 5 - 4   LM of neutrophils

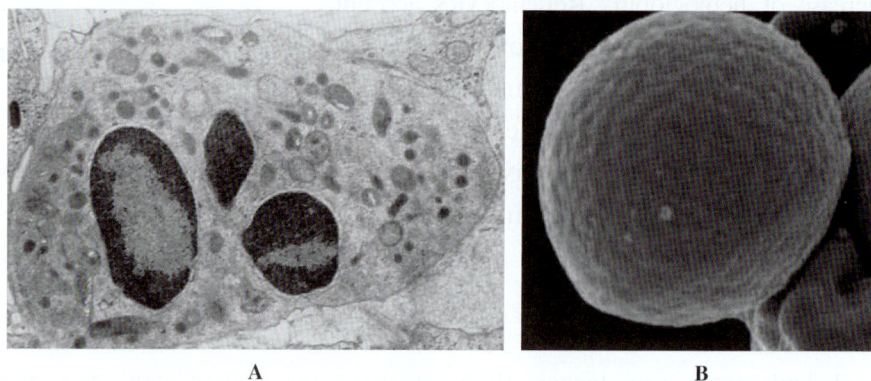

A   B

Figure 5 - 5   EM of neutrophils
A. TEM of neutrophils; B. SEM of neutrophils

Neutrophils show active amoeboid movement and phagocytosis. When bacterial invasion happens in some part of the body, bacterial products and infected tissue will release some chemical substances that attract neutrophils. Neutrophils will pass through the capillaries to the location that bacterial invaded, then surround and engulf bacterial with the pseudopod extension, and finally the enzymes in the granules will digest bacterial. Following phagocytosis, neutrophils will die and become pus cells. Therefore, the percentage of neutrophils and the total number of leukocytes increase in the acute inflammation. Neutrophils have a lifespan of 6 - 7 hours in blood and 1 - 3 days in tissue.

2.2 Eosinophil

Spherical eosinophils are $10 - 15 \mu$m in diameter, and contain bilobed nucleus mostly. The major characteristic of eosinophils is the even distribution of many large, refractive eosinophilic granules in the cytoplasm, which can be stained orange. Under the electron microscope, the granules are round or oval with rectangular crystalline cores and dense fine-grained matrix (Figure 5 – 6). There are histamine, aromatic sulfatase, acid phosphatase, peroxidase and cationic protein in the granules. The granules are specialized lysosomes.

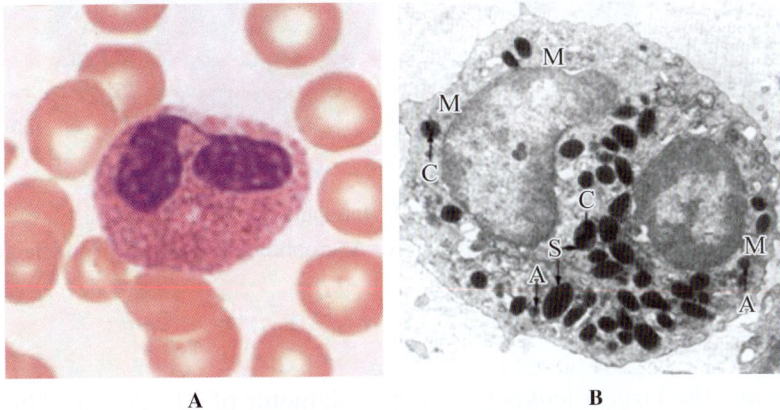

Figure 5 – 6   EM of eosinophils
A. LM of eosinophils; B. TEM of eosinophils (A. Azurophilic granules; C. Crystal; M. Mitochondria; S. Specifc granules)

Eosinophils can also do ameboid movement and have chemotaxis. They will be attracted by the eosinophil chemotactic factor of anaphylaxis released by mast cells, pass through the blood vessels into tissue, and reach the location that allergic reaction happens. Eosinophils can phagocytize antigen-antibody complexes, release histaminase to decompose histamine, release aromatic sulfatase to inactivate leukotrienes, thereby inhibiting allergic reactions. Eosinophils can also bind to some parasitic larvae with the help of antibodies or complements, and release substances inside the granules to kill parasitic worms. Eosinophils have a lifespan of 6 – 8 hours in blood, and 8 – 12 days in tissue.

2.3   Basophil

Basophils are the least common type of leukocytes. They are spherical and 10 – 12 μm in diameter. The nucleus is divided into S-shaped or irregular lobes with lighter staining. There are various size and uneven distribution of basophilic granules in the cytoplasm that can be stained bluish violet. Because the granules will cover the nuclei, the outline of nuclei might be unclear. Under the electron microscope, basophilic granules contain fine particles that are evenly distributed (Figure 5 – 7). The heparin and histamine in the granules, and the leukotrienes in the cytoplasm can induce smooth muscle contraction, increase the permeability of small blood vessels, thereby inducing allergic reactions. This is similar to mast cells. The lifespan of basophils in tissue is 10 – 15 days.

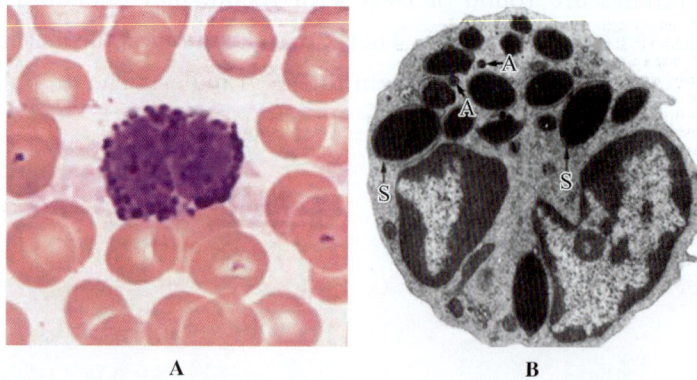

Figure 5 – 7   Basophils
A. LM of basophils; B. TEM of basophils (A. Azurophilic granules; S. Specific granules)

2.4   Monocyte

Monocytes are the largest leukocytes with a diameter of $14 - 20\,\mu$m. They are round or oval. The nucleus is kidney-shaped or horseshoe-shaped. The chromatin shows fine reticulation and lighter staining. Rich cytoplasm is weakly basophilic, stained dusty blue, and contains few azurophilic granules. Under the electron microscope, there are ruffles and short microvilli on the surface of cells. There are many phagocytic vesicles and membrane-coating granules in the cytoplasm. Azurophilic granules are lysosomes containing acid phosphatase, peroxidase, nonspecific esterase and lysozyme (Figure $5 - 8$).

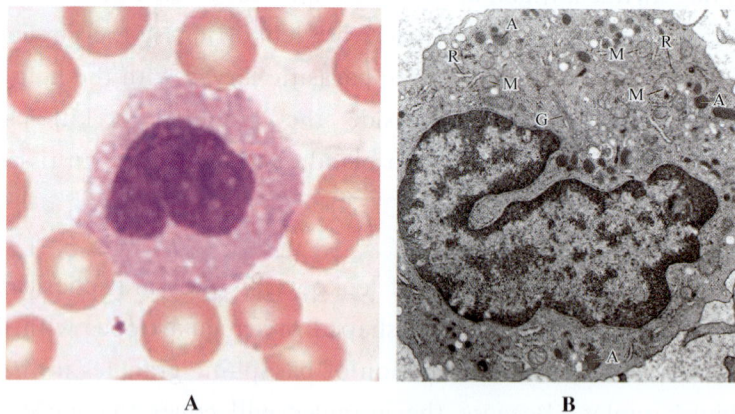

Figure 5 – 8   Monocytes
A. LM of monocytes; B. TEM of monocytes (A. Azurophilic granules; G. Golgi apparatus; M. Mitochondria; R. Ribosome)

Monocytes have active ameboid movement, obvious chemotaxis and robust phagocytic function. The monocytes produced in the bone marrow enter the bloodstream and stay for $1 - 5$ days, then pass through the blood vessels into the tissue and differentiate into various types of macrophages. Monocytes in the blood and bone marrow and macrophages in the organs and tissue constitute mononuclear phagocyte system. Monocytes and macrophages both can pathogenic microorganisms that invade the body, phagocytize foreign particles, discard aging and damaged cells in the body, and are involved in the immune response.

2.5 Lymphocyte

Lymphocytes are spherical, and have different sizes with different diameters including $6 - 8 \mu m$ (small lymphocytes), $9 - 12 \mu m$ (medium sized lymphocytes), and $13 - 20 \mu m$ (large lymphocytes). There are the largest number of small lymphocytes in the peripheral blood. The nuclei of small lymphocytes are round, and there are often dimples on one side. The chromatin is condensed and stained deeply. More nuclei and less cytoplasm make the cytoplasm form a thin rim around the nucleus, which can be stained blue. The nuclei contain a few azurophilic granules. The nuclei of medium sized lymphocytes and large lymphocytes are oval. There are loose chromatin with light staining, more cytoplasm, and a few azurophilic granules in the cells. Under the electron microscope, abundant free ribosomes, a little mitochondria and Golgi complex, and nucleoli can be observed in the cytoplasm of lymphocytes (Figure $5 - 9$).

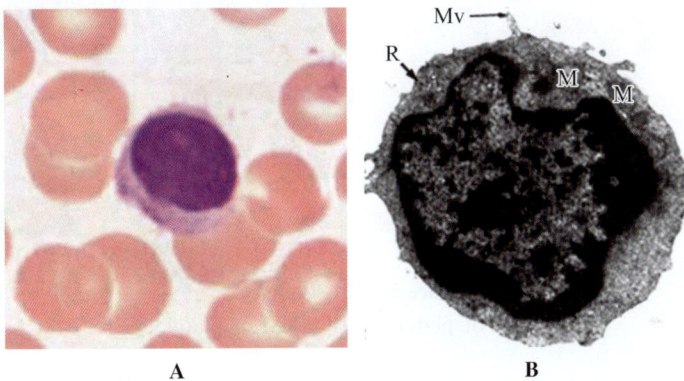

Figure 5 – 9 Lymphocytes
A. LM of lymphocytes; B. TEM of lymphocytes (M. Mitochondria; Mv. Microvilli; R. Ribosome)

Lymphocytes are a kind of cell population with the most complicated functions and classifications in vivo. According to the differences in the developmental process, morphology, surface markers and immune functions, lymphocytes can be classified into 3 types: thymus dependent lymphocytes (T cells), bone marrow dependent lymphocytes (B cells) and natural killer cells (NK cells). T cells mediate cellular immunity and B cells mediate humoral immunity. NK cells can non-specifically kill certain tumor cells and virus-infected cells. Lymphocytes are the only type of leukocytes in the body that can return to the blood from the tissue, and play an important role in the immune defense.

3 Platelet

Platelets, also known as thrombocytes, are cytoplasmic fragmentations of megakaryocytes.

They are biconcave disks with thick center and thin edge, and $2-4\,\mu$m in diameter. When stimulated mechanically or chemically, platelets will protrude into irregular shapes. They are nonnucleated and covered by the intact cell membrane. There are bluish violet platelet granules in the center of platelets, which are called granulomere. These granules are special granules, dense granules and a few lysosomes. The special granules contain platelet factor 4, fibrinogen, thrombospondin, and platelet-derived growth factor, etc. The dense granules contain Ca^{2+}, pyrophosphate, ADP, ATP and serotonin. The cytoplasm near the granulomere is weakly basophilic and stained light blue, called the transparent zone. Blood smears show that platelets are often polygonal and clustered together. Under the electron microscope, thick sugar-coating on the surfaces of platelets can be observed. Microtubules form a ring around the cells, which is beneficial to maintaining the morphology of platelets (Figure 5 - 10).

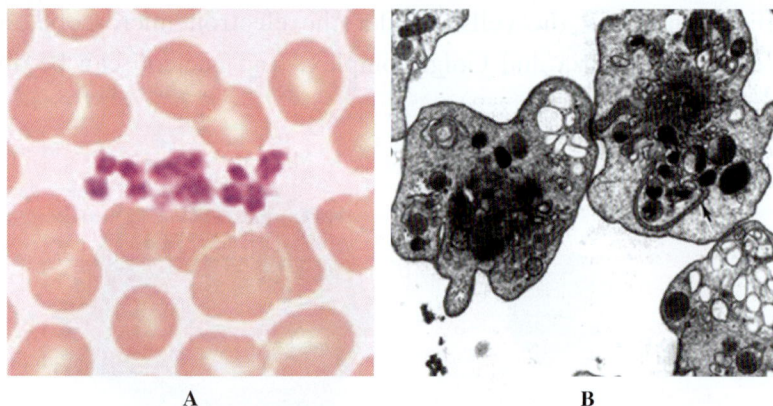

A   B

Figure 5 - 10 Platelets
A. LM of platelets; B. TEM of platelets

There are 2 tubular systems in the platelets: the open canalicular system and the dense tubular system. The open canalicular system is connected with the platelet surface, which is beneficial to the release of particle content. Dense tubules are located in the transparent area. They are irregular closed tubules with dense electrons, and equivalent to smooth endoplasmic reticulum and have the functions of collecting Ca^{2+} and synthesizing prostaglandins. Platelets are involved in the process of hemostasis and coagulation. When the vascular endothelium ruptures, platelets will rapidly release particle content that adheres and gathers at the damaged place, forms thrombosis, blocks the rupture and even the lumen of small blood vessels. Serotonin in the particle content released by platelets can induce vasoconstriction. Platelet factor 4 can resist the anticoagulant effect of histamine. Thrombin-sensitive protein can promote platelet aggregation. Platelet-derived growth factor can stimulate proliferation of endothelial cells and repairment of blood vessels. The lifespan of the platelet is 7 - 14 days.

4　Hematopoiesis

All blood cells have a certain lifespan. The continuous aging and dying of blood cells and the continuous production of new blood cells maintain the homeostasis of number and quality of blood cells.

4.1　Red Bone Marrow

Red bone marrow is mainly distributed in the flat bones, irregular bones, and cancellous bones in the epiphysis of long bones (Figure 5 - 11). It consists of hematopoietic tissue and blood sinuses. The hematopoietic tissue consists of reticular tissue and hematopoietic cells. There are multiple blood cells at different development stages in the mesh formed by reticular cells and fibers, as well as few hematopoietic stem cells, macrophages, etc. The environment for the growth and development of hematopoietic cells is hematopoietic-inductive microenvironment. Reticular cells, macrophages, fibroblasts, sinusoidal endothelial cells are called stromal cells. Stromal cells are an important part of the hematopoietic-inductive microenvironment, which can support cells and secret cytokines to regulate proliferation and differentiation of hematopoietic cells. Blood sinuses are capillaries with large and irregular lumen, and thin walls. Large endothelial cell gaps and incomplete endothelial basement membranes of blood sinuses are beneficial to the entry of mature blood cells into the blood.

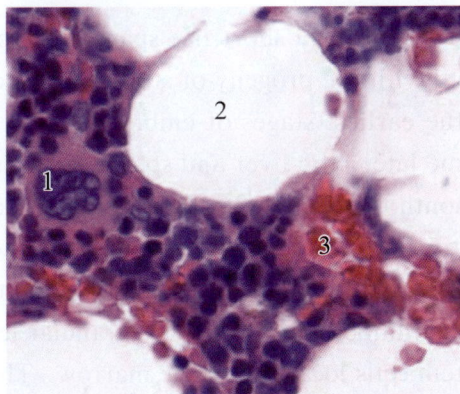

1. Megakaryocyte; 2. Adipose; 3. Sinusoid

Figure 5 - 11　LM of red bone marrow

4.2　Hematopoietic Stem Cell and Hematopoietic Progenitor

Hematopoietic stem cells are primitive cells that can differentiate into various blood cells. They are also known as pluripotent stem cells and originate from the yolk sac of human embryos. After birth, most hematopoietic stem cells can be found in the red bone marrow, and less cells are found in the spleen, liver, lymph nodes and peripheral blood. The morphology of hematopoietic stem cells is similar to that of small lymphocytes. They are small with large nuclei, and have the cytoplasm rich in ribosomes. The characteristics of hematopoietic stem cells are: ①High proliferative potential. Under normal conditions, most stem cells are in a quiescent state in G_0 phase, only 10% stem cells are in a proliferating state. ②Multipotential differentiation. They can differentiate into different progenitors. ③ Self-renewal. They can self-renew to maintain the homeostasis of cell number. The hematopoietic stem cells have multiple cell populations with different differentiation levels. For example, myeloid lineage can differentiate into erythrocytes, granulocyte-monocytes, megakaryocytes and so on. Lymphoid lineage can differentiate into different kinds of lymphocytes.

Hematopoietic progenitor cells are differentiated hematopoietic stem cells, and also known as committed stem cells. The defined hematopoietic progenitor cells are: ① Erythroid progenitor cell. They can differentiate into erythrocytes with the supplementation of erythropoietin. ② Granulocyte-monocyte progenitor cell. They can differentiate into neutrophils and monocytes. When inflammation occurs in the body, the interleukins released by macrophages can activate the proliferation of neutrophils and monocytes, and induce the migration of these 2 cells from the bone marrow into the peripheral blood. ③Megakaryocyte progenitor cell. With the stimulation of thrombopoietin, megakaryocyte colonies are formed and finally platelets are produced.

4.3 Hemopoiesis

Mature blood cells have a relatively short life span, and consequently the population must be continuously replaced with the progeny of stem cells produced in the hematopoietic organs (Figure 5 - 12). In the earliest stages of embryogenesis, blood cells arise from the yolk sac mesoderm. Sometime later, the liver and spleen serve as temporary hematopoietic tissues, but by the second month the clavicle has begun to ossify and begins to develop bone marrow in its core. As the prenatal ossification of the rest of the skeleton accelerates, the bone marrow becomes an increasingly important hematopoietic tissue.

After birth and on into childhood, erythrocytes, granular leukocytes, monocytes, and platelets are derived from stem cells located in bone marrow. The origin and maturation of these cells are termed erythropoiesis, granulopoiesis, monocytopoiesis, and megakaryocytopoiesis, respectively (Figure 5 - 12). The bone marrow also produces cells that migrate to the lymphoid organs, producing various types of lymphocytes.

Before attaining maturity and being released into the circulation, blood cells go through specific stages of differentiation and maturation. Because these processes are continuous, cells with characteristics that lie between the various stages are frequently encountered in smears of blood or bone marrow.

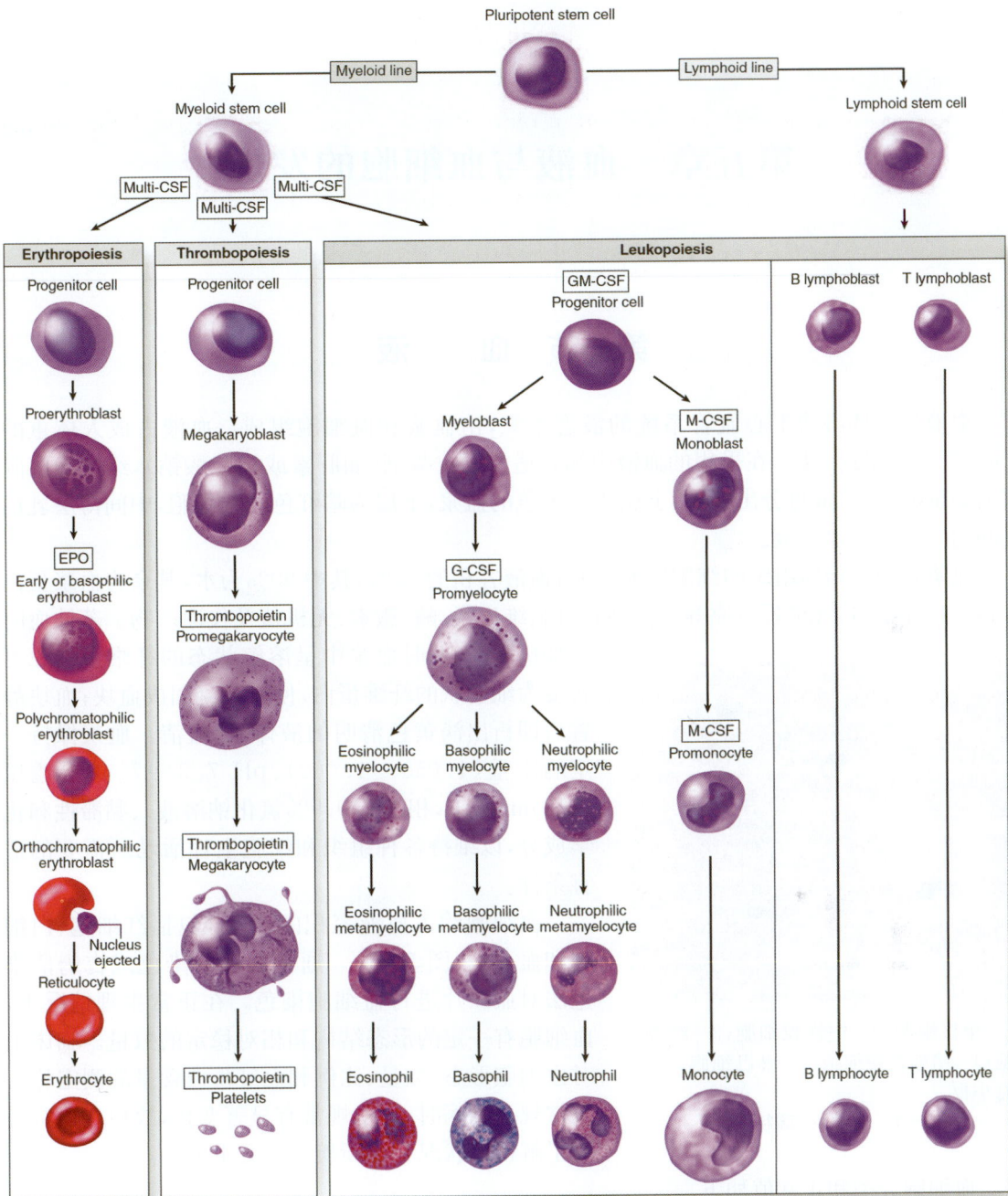

Figure 5 – 12　Diagram of hemopoiesis

(Xu Wenhua, Yang Fan)

第五章　血液与血细胞的发生

第一节　血　液

血液是循环流动于心血管系统的液态组织,由血浆和血细胞组成。血液占成人体重的7%～8%,总量约5L。在采集的血液中加入适量的抗凝剂(如肝素或枸橼酸钠),经自然沉降或离心沉淀后,血液可分出三层:上层为淡黄色的血浆,下层为暗红色的红细胞,中间薄层乳白色的为白细胞和血小板。

血浆相当于结缔组织的细胞间质,约占血液容积的55%,其中90%为水,其余为血浆蛋白(白蛋白、球蛋白、纤维蛋白原等)、糖、脂蛋白、维生素、酶、激素、无机盐及代谢产物。若抽血时不加抗凝剂,此时血浆中呈溶解状态的纤维蛋白原可转变为细丝状的纤维蛋白,使血液凝固成血块;血块静置后即析出淡黄色清明的液体,称血清。血浆保持一定的比重(1.050～1.060)、pH 7.3～7.4、渗透压(313 mmol/L,相当于0.9%氯化钠溶液)、黏滞性和化学成分,以维持各种组织和细胞生理活动所需要的适宜条件。

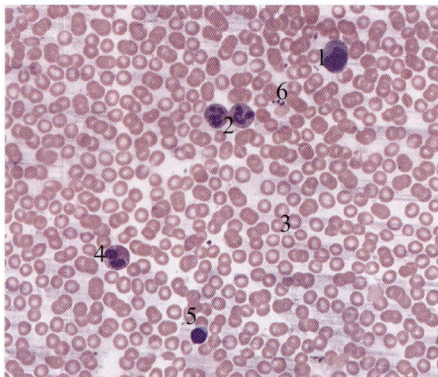

1—单核细胞;2—中性粒细胞;3—红细胞;4—嗜酸性粒细胞;5—淋巴细胞;6—血小板

图5-1　血涂片(瑞特染色)

血细胞约占血液容积的45%,包括红细胞、白细胞和血小板(图5-1)。通常用瑞特染色或吉姆萨染色法对血涂片进行血细胞染色。在正常生理情况下,血细胞有一定的形态结构和相对稳定的数量。临床上对血细胞形态、数量、比例和血红蛋白含量的测定称为血常规。患病时,血常规常有显著变化,故检查血常规对了解机体状况和诊断疾病十分重要。

血细胞分类和正常值如下:

血细胞
- 红细胞 $(3.5\sim5.5)\times10^{12}/L$
- 白细胞 $(4\sim10)\times10^{9}/L$
  - 中性粒细胞　　50%～70%
  - 嗜酸性粒细胞　0.5%～3%
  - 嗜碱性粒细胞　0～1%
  - 淋巴细胞　　　25%～30%
  - 单核细胞　　　3%～8%
- 血小板 $(1.0\sim3.0)\times10^{11}/L$

一、红细胞

红细胞直径为 $7.5 \sim 8.5\,\mu m$,呈双凹圆盘状,中央较薄,周缘较厚,故在血涂片上,可见中央染色淡,周缘染色深(图5-2)。红细胞的这种形态特点增加了红细胞的表面积,有利于细胞内外气体的交换。

成熟的红细胞无细胞核,也无细胞器,细胞质内充满血红蛋白,使红细胞呈红色。血红蛋白是含铁的蛋白质,约占红细胞重量的33%。血红蛋白具有结合与运输 O_2 和 CO_2 的功能,为组织细胞提供 O_2,带走产生的部分 CO_2。当血液流经肺时,肺泡内的氧分压高,二氧化碳分压低,血红蛋白就释放 CO_2 而与 O_2 结合;当血液流经其他组织和器官时,由于该处的二氧化碳分压高而氧分压低,血红蛋白就释放 O_2 供局部代谢所需,并带走部分 CO_2。血红蛋白对 CO 的亲和力比 O_2 大,而且与 CO 结合后不易分离。如果空气中 CO 较多,血红蛋白与大量 CO 结合后,可出现组织和细胞缺氧,严重时可导致死亡,此类情况多见于煤气中毒。

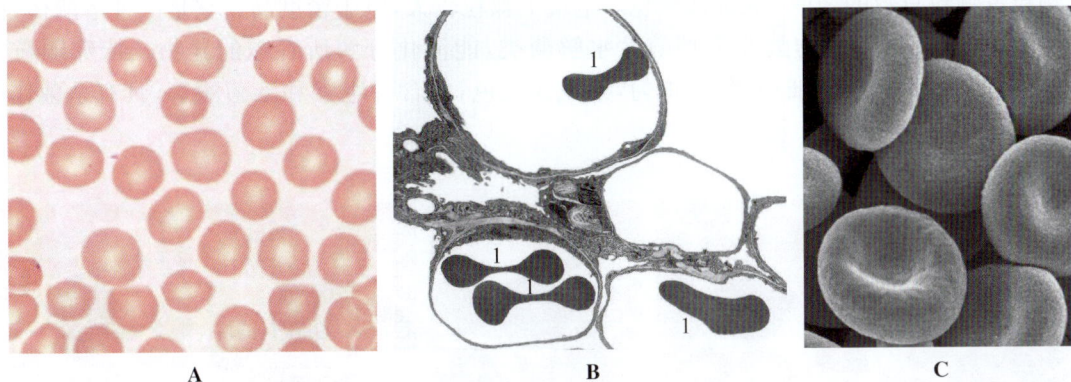

图5-2 红细胞
A.红细胞光镜结构;B.红细胞透射电镜结构(1—红细胞);C.红细胞扫描电镜结构

成人血液中红细胞的平均值,男性为 $(4.0 \sim 5.5) \times 10^{12}/L$,女性为 $(3.5 \sim 5.0) \times 10^{12}/L$。每升血液内血红蛋白的平均含量,男性为 $120 \sim 150\,g/L$,女性为 $110 \sim 140\,g/L$。红细胞和血红蛋白的数值可因生理或病理状态的变化而改变。一般情况下,血红蛋白低于 $100\,g/L$ 则为贫血。贫血时常伴有红细胞大小和形态的改变。

从骨髓进入血液,尚未完全成熟的红细胞称为网织红细胞,这些细胞内尚残留部分核糖体,在常规染色的血涂片中不能与成熟红细胞区别,用煌焦油蓝染色可见网织红细胞内有染成蓝色的细网或颗粒,它是细胞内残留的核糖体,说明该细胞仍有合成血红蛋白的功能(图5-3)。网织红细胞进入外周血 $1 \sim 3$ 天后,核糖体消失,血红蛋白不再增加,变成成熟的红细胞。成人网织红细胞占红细胞总数的 $0.5\% \sim 1.5\%$,新生儿可达 $3\% \sim 6\%$。该细胞数值的变化,可作为衡量骨髓造血功能的一种指标。

红细胞的平均寿命约为120天。衰老的红细胞在

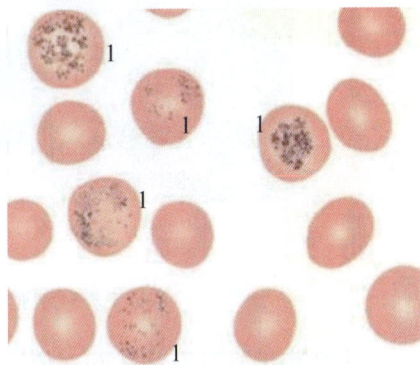

1—网织红细胞
图5-3 网织红细胞光镜结构

肝、脾和骨髓等处被巨噬细胞吞噬。

二、白细胞

白细胞为有核的球形细胞,较红细胞大,能以变形运动方式穿过毛细血管壁进入周围组织,发挥防御和免疫功能。在光镜下,根据白细胞胞质内有无特殊颗粒,可将其分为有粒白细胞和无粒白细胞。根据其特殊颗粒的染色性,有粒白细胞可分为中性粒细胞、嗜酸性粒细胞和嗜碱性粒细胞三种。无粒白细胞有单核细胞和淋巴细胞两种。

1. 中性粒细胞

中性粒细胞是白细胞中数量最多的一种。细胞呈球形,直径 $10 \sim 12\ \mu m$。核染色质呈团块状,着色深。核的形态多样化,有的呈腊肠状,称杆状核;有的呈分叶状,叶间有细丝相连,称分叶核,一般分 $2 \sim 5$ 叶,正常人以 $2 \sim 3$ 叶者居多。胞质染成粉红色,含有许多细小的浅紫色和浅粉红色的中性颗粒,分布均匀。颗粒可分为嗜天青颗粒和特殊颗粒两种(图 5-4)。嗜天青颗粒占颗粒总数的 20%,染成浅紫色。电镜下颗粒较大,电子密度高。它是一种溶酶体,内含酸性磷酸酶、过氧化物酶及多种酸性水解酶类,能消化分解所吞噬的异物。特殊颗粒占颗粒总数的 80%,颗粒细小,分布均匀,染成浅红色,内含吞噬素和溶菌酶等,具有杀菌作用(图 5-5)。

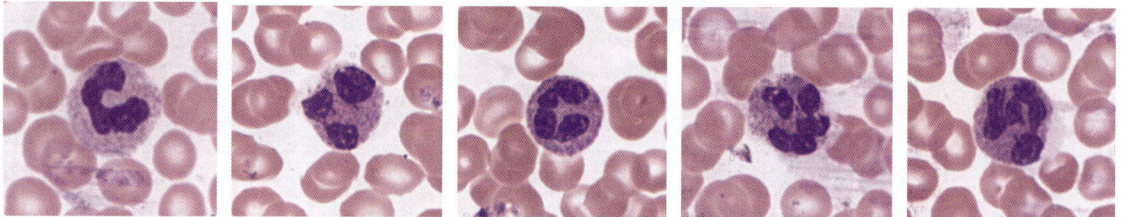

图 5-4　中性粒细胞光镜结构

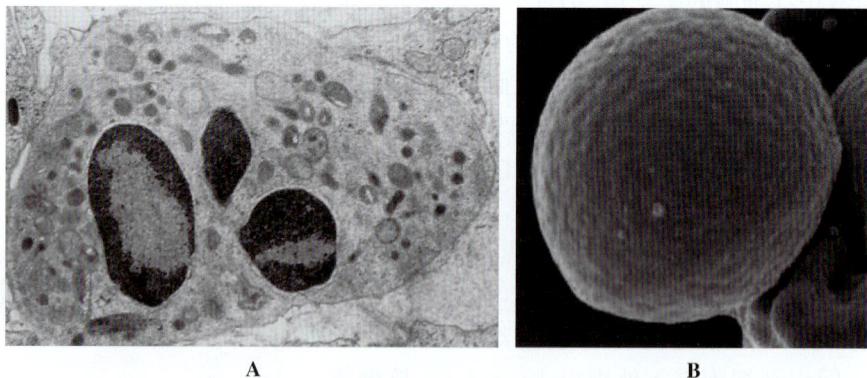

A　　　　　　　　　　　　　　B

图 5-5　中性粒细胞
A. 中性粒细胞透射电镜结构;B. 中性粒细胞扫描电镜结构

中性粒细胞具有活跃的变形运动和吞噬功能。当机体某部位受到细菌侵入时,中性粒细胞对细菌产物及受感染组织释放的某些化学物质具有趋化性,能以变形运动穿过毛细血管,聚集到细菌侵入部位,伸出伪足包围并吞噬细菌,颗粒内的酶类物质对细菌进行分解消化。同时,中性粒细胞吞噬、处理大量细菌后,自身也死亡,成为脓细胞。故中性粒细胞在体内起着重要的防御作用。在急性炎症时,中性粒细胞百分比和白细胞总数均升高。中性粒细胞在血液中停留 6～7 h,在组织中存活 1～3 天。

2. 嗜酸性粒细胞

嗜酸性粒细胞呈球形,直径为 10～15 μm,核多为 2 叶,其主要特征为胞质内充满粗大、分布均匀、有折光性的嗜酸性颗粒,染成橘红色。电镜下颗粒为圆形或椭圆形膜包颗粒,内有长方形结晶体和致密的细颗粒状基质(图 5-6)。颗粒内含有组胺酶、芳香硫酸酯酶、酸性磷酸酶、过氧化物酶和阳离子蛋白等,它是一种特化的溶酶体。

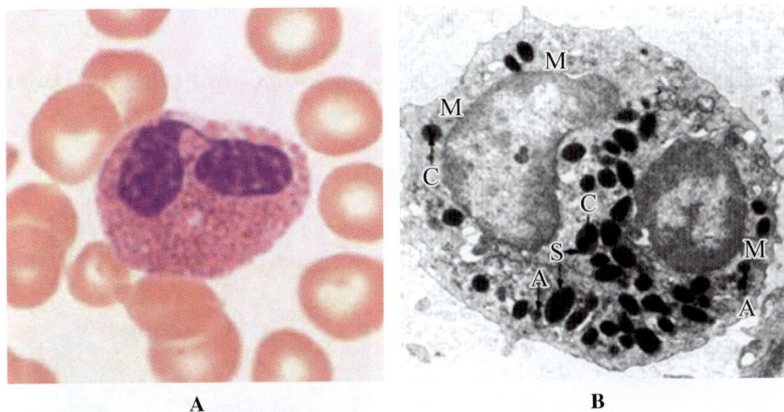

图 5-6　嗜酸性粒细胞
A.嗜酸性粒细胞光镜结构;B.嗜酸性粒细胞电镜结构(A—嗜天青颗粒;C—结晶体;M—线粒体;S—特殊颗粒)

嗜酸性粒细胞也能做变形运动,并具有趋化性,可受肥大细胞释放的嗜酸性粒细胞趋化因子的作用,穿越血管壁进入组织,到达发生过敏反应的部位。嗜酸性粒细胞能吞噬抗原抗体复合物,释放的组胺酶能分解组胺,芳香硫酸酯酶能灭活白三烯,从而抑制过敏反应。嗜酸性粒细胞还能借助抗体或补体与某些寄生虫幼体结合,释放颗粒内物质,杀死寄生虫。嗜酸性粒细胞在血液中一般仅停留 6～8 h,在组织中可存活 8～12 天。

3. 嗜碱性粒细胞

嗜碱性粒细胞在白细胞中数量最少。细胞呈球形,直径为 10～12 μm。胞核分叶,或呈 S 型或不规则形,着色较浅。胞质内含有大小不等、分布不均、染成蓝紫色的嗜碱性颗粒。颗粒可覆盖在核上,故胞核轮廓常不清楚。电镜下,嗜碱性颗粒内含细小微粒,均匀分布(图 5-7),颗粒内含肝素、组胺等。而细胞胞质中含白三烯,这些物质的释放可以使平滑肌收缩,小血管通透性增高,导致过敏反应,这与肥大细胞很相似。嗜碱性粒细胞在组织中可存活 10～15 天。

4. 单核细胞

单核细胞是体积最大的白细胞,直径为 14～20 μm,呈圆形或椭圆形。胞核呈肾形或马蹄形,染色质呈细网状,着色较浅。胞质丰富,呈弱嗜碱性,常染成灰蓝色,内含少量嗜天青颗粒。电镜下,细胞表面有皱褶和短的微绒毛,胞质内有许多吞噬泡和膜包颗粒。嗜天青颗粒为溶酶体,内含酸性磷酸酶、过氧化物酶、非特异性酯酶和溶菌酶(图 5-8)。

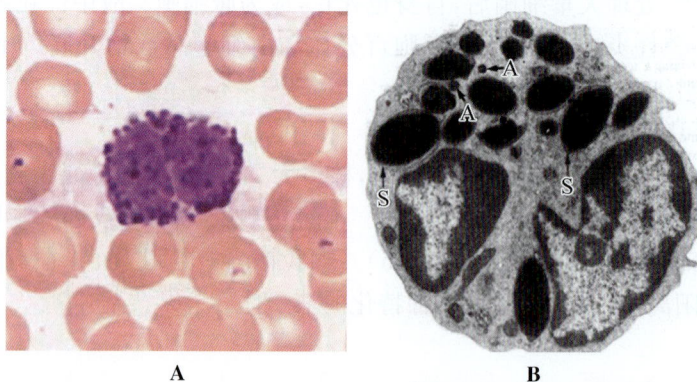

图 5-7 嗜碱性粒细胞
A.嗜碱性粒细胞光镜结构；B.嗜碱性粒细胞电镜结构(A—嗜天青颗粒；S—特殊颗粒)

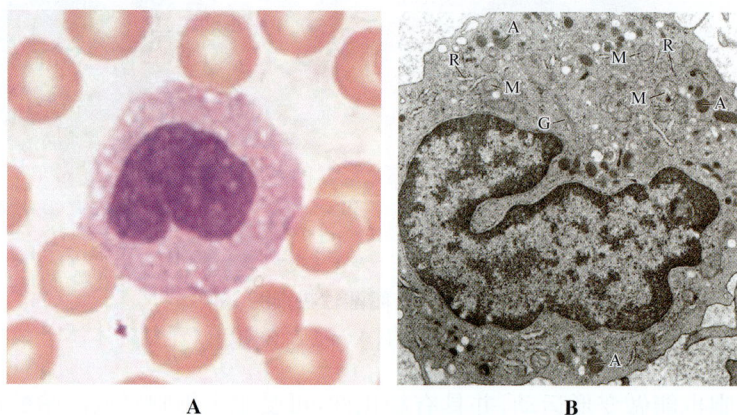

图 5-8 单核细胞
A.单核细胞光镜结构；B.单核细胞电镜结构(A—嗜天青颗粒；G—高尔基体；M—线粒体；R—核糖体)

单核细胞具有活跃的变形运动、明显的趋化性和很强的吞噬功能。骨髓生成的单核细胞进入血液循环,停留1~5天后穿出血管进入组织分化成各种类型的巨噬细胞。血液、骨髓中的单核细胞和器官组织内的巨噬细胞共同构成单核吞噬细胞系统。单核细胞与巨噬细胞都能消灭入侵机体的病原微生物,吞噬异物颗粒,消除体内衰老损伤的细胞,并参与免疫应答。

5. 淋巴细胞

淋巴细胞呈球形,大小不等,直径6~8 μm的为小淋巴细胞,直径9~12 μm的为中淋巴细胞,直径13~20 μm的为大淋巴细胞。外周血中小淋巴细胞数量最多。小淋巴细胞的核占细胞的大部分,为圆形,一侧常有浅凹,染色质浓密呈块状,着色深;胞质很少,在核周形成一窄缘,染成蔚蓝色,含少量嗜天青颗粒。大、中淋巴细胞的核椭圆形,染色质较疏松,着色较浅,胞质较多,可见少量嗜天青颗粒。电镜下,淋巴细胞胞质内含丰富的游离核糖体,少量线粒体和高尔基复合体(图5-9)。

淋巴细胞是体内功能与分类最为复杂的细胞群。根据淋巴细胞的发生过程、形态特点、细胞表面标志和免疫功能等不同,可将其分为三类:胸腺依赖淋巴细胞(thymus dependent lymphocyte,T细胞)、骨髓依赖淋巴细胞(bone marrow dependent lymphocyte,B细胞)和

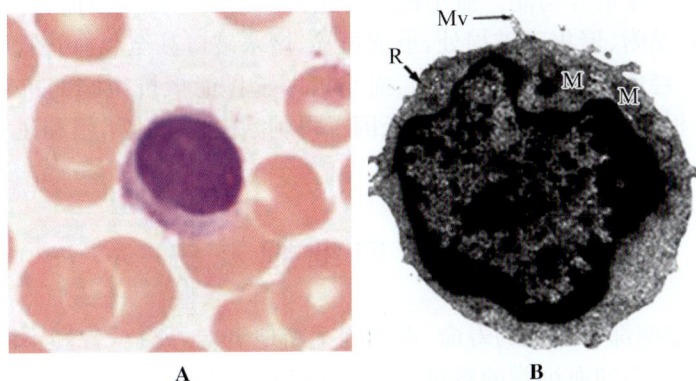

图5-9 淋巴细胞
A.淋巴细胞光镜结构;B.淋巴细胞电镜结构(Mv—微绒毛;M—线粒体;R—核糖体)

自然杀伤细胞(natural killer cell，NK 细胞)。T 细胞介导细胞免疫,B 细胞介导体液免疫。NK 细胞能非特异杀伤某些肿瘤细胞和病毒感染细胞。淋巴细胞是机体内唯一可从组织中返回血液的白细胞,在机体的免疫防御过程中发挥重要作用。

三、血小板

血小板又称血栓细胞,是骨髓巨核细胞胞质脱落下来的细胞质小块。血小板呈双凸圆盘状,大小不一,直径为 2~4 μm;当受到机械或化学刺激时,则伸出突起,呈不规则形。血小板无核,表面有完整的细胞膜。血小板中央部有蓝紫色的血小板颗粒,称为颗粒区,其中有特殊颗粒、致密颗粒和少量溶酶体。特殊颗粒内含血小板因子Ⅳ、纤维蛋白原、凝血酶敏感蛋白和血小板源性生长因子等。致密颗粒内含 Ca^{2+}、焦磷酸盐、腺苷二磷酸(adenosine diphosphate，ADP)、腺苷三磷酸(adenosine triphosphate，ATP)和5-羟色胺等。周边胞质呈弱嗜碱性,呈均质浅蓝色,称为透明区。在血涂片上,血小板常呈多角形,聚集成群。电镜下,血小板表面有较厚的糖衣,微管在细胞周边形成环状,有利于保持血小板的形态(图5-10)。血小板内有开放小管系和致密小管系两套小管系统。开放小管系的管道与血小板表面连通,有利于颗粒内容物的释放。致密小管系位于透明区,呈电子致密的不规则封闭小管,相当于滑面内质网,有

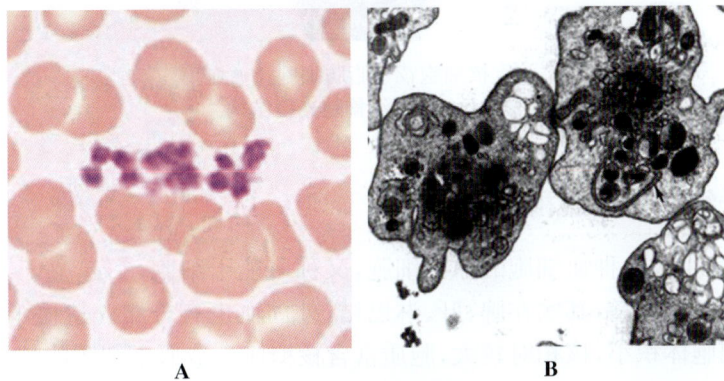

图5-10 血小板
A.血小板光镜结构;B.血小板电镜结构

收集 Ca^{2+} 和合成前列腺素等功能。血小板参与止血和凝血过程。当血管内皮破裂,血小板迅速释放颗粒内容物,黏附、聚集于破损处,形成血栓,堵塞破口甚至小血管管腔。血小板释放的颗粒内容物中的 5-羟色胺能使血管收缩。血小板因子 IV 能抵抗组胺的抗凝血作用。凝血酶敏感蛋白促进血小板聚集。血小板源性生长因子可刺激内皮细胞增殖和血管修复。血小板寿命为 7~14 天。

第二节 血细胞发生

血液内各种血细胞都有一定的寿命,血细胞不断地衰老、死亡,骨髓不断地产生新的血细胞进入血流,使外周血中的血细胞的数量和质量维持动态平衡。

一、红骨髓的结构

成人红骨髓主要分布于扁骨、不规则骨及长骨骨骺端的松质骨内,由造血组织和血窦构成(图 5-11)。造血组织主要由以网状组织和造血细胞组成。网状细胞和网状纤维作为造血组织的网架,网孔中充满不同发育阶段的各种血细胞,以及少量造血干细胞、巨噬细胞等。造血细胞赖以生长发育的环境被称为造血诱导微环境。骨髓内的网状细胞、巨噬细胞、成纤维细胞、血窦内皮细胞等细胞统称为基质细胞,是造血微环境中的重要成分,不仅起支持作用,还分泌细胞因子,调节造血细胞的增殖与分化。血窦为腔大、壁薄、腔形不规则的毛细血管,内皮细胞间隙较大,内皮基膜不完整,有利于成熟血细胞进入血液。

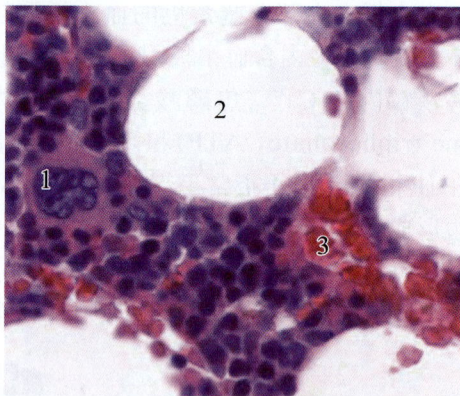

1—巨核细胞;2—脂肪细胞;3—血窦
图 5-11 红骨髓光镜结构

二、造血干细胞和造血祖细胞

造血干细胞是生成各种血细胞的原始细胞,又称多能干细胞,它起源于人胚卵黄囊血岛。出生后,主要存在于红骨髓,其次在脾、肝、淋巴结、外周血也有分布。造血干细胞的形态类似小淋巴细胞,即细胞体积小,核相对较大,胞质富含核糖体。造血干细胞的特性是:①很强的增殖潜能。在正常情况下,多数干细胞处于 G_0 期静止状态,仅有 10% 的造血干细胞处于增殖状态。②具有多向分化能力,能分化形成不同的祖细胞。③可自我复制能力。细胞分裂后的部分子细胞仍具原有特性，故造血干细胞可终身保持恒定的数量。造血干细胞中存在不同分化等级的细胞群体，如髓性造血干细胞可分化为红细胞系、粒细胞单核细胞系、巨核细胞系等细胞系的造血祖细胞；淋巴性造血干细胞可分化为各种淋巴细胞。

造血祖细胞是由造血干细胞分化而来、其分化方向确定的干细胞，也称定向干细胞。目前已确认的造血祖细胞有：①红细胞系造血祖细胞，在红细胞生成素作用下生成红细胞。②粒细胞单核细胞系造血祖细胞，是中性粒细胞和单核细胞共同的祖细胞，在机体发生炎症时，炎症部位的巨噬细胞释放的白细胞介素能刺激骨髓中这两种细胞的增殖和释放入外周血。③巨核细胞系造血祖细胞，在血小板生成素作用下形成巨核细胞集落，最终产生血小板。

三、血细胞发生过程的形态演变

血细胞的发生从幼稚走向成熟可分为原始阶段、幼稚阶段和成熟阶段 3 个时期（图 5-12）。每个时期都有各自的形态结构特点，是血液病诊断的重要依据。一般的变化规律如下：①胞核由大变小，红细胞核最后消失，粒细胞核由圆形逐渐变为杆状，直至分叶状，巨核细胞的核由小变大呈分叶状。染色体逐渐变粗密，核仁渐消失。②胞质由少变多，嗜碱性逐渐变弱，但单核细胞和淋巴细胞仍保持弱碱性。胞质内的特殊结构如血红蛋白、特殊颗粒、嗜天青颗粒等均由无到有，并逐渐增多。③胞体由大变小，而巨核细胞的发生则由小变大。④细胞分裂能力逐渐减弱至消失，但淋巴细胞仍有很强的潜在分裂能力。

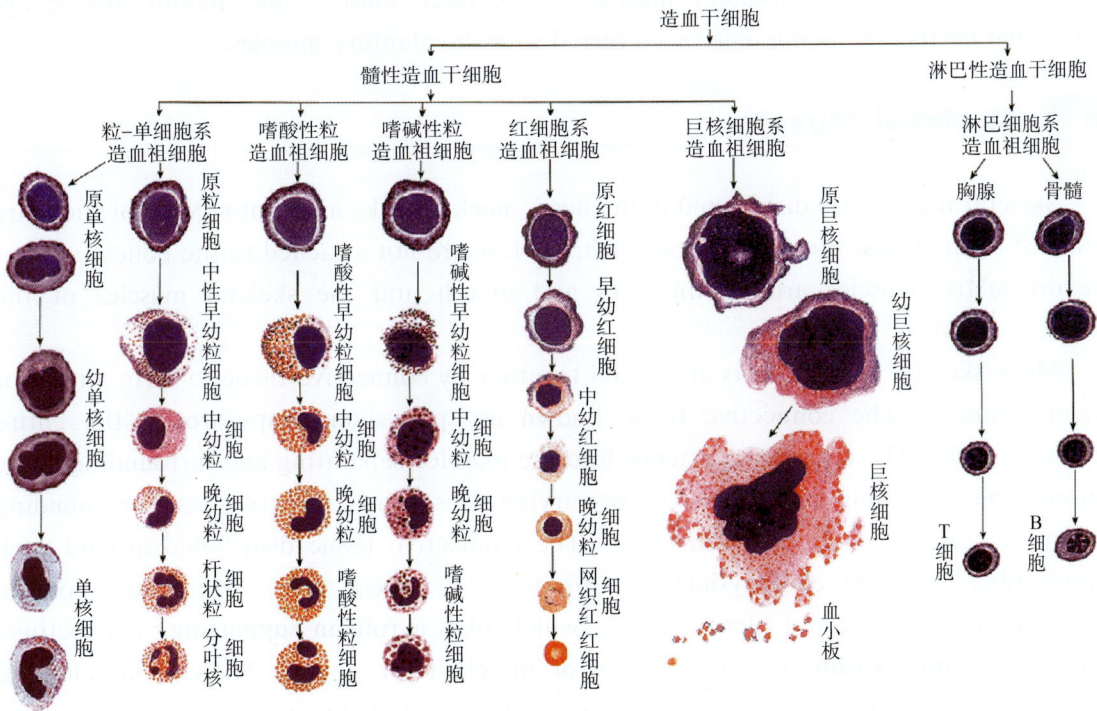

图 5-12　血细胞发生模式图

（郑　英　牛长敏）

Chapter 6

Muscle Tissue

Muscle tissue is composed of muscle cells, with a little connective tissue and a few blood vessels, lymphatic vessels, and nerves between them. Muscle cells are also called muscle fibers because they have an elongated and thread-like shape. The cytoplasm of the skeletal muscle is often called sarcoplasm; and its smooth endoplasmic reticulum is called sarcoplasmic reticulum; and its cell membrane is called sarcolemma. According to the structure and function, muscle tissues are classified into three major categories: skeletal muscle, cardiac muscle and smooth muscle. Skeletal muscle and cardiac muscle are striated muscles because they have cross striations. Skeletal muscles are innervated by somatic nerves, referred to as voluntary muscle; the cardiac muscle and smooth muscle are innervated by the autonomic nerves, referred to as involuntary muscles.

1 Skeletal Muscle

Skeletal muscles are distributed in the head, neck, trunk, and limbs. Most of them are attached to the bones through tendons, while a few are not attached to the bones, such as the orbicularis muscles around the eyes and mouth and the skeletal muscles of the esophageal wall.

Many skeletal muscle fibers are bound together by connective tissue to form a mass of skeletal muscle. The connective tissue known as epimysium wraps around the entire skeletal muscle. The epimysium extends into the muscle, separating and surrounding many muscle fibers, forming muscle fascicles of varying sizes. The connective tissue surrounding the muscle fascicle is called perimysium. The connective tissue distributed around each muscle fiber is called endomysium (Figure 6 - 1). These connective tissues contain abundant nerve fibers and blood vessels, which play a role in supporting, connecting, nourishing, and coordinating the activity of muscle fiber groups. Skeletal muscles are connected to tendons, periosteum, or dermis through the epimysium, perimysium and endomysium.

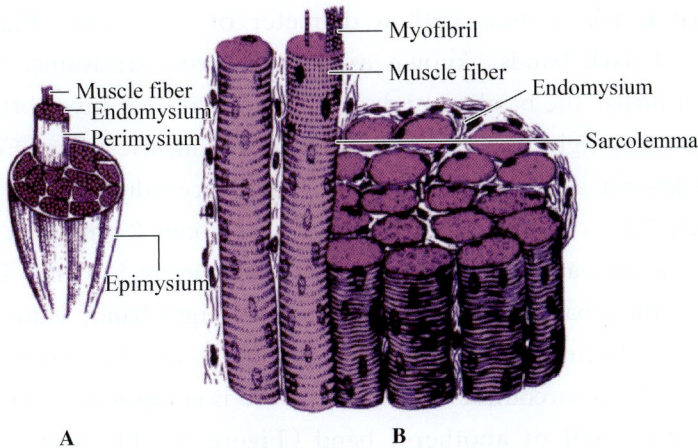

Figure 6 – 1   Drawing showing the structure of skeletal muscle
A. A mass of skeletal muscle; B. A muscle fascicle

1.1   LM Structure of Skeletal Muscle Fibers

A skeletal muscle fiber is slender cylindrical (Figure 6 – 2), with a diameter of 10 – 100 μm and a length of 1 – 40 mm. Except a few muscle fibers, such as those in tongue, skeletal muscle fibers have very few branches. There is a basement membrane attached outside the sarcolemma. There are flat and protuberant muscle satellite cells between the sarcolemma and the basement membrane, serving as stem cells. When muscle fibers are damaged, muscle satellite cells can proliferate and differentiate, participating in the repair of muscle. The skeletal muscle fiber is a multinucleated cell, with dozens to hundreds of nuclei. The nuclei are flat, oval, and palely stained, which are located beneath the sarcolemma (Figure 6 – 2). The sarcoplasm is eosinophilic and contains many myofibrils arranged parallel to the long axis of the muscle fibers (Figure 6 – 1), which appear punctate in cross-sections (Figure 6 – 3).

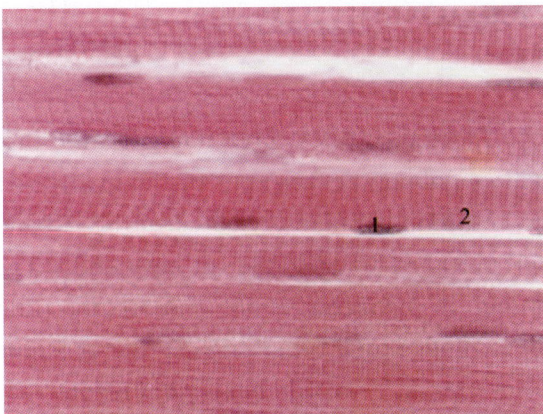

1. Nucleus; 2. Cross striation
Figure 6 – 2   Light micrograph of the skeletal muscle in longitudinal section (HE)

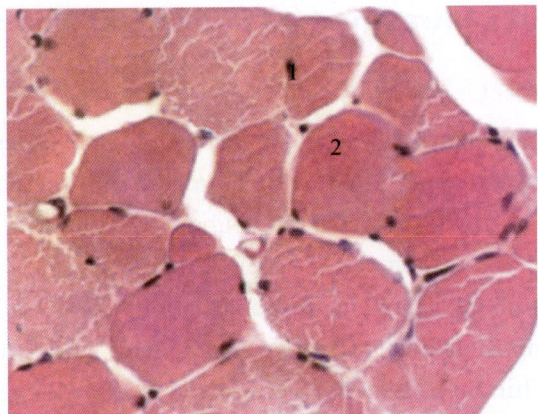

1. Nucleus; 2. Myofibril
Figure 6 – 3   Light micrograph of the skeletal muscle in cross-section (HE)

The myofibril is filamentous with a diameter of $1 - 2 \mu$m. Each myofibril has alternating light and dark bands, known as periodic cross striations. Due to the tight aggregation of myofibrils, the bright and dark bands of adjacent myofibrils are aligned, so there are also alternating light and dark striations on the muscle fiber (Figure 6 - 1). The bright band, also known as I band, varies in length according to the contraction and relaxation of muscle fiber, with a maximum value of about 2μm; The dark band, also known as the A band, has a constant length of approximately 1.5μm. There is a dark Z line in the center of the I band. The H band, a narrow light band, is in the middle of the dark band, and a dark M line bisects the H band. The segment of myofibril between two adjacent Z lines is called a sarcomere. Each sarcomere is composed of a half of an I band, a whole A band, and a half of another I band (Figure 6 - 4), with a length of $1.5 - 3.5 \mu$m. It is the basic structural unit for the contraction and relaxation of skeletal muscle fiber.

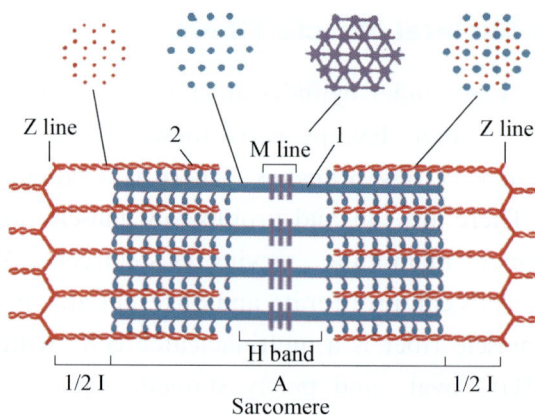

1. Thin myofilament; 2. Thick myofilament
Figure 6 - 4 Drawing showing the ultrastructure of myofibil

1.2 Ultrastructure of Skeletal Muscle Fibers

1.2.1 Myofibrils

Myofibrils are composed of two types of filaments, thick myofilament and thin myofilament, which are arranged in a regular pattern along the long axis of the myofibril. The thick myofilament is about 1.5μm long and 15 nm in diameter, located in the A band of the sarcomere. The thick myofilament is fixed on the M line and free at both ends. The thin myofilament is about 1μm long and 5 nm in diameter. One end of the thin myofilament is fixed on the Z line, while the other ends at the outer edge of the H band. Thin myofilaments are inserted in parallel between the thick myofilaments. Therefore, the I band is only composed of thin myofilaments, and the H band is only composed of thick myofilaments, and the remaining A band is composed of both thick myofilaments and thin myofilaments. On the transverse section, there are 6 thin myofilaments surrounding one thick myofilament, while there are 3 thick myofilaments surrounding one thin myofilament (Figure 6 – 4).

Molecular Configuration of Myofilaments

The thick myofilaments are bundles of myosin (Figure 6 – 5). The myosin molecule is polarized and has a globular head and a rod region, thus looking like a bean sprout. The myosin heads can bind actin, forming transient cross bridges between the thick and thin myofilaments. The head contains an ATPase that facilitates the binding to actin to move the head and produce a power stroke. Myosin heads are oriented at the Z line; the pods are oriented at the M line. Myosin heads bind to actin and draw the thin filament a short distance passed the thick filament.

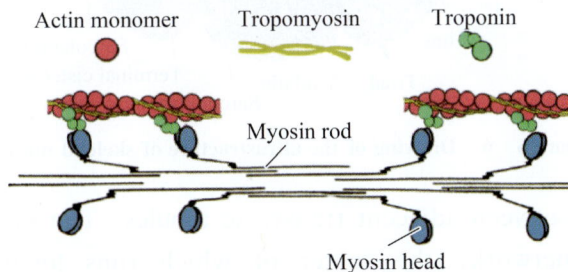

Figure 6 – 5   Drawings showing the molecular structure of thick and thin myofilaments

The thin myofilaments are composed of three molecules: actin, tropomyosin and troponin (Figure 6 – 5). Actin monomers are spherical, and each monomer owns a binding site with myosin. Actin monomers are connected into bead-like chains and intertwine with each other to form double helix chains. Tropomyosin is composed of a short double helix of polypeptide chains, connected head to tail and embedded in shallow grooves on both sides of the actin double helix. During the relaxation of muscle fibers, tropomyosin covers the binding site between actin and myosin. Each tropomyosin binds to a troponin. Troponin is composed of three subunits, TnT, TnI and TnC. TnC immobilizes troponin onto tropomyosin. TnI inhibits the interaction between actin and myosin. TnC binds to Ca^{2+} and causes conformational changes in troponin.

1.2.2   Transverse Tubules

The transverse tubule (also called T tubule) is a small tube formed by the depression of the sarcolemma into the sacroplasm, which is perpendicular to the long axis of the muscle fibers. The transverse tubules of skeletal muscle are located at the junction of the I band and the A band (Figure 6 – 6). The transverse tubules at the same horizontal level anastomose and surround each myofibril. The function of the transverse tubule is to rapidly transmit the excitation of the sarcolemma to the interior of the cell.

1.2.3   Sarcoplasmic Reticulum

The sarcoplasmic reticulum is a specialized smooth endoplasmic reticulum within

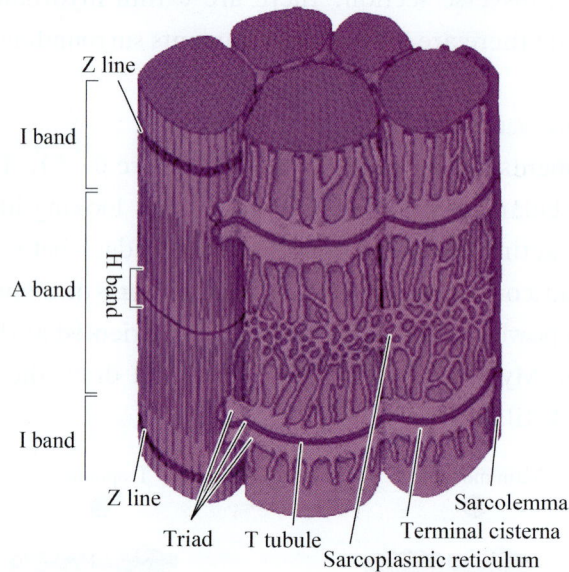

Figure 6 – 6   Drawing of the ultrastructure of skeletal muscle

muscle fibers, located between adjacent transverse tubules. The sarcoplasmic reticula are interwovened into a network, the center of which runs longitudinally around the myofibrils, called longitudinal tubule. The sarcoplasmic reticulum adjacent to both sides of the transverse tubules expands into a circular and flattened sac called terminal cisterna, transmitting the excitation from the sarcolemma to the sarcoplasmic reticulum membrane. A transverse tubule and the two adjacent terminal cisternae form a triad. There are abundant calcium pumps on the membrane of the sarcoplasmic reticulum, which can pump Ca^{2+} from the sarcoplasm into the sarcoplasmic reticulum, thus playing a role in storing and regulating Ca^{2+} concentration in the sarcoplasm. When the membrane of the transverse tubules is excited, it causes a rapid release of Ca^{2+} stored in the sarcoplasmic reticulum into the sarcoplasm, resulting in an increase in Ca^{2+} concentration in the sarcoplasm. After the excitation, the calcium pump on the sarcoplasmic reticulum can pump Ca^{2+} back into the sarcoplasmic reticulum, thereby reducing the concentration of Ca^{2+} in the sarcoplasma.

In addition, the sarcoplasm among the myofibrils also contains mitochondria, glycogens, lipid droplets, oxygen-binding myoglobins, etc.

1.3 Mechanism of Contraction

At present, it is generally believed that the contraction of the skeletal muscle fiber can be explained by the myofilament sliding theory. The following is a brief description of this theory. When nerve impulses are transmitted to the sarcolemma through the motor end plate, the excitation is transmitted through the transverse tubules to the terminal cisterna. Ca^{2+} is then rapidly released into the sarcoplasmic reticulum. As a result, the binding of the TnC subunit of troponin to Ca^{2+} triggers the conformational change of tropomysin, which in turn alters the position of tropomyosin and the binding sites on actin are exposed. The myosin head immediately binds to actin, activating myosin ATPase and hydrolyzing ATP to release energy. Myosin heads undergo bending and rotation, pulling actin towards the M line. The thin myofilaments slide towards the M line between thick myofilaments, causing narrowing of the I and H bands, while the length of the A band remains unchanged. Thus, the sarcomere is shortened and the muscle fiber contracts (Figure 6-7). After the contraction is completed, Ca^{2+} is pumped back into the sarcoplasmic reticulum, decreasing the concentration of Ca^{2+} in the sarcoplasma, so troponin and the tropomyosin recover. The myosin heads are disengaged from actin, and the muscle fiber relaxes (Figure 6-7).

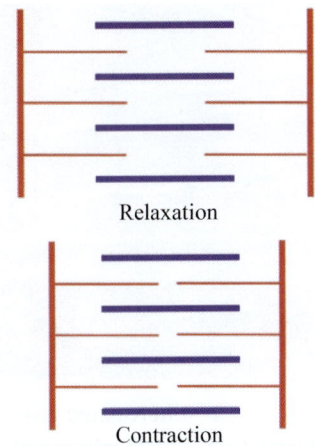

Figure 6-7 Drawings showing the changes in a sarcomere when a skeletal muscle fiber contracts

2 Cardiac Muscle

Cardiac muscles are distributed on the walls of the heart and adjacent large blood vessels. Their contractions are rhythmic, slow and persistent.

2.1 LM Structure of Cardiac Muscle Fibers

The cardiac muscle fiber is short and cylindrical, mostly with branches that connect to each other to form a network (Figure 6-8), with a diameter of $6-15\,\mu$m and a length of $20-100\,\mu$m. The nucleus is oval and located at the center of the cell. Most cardiac muscle fibers have one nucleus, but few have two nuclei (Figure 6-8, Figure 6-9). The connection between cardiac muscle fibers is stained darker, called intercalated disk (Figure 6-8). The sarcoplasm is eosinophilic and relatively abundant, containing a small amount of lipid droplets and lipofuscins. Lipofuscin increases with age. The myocardial fiber also has periodic cross striations, but the striations are not as obvious as those in the skeletal muscle (Figure 6-8). On the cross-section of the cardiac muscle, the area around the nucleus is palely stained, and the myofibrils are radially distributed around the nucleus (Figure 6-9). Of the three kinds of muscle tissue, cardiac muscle is the most richly vascularized. Cardiac muscle lacks satellite cells and shows very little regenerative capacity beyond early childhood. Defects or damage to heart muscle are generally replaced by proliferating fibroblasts and the growth of connective tissue, forming myocardial scars.

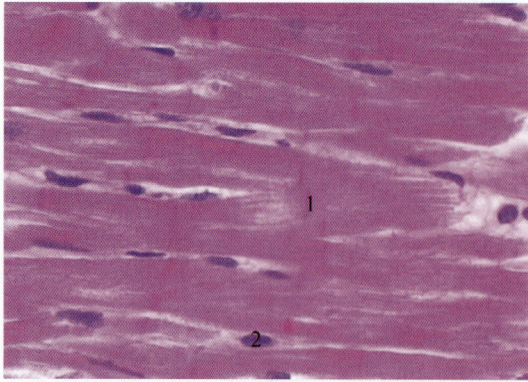

1. Intercalated disk; 2. Nucleus

Figure 6 – 8　Light micrograph of the cardiac muscle in longitudinal section (HE staining)

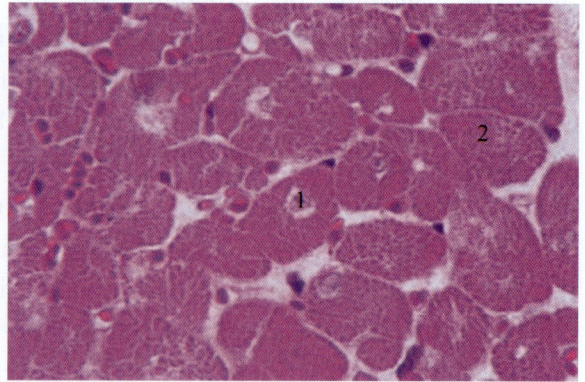

1. nucleus; 2. myofibril

Figure 6 – 9　Light micrograph of the cardiac muscle in cross-section (HE staining)

2.2　Ultrastructure of Cardiac Muscle Fibers

The ultrastructure of cardiac muscle fibers is similar to that of skeletal muscle, containing both thick myofilaments and thin myofilaments, and regularly forming sarcomeres. Compared with skeletal muscle fibers, myocardial fibers have the following characteristics.

2.2.1　Myofibrils

Many vertically arranged myofilaments form the myofibrils of varying thickness and indistinct boundaries (Figure 6 – 9, 6 – 10).

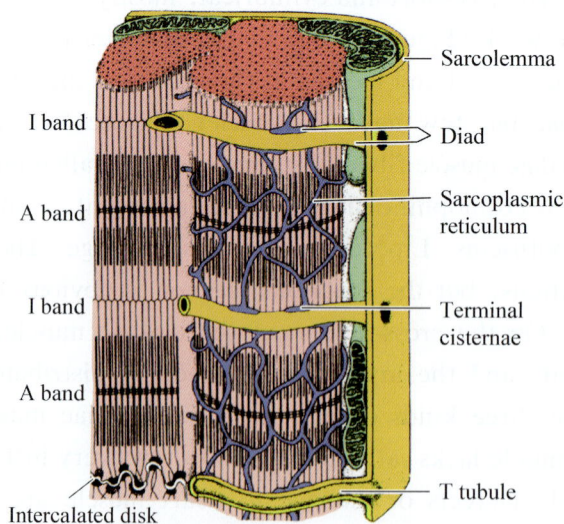

Figure 6 – 10　Drawing showing the ultrastructure of cardiac muscle

2.2.2   Mitochondria

There are numerous mitochondria arranged longitudinally between myofibrils. (Figure 6 – 10).

2.2.3   Transverse Tubules

T tubule diameters are larger than those in skeletal muscle. T tubules sit at Z band levels of sarcomeres (Figure 6 – 10).

2.2.4   Sarcoplasmic Reticulum

The longitudinal tubules are relatively sparse, and the terminal cistern is few and small. A T tubule is usually associated with one expanded terminal cistern of the sarcoplasmic reticulum, forming diad rather than the triad (Figure 6 – 10). The sarcoplasmic reticulum is underdeveloped, resulting in poor Ca^{2+} storage capacity. Before the contraction, Ca^{2+} needs to be taken up from the extracellular space.

2.2.5   Intercalated Disks

The ends of the cardiac muscle fibers in the intercalated disk are shown in a stepped shape. The transverse regions of the intercalated disk sit at the Z-line level (Figure 6 – 10), in which there are desmosomes and zonula adherens, increasing the contact surface between adjacent cells, strengthening the connections between cells, and transmitting tension. In the longitudinal regions, there are gaps connecting the adjacent muscle fibers (Figure 6 – 11), facilitating the exchange of chemical information between cells and the conduction of electrical impulses, which ensures the synchronization of contraction and relaxation of muscle fibers.

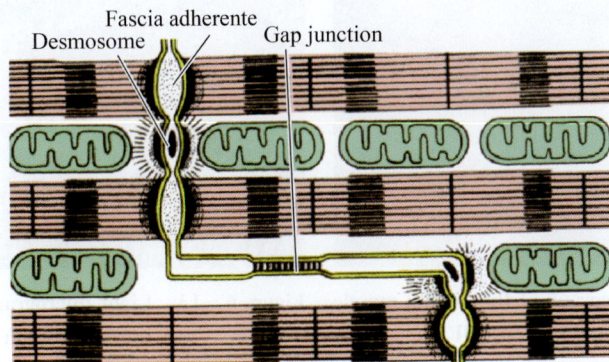

Figure 6 – 11   Drawing showing the ultrastructure of intercalated disk

2.2.6   Atrial Muscle Fibers

The atrial muscle fibers are shorter and slender than ventricle muscle fibers, some of which have endocrine function. Excretory granules are present in the sarcoplasm. The granules contain a peptide hormone, atrial natriuretic factor, which acts on target cells in the kidney to excrete sodium and water.

2.3 Mechanism of Contraction

The mechanism of contraction of the cardiac muscle fiber is essentially the same as that in the skeletal muscle.

3 Smooth Muscle

Smooth muscles are widely distributed in walls of viscera and blood vessels. Their contractions are slow and persistent.

3.1 LM Structure of Smooth Muscle Fibers

A smooth muscle fiber is spindle (Figure 6 - 12), with a diameter of approximately 8 μm and a length of 20 - 500 μm. The muscle fiber has only one nucleus, which is rod-shaped or oval and located in the center of the cell. The eosinophilic sarcoplasm is abundant at both ends of the nucleus (Figure 6 - 12). In the cross-sectioned specimen, smooth muscle fibers appear as oval profiles of varying sizes. The nucleus is only visible in the center of larger profiles (Figure 6 - 13). Except a few that exist alone in viscera, smooth muscle fibers are mostly distributed in bundles or layers, with the narrow part of one cell lying adjacent to the broad part of neighboring cells.

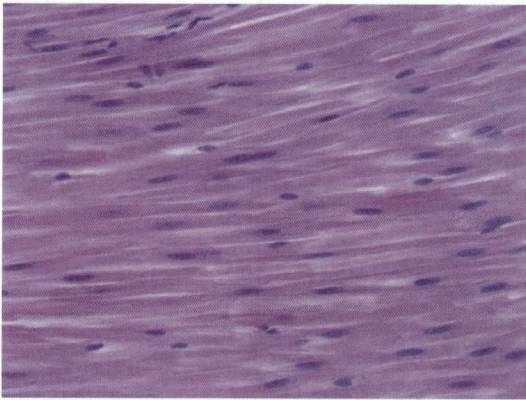

Figure 6 - 12　Light micrograph of the smooth muscle in longitudinal section (HE)

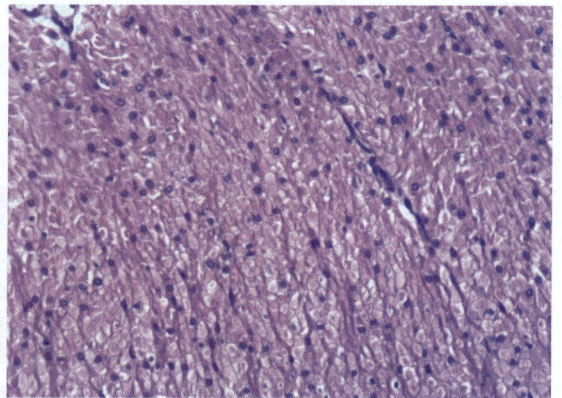

Figure 6 - 13　Light micrograph of the smooth muscle in cross-section (HE)

3.2 Ultrastructure of Smooth Muscle Fibers

Most organelles are located at poles of the cell, including mitochondria, Golgi complexes, rough endoplasmic reticula, glycogen granules, lipid droplets, etc. Smooth muscle fibers have rudimentary sarcoplasmic reticulum, so their contraction also needs the influx of the extracellular Ca^{2+}.

There are no myofibrils in smooth muscle fibers. However, there are many dense bodies, dense patches, intermediate filaments, and myofilaments in the cell. The dense bodies and dense patches, unique to smooth muscle fibers, show higher electron densities. Dense patches are attached to the sarcolemma, and dense bodies are scattered in the cytoplasm. The intermediate filaments are connected to the dense bodies and dense patches, which are composed of desmin and are 10 nm in diameter, forming an intersecting cytoskeletal network.

Sets of myofilaments that are oriented obliquely and longitudinally in the sarcoplasm, in which thick myofilaments consisting of myosin, are 12 - 16 nm in diameter and thin myofilaments mainly composed of actin, are 5 - 7 nm in diameter. There are rows of cross bridges arranged on the surface of the thick myofilaments, and the adjacent rows of cross bridges bend in opposite directions. The thin myofilaments are connected to the dense patches or dense bodies. Some thick myofilaments run parallel to thin myofilaments, forming a contractile unit with the amount ratio of 1 : 12.

Many flask-shaped invaginations, called caveolae, are found in the sarcolemma, which may act as the T tubules in striated muscles. There are gap junctions and zonula adherens between the muscle fibers. The gap junctions can make the muscle fibers function synchronously, while the zonula adherents can provide adhesion and anchors during contraction.

3.3 Mechanism of Contraction

The contraction of smooth muscle fibers is also accomplished through the sliding between thick and thin myofilaments. However, due to the spiral arrangement of the two ends of the contraction unit on the inner side of the muscle membrane, and the opposite bending directions of the adjacent cross bridges, smooth muscle fibers become shorter, thicker, and twisted in a spiral shape during contraction.

(Yue Haiyuan)

第六章 肌 组 织

肌组织主要由具有收缩功能的肌细胞构成。肌细胞之间有少量结缔组织、血管、淋巴管和神经。肌细胞呈细长纤维状,故又称肌纤维,其细胞膜称肌膜,细胞质称肌质,滑面内质网称肌质网。根据结构和功能特点,肌组织可分为骨骼肌、心肌和平滑肌三种类型。骨骼肌和心肌均具有明显的横纹,属于横纹肌。骨骼肌由躯体神经支配,为随意肌;而心肌和平滑肌则由自主神经支配,为不随意肌。

第一节 骨 骼 肌

骨骼肌分布于头、颈、躯干和四肢,大多数通过肌腱附着于骨骼上,但也有少数不附着于骨骼上,如眼和口周围的轮匝肌以及食管壁的骨骼肌。

许多骨骼肌纤维通过结缔组织结合在一起,形成一块骨骼肌。包裹在整块骨骼肌外面的结缔组织膜称肌外膜。肌外膜的结缔组织伸入肌肉内,分隔并包围许多肌纤维,形成大小不一的肌束,肌束周围的结缔组织称肌束膜。分布在每条肌纤维周围的结缔组织称肌内膜(图 6-1)。肌内膜、肌束膜和肌外膜内含有丰富的神经纤维和血管,起支持、连接、营养和协调肌纤维群体活动的作用。骨骼肌通过肌内膜、肌束膜和肌外膜与肌腱、骨外膜或真皮相连。

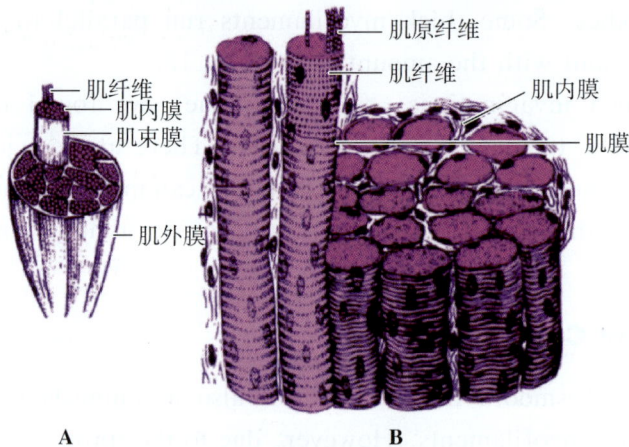

图 6-1 骨骼肌构造示意图
A.一块骨骼肌;B.一个肌束

一、骨骼肌纤维的光镜结构

骨骼肌纤维呈细长的圆柱形(图 6-2),直径为 10~100 μm,长 1~40 mm。除舌肌等少数肌纤维外,骨骼肌纤维极少有分支。肌膜外有基膜贴附。肌膜与基膜之间有一种扁平、有突起的肌卫星细胞,具有干细胞的性质。当肌纤维受损时,肌卫星细胞可增殖分化,参与肌纤维的修复。骨骼肌纤维为多核细胞,一条肌纤维含几十个到几百个细胞核,核呈扁椭圆形,染色较浅,位于肌膜下方。肌质嗜酸性,内含有大量与肌纤维长轴平行排列的肌原纤维,在横切面上呈点状排列(图 6-3)。

肌原纤维呈细丝状,直径 1~2 μm。每条肌原纤维上都有明暗相间排列的条带,即周期性横纹。肌原纤维紧密聚集,相邻肌原纤维的明、暗又排列在同一平面上,所以肌纤维上也呈现明暗交替的横纹。明带又称 I 带,长度依骨骼肌的收缩和舒张状态而异,最长可达约 2 μm;暗带又称 A 带,长度恒定,约 1.5 μm。明带中央有一条深色的 Z 线,暗带中部有浅色窄带称 H 带,H 带中央还有一条深色的 M 线。相邻两条 Z 线之间的一段肌原纤维称肌节。每个肌节由 1/2 I 带＋A 带＋1/2 I 带组成(图 6-4),长度介于 1.5~3.5 μm 之间,它是骨骼肌纤维

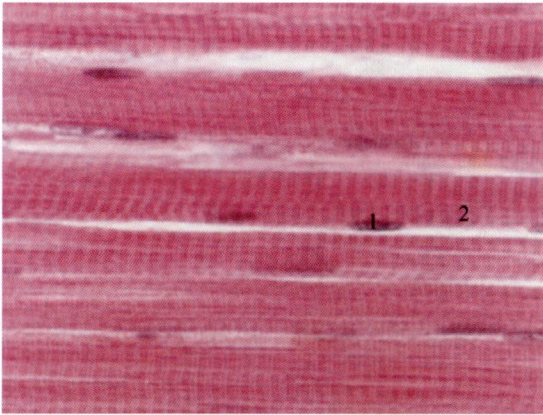

1—细胞核；2—横纹
图6-2 骨骼肌纵切面光镜图(HE染色)

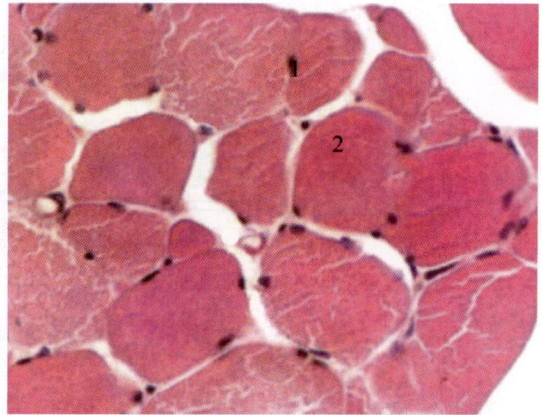

1—细胞核；2—肌原纤维
图6-3 骨骼肌横切面光镜图(HE染色)

收缩和舒张功能的基本结构单位。

二、骨骼肌纤维的超微结构

1. 肌原纤维

由粗、细两种肌丝构成，两种肌丝沿肌原纤维的长轴有规律地排列。粗肌丝长约 $1.5\,\mu m$，直径 $15\,nm$，位于肌节 A 带，中央固定于 M 线上，两端游离。细肌丝长约 $1\,\mu m$，直径 $5\,nm$，一端固定于 Z 线上，另一端游离，插入粗肌丝之间，与之平行，止于 H 带外缘。因此，I 带由细肌丝组成，而 H 带由粗肌丝组成，H 带两侧的 A 带则由粗、细两种肌丝共同组成。在横切面上，每根粗肌丝周围排列有 6 根细肌丝，而每根细肌丝周围则有 3 根粗肌丝排布(图6-4)。

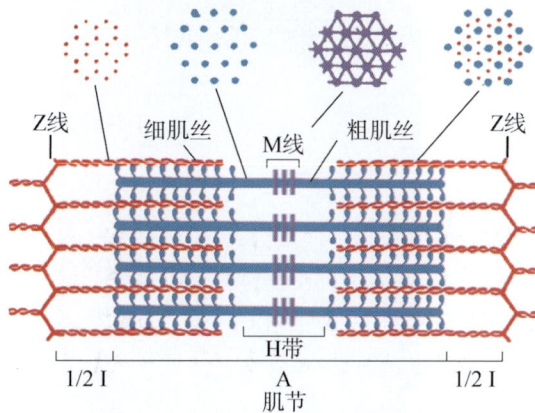

图6-4 骨骼肌肌原纤维结构模式图

粗肌丝主要由肌球蛋白分子组成(图6-5)。肌球蛋白分子平行排列，集合成束，形成一条粗肌丝。肌球蛋白形如豆芽状，分为头部和杆部。M 线两侧的肌球蛋白分子对称排列，杆部朝向 M 线，头部则朝向 Z 线。肌球蛋白头部突出于粗肌丝表面形成横桥，它们具有 ATP 酶活性，并具有与细肌丝的肌动蛋白结合的能力。当横桥与肌动蛋白接触时，头部 ATP 酶被激活，水解 ATP 释放出能量，横桥随即发生屈曲运动，拉动细肌丝向 M 线方向滑动一小段距离。

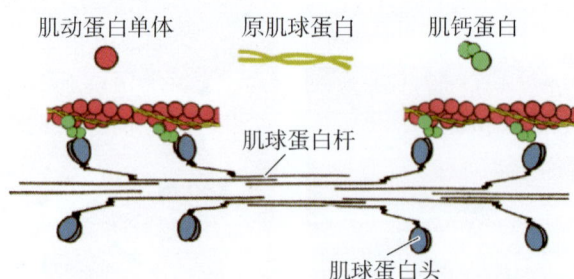

图 6-5　粗肌丝和细肌丝分子结构模式图

　　细肌丝由肌动蛋白、原肌球蛋白和肌钙蛋白 3 种分子组成。肌动蛋白单体呈球形,每个单体上都有一个与肌球蛋白结合的位点。肌动蛋白单体连接成串珠状并相互缠绕形成双股螺旋链。原肌球蛋白由较短的双股螺旋多肽链组成,首尾相连,嵌于肌动蛋白双螺旋两侧的浅沟内。当肌纤维处于舒张期时,原肌球蛋白遮盖肌动蛋白与肌球蛋白结合的位点。每个原肌球蛋白上结合有一个肌钙蛋白。肌钙蛋白由三个亚单位组成:TnT 亚单位将肌钙蛋白固定于原肌球蛋白上;TnI 亚单位抑制肌动蛋白和肌球蛋白的相互作用;TnC 亚单位与 Ca^{2+} 结合而引起肌钙蛋白构象改变。

2. 横小管

　　横小管又称 T 小管,是肌膜向肌质内凹陷形成的小管,它与肌纤维的长轴垂直。骨骼肌的横小管位于 I 带与 A 带的交界处(图 6-6),同一水平的横小管相互吻合,环绕在每条肌原纤维周围。横小管的功能是将肌膜的兴奋迅速传导至肌纤维内部。

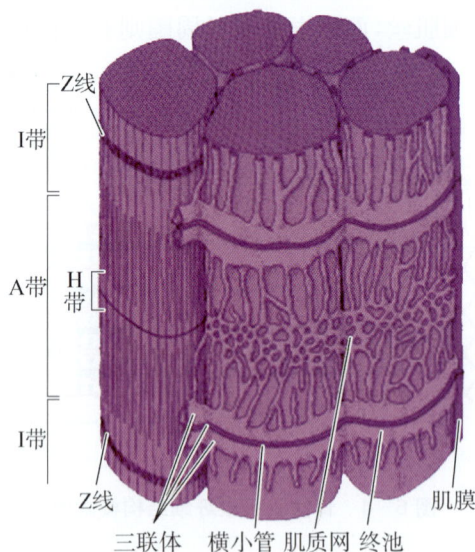

图 6-6　骨骼肌纤维超微结构模式图

3. 肌质网

　　肌质网是肌纤维内特化的滑面内质网,位于相邻的横小管之间,交织成网。其中部纵行环绕在肌原纤维周围,称纵小管。紧靠横小管两侧的肌质网扩大成环行的扁囊,称终池。每条横小管与其两侧的两个终池组成三联体(图 6-6),将兴奋从肌膜传递到肌质网膜。肌质网的膜上含有丰富的钙泵,能够将肌质中的 Ca^{2+} 泵入肌质网,从而起到储存和调节肌质中 Ca^{2+} 浓度的作用。横小管膜的兴奋会引起肌质网内储存的 Ca^{2+} 迅速释放到肌质中,从而使肌质内 Ca^{2+} 浓度升高。兴奋过后,肌质网膜上的钙泵将肌质内的 Ca^{2+} 再泵回到肌质网内,从而降低肌质内 Ca^{2+} 浓度。

此外,肌原纤维之间含有线粒体、糖原、脂滴以及可与氧结合的肌红蛋白等。

三、骨骼肌纤维的收缩原理

目前普遍认为,骨骼肌收缩的机制可以用肌丝滑动理论来解释。其简要过程如下:①神经冲动经运动终板传递至肌膜。②肌膜的兴奋通过横小管传导至终池。③肌质网内的 Ca^2 迅速释放入肌质中。④肌钙蛋白 TnC 亚单位与 Ca^{2+} 结合,引发原肌球蛋白的构象改变,进而使原肌球蛋白的位置发生改变,暴露出肌动蛋白上的结合位点。⑤肌球蛋白的头部迅速与肌动蛋白结合,激活横桥 ATP 酶,ATP 被水解并释放能量。⑥肌球蛋白的头部屈动,将细肌丝向 M 线方向牵引。⑦细肌丝在粗肌丝之间向 M 线滑动,I 带和 H 带缩窄,A 带长度不变,肌节缩短,肌纤维收缩(图 6-7)。⑧收缩结束后,肌质网膜的钙泵将肌质内的 Ca^{2+} 泵回到肌质网内,肌质内 Ca^{2+} 浓度降低,肌钙蛋白恢复原状,原肌球蛋白的构象复原且其位置也回到原位,肌球蛋白头部与肌动蛋白分离,肌纤维舒张(图 6-7)。

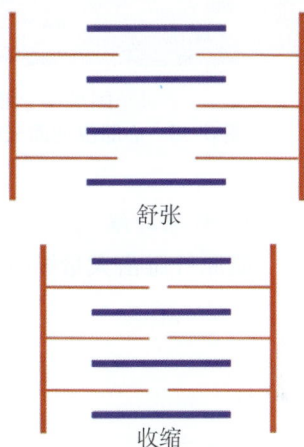

图 6-7 骨骼肌收缩时肌节变化示意图

第二节 心 肌

心肌分布于心壁及与邻近心脏的大血管壁上。心肌的收缩具有节律性,缓慢而持久。

一、心肌纤维的光镜结构

心肌纤维呈短圆柱状,多数具有分支,通过分支互连成网,其直径为 6~15 μm,长 20~100 μm(图 6-8)。心肌纤维的细胞核呈卵圆形,位于细胞的中央,多数细胞只有一个核,少数细胞则为双核。心肌纤维间的连接处染色较深,称闰盘。肌质呈嗜酸性,较丰富,内含少量脂滴和脂褐素。脂褐素的含量随年龄增长而增多。心肌纤维也有周期性横纹,但不如骨骼肌明显。在心肌的横切面上,细胞核周围染色浅,肌原纤维在核周围呈放射状分布(图 6-9)。在三种肌组织中,心肌的血管最为丰富。心肌缺乏肌卫星细胞,幼儿期之后几乎没有再生能力。心肌的缺陷或损伤通常被增殖的成纤维细胞和生长的结缔组织所取代,形成瘢痕。

二、心肌纤维的超微结构

心肌纤维的超微结构与骨骼肌相似,也含有粗肌丝和细肌丝,也有规律地形成肌节。与骨骼肌纤维相比,心肌纤维有以下特点。

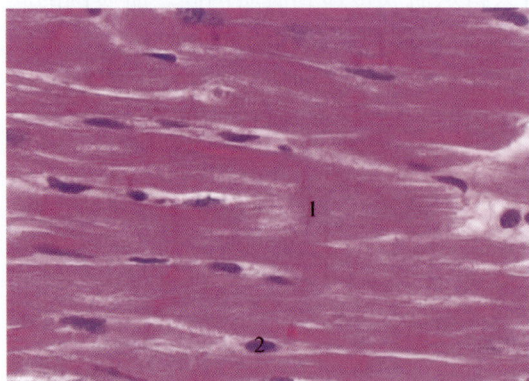

1—闰盘;2—细胞核
图 6-8 心肌纵切面光镜图(HE 染色)

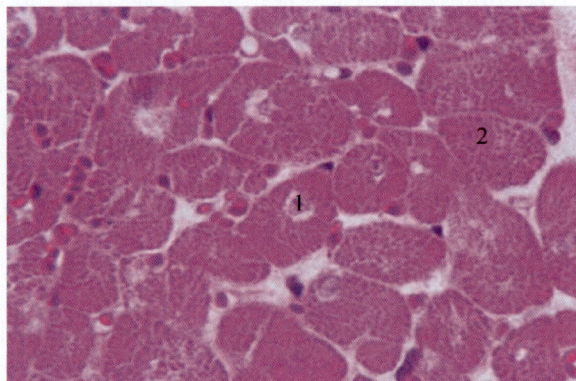

1—细胞核;2—肌原纤维
图 6-9 心肌横切面光镜图(HE 染色)

1. 肌原纤维

肌原纤维由大量纵行排列的肌丝组成,粗细不一,界限并不很明显(图 6-10)。

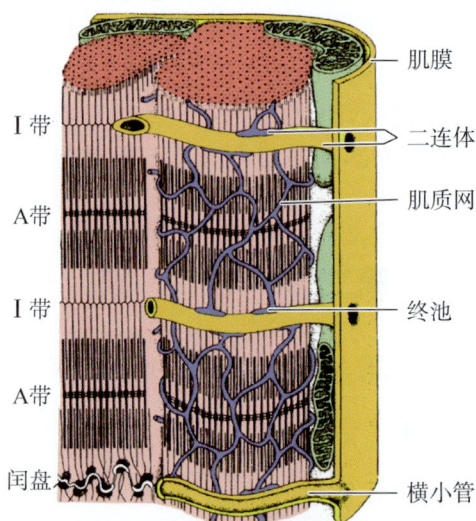

图 6-10 心肌纤维超微结构立体模式图

2. 线粒体

肌原纤维之间含有大量纵行排列的线粒体。

3. 横小管

横小管较粗,位于 Z 线水平。

4. 肌质网

纵小管较稀疏,终池少而且体积小,常见横小管与其一侧的终池紧贴,组成二联体(图 6-10)。因此,心肌纤维储存 Ca^{2+} 能力较弱,收缩前尚需从细胞外摄取 Ca^{2+}。

5. 闰盘

闰盘处的心肌纤维末端呈阶梯状。阶梯的横向部分位于 Z 线水平,有黏合带和桥粒,增强细胞间的连接,传递张力;在阶梯的纵向部分,相邻心肌纤维的侧面存在缝隙连接(图 6-11),便于细胞间化学信息的交流和电冲动的传导,使心肌整体的收缩和舒张同步化。

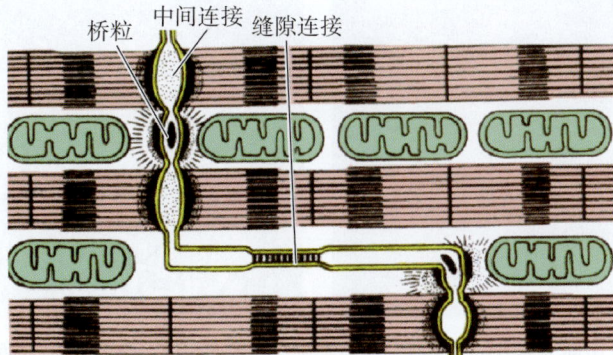

图 6-11 闰盘超微结构模式图

6. 心房肌纤维

心房肌纤维比心室肌纤维短而细。部分心房肌纤维还具有内分泌功能,其肌质中含有分泌颗粒,能够分泌心房钠尿肽,具有排钠、利尿的作用。

三、心肌纤维的收缩原理

心肌的收缩原理与骨骼肌相似。

第三节 平 滑 肌

平滑肌广泛分布于内脏器官和血管壁,其收缩缓慢而持久。

一、平滑肌纤维的光镜结构

平滑肌纤维呈长梭形(图 6-12),直径约 $8\mu m$,长 $20\sim500\mu m$。一条肌纤维仅有一个细胞核,核呈杆状或椭圆形,位于细胞中央,核两端富含嗜酸性肌质(图 6-12)。在平滑肌横切面上,平滑肌纤维呈大小不等的卵圆形断面,只有较大的断面中央可见细胞核(图 6-13)。在内脏器官中,平滑肌纤维除了少数可以单独存在外,绝大部分以束状或层状分布,每个肌纤维的粗部与邻近肌纤维的细部相嵌合。

二、平滑肌纤维的超微结构

细胞核两端的肌质含有线粒体、高尔基复合体、粗面内质网、游离核糖体、糖原和脂滴等。由于肌质网不发达,细胞在收缩时也需要从细胞外摄取 Ca^{2+}。

细胞内没有肌原纤维,但可见较多的密斑和密体,以及中间丝和肌丝。密斑和密体都是电子致密小体,前者位于肌膜下,后者位于肌质内。中间丝由结蛋白组成,直径为 10 nm,连接于密斑与密体之间,形成细胞骨架。

肌质内也含有粗、细两种肌丝。细肌丝主要由肌动蛋白组成,直径为 $5\sim7$ nm,一端固定于密斑或密体上,另一端是游离的。粗肌丝由肌球蛋白组成,直径为 $12\sim16$ nm,均匀地分布

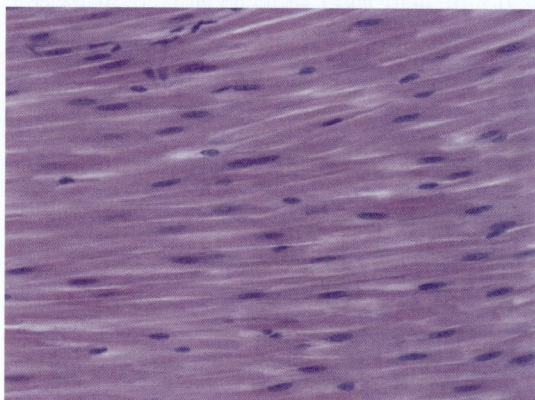

图 6-12　平滑肌纵切面光镜图(HE 染色)

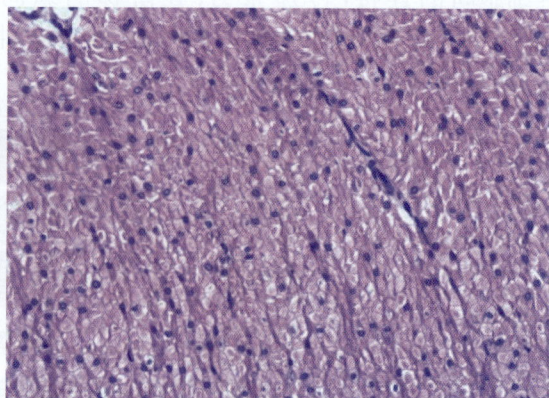

图 6-13　平滑肌横切面光镜图(HE 染色)

在细肌丝之间。粗肌丝表面有成行排列的横桥,相邻两行横桥屈动方向相反。粗、细肌丝的数量比约为 1∶12。若干条粗肌丝和细肌丝聚集形成收缩单位。

肌膜向肌质内凹陷,形成了数量众多的小凹,这些小凹可能相当于横纹肌的横小管。相邻肌纤维之间存在大量的缝隙连接,便于细胞间的信息传递,使相邻的肌纤维能够同步收缩;也存在黏合带,在收缩过程中起黏附和锚定的作用。

三、平滑肌纤维的收缩原理

平滑肌纤维的收缩也是通过粗肌丝和细肌丝之间的滑动实现的。然而,由于收缩单位的两端在肌膜内侧呈螺旋形排布,且相邻两行横桥屈动方向相反,故平滑肌纤维在收缩时会变短、增粗,并呈现出螺旋形的扭曲。

(岳海源)

Chapter 7

Nervous Tissue

Nervous tissue is the principal element of the nervous system, consisting of two major cell types: nerve cells and glial cells. Nerve cells, also known as neurons, have the function of receiving stimuli, integrating information, and conducting impulses. Neurons connect with each other through special cellular connections, analyzing and storing the received information, and may transmit the information to effector cells such as muscle fibers and glandular cells to produce an effect. In addition, neurons are also the basis for the regulation of consciousness, memory, thinking, and behavior. Some neurons having endocrine function are called neuroendocrine cells. Glial cells are more abundant, which play a role in support, protection, nutrition, defense, and insulation for neurons, as well as participating in the metabolism of neurotransmitters and active compounds.

1   Neurons

Neurons are usually morphologically diverse, consisting of two parts: the cell body (also called soma) and the processes. Neurons have two types of processes: dendrites and axons (Figure 7 - 1).

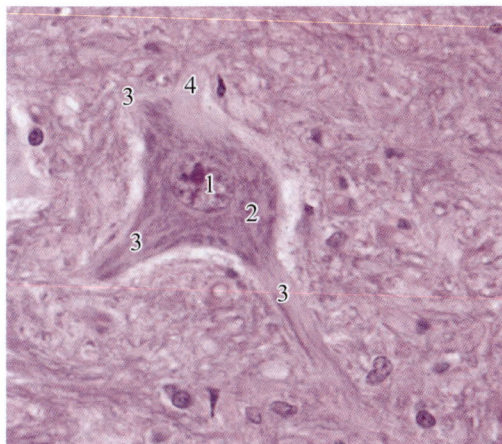

1. Nucleus; 2. Nissl body; 3. Dendrite; 4. Axon

Figure 7 - 1　Light micrograph of a neuron in spinal cord ventral horn (HE)

1.1 Structure of Neurons

1.1.1 Cell Body

The cell bodies are highly variable in size, with diameters of 4 – 150 μm, appearing round, pyramidal, pear-shaped, etc. They are distributed in the gray matter of the central nervous system, such as the cerebral cortex, cerebellar cortex, the grey matter of brainstem, and spinal cord, as well as in the ganglia of the peripheral nervous system, such as the cerebral ganglia, spinal ganglia, and autonomic ganglia. The cell body is composed of the cell membrane, cytoplasm and nucleus, and is the metabolic and nutritional center of the entire neuron.

1.1.1.1 Cell Membrane

The cell membrane of a neuron is excitable and can receive stimuli, process information, and generate and transmit nerve impulses. Like that of other cells, the neuronal membrane also consists of a double layer of phospholipids and embedded proteins. The properties of the membrane of neurons depend on the embedded proteins. Some proteins are receptors that interact with neurotransmitters, and some proteins are ionic channels that are responsible for the flow of specific ions through the membrane. When a neuron is in a resting condition, the concentrations of ions inside and outside the membrane are different, forming a certain potential difference. Various stimuli from the internal and external environment can cause a rapid reversible change of the potential difference, thereby forming the nerve impulse.

1.1.1.2 Nucleus

The neuronal nucleus is large, round, and located in the center of the neuron. The nuclear envelope is prominent. It is palely stained because heterochromatin is finely dispersed. The nucleolus is big and round.

1.1.1.3 Cytoplasm

The cytoplasm of the cell body is also called perikaryon. Under a light microscope, its characteristic structures are Nissl bodies and neurofibrils.

Under a light microscope, Nissl bodies are basophilic spot-liked or granule-liked structures, present throughout the cytoplasm of the cell body and dendrites, but absent from the axons (Figure 7 – 1). The form, size, and number of the Nissl bodies vary according to neuronal type and functional state. For instance, Nissl bodies are coarser and more abundant in motor neurons of the spinal cord, whereas they are very fine and uniformly distributed in neurons of the dorsal root ganglion. Under an electron microscope, Nissl bodies are composed of a large number of rough endoplasmic reticula and free ribosomes, indicating that neurons have the function of synthesizing proteins. The synthesized proteins include structural proteins needed for organelle renewal, enzymes needed to produce neurotransmitters and peptide neuromodulators. The neurotransmitter refers to a special chemical compound released by nerve endings that act on receptors on the membranes of innervated neurons or effector cells, thereby completing information transmission. The neuromodulator refers to another type of chemical compound produced by neurons, which can regulate the efficiency of information transmission, either enhance or weaken the effects of neurotransmitters.

Under a light microscope, the neurofibrils are shown as brown-black filaments that are interwoven into a network in the silver-impregnation stained sections. Neurofibrils are distributed in the cell body and extend into dendrites and axons (Figure 7 – 2). Under an electron microscope, the neurofibril is composed of neurofilaments and microtubules. Neurofibrils help maintain cell shape and structural stability and play a role in substance transport.

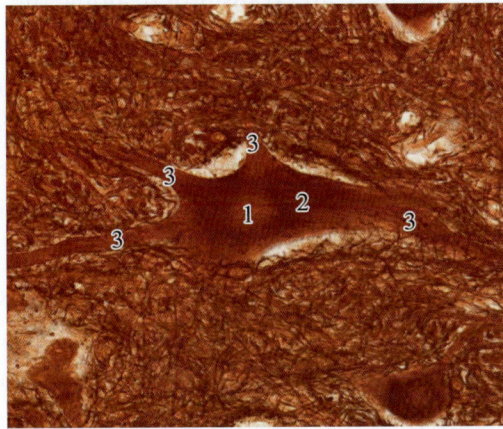

1. Nucleus; 2. Neurofibril; 3. Process
Figure 7 – 2   Light micrograph of a neuron in spinal cord ventral horn (silver-impregnation staining)

Neuronal cytoplasm also contains mitochondria, Golgi complexes, smooth endoplasmic reticula, lysosomes, lipofuscin, etc. In addition, endocrine neurons also contain secretory granules.

1.1.2   Dendrites

Each neuron has one or more dendrites, which branch repeatedly and gradually taper into a dendritic shape (Figure 7 – 1). Similar to the cell body, the dendrites also contain Nissl bodies and neurofibrils. There are many small and short processes on the surface of dendritic branches, called dendritic spines. The dendrite is specialized in receiving stimuli and conducting nerve impulses to the cell body. Dendritic spines and dendritic branches considerably increase the receptive area of the neuron.

1.1.3   Axon

One neuron has only one axon (Figure 7 – 1). The axon is a fine cylindrical process that varies in length (from several mm to more than 100 cm) and diameter according to the type of neuron. Axons originate from a pyramid-shaped cell body region called axon hillock. Under a light microscope, there is no Nissl body in this area, so the staining is pale. Axons are generally thinner and have a more uniform diameter than dendrites, with collaterals branching out at right angles. Axon terminals often have multiple branches, forming axon terminals. The plasma membrane of an axon is often called axolemma and its cytoplasms are known as axoplasm. Axoplasm contains mitochondria, microfilaments, neurofilaments, and smooth endoplasmic reticulua, but essentially no rough endoplasmic reticula or Golgi complexes.

The axons are frequently surrounded by myelin sheaths. The portion of axon that extends from the axon hillock to the beginning of the myelin sheath is termed initial segment, a site of forming nerve impulses. Under electron microscopy, it can be seen that the axolemma here is relatively thick, and there is a dense layer with high electron density under the membrane. Nerve impulses are transmitted along the axolemma. The axon is specialized in generating and conducting nerve impulses.

The transport of substances within axons is called axonal transport. The process of transporting from the cell body to the axon terminal is called anterograde axonal transport, while the opposite is called retrograde axonal transport. The network composed of microfilaments, microtubules, and neurofilaments synthesized inside the cell slowly moves towards the axon terminals ($1-4$ mm/d), indicating slow axonal transport. The proteins required for axonal renewal, synaptic vesicles, and enzymes required for synthesizing neurotransmitters are transported from the cell body to the axon terminals at a speed of $100-400$ mm/d, known as rapid axonal transport. The metabolic products of axon terminals or substances (e. g., proteins, small molecules, or neurotrophic factors, etc.) taken up by the axon terminals are transported to the cell body at a speed of half of that in rapid retrograde transport, known as rapid retrograde axonal transport. Certain viruses and toxins, such as rabies virus, poliovirus, and tetanus toxin, can also rapidly invade neuronal cell bodies through retrograde axonal transport. Microtubules play an important role in axonal transport.

1.2 Classification of Neurons

There are multiple classification methods for neurons. Neurons can be classified based on the number of their cytoplasmic processes, functions, length of the axons, and chemical properties of the neurotransmitters or neuromodulators that they release.

Based on the number of processes, most neurons can be classified into 3 categories (Figure 7 - 3). Pseudounipolar neurons (e. g., dorsal root ganglion neuron) emit a process from the cell body, which is divided into two branches not far from the cell body in the shape of T. One branch is distributed to peripheral tissues and organs, called peripheral process, and the other branch enters the central nervous system, called central process. The central process sends out nerve impulses and has the function of axons; the peripheral process is stimulated and has the function of dendrites. Bipolar neurons have two processes, an axon and a dendrite, found in the retina, olfactory mucosa, and the cochlear and vestibular ganglia. Multipolar neurons are the most common and have one axon and two or more dendrites. They are present in the brain, spinal cord and automatic ganglia.

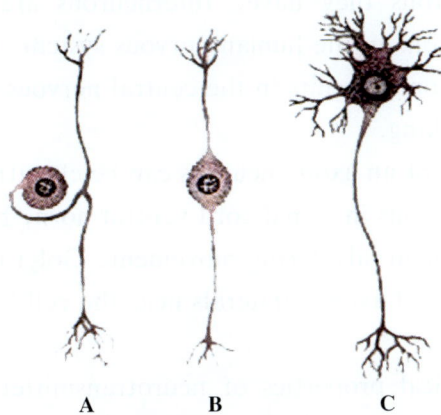

Figure 7 – 3   Classification of neurons based on the process number
A. Pseudounipolar neuron; B. Bipolar neuron; C. Multipolar neuron

According to the functional roles, neurons can be classified into 3 types (Figure 7 – 4). Sensory neurons, also known as afferent neurons, receive the chemical or physical stimulation of the internal and external environment and transmit the information to the center. Sensory neurons are generally bipolar neurons. The cell bodies are located within the spinal ganglia of the brain, and its peripheral protrusions are distributed in the skin, muscles, and viscera. Motor neurons, also known as efferent neurons, send impulses to effector organs such as muscle fibers and glands. Motor neurons are generally multipolar neurons. The cell bodies are mainly located in the gray matter and autonomic ganglia. Interneurons

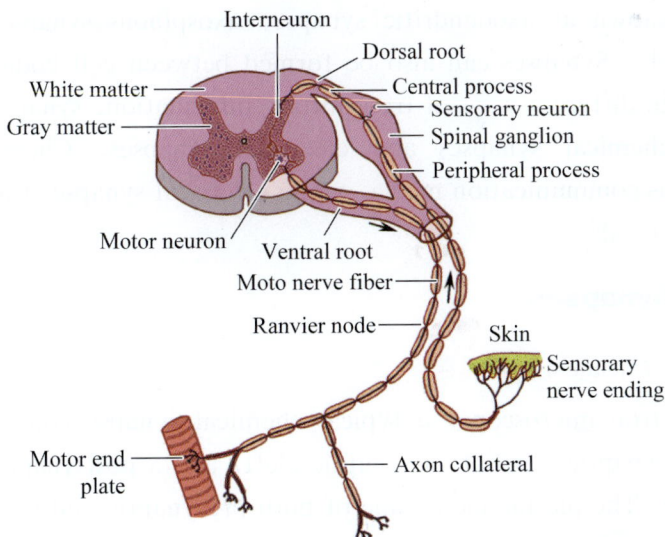

Figure 7 – 4   Drawing of the spinal cord and spinal nerve

establish relationships among other neurons, forming complex functional networks or circuits. Interneurons can modify and integrate nerve impulses. The more animals evolve, the more intermediate neurons they have. Interneurons are generally multipolar and account for 99% of the neurons in the human nervous system. In addition, the formation of the complex neural functional circuits in the central nervous system may be the basis of learning, memory, and thinking.

According to the length of an axon, neurons can be classified into 2 types. Golgi type Ⅰ neurons, e.g., motor neurons in spinal cord ventral horn, have large cell bodies, long axons, and send out axon collaterals during movement. Golgi type Ⅱ neurons have small cell bodies with short axons and axon collaterals near the cell body, e.g., interneurons in the cerebral cortex.

According to the chemical properties of neurotransmitters or neuromodulators that they release, neurons can be classified into various types. Cholinergic neurons release acetylcholine. Aminergic neurons release dopamine, serotonin, etc. Amino acidergic neurons release amino acids, such as glutamate, glycine, γ-aminobutyric acid (GABA), etc. Peptidergic neurons release neuropeptides such as substance P, neurotensin, enkephalin, etc. NOergic neurons release NO. COergic neurons release CO.

2　Synapse

Synapse is the specialized cellular junction between two neurons, or a neuron and an effector cell, for transmitting information. The most common synapses are those formed by an axon terminal of a neuron and the dendrite, dendrite spine, or the cell body of another neuron, known as axodendritic synapse, axospinous synapse, and axosomatic synapse, respectively. Synapses can also be formed between cell bodies, dendrites, and axons. According to different ways of transmitting information, synapses are divided into two categories: chemical synapses and electrical synapses. Chemical synapses use neurotransmitters as communication media, while electrical synapses transmit information through electrical signals.

2.1　Chemical Synapses

2.1.1　Structure of Chemical Synapses

Under an electron microscope, a typical chemical synapse consists of three major components: a presynaptic element, a synaptic cleft, and a postsynaptic element (Figure 7-5, Figure 7-6). The plasma membrane of both presynaptic and postsynaptic elements at the synaptic contact regions are called presynaptic and postsynaptic membrane, respectively. The synaptic cleft is the extracellular space between the presynaptic and postsynaptic membranes and is about 15-30 nm wide.

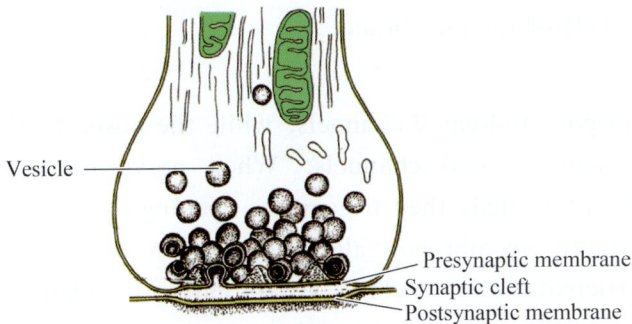

Figure 7 - 5　Drawing of the ultrastructure of synapse

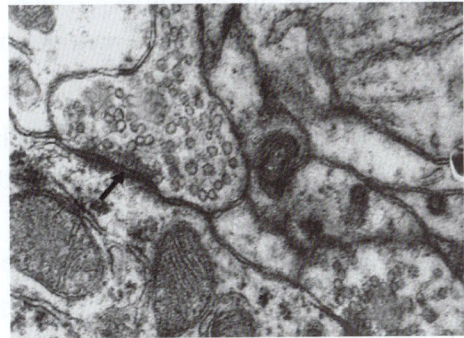

Figure 7 - 6　Electron micrograph of synapse

The presynaptic element is usually formed by the enlargement of an axon terminal. The terminal is shown as a dark brown knob attached to the cell body or dendrites of another neuron by silver-impregnation staining, which is called synaptic knob (also called synaptic bouton) (Figure 7 - 7). Presynaptic elements always contain many synaptic vesicles, mitochondria, microtubules, and neurofilaments. Synaptic vesicles vary in size and shape and contain neurotransmitters or neuromodulators. Most of the synaptic vesicles containing acetylcholine are small round clear vesicles; the ones containing amino acid transmitters are flat clear vesicles; the ones containing monoamine transmitters are small granular vesicles; and those containing neuropeptides are mostly large granular vesicles. On the outside of the synaptic vesicles, there is a protein known as synapsin that links the vesicles to the cytoskeleton. The cytoplasmic surface of the presynaptic membrane also has cone-shaped dense protrusions with high electron density, between which synaptic vesicles are accommodated.

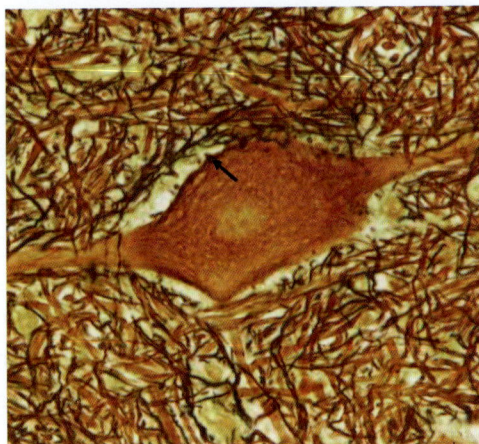

Figure 7 - 7　Electron micrograph of the synaptic knob (silver-impregnation staining)

The postsynaptic element is mainly the postsynaptic membrane, which contains receptors for specific neurotransmitters or neuromodulators. Both of the presynaptic and postsynaptic membranes appear thicker and denser than the adjacent membranes because of some dense materials on the cytoplasmic side of the membrane.

2.1.2 Chemical Synapse Transmission

The presynaptic membrane is rich in potential-gated channels, while the postsynaptic membrane is rich in receptors and chemical-gated channels. When nerve impulses propagate along the axolemma to the axon terminal, they trigger the opening of voltage-gated calcium channels on the presynaptic membrane, allowing Ca^{2+} to enter the presynaptic terminal. With the participation of ATP, synaptophysin undergoes phosphorylation that reduces its affinity with vesicles, causing them to detach from the cytoskeleton and attach to the presynaptic membrane. Through exocytosis, neurotransmitters inside the vesicles are released into the synaptic cleft. Some neurotransmitters bind to corresponding receptors on the postsynaptic membrane, causing the receptor coupled chemical-gated channels to open, allowing corresponding ions to enter and exit, changing the distribution of ions inside and outside the postsynaptic membrane, producing excitatory or inhibitory changes, and thereby affecting the activity of postsynaptic neurons or effector cells. The chemical synapse transmission is unidirectional.

A neuron can transmit information to many other neurons or effector cells through synapses, e.g., a motor neuron that can simultaneously control thousands of skeletal muscles. And a neuron can also receive information from many other neurons through synapses, e.g., hundreds of thousands of synapses on the dendrites of Purkinje cells in the cerebellum. The synaptic information is either excitatory or inhibitory. If the sum of excitatory information exceeds the sum of inhibitory information and is sufficient to stimulate the axon initiation segment of the neuron to produce nerve impulses, the neuron exhibits excitation; otherwise, the neuron exhibits inhibition.

2.2 Electrical Synapses

Electrical synapses are gap junctions that do not require neurotransmitters to transmit nerve impulses, and the transmission is generally bidirectional.

3 Glial Cells

Glial cells are widely distributed in the central and peripheral nervous systems. They are 10 - 50 times more abundant than neurons. They also have processes, but the processes are not defined as dendrites and axons. Except for ependymal cells, routine HE staining can only display their nuclei, while silver-impregnation staining or immunohistochemistry can show their panoramas.

3.1 Glial Cells in Central Nervous System

There are four types of glial cells in the central nervous system: astrocytes, oligodendrocytes, microglial cells, and ependymal cells (Figure 7 - 8).

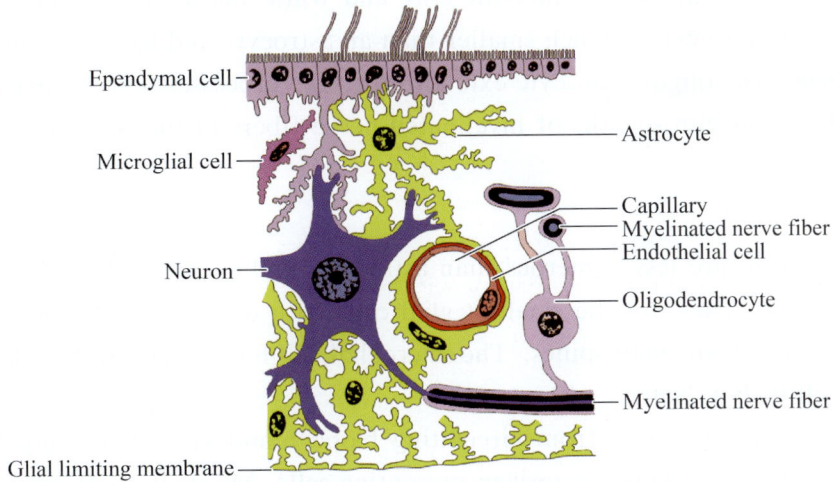

Figure 7 - 8   Drawing of the glial cells in central nervous system

3.1.1   Astrocytes

Astrocytes are the largest and most numerous glial cells in the central nervous system. Astrocytes are star-shaped cells with multiple radiating processes. The nucleus of the astrocyte is large, round or oval, and palely stained. The cytoplasm is replete with glial filaments, which are tightly packed intermediate filaments made of glial fibrillary acidic protein. Glial filaments are the main constituent of the cytoskeleton.

There are two forms of astrocytes: fibrous astrocytes and protoplasmic astrocytes. Fibrous astrocytes have long, thin processes with fewer branches and are mainly located in the white matter of the brain and spinal cord. The cytoplasm contains more glial filaments. Protoplasmic astrocytes have short, thick processes with more branches and are distributed predominantly in the gray matter of the brain and spinal cord. The cytoplasm contains relativity fewer glial filaments.

The processes of the astrocytes stretch and fill between the cell bodies and processes of neurons. They often form terminal expansions, known as end-feet (also called foot plates). Some end-feet, known as perivascular end-feet, attach to the wall of blood capillaries and completely enclose all capillaries, forming the neuroglia membrane of the blood-brain barrier (Figure 7 - 8). Others are aligned along the internal surface of the pia mater to form a membrane-like glia limitans, which separates the connective tissue of the pia mater from neurons.

Astrocytes can secrete neurotrophic factors and various growth factors, maintain the survival and functional activity of neurons, and have an important impact on the plasticity changes of neurons after trauma. The damaged parts of the central nervous system are often repaired by glial scar formation caused by the proliferation of astrocytes.

3.1.2　Oligodendrocytes

Oligodendrocytes are found in both gray and white matter of the brain and spinal cord. The oligodendrocyte is much smaller than an astrocyte and has fewer processes with an oval nucleus. The oligodendrocyte extends sheet-like processes that wrap around several axons, producing myelin sheaths of myelinated nerve fibers in the central nervous system (Figure 7 - 8).

3.1.3　Microglial Cells

Microglial cells are less numerous than astrocytes and evenly distributed in both gray and white matter. They are the smallest glial cells with elongated cell bodies and short, irregular processes with small spines. The microglial cell has a small oval nucleus along the axis of the cell body (Figure 7 - 8).

Microglial cells originate from circulating blood monocytes, belonging to the same family as macrophages and other antigen-presenting cells. Microglial cells protect the brain from invading microorganisms. When activated by damage or invaders, microglial cells act as phagocytes and remove unwanted cellular debris caused by the central nervous system lesions.

3.1.4　Ependymal Cells

Ependymal cells are epithelial-like cells that form a single layer of ependyma lining the ventricles of the brain and central canal of the spinal cord. They are columnar or cuboidal cells with a large number of apical microvilli (Figure 7 - 8). In some locations, the apical ends of ependymal cells have cilia, which beat to facilitate the movement of cerebrospinal fluid. The basal ends of ependymal cells are elongated, extending processes that branch and penetrate into the surrounding parenchyma of the brain and spinal cord. Ependymal cells mainly support and protect neurons and are responsible for the production of cerebrospinal fluid.

3.2　Glial Cells in Peripheral Nervous System

There are two types of glial cells in the peripheral nervous system: Schwann cells and satellite cells.

3.2.1　Schwann Cells

Schwann cells are the main protective and insulating cells of the peripheral nervous system. They exist in both of the myelinated and unmyelinated nerve fibers of the peripheral nervous system. Like oligodendrocytes, Schwann cells produce myelin sheaths by wrapping around axons, however, one Schwann cell forms myelin around one axon segment. The outer surface of the Schwann cell is covered by a basement membrane. Schwann cells can also secrete neurotrophins, promoting the survival of damaged neurons and the regeneration of their axons.

3.2.2 Satellite Cells

Satellite cells are also known as capsular cells. They are a layer of flat or cuboidal cells surrounding the cell bodies of neurons in the ganglia. The nucleus is flat or round and deeply stained. There is a basement membrane on the outer surface of the cell. Satellite cells have nutritional and protective effects on ganglion neurons.

4   Nerve Fibers and Nerves

4.1 Nerve Fibers

Nerve fibers are made up of axons and glial cells surrounding them. According to whether the glial cells form myelin sheath, they are divided into two types: myelinated nerve fibers and unmyelinated nerve fibers.

4.1.1 Myelinated Nerve Fibers

In the peripheral nervous system, myelinated nerve fibers are composed of axons of neurons and the myelin sheath of Schwann cells. The adjacent Schwann cells do not connect, causing narrow parts of the nerve fibers, whereas the axolemma is exposed without myelin sheaths; the exposed region of the nerve fiber is called Ranvier node (figure 7 – 9). The nerve fiber between the adjacent Ranvier nodes is called internode. The peripheral part of an internode is a Schwann cell. On the cross-section of myelinated nerve fibers, Schwann cells can be divided into three layers. The middle layer is the myelin sheaths formed by concentric winding of multi-layer cell membranes (up to 50 layers). With the myelin sheaths as the boundary, the cytoplasm is divided into medial and lateral cytoplasm. The medial cytoplasm is tightly attached to the axial membrane, extremely thin, and difficult to distinguish under a light microscope; the lateral cytoplasm is slightly thick, with the nucleus located within it, forming a crescent shape. Under electron microscopy, the myelin sheath appears as a layered structure with alternating light and dark layers.

The chemical composition of myelin sheath is mainly lipoproteins, known as myelin. In the preparations of HE staining, lipids in the myelin are dissolved, leaving only a small amount of residual protein in a pink mesh-like structure. If fixed and stained with osmium acid, myelin can be preserved, making the myelin sheath appear black. An uncolored funnel-shaped fissure can be seen on the longitudinal section of the myelin sheath, called Schmidt-Lanterman incisures (Figure 7 – 9), which are channels between the median and lateral cytoplasm of Schwann cells. Under the electron microscope, the myelin sheath is seen as a series of concentrically arranged light and dark lamellae. The outer surface of the myelin sheath is covered by a basement membrane.

In the process of the formation of myelinated nerve fibers, the surface of Schwann cells is sunken to form a longitudinal groove, the axons are trapped in the longitudinal

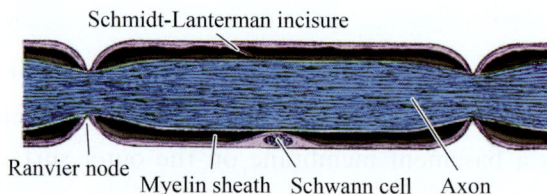

Schmidt-Lanterman incisure

Ranvier node   Myelin sheath   Schwann cell   Axon

Figure 7 - 9   Drawing of the myelinated axon in peripheral nervous system

groove, and the cell membranes on both sides of the groove are attached to each other to form mesaxons. The mesaxon stretches and rotates around the axon, forming many concentric circles of the spiral lamellar membrane, the myelin sheath (Figure 7 - 10). The myelin sheath is composed of the membrane of Schwann cells, and the cytoplasm is squeezed to the median and lateral sides and both ends.

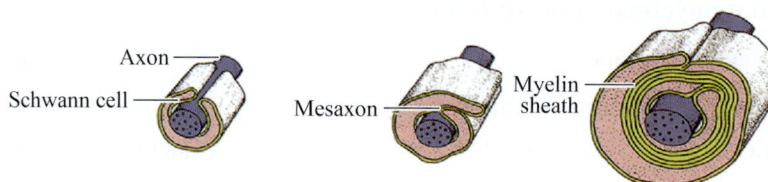

Axon

Schwann cell

Mesaxon

Myelin sheath

Figure 7 - 10   Drawings showing the formation of myelin sheath in the peripheral nervous system

In the central nervous system, myelinated nerve fibers are composed of axons and the myelin sheath of processes of oligodendrocytes (Figure 7 - 11). An oligodendrocyte has multiple processes, and the end of each process is a flat membrane, each wrapped around an axon to form a myelin sheath. The cell bodies of oligodendrocytes are located between nerve fibers. In addition, the myelin sheath formed by adjacent oligodendrocytes is not arranged as close as Schwann cells, so the Ranvier node is wider. The outer surface of the myelin sheath is not covered by a basal lamina. There are no Schmidt-Lanterman clefts in the myelin sheath.

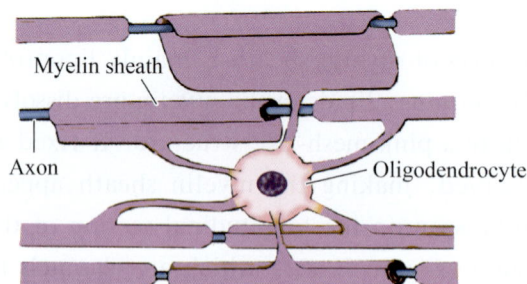

Myelin sheath

Axon

Oligodendrocyte

Figure 7 - 11   Drawing of myelinated nerve fibers in the central nervous system

The nerve impulses of myelinated nerve fibers only occur at the axon membrane of the Ranvier node, so the nerve impulse transmission is saltatory conduction with a faster speed. This is because the myelin sheath of myelinated nerve fibers contains a large amount of lipids and is hydrophobic, providing insulation between the tissue fluid and the axon. In addition, the resistance of the myelin sheath is higher than that of the axon membrane, while its capacitance is very low. The current can only excite the axon membrane (directly contacting with tissue fluid) at the node. Therefore, the nerve impulse generated by the initial segment of the axon must be transmitted through the axon membrane, jumping from one Ranvier node to the next. In general, the thicker the myelin sheath, the greater the internodal distance and the higher the conduction velocity.

4.1.2 Unmyelinated Nerve Fibers

In the peripheral system, unmyelinated axons with small diameters are enveloped within simple clefts of the Schwann cells. Under an electron microscope, there are different numbers and depths of longitudinal grooves on the surface of Schwann cells, and the axons are located in the grooves of Schwann cells. Schwann cells are arranged continuously along the axons, but there are no myelin sheaths and no Ranvier nodes. A Schwann cell can wrap many axons (Figure 7 – 12). There is also a basement membrane outside the Schwann cells. In the central nervous system, many short axons are not myelinated at all and run free among myelinated nerve fibers and glial cells.

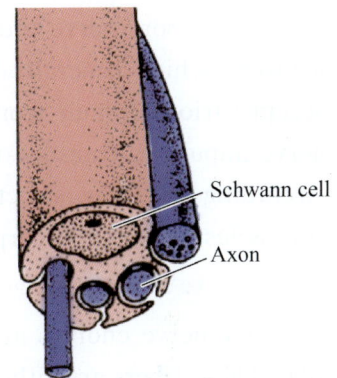

Figure 7 – 12 Drawing of unmyelinated axons in peripheral nervous system

Without myelin sheaths or Ranvier nodes, the nerve impulses unmyelinated fibers are conducted along the entire length of the axon, thus traveling slowly.

4.2 Nerves

In the peripheral nervous system, nerve fibers gather to form nerve fiber fascicles, and several nerve fiber fascicles form nerves. Big nerves (e. g., the sciatic nerve) are composed of dozens of nerve fascicles, while many small nerves within tissues are composed of a single nerve fiber fascicle. Most nerves contain motor nerve fibers, sensory nerve fibers, and autonomic nerve fibers. Except for very thin nerves that only contain unmyelinated fibers, nerves usually contain myelinated nerve fibers. Due to the presence of myelin in myelinated nerve fibers, nerves appear white.

Nerves are rich in connective tissue, which contains blood vessels and lymphatic vessels. The dense connective tissue surrounding the surface of a nerve is called the epineurium. The connective tissue of the epineurium extends between nerve fiber fascicles. Several layers of flat epithelioid cells and connective tissue surrounding the nerve fiber fascicle form the perineurium. There are tight connections between the flat cells, which act as a barrier for large molecules entering nerve fiber fascicles. There is only a thin layer of connective tissue around each nerve fiber, called endometrium.

5 Nerve Endings

The nerve endings are the terminal parts of peripheral nerve fibers, distributed in various tissues and organs throughout the body, forming various terminal devices. They can be divided into sensory nerve endings (also called efferent endings) and motor nerve endings (also called afferent endings) according to different functions.

5.1 Sensory Nerve Endings

The sensory nerve endings are the terminal parts of the peripheral processes of sensory neurons, which generally form receptors together with other surrounding tissues. It can accept various stimuli from both internal and external environments, convert them into nerve impulses, transmit them to the central nervous system, and generate sensations. According to their structure, they can be divided into free nerve endings, tactile corpuscles, lamellated corpuscles, and muscle spindles.

5.1.1 Free Nerve Endings

Free nerve endings are terminal branches of naked afferent nerve fibers (Figure 7 – 13). These fibers are either unmyelinated or finely myelinated in type. Free nerve endings are particularly abundant in the epithelia of the epidermis, cornea, hair follicles, and connective tissue (e. g., the dermis, periosteum of bone, joint capsules, dental pulp, etc.), responding primarily to temperatures, pain, and light touch. Free nerve endings are physiologically specific; each free nerve ending responds to only one particular sensation.

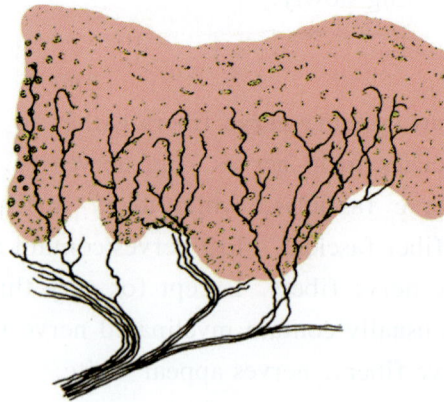

Figure 7 – 13   Drawing of the free nerve ending in skin epidermis

5.1.2 Tactile Corpuscles

Tactile corpuscles (also called Meissner's corpuscles) are encapsulated receptors located in the dermal papillae of the skin, especially in the tips of fingers or toes, palms of the hands and soles of the feet. Tactile corpuscles are elliptical structures with their long axes perpendicular to the skin surface. The corpuscle is surrounded by a special connective tissue capsule. Within the capsule there are multiple transverse stacks of flattened cells (Figure 7 - 14). When the nerve fibers approach their respective capsules, they generally lose their myelin sheaths and enter the capsules as naked endings. The unmyelinated nerve terminals enter into the capsule, branching repeatedly and winding spirally through the flattened cells. Tactile corpuscles are specialized for sensing touch.

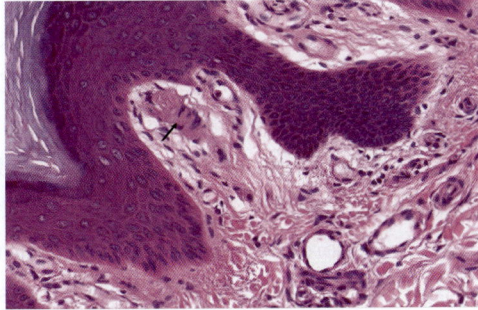

Figure 7 - 14   Light micrograph of the tactile corpuscle (HE staining)

5.1.3   Lamellated Corpuscles

Lamellated corpuscles (also called Pacinian corpuscles) are also encapsulated receptors and are widely distributed in subcutaneous tissue, mesentery, ligaments, joint capsules, and loose connective tissue. Lamellated corpuscles are large, oval or spherical. The corpuscle is characterized by a highly developed connective tissue capsule, which comprises a large number of concentric lamellae of flattened cells surrounding a homogenous cylinder (Figure 7 - 15). One or more myelinated sensory nerve fibers lose their myelin sheath and enter the capsules as free endings, lying in the cylinder. Lamellated corpuscles are sensory receptors responsive to pressure and vibration.

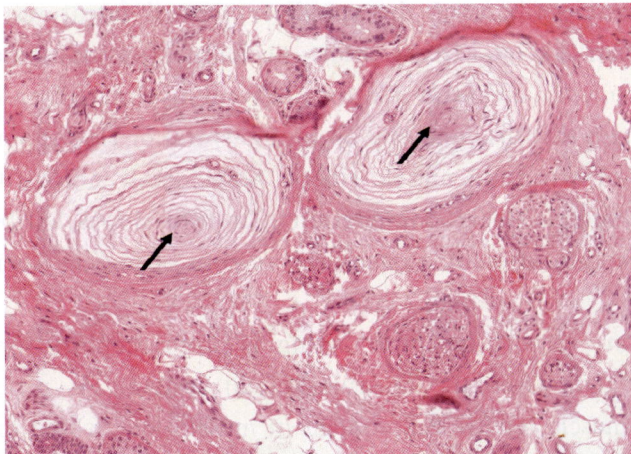

Figure 7 - 15   Light micrograph of lamellated corpuscles (HE staining)

5.1.4　Muscle Spindles

Muscle spindles are distributed within skeletal muscles with a length of 1 − 6 mm. There are a connective tissue capsule, and several relatively small skeletal muscle fibers called intrafusal muscle fibers in the muscle spindle. The nuclei of the intrafusal muscle fibers are concentrated in the center of the fibers, causing the middle segment to expand. When the nerve fibers enter the muscle spindle, they lose the myelin sheath, and their exposed terminal branches surround the nuclear containing part of the middle segment of the muscle fibers in the spindle or attach to the adjacent middle segment in a flower-spray-like manner. There are motor nerve endings inside the muscle fibers, distributed at both ends of the fibers (Figure 7 − 16). The muscle fibers within the spindle contract or relax together with the skeletal muscle fibers around the spindle, and changes in their tension can stimulate sensory nerve endings to produce nerve impulses that are transmitted to the central nervous system, producing a perception of the contraction or relaxation of skeletal muscles, that is, the flexion and extension status of various parts of the body. Therefore, the muscle spindle is a proprioceptor that plays an important role in regulating skeletal muscle activity.

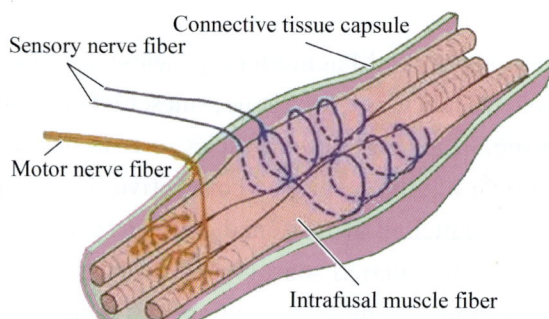

Figure 7 − 16　Drawing of muscle spindle

The modified muscle fibers of the spindles, termed intrafusal muscle fibers, are thinner than the ordinary skeletal fibers. Many nuclei of intrafusal muscle fibers can either be closely aligned or piled in a central dilation. Several myelinated sensory fibers penetrate the capsule, lose myelin sheaths, and end as annulo-spiral or flower-spray endings, rolling up the central areas of intrafusal muscle fibers. Some small motor fibers innervate both ends of the intrafusal muscle fibers. Stimulation of intrafusal muscle fibers by motor nerves elicits contraction, thereby stretching equatorial regions of muscle fibers and their sensory endings.

Muscle spindles are sensory receptors acting as proprioceptors, providing the central nervous system with data from the musculoskeletal system. As proprioceptors, muscle spindles detect both muscle length and change in muscle length and are important in the reflex regulation of muscle tone. Muscle spindles contribute to control of posture, muscle tone, position sense, and movement.

5.2 Motor Nerve Endings

Motor nerve endings (or efferent endings) are terminal structures of the axons of motor neurons. They regulate the contraction of muscle tissue and the secretion of glandular epithelium. Motor nerve endings and the tissues that they innervate together constitute effectors. There are two types of motor nerve endings: somatic motor nerve endings and visceral motor nerve endings.

5.2.1 Somatic Motor Nerve Endings

Somatic motor nerve endings are distributed in skeletal muscles. Myelinated motor nerves branch out within the perimysium connective tissue, where each nerve gives rise to several unmyelinated terminal branches that pass through the endomysium and form synapses with individual muscle fibers. This synaptic structure between the motor axon and the muscle fiber is called motor end-plate (or called neuro-muscular junction) (Figure 7 – 17).

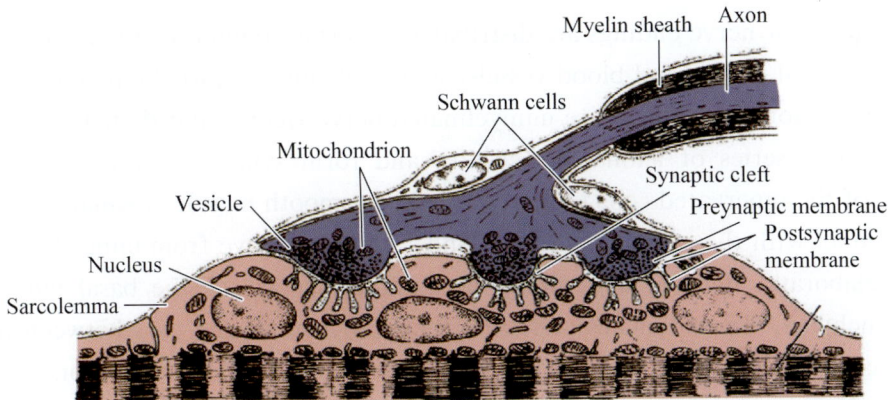

Figure 7 – 17　Drawing of the ultrastructure of motor end-plate

Each axonal branch forms a dilated termination within a trough on the muscle cell surface. Within the axon terminal there are mitochondria and numerous synaptic vesicles, containing the neurotransmitter acetylcholine. Between the axon and the muscle is a space, the synaptic cleft.

The sarcolemma is the postsynaptic membrane, which is thrown into numerous deep junctional folds that markedly increase the postsynaptic surface area of the muscle fiber (Figure 7 – 17). The acetylcholine receptors are concentrated at the margins of deep junctional folds of the sarcolemma. These folds of the sarcolemma also increase the number of transmembrane acetylcholine receptors.

An axon from a single motor neuron can form motor end-plates with one or many muscle fibers. Innervation of single muscle fibers by single motor neurons provides precise control of muscle activity and occurs, for example, in the extraocular muscles for eye movements. Larger muscles with coarser movements have motor axons that branch profusely and innervate 100 or more muscle fibers. In this case, the single axon and all the muscle fibers in contact with its branches make up a motor unit.

When an action potential (i. e. , nerve impulse) invades the motor end-plate, the synaptic vesicles from the axon terminal release the acetylcholine. The acetylcholine diffuses through the cleft and binds to acetylcholine receptor sites on the sarcolemma of the secondary synaptic cleft, resulting in the generation of an action potential. This action potential passes over the sarcolemma and into the T-tubules, causing the release of Ca^{+2} from the endoplasmic reticulum and triggering contraction of the muscle fibers. When contraction ceases, the Ca^{+2} is transported back into the sarcoplasmic reticulum cisternae, and the muscle relaxes.

Acetylcholinesterase, the hydrolytic enzyme of acetylcholine, present along the inner aspect of the secondary clefts, rapidly breaks down the acetylcholine between successive nerve impulses, limiting the duration of contraction and permitting repetitive stimulation.

5.2.2 Visceral Motor Nerve Endings

Visceral motor nerve endings are distributed in certain regions of the heart, in smooth muscles of visceral organs and blood vessels, and in glandular epithelium, etc.

Visceral motor nerve fibers are unmyelinated nerve fibers, and their terminations are distended into a series of axonal varicosities and form synaptic contacts with the cell membrane of the innervated cells (Figure 7 – 18). In smooth muscle, axonal varicosities lie in close contact with the sarcolemma. In glands, endings derive from unmyelinated nerves and form elaborate, delicate nets along the external surface of the basal lamina of the gland parenchyma. Fine branches penetrate the basal lamina and pass between individual epithelial cells. The axonal varicosity typically contains focal accumulations of synaptic vesicles of various sizes and electron densities, microtubules, and mitochondria. The synaptic vesicles typically contain round vesicles containing acetylcholine or granular vesicles containing norepinephrine.

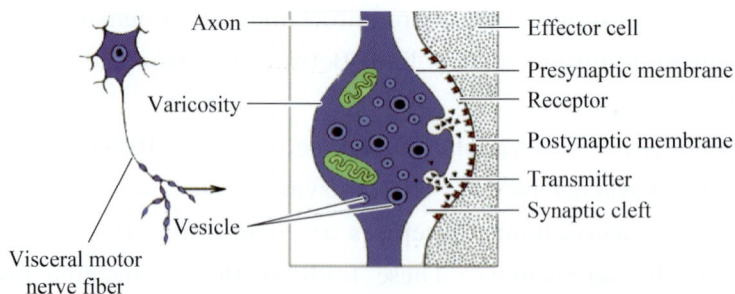

Figure 7 – 18   Drawings of the visceral motor nerve fiber and axonal varicosity

(Yue Haiyuan)

第七章 神 经 组 织

　　神经组织是组成神经系统的主要组成部分,由神经细胞和神经胶质细胞组成。神经细胞也称神经元,约有 10^{11} 个,具有接受刺激、整合信息和传导冲动的功能。神经元之间通过特殊的细胞连接相互联系,分析和贮存接收到的信息,并将其传递给肌细胞、腺细胞等效应细胞以产生相应的效应。神经元也是意识、记忆、思维和行为调节的基础。有些神经元具有内分泌功能,称为神经内分泌细胞。神经胶质细胞,数量众多,主要起到支持、保护、营养、防御和绝缘等作用,同时也参与神经递质和活性物质的代谢。

第一节 神 经 元

　　神经元形态多种多样,但都具有胞体和突起。突起又分为树突和轴突两种。

一、神经元的形态结构

(一) 胞体

　　神经元的胞体大小差异很大(直径为 $4\sim150\,\mu m$),呈圆形、锥形和梨形等,主要分布在中枢神经系统的灰质中,如大脑皮质、小脑皮质、脑干和脊髓灰质,也存在于周围神经系统的神经节内,如脑神经节、脊神经节和自主神经节。胞体由细胞膜、细胞质和细胞核构成,是整个神经元的代谢和营养中心。

1. 细胞膜

　　细胞膜是可兴奋膜,具有接受刺激、处理信息、产生和传导神经冲动的功能。与其他细胞的膜相似,神经元细胞膜也是脂质双层膜性结构,膜上镶嵌有不同功能的蛋白质。细胞膜的性质主要取决于膜蛋白。膜蛋白中有些是特异的化学信号的受体,有些是控制特定离子通过的离子通道。细胞在静息状态下,膜内、外离子的浓度不同,形成一定的电位差。内、外环境的各种刺激,可引起膜内、外电位差发生快速的可逆性变化,从而形成神经冲动。

2. 细胞核

　　细胞核大而圆,位于细胞中央,核被膜明显,核内异染色质少,故着色浅,核仁大而圆。

3. 细胞质

　　胞体的细胞质又称核周质,在光镜下,其特征性结构为尼氏体和神经原纤维。

　　光镜下,尼氏体是嗜碱性斑点状或颗粒状结构,存在于神经元胞体和树突的细胞质中,但不存在于轴突中(图 7 - 1)。尼氏体的形状、大小和数量因神经元类型和功能状态而异。例如,脊髓的运动神经元中的尼氏体粗大且丰富,而背根神经节神经元中的尼氏体则非常细小且分布均匀。电镜下,尼氏体由发达的粗面内质网和游离核糖体组成,这表明神经元具有蛋白质合成的功能。合成的蛋白质包括细胞器更新所需的结构蛋白、产生神经递质所需的酶及肽类神经调质。神经递质是指神经末梢释放的特殊化学物质,它们作用于支配的神经元或效应细胞膜上的受体,从而完成信息传递功能。神经调质则是神经元产生的另一类化学物质,它能调节信息传递的效率,增强或削弱递质的效应。

光镜下,神经原纤维在镀银染色切片中呈棕黑色细丝,交织成网,并伸入树突和轴突(图7-2)。电镜下,神经原纤维由神经丝和微管聚集而成。神经原纤维有助于维持神经元形状结构的稳定,并在物质运输中发挥作用。

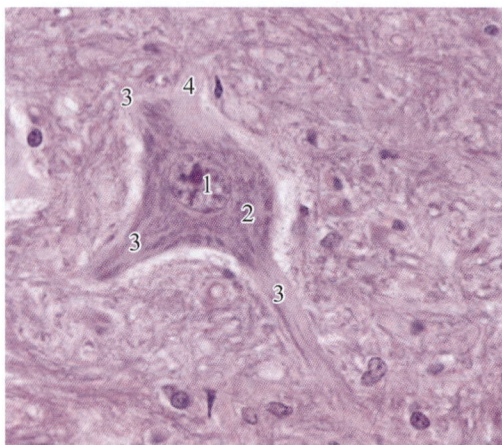

1—细胞核;2—尼氏体;3—树突;4—轴突
图7-1 脊髓前角运动神经元光镜图(HE 染色)

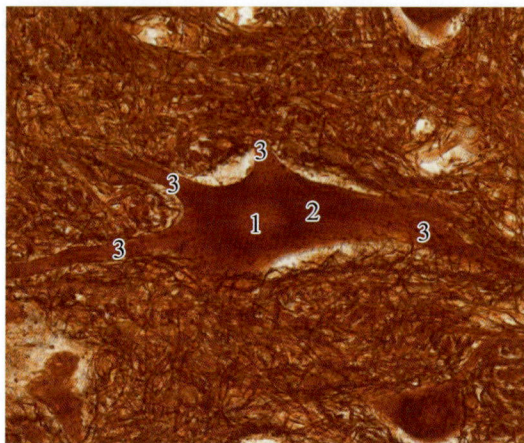

1—细胞核;2—神经原纤维;3—突起
图7-2 脊髓前角运动神经元光镜图(镀银染色)

神经元胞质内还含有线粒体、高尔基复合体、滑面内质网、溶酶体和脂褐素等。此外,内分泌神经元也含有分泌颗粒。

(二) 突起

1. 树突

一个神经元有一个或多个树突,一般自胞体发出后即反复分支,逐渐变细,形如树枝状。与胞体相似,树突内也含有尼氏体和神经原纤维。树突分支表面有许多短小突起,称树突棘。树突的主要功能是接受刺激,并将神经冲动传向神经元胞体。树突棘和树突的分支可显著扩大接受刺激的表面积。

2. 轴突

一个神经元只有一个轴突,由胞体发出,短的仅数微米,长的可达 100 cm 以上,粗细也不一。胞体中发出轴突的部位呈圆锥形,称轴丘。光镜下该区无尼氏体,染色淡。轴突一般比树突细,直径较均一,有侧支呈直角分出。轴突末端常分支较多,形成轴突终末。轴突表面的细胞膜称轴膜,内含的细胞质称轴质。轴质内含有大量的神经丝和微管,还含有微丝、线粒体、滑面内质网和小泡,但基本没有粗面内质网和高尔基复合体。轴突通常被髓鞘包围,从轴丘延伸到髓鞘的起点部分称为起始段,是神经元产生神经冲动的部位。电镜下见此处轴膜较厚,膜下有电子密度高的致密层。神经冲动产生后沿着轴膜传导。轴突的主要功能是产生和传导神经冲动。

轴突内物质经轴质运送，称为轴突运输。由胞体运向轴突终末的过程称顺向轴突运输，反之称逆向轴突运输。胞体内合成的微丝、微管和神经丝组成的网架缓慢移向轴突终末（1～4 mm/d），为慢速轴突运输。轴膜更新所需蛋白质、突触小泡及合成递质所需的酶等，以 100～400 mm/d 的速度由胞体运向轴突终末，称快速顺向轴突运输。轴突终末代谢产物或轴突终末摄取的物质（蛋白质、小分子物质或神经营养因子等）以 1/2 快速逆向运输的速度运向胞体，称快速逆向轴突运输。某些病毒和毒素，如狂犬病毒、脊髓灰质炎病毒和破伤风毒素等，也可经逆向轴突运输迅速侵入神经元胞体。微管在轴突运输中起重要作用。

二、神经元的分类

神经元有多种分类方法，可根据神经元突起的数量、突起的长短、神经元的功能及释放的神经递质或神经调质的化学性质等进行分类。

根据突起的数量可将神经元分为三类（图 7-3）。①假单极神经元：如神经节细胞，从胞体发出一个突起，距胞体不远呈"T"形分为两支，一支分布到外周的其他组织和器官，称周围突；另一支进入中枢神经系统，称中枢突。假单极神经元的这两个突起，按神经冲动的传递方向，中枢突传出神经冲动，具有轴突的功能；周围突接受刺激，具有树突的功能。②双极神经元：由胞体发出两个突起，一个是树突，一个是轴突。它们存在于视网膜、嗅黏膜、耳蜗和前庭神经节中。③多极神经元：从胞体发出一个轴突，多个树突，为体内数量最多的一类神经元。它们存在于大脑、脊髓和自主神经节中。

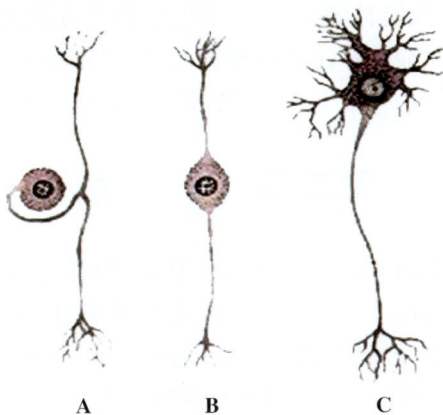

图 7-3 根据突起数量神经元分类示意图
A.假单极神经元；B.双极神经元；C.多极神经元

根据神经元的功能将神经元分为三类。①感觉神经元：又称传入神经元，多为假单极神经元。胞体位于脑脊神经节内，其周围突的末梢分布在皮肤、肌肉和内脏等处，可接受内、外环境的化学或物理性刺激，并将信息传向中枢。②运动神经元：又称传出神经元，多为多极神经元。胞体主要位于中枢神经系统的灰质及自主神经节内，其轴突将神经冲动传给肌肉或腺体，产生效应。③中间神经元：多为多极神经元。联络前两种神经元，起信息加工和传递作用。动物越进化，其中间神经元越多。人类的中间神经元占神经元总数的 99% 以上，在中枢神经系统内构成复杂神经网络，是学习、记忆和思维的基础（图 7-4）。

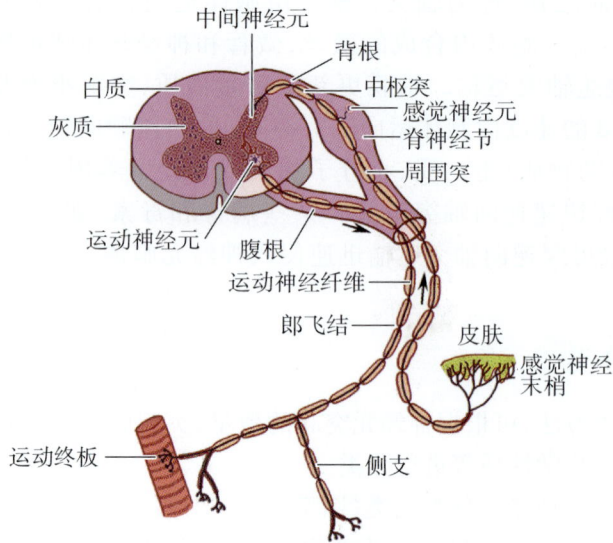

图 7-4　脊髓与脊神经模式图

根据轴突的长短将神经元分为两类。①高尔基 I 型神经元：胞体大，轴突长，在行径途中发出侧支，如脊髓前角运动神经元。②高尔基 II 型神经元：胞体小，轴突短，在胞体附近发出侧支，如大脑皮质内的中间神经元等。

根据神经元释放的神经递质或神经调质的化学性质将神经元主要分为以下几类。①胆碱能神经元：释放乙酰胆碱。②胺能神经元：释放多巴胺和 5-羟色胺等。③氨基酸能神经元：释放 γ-氨基丁酸、甘氨酸和谷氨酸等。④肽能神经元：释放脑啡肽、P 物质和神经降压素等神经肽。⑤一氧化氮能神经元：释放 NO。⑥一氧化碳能神经元：释放 CO。

第二节　突　　触

突触是神经元与神经元之间或神经元与效应细胞之间传递信息的一种特化的细胞连接。最常见的突触是一个神经元的轴突与另一个神经元的树突、树突棘或胞体形成的轴-树突触、轴-棘突触和轴-体突触。此外，胞体与胞体、树突与树突以及轴突与轴突之间也可形成突触。按信息传递方式不同，突触分为化学突触和电突触两大类。化学突触以神经递质作为通信媒介，电突触以电信号传递信息(图 7-5)。

一、化学突触

(一) 化学突触的结构

电镜下，化学突触的结构分为突触前成分、突触间隙和突触后成分三部分。突触前、后成分中彼此相对的细胞膜分别称为突触前膜和突触后膜，两者之间相隔 15～30 nm 的狭窄间隙称为突触间隙(图 7-6)。

突触前成分通常是神经元的轴突终末，呈囊状膨大，在镀银染色标本中呈现为棕黑色的圆形颗粒，附着在另一神经元的胞体或树突上，称突触扣结，又称突触小体(图 7-7)。

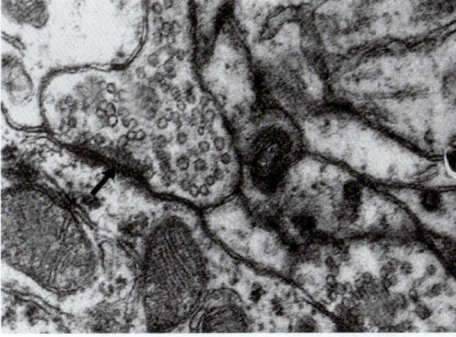

图 7-5　突触电镜图

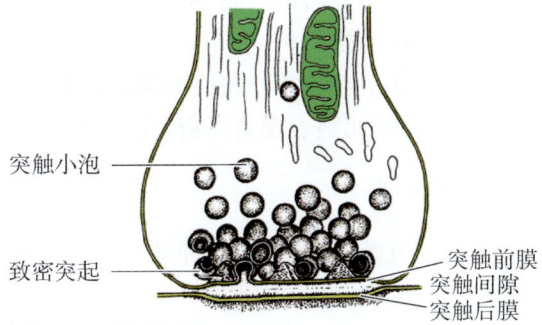

图 7-6　突触超微结构示意图

突触小泡

致密突起

突触前膜
突触间隙
突触后膜

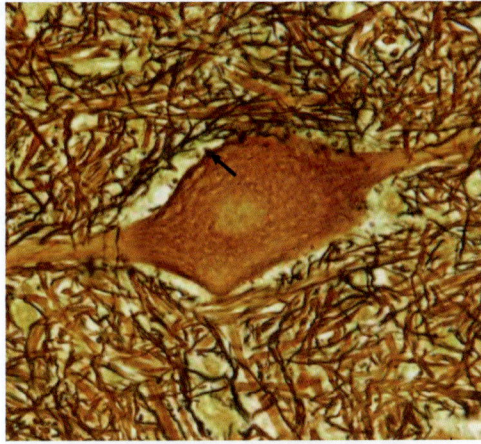

图 7-7　突触小结光镜图(镀银染色)

突触前成分内含有许多突触小泡,还有少量线粒体、微管和微丝等。突触小泡的大小和形状不一,内含神经递质或神经调质。含有乙酰胆碱的突触小泡多呈小圆形清亮小泡,含氨基酸类递质的多是扁平清亮小泡,含单胺类递质的则呈小颗粒型小泡,含神经肽的多是大颗粒型小泡。突触小泡表面附有一种蛋白质,称突触素,它将小泡与细胞骨架连接在一起。突触前膜胞质面还有排列规则的电子密度高的锥形致密突起,其间容纳突触小泡。突触后成分主要为突触后膜,膜上有特异性神经递质或神经调质的受体。突触前膜和突触后膜比一般细胞膜略厚,这是由于其胞质面均附有一些致密物质。

(二) 化学突触传递

突触前膜上富含电位门控通道,突触后膜上则富含受体和化学门控通道。当神经冲动沿轴膜传至轴突终末时,触发突触前膜上电位门控钙通道开放,Ca^{2+}进入突触前成分,在 ATP 参与下,突触素发生磷酸化。磷酸化的突触素与小泡亲和力降低致使小泡脱离细胞骨架,使突触小泡移附在突触前膜上,通过出胞作用将小泡内神经递质释放到突触间隙内。部分神经递质与突触后膜上相应受体结合,引起与受体耦连的化学门控通道开放,使相应离子进出,改变突触后膜内、外离子的分布,产生兴奋或抑制性变化,进而影响突触后神经元或效应细胞的活动。化学突触传递是单向性的。

一个神经元可以通过突触把信息传递给许多其他神经元或效应细胞,如一个运动神经元可同时支配上千条骨骼肌。而一个神经元也可以通过突触接受来自许多其他神经元的信息，如小脑的浦肯野细胞的树突上数十万个突触。在这些突触信息中，有兴奋性的，也有抑制性的。如果兴奋性信息的总和超过抑制性信息的总和，并足以刺激该神经元的轴突起始段产生神经冲动，该神经元则表现为兴奋；反之，则为抑制。

二、电突触

电突触是缝隙连接，在传导冲动时不需要神经递质，冲动的传导一般是双向性的。

第三节 神经胶质细胞

神经胶质细胞广泛分布于中枢和周围神经系统中，其数目与神经元数目之比为 10：1～50：1。神经胶质细胞也具有突起，但突起无树突和轴突之分。除室管膜细胞外，常规 HE 染色只能显示其细胞核，而镀银染色或免疫组织化学方法则可显示其全貌。

一、中枢神经系统的神经胶质细胞

中枢神经系统的神经胶质细胞主要有星形胶质细胞、少突胶质细胞、小胶质细胞和室管膜细胞 4 种(图 7-8)。

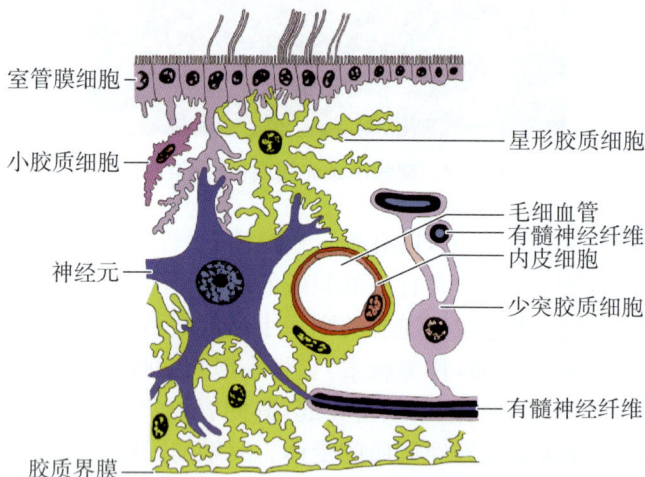

图 7-8 中枢神经系统的神经胶质细胞示意图

1. 星形胶质细胞

星形胶质细胞是胶质细胞中体积最大、数量最多的一种，胞体呈星形，突起很多，细胞核较大，圆形或卵圆形，染色浅。胞质内含有胶质丝，是由胶质原纤维酸性蛋白组成的一种中间丝，参与细胞骨架的组成。星形胶质细胞分为两种：①纤维性星形胶质细胞：多分布在脑和脊髓的白质内，突起较长，分支较少，胞质内胶质丝丰富。②原浆性星形胶质细胞：多分布在脑和脊髓的灰质内，细胞突起较粗短，分支多，胞质内胶质丝较少。

星形胶质细胞的突起伸展充填在神经元胞体及其突起之间，突起末端膨大形成脚板，有些附在毛细血管壁上，如构成血-脑屏障的神经胶质膜，有些附在脑和脊髓表面形成胶质界膜，将软脑(脊)膜的结缔组织与神经元分开。

星形胶质细胞能分泌神经营养因子和多种生长因子,维持神经元的生存及其功能活动,并对创伤后神经元的可塑性变化有重要的影响。中枢神经系统受损伤部位,常由星形胶质细胞增生形成胶质瘢痕修复。

2. 少突胶质细胞

少突胶质细胞分布于中枢神经系统的灰质与白质内。胞体较星形胶质细胞小,细胞核也较小,呈卵圆形,突起细而少,分支也少。少突胶质细胞延伸出片状突起,包裹在几个轴突的周围,形成中枢神经系统有髓神经纤维的髓鞘(图7-8)。

3. 小胶质细胞

小胶质细胞数量较少,分布于中枢的灰质和白质中,是神经胶质细胞中胞体最小的一种,胞体细长,核小,呈卵圆形,突起短而不规则,有小棘突(图7-8)。小胶质细胞来源于循环血液中的单核细胞。小胶质细胞保护大脑免受微生物入侵,当被损伤或入侵者激活时,小胶质细胞形成巨噬细胞,清除中枢神经系统损伤引起的不需要的细胞碎片。

4. 室管膜细胞

室管膜细胞呈单层立方或柱状,分布于脑室和脊髓中央管的腔面,构成上皮样室管膜。室管膜细胞表面有许多微绒毛,有些细胞表面有纤毛,其摆动有助于脑脊液流动(图7-8)。有些细胞基底面有一特别长的突起伸向深部。室管膜细胞具有支持和保护功能,并参与脑脊液形成。

二、周围神经系统的神经胶质细胞

1. 施万细胞

施万细胞是周围神经系统的主要的支持和绝缘细胞,参与有髓和无髓神经纤维的形成。与少突胶质细胞一样,施万细胞包裹轴突产生髓鞘,但一个施万细胞只在一段轴突周围形成髓鞘。施万细胞的外表面有基膜。施万细胞也能分泌神经营养因子,可促进受损伤的神经元存活及其轴突的再生。

2. 卫星细胞

卫星细胞又称被囊细胞,是神经节内围绕神经元胞体的一层扁平或立方形细胞。细胞核扁平或圆形,染色较深。细胞外表面有基膜。卫星细胞对神经节细胞有营养和保护作用。

第四节　神经纤维和神经

一、神经纤维

神经纤维由神经元的轴突和包在其外面的神经胶质细胞所构成。根据包裹轴突的神经胶质细胞是否形成髓鞘,分为有髓神经纤维和无髓神经纤维两种。

(一) 有髓神经纤维

1. 周围神经系统的有髓神经纤维

在周围神经系统中,有髓神经纤维由神经元的轴突和施万细胞的髓鞘组成(图7-9)。相邻的施万细胞不连接,导致神经纤维部分狭窄,轴膜暴露在外,没有髓鞘。这些暴露区域称为郎飞结(图7-9)。相邻郎飞结之间的神经纤维称为节间体。节间体的外围部分是一个施万细胞。在有髓神经纤维的横截面上,施万细胞可分为三层。中间层是由多层细胞膜(多达50层)同心缠绕形成的髓鞘。以髓鞘为界,细胞质分为内侧细胞质和外侧细胞质。内侧胞质紧贴轴膜,极薄,在光镜下难于分辨;外侧胞质略厚,细胞核位于其中,呈新月形。在纵切面上,施万细胞的细胞核多位于胞体中段,呈长椭圆形,长轴与轴突平行。电镜下,髓鞘呈明暗相间的板层样结构。髓鞘的化学成分主要是脂蛋白,称为髓磷脂。在常规 HE 染色组织标本制备过程中,髓鞘中类脂被溶解,仅见少量残留的蛋白质而呈粉红色细网状。若用锇酸固定和染色,则能保存髓磷脂,使髓鞘呈黑色,并在纵切面上可见髓鞘上有不着色的漏斗形裂隙,称施-兰切迹,它们是施万细胞内、外侧胞质间的通道(图 7-9)。电镜下,髓鞘显示为一系列同心排列的浅色和深色薄片。髓鞘的外面有基膜覆盖。

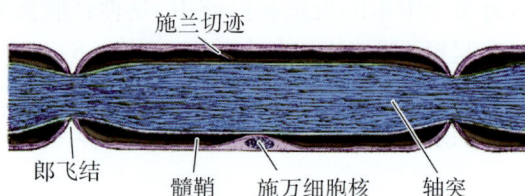

图 7-9　周围神经系统有髓神经纤维示意图

在有髓神经纤维的形成过程中,伴随轴突一起生长的施万细胞表面凹陷形成一条纵沟,轴突陷入纵沟内,沟缘两侧的细胞膜相贴合形成轴突系膜。轴突系膜不断伸长并旋转卷绕轴突,形成同心圆样板层结构,即髓鞘。施万细胞的胞膜构成髓鞘,而胞质则被挤至髓鞘的内外两侧及两端(图 7-10)。

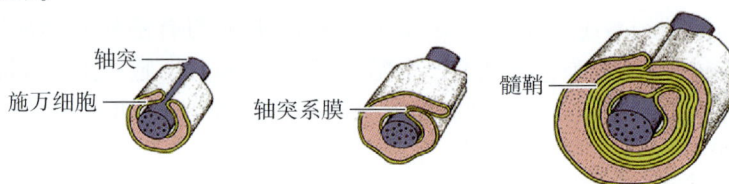

图 7-10　周围神经系统髓鞘形成过程示意图

2. 中枢神经系统的有髓神经纤维

中枢神经系统的有髓神经纤维由少突胶质细胞的突起缠绕轴突所形成(图 7-11)。一个少突胶质细胞有多个突起,突起末端呈扁平薄膜,可缠绕几个轴突形成髓鞘,其胞体位于神经纤维之间。此外,相邻少突胶质细胞的胞突不像施万细胞一样靠拢排列,故郎飞结较宽。中枢有髓神经纤维的外表面没有基膜包裹,髓鞘内也无施-兰切迹。

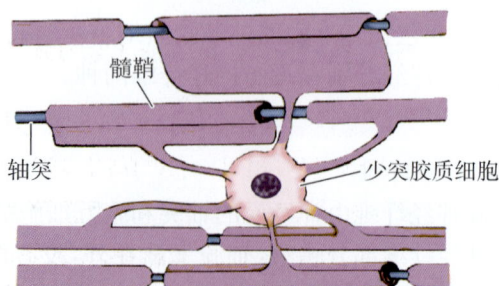

图 7-11　中枢神经系统髓鞘形成示意图

有髓神经纤维的神经冲动只发生在郎飞结处的轴膜,故其神经冲动呈跳跃式传导,速度较快。这是由于有髓神经纤维的髓鞘含大量类脂而具有疏水性,在组织液与轴膜间起绝缘作用。另外髓鞘的电阻比轴膜高,而电容却很低,电流只能使郎飞结处轴膜(与组织液直接接触)产生兴奋。故轴突的起始段产生的神经冲动,必须通过郎飞结处的轴膜传导,从一个郎飞结跳到下一个郎飞结。一般有髓神经纤维的轴突越粗,其髓鞘越厚,结间体越长,神经冲动跳跃的距离便越大,传导速度越快。

(二) 无髓神经纤维

1. 周围神经系统的无髓神经纤维

周围神经系统的无髓神经纤维由较细的轴突及其外面的施万细胞构成。电镜下观察,施万细胞表面有数量不等、深浅不一的纵形沟槽,轴突位于施万细胞沟槽中,施万细胞沿轴突连续排列,不形成髓鞘,也无郎飞结。一个施万细胞可包裹许多条轴突(图7-12)。施万细胞外亦包有基膜。

2. 中枢神经系统的无髓神经纤维

中枢神经系统的无髓神经纤维轴突外面无明显的神经胶质细胞包裹,裸露地走行于有髓神经纤维或神经胶质细胞之间。无髓神经纤维因无髓鞘和郎飞结,神经冲动只能沿着轴膜连续传导,故其传导速度慢。

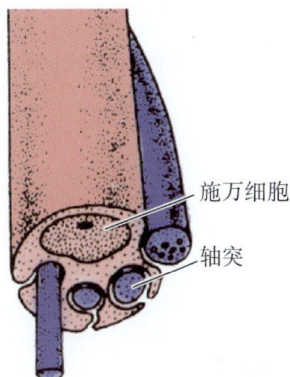

施万细胞
轴突

图7-12 周围神经系统无髓神经纤维示意图

二、神经

在周围神经系统中,神经纤维集合形成神经纤维束,若干条神经纤维束组成神经。粗的神经(如坐骨神经)由数十个神经纤维束组成,而许多组织内的细小神经由一个神经纤维束构成。大多数神经兼含运动神经纤维、感觉神经纤维和自主神经纤维。除了只含有无髓鞘纤维的非常细的神经外,神经通常含有有髓神经纤维。由于有髓神经纤维含有髓鞘磷脂,故外观呈白色。

神经中富含结缔组织,其中存在血管和淋巴管。神经表面包绕着的致密结缔组织,称神经外膜。神经外膜的结缔组织延伸到神经纤维束之间。包绕在神经纤维束周围的数层扁平上皮样细胞及其外的结缔组织形成神经束膜,这些扁平细胞间有紧密连接,对进入神经纤维束的大分子物质起一定的屏障作用。每条神经纤维周围仅有一层薄层结缔组织,称为神经内膜。

第五节 神经末梢

神经末梢是周围神经纤维的终末部分,分布于全身各组织和器官内,形成各种末梢装置,按功能不同可分为感觉神经末梢和运动神经末梢两类。

一、感觉神经末梢

感觉神经末梢是感觉神经元的周围突的终末部分,一般与其周围的其他组织共同构成感受器。它能接受内、外环境的各种刺激,并将刺激转化为神经冲动,传向中枢,产生感觉。按其结构可分为游离神经末梢、触觉小体、环层小体和肌梭。

1. 游离神经末梢

游离神经末梢为有髓或无髓神经纤维的终末,以裸露的分支分布于表皮(图7-13)、角膜和毛囊的上皮细胞间,或分布在结缔组织内,如骨膜、脑膜、关节囊、肌腱、韧带和牙髓等处,感受冷、热和疼痛等刺激。游离神经末梢具有生理特异性:每个自由神经末梢只对一种特定的感觉做出反应。

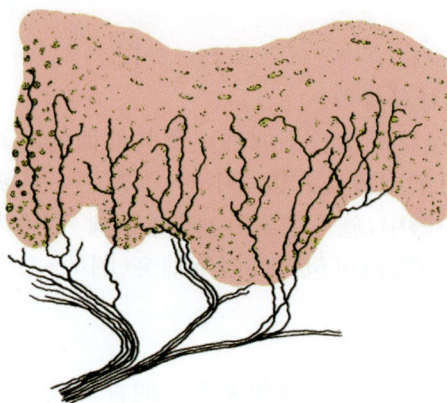

图7-13 表皮中游离神经末梢示意图

2. 触觉小体

触觉小体又称梅斯纳小体,分布在皮肤真皮乳头层,以手指、足趾的掌侧皮肤居多。触觉小体呈卵圆形,长轴与表皮垂直,外包有结缔组织被囊,囊内有许多横列的扁平细胞(图7-14)。有髓神经纤维进入被囊前失去髓鞘,裸露的终末分成细支盘绕在扁平细胞之间。触觉小体的功能为感受触觉。

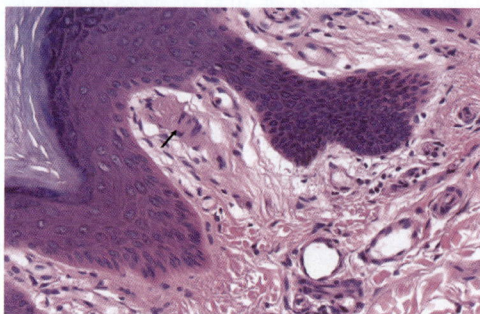

图7-14 触觉小体光镜图(HE染色)

3. 环层小体

环层小体又称帕西尼小体,分布于皮下组织、肠系膜、韧带、关节囊和疏松结缔组织中。环层小体体积较大,呈球形或卵圆形,小体被囊由数十层同心圆排列的扁平细胞构成,小体的中轴为一均质性圆柱体(图7-15)。有髓神经纤维进入被囊前失去髓鞘,裸露的终末穿行于小体中央的圆柱体内。环层小体感受压觉和振动觉。

4. 肌梭

肌梭为分布于骨骼肌内的梭形小体,长1~6 mm。外有结缔组织被囊,内含数条较细小的

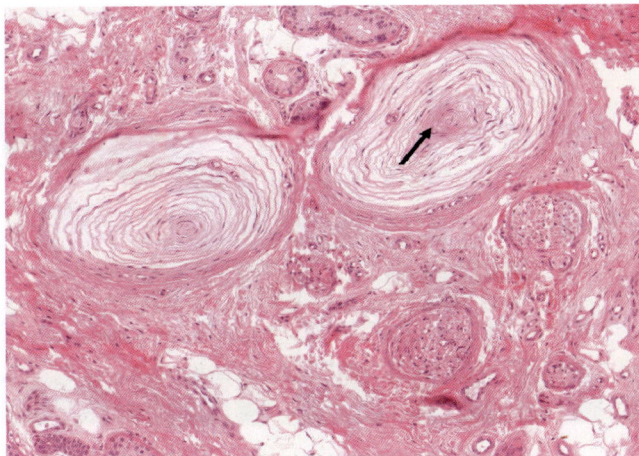

图 7‑15　环层小体光镜图(HE 染色)

骨骼肌纤维,称梭内肌纤维。梭内肌纤维的细胞核集中于肌纤维中央而使中段膨大。感觉神经纤维进入肌梭时失去髓鞘,其裸露的终末分支环绕梭内肌纤维中段含核部分,或呈花枝样附着于邻近中段处。肌梭内还有运动神经末梢,分布在梭内肌纤维的两端。梭内肌纤维与肌梭周围的骨骼肌纤维一同收缩或舒张,其张力的变化可刺激感觉神经末梢产生神经冲动传入中枢,产生对骨骼肌收缩或舒张,即身体各部位屈伸状态的感知,因此肌梭是一种本体感受器,在调节骨骼肌活动中起重要作用(图 7‑16)。

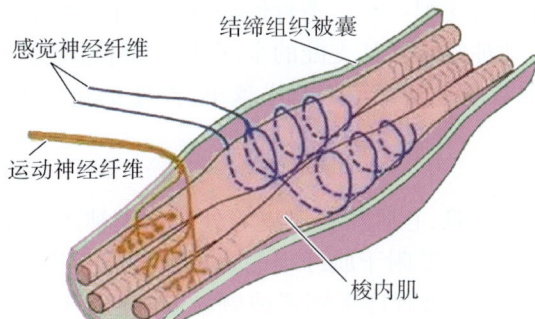

图 7‑16　肌梭模式图

二、运动神经末梢

运动神经末梢是运动神经元的长轴突分布于肌组织和腺体内的终末结构。它与邻近组织共同组成效应器,支配肌纤维收缩和调节腺的分泌。轴突终末运动神经末梢分为躯体运动神经末梢和内脏运动神经末梢两类。

1. 躯体运动神经末梢

分布于骨骼肌内。神经元的胞体位于脊髓前角或脑干,轴突很长,离开脑和脊髓后成为躯体运动神经纤维,到达所支配的骨骼肌纤维时失去髓鞘,其轴突反复分支,每一条分支形成葡萄状终末与一条骨骼肌纤维形成突触连接,躯体运动神经末梢与骨骼肌纤维接触区呈椭圆形板状隆起,称神经-肌连接或称运动终板(图 7‑17)。

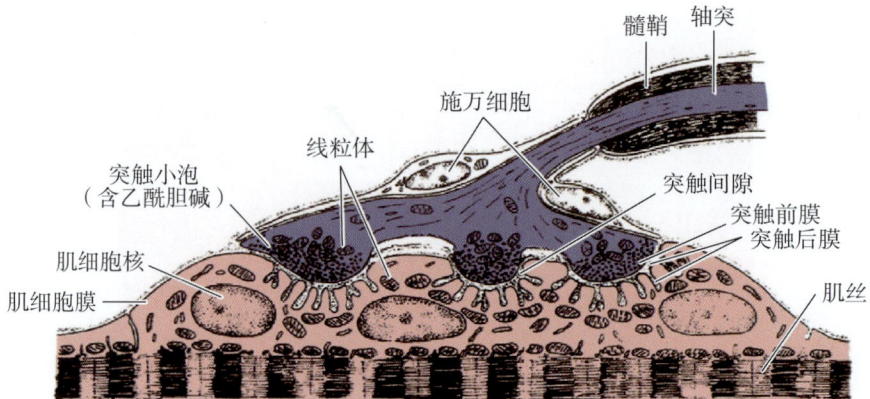

图 7-17　运动终板超微结构模式图

电镜下,运动终板处的骨骼肌纤维内含有较多的细胞核和线粒体,肌膜向内凹陷成浅槽,槽底肌膜(即突触后膜)又凹陷形成许多深沟和皱褶,使突触后膜的表面积增大。轴突终末(即突触前成分)嵌入浅槽内,其内有许多含乙酰胆碱的突触小泡。与之对应的肌膜(突触后膜)上含有乙酰胆碱 N 型受体。当神经冲动达到运动终板时,突触前膜的电位门控钙通道开放,Ca^{2+} 进入轴突终末内,使突触小泡移向突触前膜,突触小泡借出胞作用释放其内的乙酰胆碱到突触间隙,与突触后膜上的乙酰胆碱 N 型受体结合,使肌膜两侧离子分布发生变化而产生兴奋。兴奋经横小管系统传至整个肌纤维,引起肌纤维收缩。

一个躯体运动神经纤维可支配一至多条骨骼肌纤维,而一条骨骼肌纤维通常只接受一个轴突分支的支配。一个运动神经元及其支配的全部骨骼肌纤维合称一个运动单位。一个运动神经元支配的骨骼肌纤维数量越少,运动单位越小,产生的运动越精细。如手指和面部的活动。

2. 内脏运动神经末梢

分布于内脏及血管的平滑肌、心肌和腺上皮等处。这类神经纤维较细,无髓鞘,其轴突终末分支呈串珠样膨大,称为膨体,贴附于肌纤维的表面或穿行于腺上皮细胞之间,与效应细胞建立突触连接(图 7-18)。膨体内有许多圆形或颗粒型突触小泡,其内含乙酰胆碱或去甲肾上腺素等神经递质。

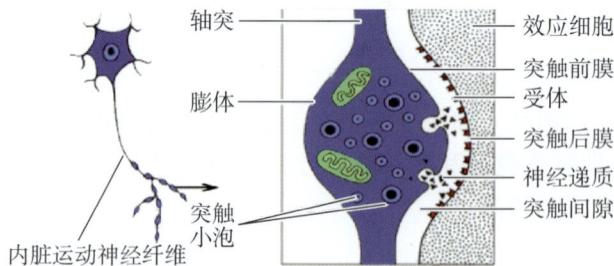

图 7-18　内脏运动神经末梢及轴突膨体超微结构示意图

（岳海源）

Chapter 8

Nervous System

The nervous system consists of the nervous tissue, which can cooperate with the endocrine system to regulate body functions. The nervous system can be divided into the central nervous system and the peripheral nervous system. The central nervous system includes the brain and spinal cord; the peripheral nervous system is composed of nerves and ganglia. In the central nervous system, the region with neuronal cell bodies is called gray matter, while the region with many nerve fibers but without any neuronal cell body is called white matter. The gray matter of the brain is also called cortex because it is located in the surface, whereas the white matter is present in more central regions where some islands of gray matter called nuclei are embedded. The gray matter of the spinal cord is in the center, which is surrounded by the white matter. In the peripheral nervous system, neuronal cell bodies are located in the ganglia.

1 Cerebral Cortex

There are lots of multipolar neurons including Golgi-type I neurons and Golgi-type II neurons in the cerebral cortex. Golgi-type I neurons include large pyramidal cells, medium pyramidal cells and fusiform cells, while Golgi-type II neurons are mainly granulosa cells, horizontal cells, astrocytes, basket cells and so forth. There are 6 layers of neurons in the cerebral cortex.

1.1 Molecular Layer

Molecular layer is the most superficial layer of the cortex and consists of many nerve fibers and a small number of neurons. Neurons are mainly horizontal cells and stellate cells. The axons and dendrites of horizontal cells run parallel to the surface of the cortex.

1.2 Outer Granular Layer

Outer granular layer is composed of many granular cells and a few small pyramidal cells. The apical dendrite of the small pyramidal cell will stretch into the molecular layer. The axon arises from the bottom of the cell body that opposite the apical dendrite, and then connect with the adjacent pyramidal cell to form the synapse.

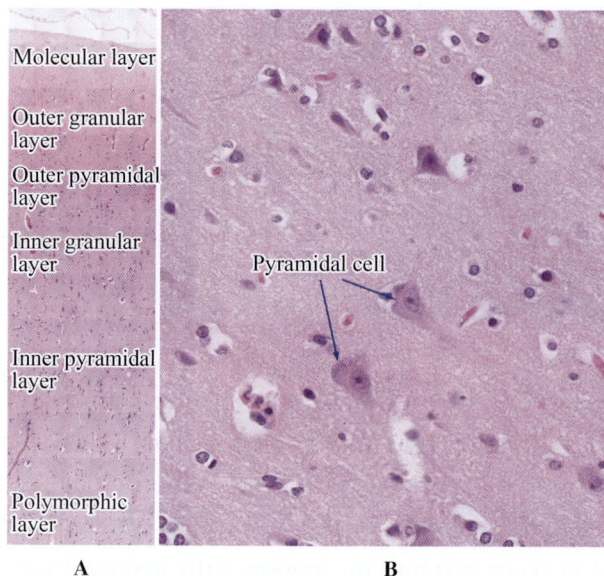

Figure 8 - 1   Micrograph of cerebral cortex
A. HE, 100×; B. HE, 400×

1.3 Outer Pyramidal Cell Layer

Outer pyramidal cell layer is thick and mainly composed of medium and small pyramidal cells, most of which are medium. The apical dendrite of the pyramidal cell will stretch into the molecular layer. The axon will form association fibers.

1.4 Inner Granular Layer

Most cells are densely packed granular cells. Their axons are short and branched in this layer.

1.5 Inner Pyramidal Cell Layer

The inner pyramidal layer is mainly composed of large and medium-sized pyramidal cells. In the motor area of the cortex, the huge pyramidal cells are known as Betz cells. The apical dendrites of the pyramidal cells in this layer will extend to the molecular layer, while their axons descend to the brainstem and the spinal cord to form projection fibers.

1.6 Polymorphic Layer

Polymorphic layer contains fusiform cells, pyramidal cells and ascending axonic cells. The dendrites of the fusiform cells extend to the surface and deep layer of the cortex. The axons will form association or projection fibers in the white matter.

The 6 layers of the cerebral cortex vary in the structure because of the different location. For example, the fourth layer in the visual cortex is developed, whereas which in the precentral gyrus is not.

The efferent nerve fibers can be divided into the projection fiber and the association fiber. The projection fiber mainly originates from the pyramidal cell in the fifth layer and the large fusiform cell in the sixth layer, and descends to the brainstem and the spinal cord. The association fiber is distributed in the ipsilateral and contralateral brain regions of the cortex, which originates from the pyramidal cell and fusiform cell in the third, fifth and sixth layers. The cells in the second, third and fourth layers of the cortex connect with other cells in each layer to construct complex neural micro-loops for analyzing, integrating and storing information. Advanced neural activity may be closely related to these micro-loops.

2　Cerebellar Cortex

The cerebellar cortex can be divided into 3 layers, which includes Purkinje cells, granular cells, stellate cells, basket cells and Golgi cells.

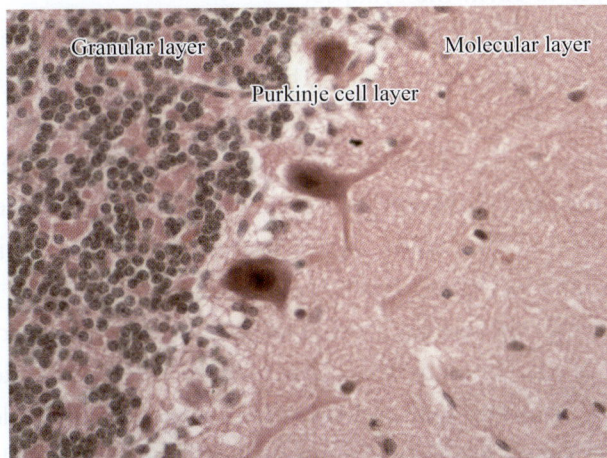

Figure 8 - 2　Micrograph of cerebellar cortex (HE, 400×)

2.1　Molecular Layer

Molecular layer is thick, and composed of many unmyelinated nerve fibers and a few scattered neurons. Neurons are mainly stellate cells and basket cells. The stellate cells are located in the shallow layer of the cortex with many protrusions. Their axons connect with the dendrites to form synapses. The basket cells are large and located in the deep of the molecular layer. Their axons descend to the lower layer, the end of which are distributed like a basket and wrap the body of Purkinje cells to form synapses.

2.2　Purkinje Cell Layer

Purkinje cell layer is composed of one layer of well-arranged Purkinje cells. These cells are the largest neurons and the only efferent neurons in the cerebellar cortex. They are pear-shaped. Two to three main dendrites from the top of the Purkinje cell branch repeatedly to extend into the molecular layer. There are many dendritic spines on the dendrites. Thin and long axons from the bottom of the Purkinje cell extend through the granular layer into the cerebellar white matter, finally terminate in the nerve nucleus.

2.3 Granular Layer

Granular layer consists of many granular cells and a few Golgi cells. Granular cells are small and round, have 4 - 5 short dendrites with claw-like endings. After entering the molecular layer, the axon shows a T-shaped distribution and parallels to the long axis of the cerebellar-folia, which is named the parallel fiber. A large number of parallel fibers pass through several layers of fan-shaped dendrites to form the synapse with the dendritic spine. Golgi cells are large in size. Their dendrites branch a lot, most of which ascend to the molecular layer to contact with the parallel fiber. The axon contacts with the granular cell in the granular layer to form the synapse.

There are 3 types of afferent fibers in the cerebellar cortex: the climbing fiber, the mossy fiber, and the noradrenaline fiber. The climbing fiber and the mossy fiber are excitatory fibers, whereas the noradrenaline fiber is inhibitory fiber. The climbing fibers are thin and mainly originate from the inferior olivary nucleus of the medulla oblongata. After entering the cortex, the climbing fiber contacts with the dendrite of the Purkinje cell to form the synapse, which can induce the excitation of the Purkinje cell directly. The mossy fibers are thick and originate from the nerve nucleus of the spinal cord and the brainstem. After entering the cortex, the end of the mossy fiber shows a moss-like distribution. The end of the branch is swollen, which forms complicated synapse group with the dendrite of the granular cell and the axon or the proximal dendrite of the Golgi cell. The noradrenaline fiber originates from the locus coeruleus of the brainstem, which shows an inhibitory effect on the Purkinje cell. The axons of the Purkinje cell constitute the only efferent fibers of the cerebellar cortex, ending at the nerve nucleus of the cerebellar white matter.

3 Gray Matter of Spinal Cord

The spinal cord is a cylindrical structure that runs through the center of the spine. Its major function is to conduct nerve impulse and reflex activity. The center of the cross section of the spinal cord is the gray matter that has the shape of butterfly, and the peripheral region is the white matter. The gray matter consists of neuronal cell bodies, dendrites, unmyelinated nerve fibers and glial cells, which can be divided into the anterior grey column, the posterior grey column and the lateral grey column.

The anterior grey column contains multipolar motor neurons with different size. The

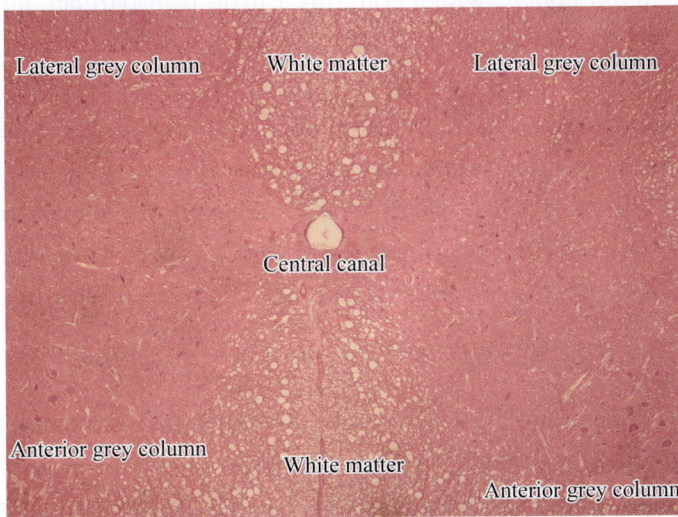

Figure 8 - 3   Micrograph of spinal cord (HE, 40×)

large motor neurons are α motor neurons, diameter of which is more than 25 μm. They have thick and long axons that are distributed in the skeletal muscles. Small motor neurons are γ motor neurons with an average diameter of 10 − 25 μm. Their axons are thin and affect muscle fibers in the muscle spindles. Additionally, there is another type of small neurons called Renshaw cells, which are inhibitory interneurons that can form synapses with the cell bodies of α motor neurons.

The neurons in the lateral grey column are visceral motor neurons, which are involved in the regulation of the sympathetic nervous system. Their axons form preganglionic nerve fibers when reaching sympathetic ganglia.

There are multi types of neurons in the posterior grey column. Some of them called tract cells have long axons that can extend into the white matter to form nerve fiber bundles. The interneurons in the spinal cord have axons with different length. Although the axons run through the white matter and terminate in neurons on the same or opposite side, they will not leave the spinal cord.

4   Meninges

Three layers of membranes known as the meninges protect the brain and spinal cord. The outer layer is called the dura mater, the middle layer is the arachnoid mater, and the inner layer is the pia mater.

4.1　Dura Mater

Dura mater is thick and composed of dense connective tissue. The internal surface is covered with simple mesothelium. There is a narrow space called subdural space between dura mater and arachnoid mater, which contains a little transparency liquid.

4.2 Arachnoid Mater

Arachnoid mater is composed of the thin connective tissue. The subarachnoid space is the space that normally exists between the arachnoid and the pia mater, which is filled with cerebrospinal fluid. Fibers of the arachnoid forms many trabeculae in the subarachnoid space, branch like a spider web, and connect with the pia mater. The surfaces of the arachnoid and formed trabeculae are all covered with the mesothelium.

4.3 Pia Mater

Pia mater is the delicate innermost layer of the meninges, the membranes surrounding the brain and spinal cord. Pia mater is composed of the thin connective tissue and covered by simple mesothelium. There are abundant blood vessels in the pia mater that can provide nutrients to the brain and spinal cord. The space between blood vessels and pia mater is named the perivascular space, which contains cerebrospinal fluid and connects to the subarachnoid space. When blood vessels branch into capillaries in the brain parenchyma, surrounding pia mater and perivascular space will disappear, the capillaries will be surrounded by the protrusions of astrocytes.

5 Blood-Brain Barrier

The blood-brain barrier is a barrier between the blood and the nervous tissue, which is composed of endothelial cells, pericytes, capillary basement membrane, and astrocyte end-feet. The blood-brain barrier can selectively allow some substances including nutrients and metabolites to enter the nervous tissue, while restrict the passage of substances that affect the homeostasis of internal environment. The capillaries in the brain and spinal cord are continuous capillaries, in which the tight junction between endothelial cells blocks cell space. Studies have shown that endothelial cells are the critical structure for the normal function of the blood-brain barrier.

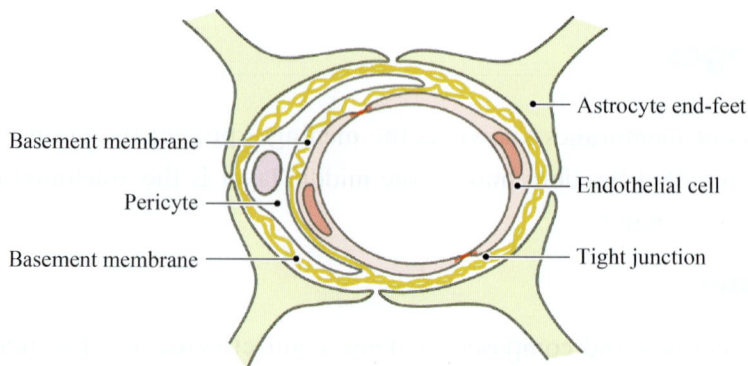

Figure 8 – 4   Diagram of blood-brain barrier.

6   Choroid Plexus

The pia mater of the third and fourth ventricles and part of the lateral ventricles penetrate the brain ventricles to form invaginated folds, which is called the choroid plexus. The ependymal epithelium will transform to the choroid plexus epithelium with secretory function, which is composed of one layer of columnar or cuboidal ependymal cells. The nucleus of the ependymal cell is large and round, with microvilli on the free surface. Under the electron microscope, a lot of mitochondria can be observed in the ependymal cell, as well as the junctional complex between adjacent cells. There are many fenestrated capillaries and macrophages in the connective tissue outside the choroid plexus epithelium.

Transparency cerebrospinal fluid secreted from the choroid plexus epithelial cells fills brain ventricles, central canals, subarachnoid space, and perivascular space to nourish and protect the brain and spinal cord. Finally, the cerebrospinal fluid will be absorbed into the blood through arachnoid granulations, forming cerebrospinal fluid circulation.

7   Ganglia

The ganglia are a part of the peripheral nervous system where the cell body of neuron aggregates. It can be divided into sensory ganglia and autonomic ganglia. The neurons in the ganglia are called ganglion cells.

7.1   Sensory Ganglia

Cranial nerve ganglia and spinal ganglia both belong to the sensory ganglia and are similar in structure. The cranial nerve ganglia are ganglia of certain cranial nerves, whereas the spinal ganglia are located in the dorsal root ganglia. There are cell body clusters of pseudo-unipolar neurons in both 2 types of sensory ganglia. Ganglion cells are round and different in size. They have central nuclei with obvious nucleoli, and granular Nissl bodies in the cytoplasm. Each ganglion cell gives rise to one process, which then divides at a T-shaped junction into 2 branches. One branch, the central dendrite, enters the spinal cord; the other one branch, peripheral dendrite, passes through the brain and spinal nerve to terminate at a sensory ending in other organs. The cell bodies of ganglion cells and nearby process are surrounded by one layer of satellite cells, which are then surrounded by Schwann cells at the T-shaped junction. There are also parallel nerve fiber bundles in the sensory ganglia, which divide ganglion cells into clusters. Most nerve fibers in the sensory ganglia are myelinated nerve fibers.

7.2   Autonomic Ganglia

Autonomic ganglia include sympathetic ganglia and parasympathetic ganglia.

Sympathetic ganglia are located at both sides of the spine, whereas parasympathetic ganglia are located near or within the organs under control.

Most ganglion cells in the autonomic ganglia are postganglionic neurons of the autonomic nerve system and belong to multipolar motor neurons. The cell bodies of ganglion cells are small and the nuclei are often partial to one side of the cell. Some cells are binuclear, and the Nissl bodies are uniformly distributed in the cytoplasm. A few satellite cells wrap cell bodies and process of the ganglion cells. Nerve fibers in the autonomic ganglia are preganglionic nerve fibers and postganglionic nerve fibers, most of them are unmyelinated. The preganglionic nerve fibers form synapses with the dendrites and cells bodies of ganglion cells. After leaving the ganglia, the nerve endings of the postganglionic nerve fibers extend to viscera, smooth muscle of blood vessels, cardiac muscle and glandular epithelial cells to form visceral motor nerve endings. Most neurons in the sympathetic ganglia are noradrenergic neuron, and a few are cholinergic neurons. Neurons in the parasympathetic ganglia normally are cholinergic neurons.

(Yang Fan)

第八章　神　经　系　统

神经系统由神经组织构成,能够与内分泌系统协同调控机体的生理活动。神经系统分为中枢神经系统和周围神经系统。中枢神经系统包括脑和脊髓;周围神经系统由神经和神经节组成。在中枢神经系统中,神经元胞体集中的部位称为灰质,大量神经纤维集中但不含神经元胞体的部位称为白质。脑中的灰质位于浅层,故又称为皮质,而其白质位于皮质下面,其中有一些灰质团块,称神经核。脊髓的灰质位于中央,被白质包围。在周围神经系统中,神经元胞体集中分布在神经节内。

第一节　大　脑　皮　质

大脑皮质中神经元数量庞大且种类繁多,均为多极神经元。其中高尔基Ⅰ型神经元有大型锥体细胞、中型锥体细胞和梭形细胞;高尔基Ⅱ型神经元主要为颗粒细胞、水平细胞、星形细胞、篮状细胞等。大脑皮质的神经元一般可分为6层(图8-1)。

一、分子层

分子层位于大脑皮质的最表面,由大量与皮质表面平行的神经纤维和少量神经元构成。

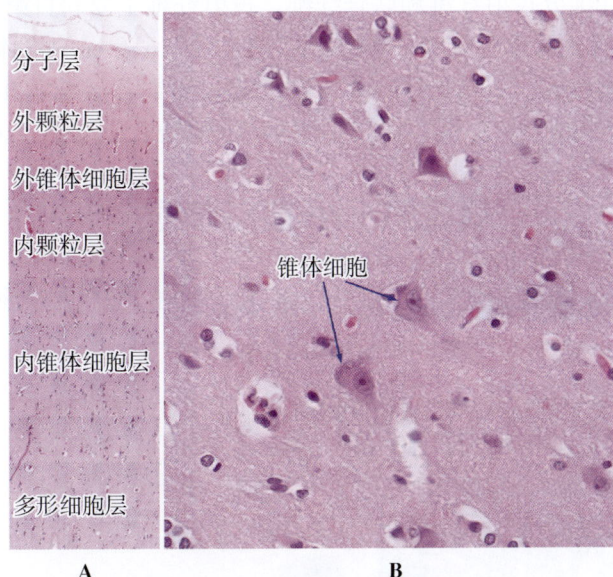

图 8-1 大脑皮质光镜图
A. HE 染色，100×；B. HE 染色，400×

神经元主要是水平细胞和星形细胞，水平细胞的轴突和树突走行与皮质表面平行。

二、外颗粒层

外颗粒层由许多颗粒细胞和少量小型锥体细胞构成。小型锥体细胞的顶树突伸入分子层，轴突从与顶树突相对的胞体底部发出，与邻近的锥体细胞形成突触。

三、外锥体细胞层

外锥体细胞层较厚，主要由中、小型锥体细胞构成，其中中型占多数。锥体细胞的顶树突伸至分子层，轴突构成联合传出纤维。

四、内颗粒层

内颗粒层细胞分布密集，多数是颗粒细胞，其轴突较短，多在本层分支。

五、内锥体细胞层

内锥体细胞层主要由大型和中型锥体细胞组成。在中央前回运动区有巨大锥体细胞，称贝兹细胞。该层锥体细胞的顶树突伸至分子层，轴突下行至脑干和脊髓，组成投射纤维。

六、多形细胞层

多形细胞层主要有梭形细胞、锥体细胞和上行轴突细胞。梭形细胞的树突从胞体两端发出，分别伸至皮质表层和深层；轴突进入白质组成联合传出纤维和投射纤维。

大脑皮质的 6 层结构因处于不同脑区会有结构差异，如第 4 层在视皮质特别发达，而在中央前回不明显。

大脑皮质的传出纤维分投射纤维和联合纤维。投射纤维主要起自第 5 层的锥体细胞和第 6 层的大梭形细胞,下行至脑干及脊髓。联合纤维起自第 3、5、6 层的锥体细胞和梭形细胞,分布于皮质的同侧及对侧脑区。皮质的第 2、3、4 层细胞主要与各层细胞相互联系,构成复杂的神经微环路对信息进行分析、整合和贮存。大脑的高级神经活动可能与这些环路有密切关系。

第二节　小 脑 皮 质

小脑皮质的神经元包括浦肯野细胞、颗粒细胞、星形细胞、篮状细胞和高尔基细胞,由表及里分为三层(图 8-2)。

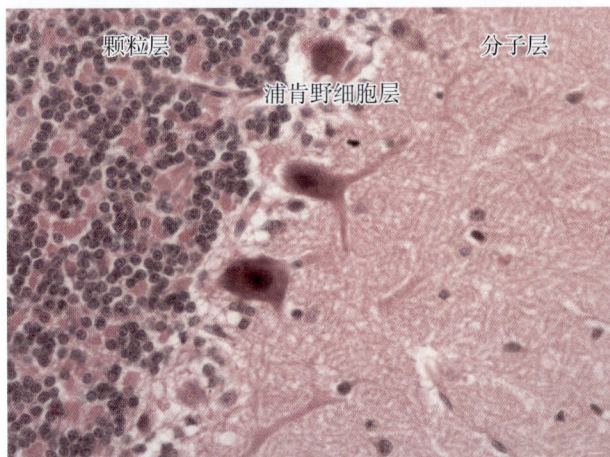

图 8-2　小脑皮质光镜图(HE 染色,400×)

一、分子层

分子层较厚,主要由大量无髓神经纤维和少量分散的神经元组成。神经元主要为星形细胞和篮状细胞。星形细胞位于浅层,突起较多,轴突与浦肯野细胞的树突形成突触。篮状细胞位于深层,胞体较大,轴突向下层延伸,末端呈篮状分布,包裹浦肯野细胞的胞体形成突触。

二、浦肯野细胞层

浦肯野细胞层由一层浦肯野细胞构成,排列规则,是小脑皮质中最大的神经元,也是唯一的传出神经元。胞体为梨形,顶端发出 2~3 条主树突,反复分支,形如扇叶状伸入分子层。树突上有大量的树突棘。细长的轴突由细胞底部发出,经颗粒层深入小脑白质,终止于其中的神经核。

三、颗粒层

颗粒层由密集的颗粒细胞和少量高尔基细胞构成。颗粒细胞胞体小,圆形,有 4~5 个短树突,末段分支如爪状。轴突进入分子层后呈 T 型分布,与小脑叶片长轴平行,称平行纤维。大量平行纤维穿过一排排浦肯野细胞的扇形树突,与其树突棘形成突触。高尔基细胞体积较大,树突分支多,大部分上行至分子层与平行纤维接触,轴突在本层与颗粒细胞形成突触。

小脑皮质的传入纤维有 3 种:攀缘纤维、苔藓纤维和去甲肾上腺素能纤维,前两者为兴奋性纤维,后者为抑制性纤维。攀缘纤维主要起源于延髓的下橄榄核,较细,进入皮质后攀附在浦肯野细胞的树突上形成突触,能直接引起浦肯野细胞兴奋。苔藓纤维主要起源于脊髓和脑干的神经核,较粗,进入皮质后纤维末端呈苔藓状分布,分支终末膨大,与颗粒细胞的树突、高尔基细胞的轴突或近端树突形成复杂的突触群,形似小球,称小脑小球。去甲肾上腺素能纤维来自脑干的蓝斑核,对浦肯野细胞有抑制作用。浦肯野细胞的轴突组成小脑皮质唯一的传出纤维,终止于与小脑白质内的神经核。

第三节　脊　髓　灰　质

脊髓位于椎管内,呈圆柱形,主要功能是传导上、下行神经冲动和进行反射活动。横切面中央为蝴蝶形状的灰质,外周是白质(图 8-3)。灰质分为前角、侧角和后角,主要由多极神经元的胞体、树突、无髓神经纤维和神经胶质细胞构成。

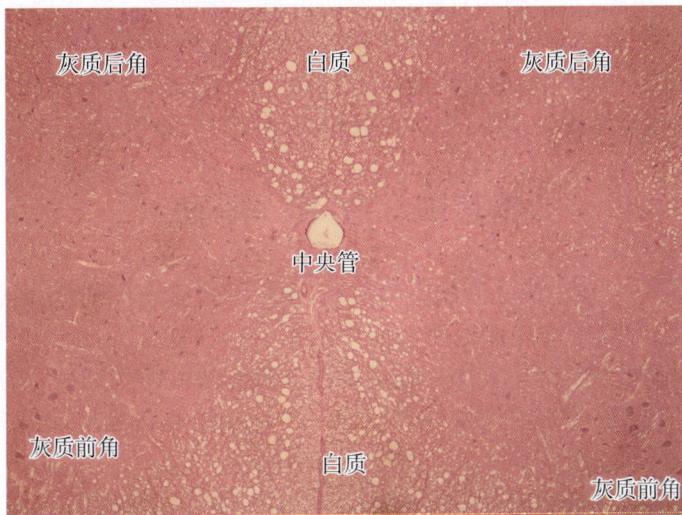

图 8-3　脊髓横切面光镜图(HE 染色,40×)

前角内多数为大小不一的多极运动神经元,大型神经元称为 α 运动神经元,胞体大,直径 25 μm 以上,轴突粗而长,分布到骨骼肌。小型神经元称为 γ 运动神经元,胞体直径 10~25 μm,轴突较细,支配肌梭内的肌纤维。另还有一种短轴突的小神经元,称闰绍细胞,其轴突与 α 运动神经元的胞体形成突触,起抑制 α 运动神经元作用。

侧角内的神经元为内脏运动神经元,是交感神经的起始神经元,其轴突经脊髓前根到达交感神经节,形成节前纤维。

后角的神经元类型较多,有些神经元轴突较长,伸入白质形成神经纤维束,上行至脑干、小脑和丘脑,称束细胞。脊髓灰质内的中间神经元轴突长短不一,可在白质内上下穿行,终止于同侧或对侧的神经元,但都不离开脊髓。

第四节　脑　脊　膜

脑和脊髓表面的结缔组织被膜称脑脊膜,共3层,由外向内分别为硬膜、蛛网膜和软膜。

一、硬膜

硬膜是致密结缔组织,较厚,内表面覆盖一层间皮。它与蛛网膜之间存在一个狭窄腔隙,为硬膜下隙,内含少量透明液体。

二、蛛网膜

蛛网膜由薄层结缔组织构成,与软膜之间有较大的空隙,称蛛网膜下隙,腔内充满脑脊液。蛛网膜的纤维形成许多小梁,在蛛网膜下隙内分支吻合成蛛网状结构,并与软膜相连。蛛网膜的内、外表面和小梁表面均被覆间皮。

三、软膜

软膜为薄层结缔组织,紧贴脑和脊髓,外表面覆盖一层间皮。软膜内含有丰富的血管,可为脑和脊髓提供营养。软膜和蛛网膜随着软膜的血管进入脑内,但软膜并不紧贴血管,两者之间有空隙,称血管周隙,与蛛网膜下隙相通,内含脑脊液。当血管在脑实质内分支形成毛细血管后,其周围的软膜和血管周隙消失,毛细血管则由星型胶质细胞突起包裹。

第五节　血　脑　屏　障

血脑屏障是血液与神经组织之间的屏障结构,由毛细血管内皮细胞及其基膜、神经胶质膜组成(图8-4)。血脑屏障可选择性地使血液中的某些物质如营养成分和代谢产物进入神经组织,而阻止影响神经组织内环境稳态的物质通过。脑和脊髓的毛细血管为连续毛细血管,内皮细胞间有紧密连接封闭了细胞间隙。研究表明,内皮细胞是血脑屏障发挥作用的主要结构基础。

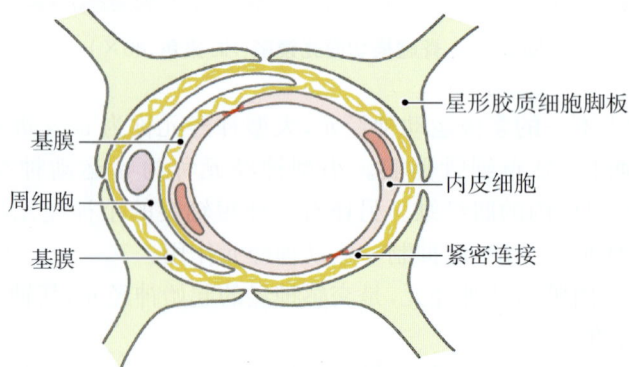

图8-4　血脑屏障模式图

第六节 脉 络 丛

第三、第四脑室和部分侧脑室壁的软膜与室管膜直接相贴,突入脑室形成的皱襞状结构即为脉络丛。室管膜转变为具有分泌功能的脉络丛上皮。脉络丛上皮由一层矮柱状或立方形的室管膜细胞构成,细胞核大而圆,游离面有微绒毛;电镜下观察胞质内存在大量线粒体,相邻细胞顶部有连接复合体。上皮外的结缔组织中含有丰富的有孔毛细血管和巨噬细胞。

脉络丛上皮细胞持续分泌无色透明的脑脊液,充满脑室、脊髓中央管、蛛网膜下隙和血管周隙,营养和保护脑与脊髓。脑脊液最后通过蛛网膜颗粒吸收入血,从而形成脑脊液循环。

第七节 神 经 节

神经节是周围神经系统中神经元胞体聚集的部位,分为感觉神经节和自主神经节。神经节中的神经元称节细胞。

一、感觉神经节

包括脑神经节和脊神经节,两者结构类似。脑神经节位于某些脑神经干上,脊神经节是脊神经背根上的膨大结构。两者均含许多假单极神经元胞体群。节细胞胞体呈圆形,大小不等。核圆形,居中,核仁明显;胞质内尼氏体呈细小颗粒状。从胞体只发出一个突起,先在胞体附近盘曲,随后呈 T 形分支,一支为中枢突进入脊髓,另一支为周围突经脑、脊神经分布到其他器官,末梢形成感受器。节细胞胞体及其附近盘曲的突起外侧由一层卫星细胞包裹,在 T 形分支处改由施万细胞包裹。感觉神经节内还有平行排列的神经纤维束,将节细胞分割成群,其内神经纤维大部分是有髓神经纤维。

二、自主神经节

包括交感神经节和副交感神经节。交感神经节位于脊柱两旁,而副交感神经节位于所支配器官附近或器官内。节细胞主要是自主神经系统的节后神经元,属多极运动神经元。胞体较小,细胞核常偏于细胞一侧,部分细胞有双核,胞质内尼氏体呈颗粒状均匀分布。卫星细胞数量较少,包裹节细胞胞体及突起。节内的神经纤维有节前纤维和节后纤维,多为无髓神经纤维。节前纤维与节细胞的树突和胞体形成突触,节后纤维离开神经节后,其神经末梢分布于内脏、血管平滑肌、心肌及腺上皮细胞,形成内脏运动神经末梢。交感神经节内多数为去甲肾上腺素能神经元,少数为胆碱能神经元。副交感神经节的神经元一般为胆碱能神经元。

（杨　凡）

Chapter 9

Circulatory System

The circulatory system consists of the blood and lymphatic vascular systems, through which blood and lymph circulate in the body. The blood vascular system (also known as the cardiovascular system) is composed of the heart and blood vessels (arteries, capillaries and veins). The lymphatic vascular system is composed of lymphatic capillaries, lymphatic vessels and lymphatic ducts.

1   General Structure of Blood Vessels

Blood vessels, except for capillaries, are usually composed of the following layers (Figure 9 – 1).

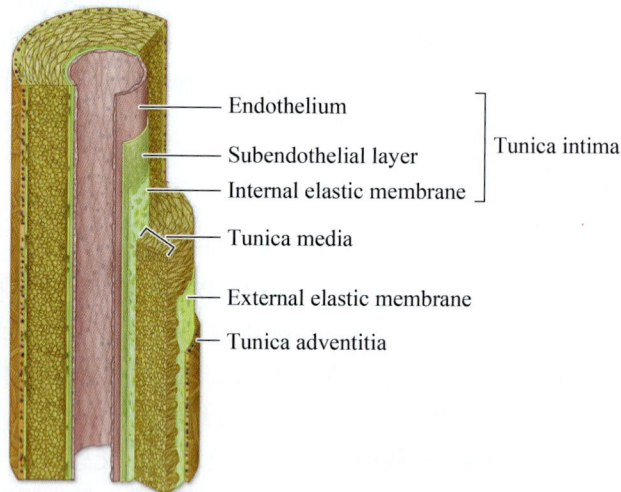

Figure 9 – 1   Schematic of the general wall structure of blood vessels

1.1   Tunica Intima

Tunica intima is located in the innermost layer of blood vessels wall, which is also the thinnest layer. It consists of the endothelium, the subendothelial layer and the internal elastic membrane arranged from inside to outside.

Endothelium is a layer of endothelial cells, lining the vessel's interior surface. Under an electron microscope, the endothelial cells were polygonal and arranged like "pebbles". They contain abundant plasmalemmal vesicles (also known as pinocytotic vesicles) in cytoplasm, whose main function is to transport substances to and from blood vessels. Otherwise, it contains a rod-like specific organelles, called Weibel-Palade body (W-P body) in cytoplasm. The function is to store the von Willebrandt factor (vWF), which participates in blood clotting.

Subendothelial layer is beneath the endothelium, consisting of loose connective tissue that may contains a small amount of collagenous fibers, elastic fibers and occasional smooth muscle fibers, etc.

Internal elastic membrane is composed of elastin, separating the intima from the media. In medium-sized arteries section stained with HE, the internal elastic membrane appears bright pink and wavy, due to tissue shrinkage (Figure 9 - 2).

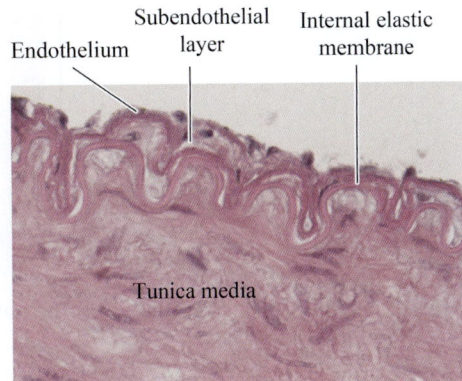

Figure 9 - 2   The tunica intima of a medium-sized artery (HE, 400×)

1.2 Tunica Media

Tunica media is composed of elastic membranes, smooth muscle cells and connective tissue, separating the intima from the adventitia.

The structure of the media varies significantly among different vessels. In large arteries, the media is predominantly composed of elastic membranes, hence they are referred to elastic arteries. In medium-sized arteries, the media is dominated by smooth muscle cells, so they are muscular arteries.

Smooth muscle cells within the tunica media are a subtype of fibroblast responsible for producing matrix and fibers. In pathological circumstances, smooth muscle cells can migrate into the tunica intima, resulting in intima thickening by the proliferation of fibers and matrix, which constitutes a crucial step in the development of atherosclerosis.

1.3 Tunica Adventitia

Tunica adventitia is the outermost layer of the blood vessel wall, comprising loose connective tissue. In some arteries, the adventitia is separated from the media by external elastic membranes, which are composed of elastin.

In general, because of no vascular distribution in the intima of blood vessels, the nutrition is supplied via blood diffusion. In the media and adventitia of some vessels with thicker diameters, there are small vessels that provide nutrition, known as vasa vasorums (Figure 9 - 3).

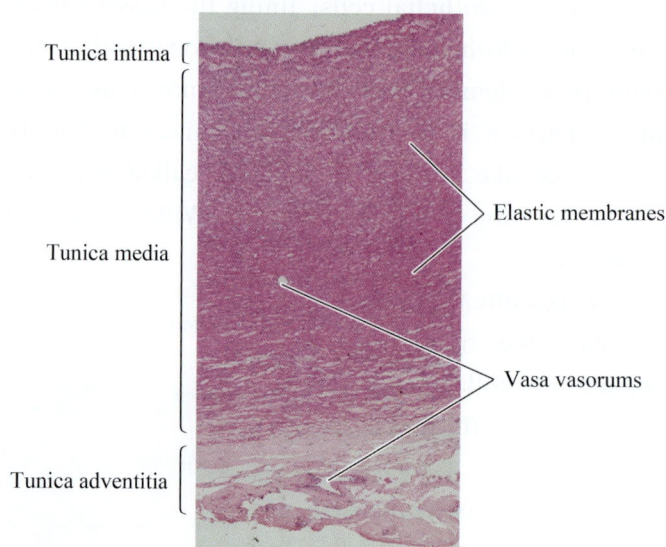

Figure 9 - 3　The wall structure of a large artery（HE，40×）

2　Arteries

Arteries flow from the heart, carrying blood to tissues. They branch step by step like a tree, and the diameter of the vessels become smaller gradually. According to their size, arteries are classified into large arteries, medium-sized arteries, small arteries and arterioles. From the largest to the smallest arteries, the diameter and wall structure of the vessels are gradually changing, and there is no obvious boundary between them. Usually, the changes of the tunica media are most apparent.

2.1　Large Arteries

The large arteries include the aorta and its major branches, such as the pulmonary artery, the innominate artery, the common carotid artery, the subclavian artery, and the common iliac artery, etc. Their diameters are typically exceed 10 mm.

Because of abundant elastic membranes and elastic fibers in tunica media, the large arteries are also called the elastic arteries. This type of artery has the following characteristics (Figure 9 - 4).

Tunica intima is about 1/6 of the thickness of the vessel wall. In endothelial cells, there are abundant W-P bodies. The subendothelial layer is thick, which composes of loose connective tissue. Internal elastic membranes, although present, may not be readily discernible, due to their similarity to the elastic membranes of the tunica media.

Tunica media is the thickest part of the vessel wall, consisting of 40 to 70 concentric layers of elastic membranes. In a cross-section of a large artery, the elastic membrane is

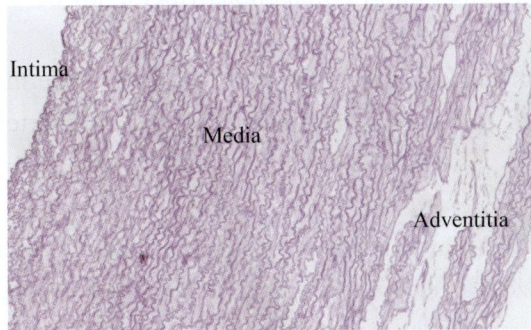

Figure 9 − 4   The vessel wall structure of a large artery (Raisocine staining, 100×)

wavy due to constriction. The elastic membranes are composed of elastin, fenestrated and interconnected by elastic fibers. Between the elastic membranes are smooth muscle cells and a small amount of collagenous fibers.

Tunica adventitia consists of loose connective tissue, which does not show obvious external elastic membranes.

2.2   Medium-Sized Arteries

Except for the large arteries, most of the named arteries in human body are medium-sized arteries, whose diameter is generally greater than 1 mm. Because containing abundant smooth muscle cells in the media, the medium-sized arteries are also named muscular arteries. The structural characteristics of the wall of the medium-sized arteries are as follows (Figure 9 − 2, 9 − 5):

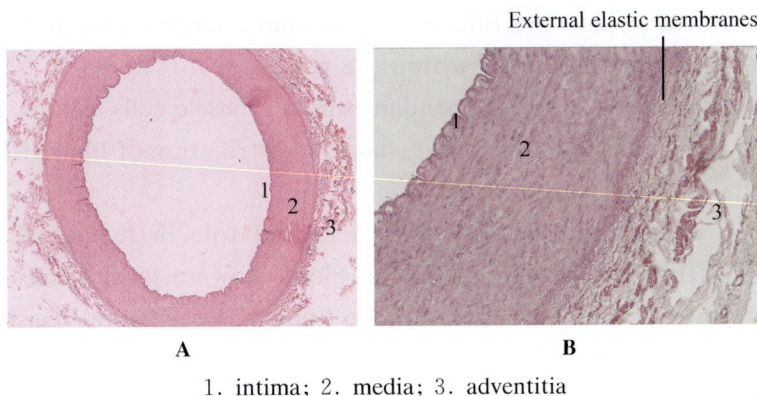

1. intima; 2. media; 3. adventitia

Figure 9 − 5   The wall structure of a medium-sized artery (HE; A. 40×; B. 100×)

Tunica intima: the W-P bodies were scarce in endothelial cells. The subendothelial layer is thin and the internal elastic membranes are prominent between the intima and media.

Tunica media: the muscular artery is characterized by a thick muscular layer with comprising up to 40 layers of smooth muscle cells. These cells are intermingled with variable numbers of elastic fibers and collagenous fibers, all of which are synthesized by the smooth muscle cells.

Tunica adventitia: its thickness is comparable to that of the media. At the junction of the two layers, there are 4 to 5 layers of thin and intermittent external elastic membranes.

2.3 Small Arteries

The diameter of the small arteries is generally between 0.3 to 1 mm. Their structure is similar to the medium-sized arteries, though all layers are thinner. The internal elastic membranes are absent except in larger arterioles. The tunica media is composed of 3 to 9 circularly arranged layers of smooth muscle cells, so small arteries are also muscular arteries. The thickness of the adventitia is similar to that of the media, and there are generally no external elastic membranes.

2.4 Arterioles

Arterioles typically have a diameter less than 0.3 mm. The media only contains 1 to 5 circularly arranged layers of smooth muscle cells. Arterioles generally show no internal or external elastic membranes.

2.5 The Relationship Between the Structure and Function of Arterial Wall

Large arteries: during the contraction phase of the cardiac cycle, the large arteries undergo passive dilation. Simultaneously, a lot of potential energy accumulates in arteries due to the abundance of elastic membranes and elastic fibers in arterial wall. During the relaxation phase of the cardiac cycle, no pressure is generated by the heart. The recoil of the dilated elastic arteries and the release of potential energy, serve to maintain arterial blood pressure and sustain blood flow within the vessels.

Medium-sized arteries: there are abundant smooth muscle cells in tunica media, which can alter the arterial diameter, thereby regulate the distribution of blood flow, so they are also called distributing arteries.

Small arteries and arterioles: they play a crucial role in regulating the peripheral resistance to blood flow, thereby regulate the blood flow to local tissues, and maintain normal blood pressure. Therefore, they are also known as peripheral resistance vessels.

3 Veins

Veins, also known as volume vessels, return blood from the capillaries back to the heart. They converge from small to large, and their diameters are gradually thickened. According to their size, veins are classified into venules, small veins, medium-sized veins, and large veins. The small and medium-sized veins are often accompanied with the same sized arteries, but more numerous.

The wall structure of veins also comprises intima, media and adventitia, but the variation is greater than that of arteries. The characteristics are as follows (Figure 9 - 6).

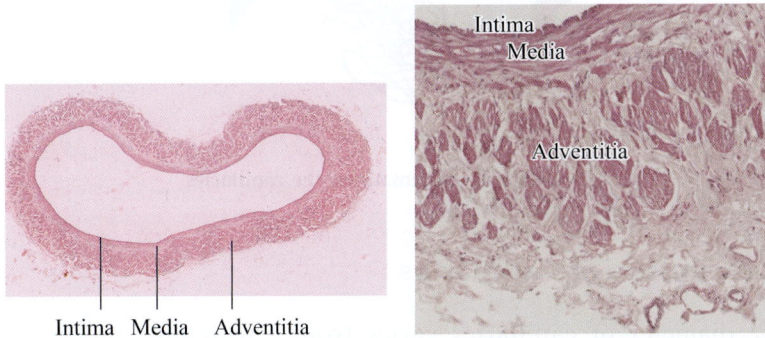

Figure 9 - 6   The wall structure of a large vein (HE; Left: 40×; Right:100×)

The wall of veins is thin, whereas the lumen is large and irregular.

The structure of veins is not as distinct as those of arteries. The internal and external elastic membranes are often underdeveloped. Usually, the media in veins is thin, whereas the adventitia is the thickest and best developed layer containing longitudinal bundles of smooth muscle cells.

Unlike arteries, medium-sized and small veins (with a diameter greater than 2 mm) have valves in their interior. The valves consist of 2 semilunar folds of the intima that protrude into the lumen, serving to prevent blood flow in the reverse direction (Figure 9 - 7).

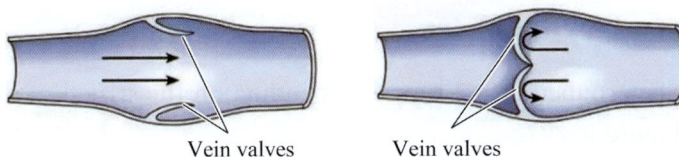

Figure 9 - 7   Schematic of the valves in the vein

4 Capillaries

Capillaries are the most widely distributed and thinnest vessels in the body. They anastomose freely, forming a rich network that interconnects the arterioles and venules (Figure 9 - 8). In different organs or tissues, the density of the capillary network varies greatly. In organs with high metabolism, such as liver, kidney, heart and lung, the capillary network is dense. Whereas in organs or tissues with a lower metabolic rate, such as smooth muscle, tendons and ligaments, the capillary network is sparse.

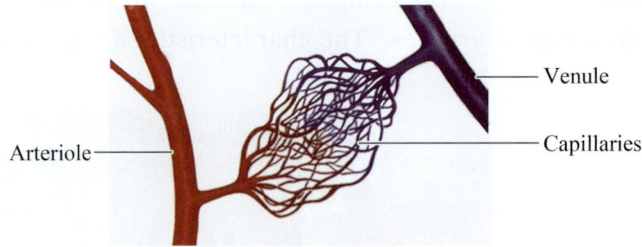

Figure 9 – 8　Schematic of the capillaries

4.1　General Structure of Capillaries

The average diameter of capillaries varies from 6 to 8 μm, only permitting one red blood cell to pass through. The wall structure of capillaries is composed of endothelium, basal lamina and pericytes.

Endothelium: when cut transversely, the wall of capillaries is observed to consist of 1 or 2 endothelial cells. These cells contain a large number of plasmalemmal vesicles, which are responsible for the transport of substances in both direction across the endothelial cells.

Basal lamina is a product of epithelial origin.

Pericytes are spaced at intervals along the outside of capillary wall, with long cytoplasmic processes that partly surround the endothelial cells. Pericytes have contractile function, which can regulate blood flow of capillaries. When capillaries are wounded, pericytes have great potential for transformation into other cells, such as endothelial cells, smooth muscle cells and fibroblasts.

4.2　Classification of Capillaries

Capillaries can be grouped into 3 types, depending on the structure of the endothelium and basal lamina (Figure 9 - 9).

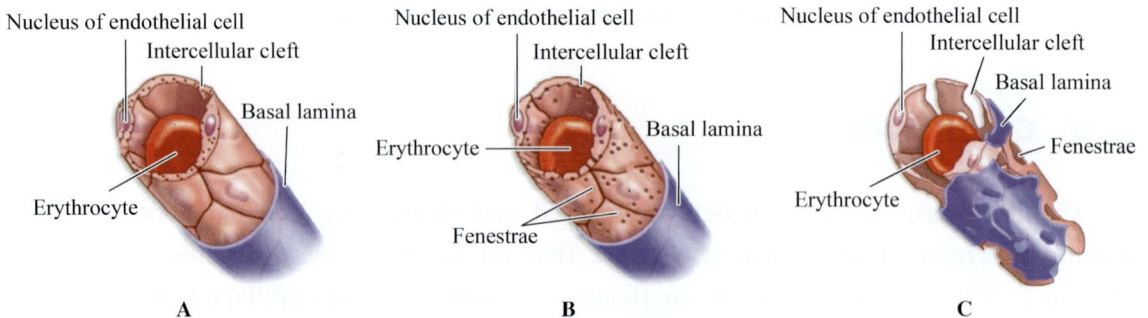

Figure 9 – 9　Schematic of the 3 types of capillaries
A. Continuous capillary; B. Fenestrated capillary; C. Sinusoid

4.2.1　Continuous Capillaries

(1) Capillaries are composed of a continuous layer of endothelial cells, and which are

held together by tight junctions.

(2) There are numerous plasmalemmal vesicles, present in the cytoplasm of endothelial cells.

(3) Basal lamina is complete.

The function of continuous capillaries is to transport metabolites between the tissues and the blood via plasmalemmal vesicles. Continuous capillaries are typically found in muscle tissue, connective tissue, exocrine glands, nervous tissue, thymus and lungs, and also act as component in various barrier structures.

4.2.2 Fenestrated Capillaries

(1) This type of capillary is also composed of continuous endothelial cells, held together by tight junctions.

(2) It is characterized by the presence of fenestrae in the thin portion of the endothelial cell walls, some of which are closed with a diaphragm.

(3) A continuous basal lamina is present.

Fenestrated capillaries are commonly found in tissues where rapid exchange of medium and small molecule substances occurs between the tissues and the blood, such as the gastrointestinal mucosa, some endocrine glands and the renal glomerulus.

4.2.3 Sinusoids or Sinusoid Capillaries, Discontinuous Capillaries

(1) This type of capillary follows a tortuous path and possess a significantly enlarged lumen.

(2) The presence of multiple fenestrae without diaphragms in the endothelial cell walls. There is an absence of a continuous lining of endothelial cells, leaving open spaces between cells through which the capillaries communicate with the underlying tissues.

(3) The basal lamina is frequently discontinuous or entirely absent.

The interchange of macromolecules between the blood and the tissue is greatly facilitated by the structure of sinusoids. This type of capillary is found mainly in the liver, spleen, bone marrow and some endocrine glands. Furthermore, the structure of sinusoid in different organs is obviously different.

5 Heart

The heart is a muscular organ and the power center of the cardiovascular system, which contracts rhythmically, pumping the blood throughout the circulatory system.

5.1 Structure of the Heart Wall

The wall of the heart is organized into the endocardium, myocardium, and epicardium (Figure 9 – 10).

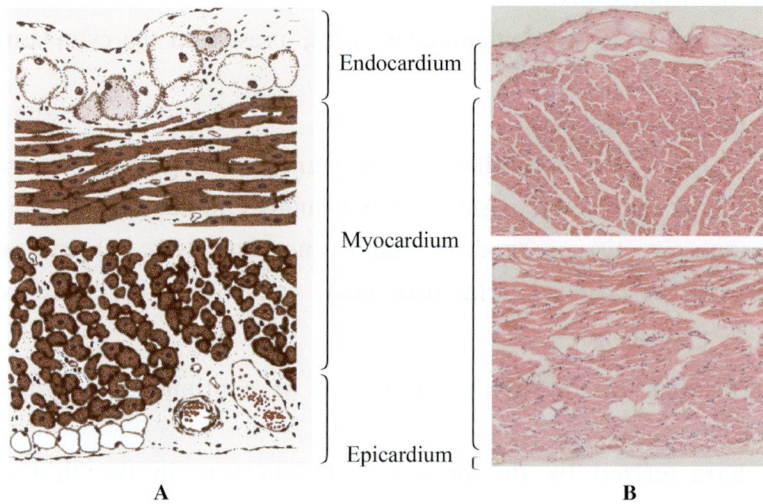

Figure 9 – 10   The structure of the heart wall
A. Schematic of the heart wall; B. Light micrograph of the heart wall (HE, 40×)

5.1.1   Endocardium

It is composed of three layers: ①Endothelium, homologous to the tunica intima, is in contact with blood vessels. ② Subendothelial layer, which comprises connective tissues containing elastic fibers and some smooth muscle cells. ③Subendocardial layer, which also comprises loose connective tissues containing veins, nerves, and branches of the cardiac conduction system, such as Purkinje fibers.

5.1.2   Myocardium

It is the thickest of the tunics of the heart, and consists mostly of cardiac muscle cells. The characteristics of myocardium are as follows: ①Cardiac muscle cells cover the heart chambers in a complex spiral manner. The arrangement of these muscle cells is extremely varied, so that in histologic section of a small area, cells are seen oriented in many directions. The muscle cells are arranged into interlacing bundles or sheets. Between them, there are a small amount of connective tissues and abundant capillaries. ②Compared to the atrium, the myocardium is much thicker in the walls of the ventricles, especially in the left ventricle. And Purkinje fibers are also located in the ventricular myocardium. Furthermore, the muscle cells in atrium are smaller than in ventricle. In the cytoplasm of atrial muscle cells, there are specific atrial granules containing atrial natriuretic peptide, which play roles in diuresis, sodium excretion, vasodilation and blood pressure reduction. ③ The cardiac skeleton is composed of dense connective tissue and forms part of the interventricular and interatrial septa, providing sturdy anchor points for the insertion of cardiac muscle.

5.1.3   Epicardium

It is the serous covering of the heart, forming the visceral layer of the pericardium.

Externally, it is covered by simple squamous epithelium (mesothelium) supported by a thin layer of loose connective tissue, containing veins, nerves and adipose tissue.

5.2 Cardiac Valves

The cardiac valves are thin folds of endocardium, the bases of which are attached to the annuli fibrosi of the cardiac skeleton. The cardiac valves consist of a central core of dense fibrous connective tissue (containing a mixture of collagen and elastic fibers, as well as occasional smooth muscle cells), lined on both sides by endothelial layers. There are four cardiac valves, including two atrioventricular valves (mitral valve and tricuspid valve), pulmonary and aortic valves, that prevent backflow of blood.

Abnormalities in the structure of heart valves can be produced by cardiovascular problems such as rheumatic heart disease, which could result in hard and deformed valves by collagenous fibers hyperplasia. Such abnormal valves may not close tightly, allowing backflow of blood.

5.3 Conducting System of the Heart

Within the wall of the heart, modified cardiac muscle cells make up the conducting system, which is composed of sinoatrial (SA) node, atrioventricular (AV) node, AV bundle of His, and the subendocardial conducting network (left and right bundle branches and following branches). The SA node is the pacemaker of the heart, located close to the entrance of the superior vena cava into the right atrium. Others of the conducting system are distributed in the subendocardial layer (Figure 9 – 11).

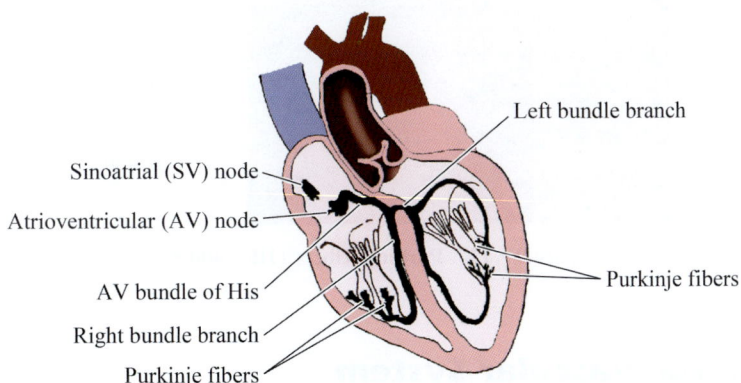

Figure 9 – 11   Schematic of conducting system of the heart

The conducting system consists of three types of modified cardiac muscle cells: pacemaker cells, transitional cells and Purkinje fibers. These cells aggregate into nodes or bundles, and are regulated by sympathetic and parasympathetic divisions of the autonomic system.

5.3.1　Pacemaker Cells

They are also called P cells, and are located in the center of the SV and AV nodes. The cells are smaller than atrial muscle cells, fusiform with branches connected into a network. The HE staining of the cells is shallow, resulting from fewer organelles, fewer myofibrils and more glycogen in cytoplasm. Impulses initiated by these cells move along the myocardial fibers of both atria, stimulating their contraction.

5.3.2　Transitional Cells

These cells are arranged around the SV node, AV node and the atrioventricular bundle, conducting the impulse from SV node. Their structure is similar to those of the SV node, but with more myofibrils, and their cytoplasmic projection branch in various directions, forming a network.

5.3.3　Purkinje Fibers

At the apex of the heart, the bundle branches are further into a subendocardial conducting network of myofibers, which are called Purkinje fibers. Compared with ordinary cardiac muscle cells, Purkinje fibers exhibit a distinctive appearance. They are larger and pale-staining, with one or two nuclei. Their cytoplasm is rich in mitochondria and glycogen. The myofibrils are sparse, and present mainly in the periphery of the cell. Purkinje fibers are tightly bound by well-developed intercalated disks (Figure 9 - 12). Purkinje fibers mingle distally with contractile fibers of both ventricles and trigger waves of contraction through both ventricles simultaneously.

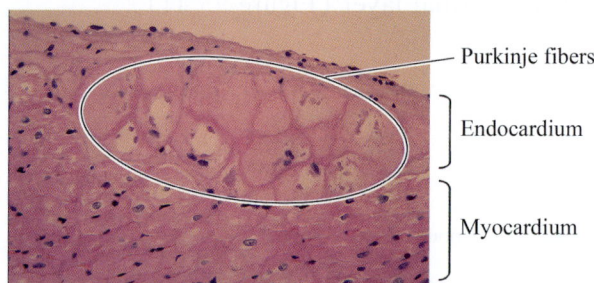

Figure 9 - 12　Purkinje fibers (HE, 400×)

6　Lymphatic Vascular System

The lymphatic vascular system includes lymphatic capillaries, lymphatic vessels, and lymphatic ducts. In addition to blood vessels, the human body has a system that collect fluid from the tissue spaces and return it to the blood. This fluid is called lymph, finally it empties into the large veins near the heart by lymphatic ducts. Except for cartilage tissue, bone tissue, bone marrow, epidermis, eyeball, inner ear and teeth, most other tissues or organs in human body have lymphatic vessels, which function is to transport water, electrolytes, and macromolecules from tissue fluid into the bloodstream.

6.1 Lymphatic Capillaries

They originate as blind-ended vessels within various tissues and subsequently anastomose to form a network. Compared with the blood capillaries, the lumen of lymphatic capillaries is larger and more irregular. Their wall of these is thinner, consisting of a single layer of endothelium and an incomplete basal lamina. They have no fenestrae in their endothelial cells and no pericytes, but larger intercellular space. This unique structure facilitates the entry of large amounts of tissue fluid, including macromolecules, into the lymphatic system.

6.2 Lymphatic Vessels

They have a structure akin to veins, but with thinner walls, and they lack a clear-cut separation between the 3 layers (intima, media, and adventitia). The wall of lymphatic vessels is composed of endothelium, a little smooth muscle cells and connective tissue. However, they possess a greater number of internal valves compared to veins.

6.3 Lymphatic Ducts

The lymphatic vessels ultimately converge and end up two large trunks: the thoracic duct, and the right lymphatic duct. They have a structure similar to that of large veins, but with thinner walls and a less distinct boundary between the three layers.

(Fu Yi)

第九章　循 环 系 统

循环系统包括心血管系统和淋巴管系统,是机体运输血液和淋巴的管道。心血管系统由心脏和血管(包括动脉、毛细血管和静脉)组成。淋巴管系统由毛细淋巴管、淋巴管和淋巴导管组成。

第一节　动脉和静脉管壁的一般结构

动脉和静脉的管壁结构由内向外,可分为内膜、中膜和外膜三层结构(图9-1)。

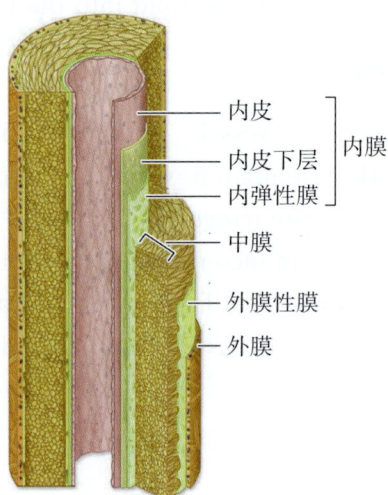

图 9-1　动脉、静脉管壁结构模式图

一、内膜

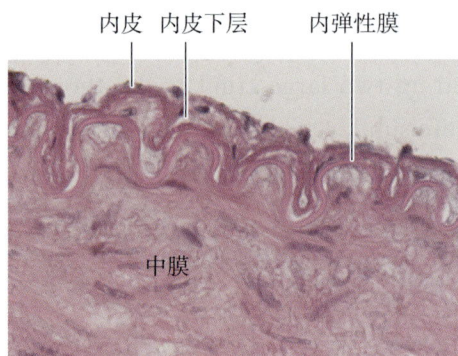

图 9-2　中动脉内膜光镜图(HE 染色，400×)

内膜位于血管壁的最内层，最薄，从内向外又可分为内皮、内皮下层和内弹性膜(图 9-2)。

1. 内皮

内皮为衬于血管腔面的单层扁平上皮。光镜下，内皮细胞很薄，只有细胞核所在部位较明显。电镜下，内皮细胞呈多边形、"鹅卵石"样镶嵌排列。胞质内含丰富的质膜小泡(也称吞饮小泡)，其主要功能是向血管内、外输送物质。此外，胞质中还可见一种长杆状的 W-P 小体，也称怀布尔-帕拉德小体，为内皮细胞所特有，其功能是储存血管性血友病因子(von Willebrand factor，vWF)，vWF 参与止血、凝血。

2. 内皮下层

内皮下层为薄层结缔组织，位于内皮和内弹性膜之间，含少量胶原纤维、弹性纤维及平滑肌纤维等。

3. 内弹性膜

由弹性蛋白构成，可作为内膜和中膜的分界。在 HE 染色的中动脉切片中，由于组织皱缩，内弹性膜呈亮粉红色、波浪状。

二、中膜

中膜位于内膜和外膜之间，由弹性膜、平滑肌和结缔组织构成。在不同的血管中，中膜的结构差异很大。比如大动脉的中膜以弹性膜为主，而中动脉的中膜以平滑肌为主。

血管壁中膜的平滑肌细胞，是成纤维细胞的一种亚型，可以产生基质和纤维。在病理情况下,平滑肌细胞可迁入内膜增生,产生更多的纤维和基质,导致内膜增厚,这是动脉粥样硬化发生过程中的重要环节。

三、外膜

外膜为血管壁的最外层,由疏松结缔组织构成。在部分动脉中膜和外膜的交界处,可见由弹性蛋白构成的外弹性膜。

一般血管的内膜无血管分布,其营养通过血液渗透来提供。在一些管径较粗的血管的中膜和外膜中,可见一些提供营养的小血管,称营养血管(图9-3)。

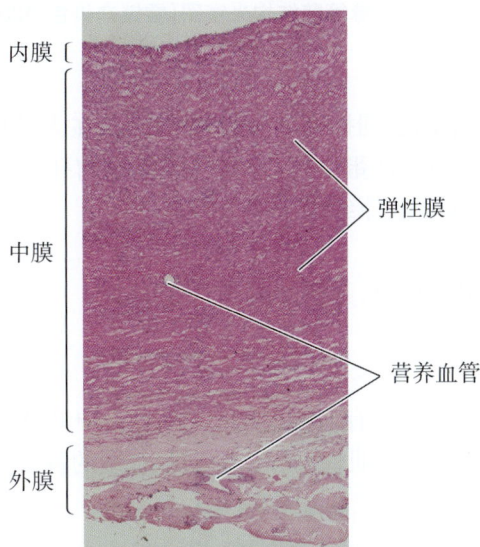

图9-3 大动脉管壁结构光镜图(HE染色,40×)

第二节 动 脉

动脉从心脏发出,向身体各器官和组织运送血液。由粗至细,逐级分支。根据管径的大小,动脉可分为大动脉、中动脉、小动脉和微动脉。从最大的动脉到最小的动脉,其管径和管壁结构是渐变的,其间没有明显的分界,而其中以中膜的变化最为明显。

一、大动脉

大动脉包括主动脉、肺动脉、无名动脉、颈总动脉、锁骨下动脉、髂总动脉等,管径通常大于10 mm。由于大动脉的中膜含有多层弹性膜和大量的弹性纤维,故大动脉又称弹性动脉。大动脉各层的结构特点如下(图9-4)。

1. 内膜

内膜占管壁厚度的1/6左右。内皮细胞中含有丰富的W-P小体。内皮下层较厚,为疏松结缔组织。由于内弹性膜与中膜的弹性膜相延续,因此内弹性膜不明显,也使内膜与中膜之间无明显界限。

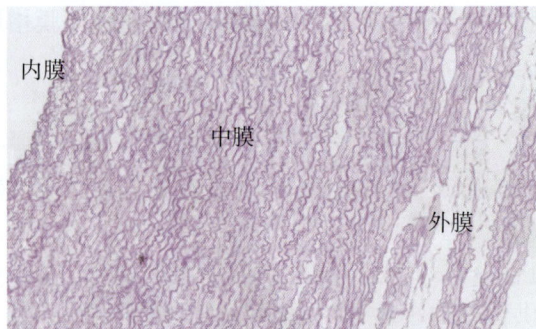

图9‑4　大动脉管壁结构光镜图(雷锁辛染色,100×)

2. 中膜

中膜最厚,由40~70层呈同心圆排列的弹性膜构成。在大动脉的横切面上,由于血管收缩,弹性膜呈波浪状。弹性膜由弹性蛋白构成,弹性膜上有窗孔,各层弹性膜由弹性纤维相连,其间还有环行平滑肌纤维及少量胶原纤维。

3. 外膜

外膜较薄,由疏松结缔组织构成,无明显外弹性膜。

二、中动脉

除大动脉以外,凡是在解剖学中有名称的动脉,大多为中动脉,管径一般大于1 mm。由于中动脉中膜的平滑肌很丰富,故又称肌性动脉。中动脉管壁的各层结构特点如下(图9‑5):

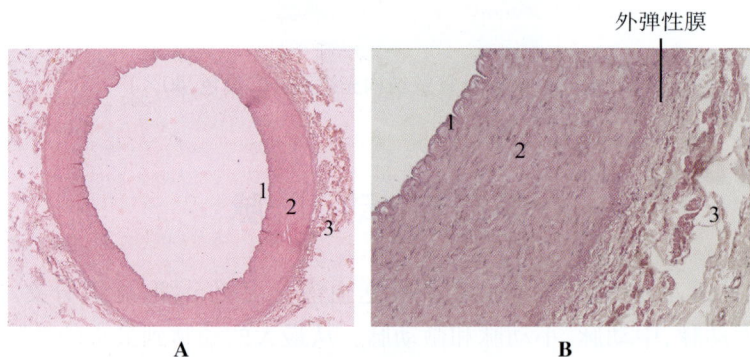

1—内膜;2—中膜;3—外膜

图9‑5　中动脉管壁结构光镜图
HE染色,A.40×,B.100×

1. 内膜

内皮细胞中W‑P小体较少,内皮下层较薄,在与中膜交界处有1~2层明显的内弹性膜。

2. 中膜

中膜较厚,由10~40层的环形平滑肌细胞组成。肌纤维之间有少量的弹性纤维和胶原纤维,均由平滑肌细胞产生。

3. 外膜

外膜厚度与中膜相近。两者交界处可见4~5层、薄而断续的外弹性膜。

三、小动脉

小动脉管径一般介于 0.3～1 mm 之间，结构与中动脉相似，但各层均更薄。较大的小动脉内弹性膜薄而明显；较小的小动脉内弹性膜则不明显或缺如。中膜含 3～9 层环行平滑肌，故小动脉也属于肌性动脉。外膜厚度与中膜相近，一般无外弹性膜。

四、微动脉

微动脉管径一般小于 0.3 mm。无内、外弹性膜，中膜仅由 1～2 层环形平滑肌组成。

五、动脉管壁结构与功能的关系

1. 大动脉

由于大动脉管壁有多层弹性膜和大量弹性纤维，当心脏收缩时，大动脉被动扩张，同时积累了强大的势能。而当心脏舒张时，大动脉反弹回缩，释放势能，使血液继续向前流动，从而保持了血流的平稳和连续性。

2. 中动脉

中动脉的中膜有大量的平滑肌，平滑肌的收缩和舒张，可改变血管管径的大小，从而调节分配到身体各部的血流量，故又称分配动脉。

3. 小动脉和微动脉

小动脉和微动脉可显著调节血流的外周阻力，从而调节局部组织的血流量，并维持正常血压，故两者又称外周阻力血管。

第三节　静　脉

静脉，又称容量血管，由小到大逐级汇合，管径逐渐增粗，管壁也逐渐增厚，把血液从毛细血管运回心脏。根据管径大小，静脉可分为大静脉、中静脉、小静脉和微静脉。中静脉和小静脉常与相应的动脉伴行，但数量比动脉多。

静脉的管壁也分内膜、中膜和外膜，但管壁结构的变异比动脉大。静脉管壁有如下特点（图 9-6）。

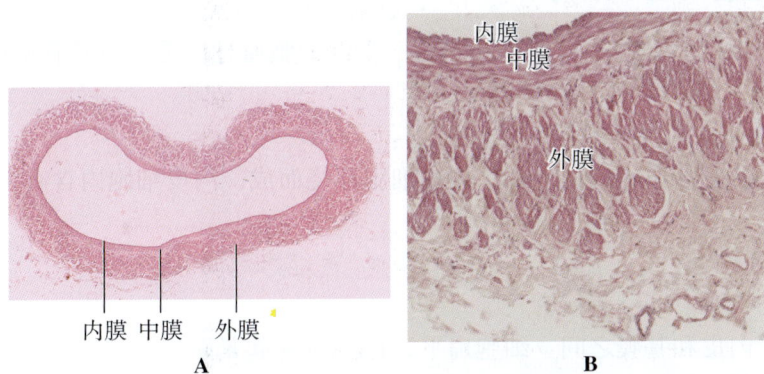

图 9-6　大静脉管壁结构光镜图
HE 染色，A. 40×，B. 100×

（1）静脉管壁薄、管腔大而不规则。

（2）血管壁的三层结构不明显，内、外弹性膜都不发达。一般中膜薄，外膜厚，外膜内有纵行的平滑肌。

（3）管径大于 2 mm 的静脉，通常有静脉瓣。静脉瓣由内膜突入管腔折叠而成，为两个彼此相对的半月形薄片，可防止静脉中的血液倒流（图 9-7）。

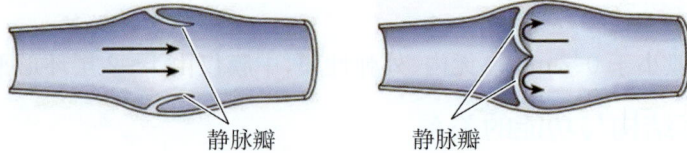

图 9-7 静脉瓣模式图

第四节 毛 细 血 管

毛细血管连接于动脉和静脉之间，是体内分布最广、管径最细的血管，其分支常吻合成网（图 9-8）。在不同的器官和组织内，毛细血管网的密度差异很大。在代谢旺盛的器官，如肝、肾、心、肺，毛细血管网很密；而在代谢较低的器官，如平滑肌、肌腱、韧带等，毛细血管网则比较稀疏。

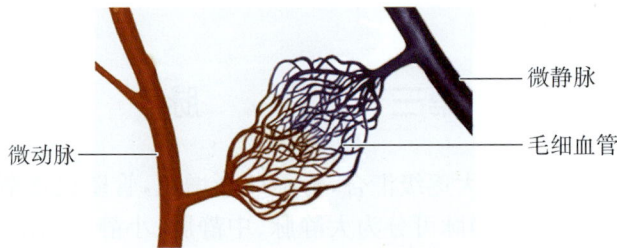

图 9-8 毛细血管模式图

一、毛细血管的基本结构

毛细血管的管径一般为 6~8 μm，仅容许一个红细胞通过。毛细血管管壁由内皮细胞、基膜和周细胞构成。

1. 内皮细胞
横断面上，毛细血管一般有 1~2 个内皮细胞环绕而成。内皮细胞内含有大量质膜小泡。

2. 基膜
仅有基板，无网板。

3. 周细胞
周细胞位于内皮和基膜之间。细胞扁平、有突起，突起紧贴内皮。周细胞具有收缩功能，可调节毛细血管的血流。当毛细血管受损时，周细胞可增殖分化为内皮细胞、平滑肌纤维和成纤维细胞。

二、毛细血管的分类

根据电镜下内皮细胞和基膜的结构特点,毛细血管可分为三类(图9-9)。

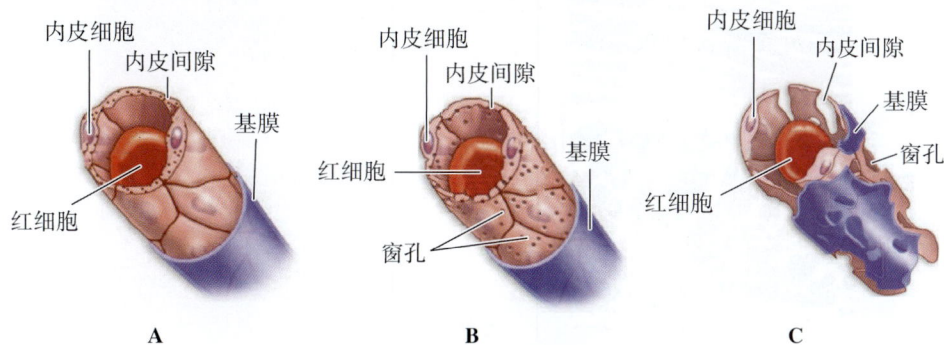

图9-9 三种毛细血管结构模式图
A.连续毛细血管;B.有孔毛细血管;C.血窦

1. 连续毛细血管

连续毛细血管的特点如下:①由一层连续的内皮细胞围成,细胞间有紧密连接。②内皮细胞的胞质中含有大量的质膜小泡。③基膜完整。连续毛细血管主要通过质膜小泡在血液和组织间进行物质交换,主要分布于结缔组织、肌组织、外分泌腺、中枢神经系统、胸腺和肺等,还可参与机体内多种屏障性结构的形成。

2. 有孔毛细血管

有孔毛细血管的特点如下:①由一层连续的内皮细胞围成,细胞间也有紧密连接。②内皮细胞不含核的部分极薄,有许多贯穿胞质的内皮窗孔。窗孔上有的有隔膜封闭,有的则没有隔膜。③基膜完整。有孔毛细血管的内皮窗孔有利于血管内外的中、小分子物质进行交换,主要分布于胃肠黏膜、某些内分泌腺和肾血管球等处。

3. 血窦

血窦也称窦状毛细血管,特点如下:①管腔大,形状不规则。②内皮细胞上常有窗孔,细胞间隙大,故又称不连续毛细血管。③基膜不完整或缺如。血窦有利于大分子物质或血细胞进出血管,主要分布于肝、脾、骨髓和某些内分泌腺。不同器官内的血窦结构差异较大。

第五节 心 脏

心脏是心血管系统的动力中心。心脏持续而有节律的收缩和舒张,使血液在血管中循环,以满足各器官和组织的血液供应。

一、心脏壁的结构

心脏壁从内向外分别由心内膜、心肌膜和心外膜三层结构组成(图9-10)。

1. 心内膜

由内向外,又可分三层:①内皮,位于心脏内表面,与血管内皮相延续。②内皮下层,位于内皮的下方,由薄层细密结缔组织构成,含丰富弹性纤维和少量平滑肌纤维。③心内膜下层,

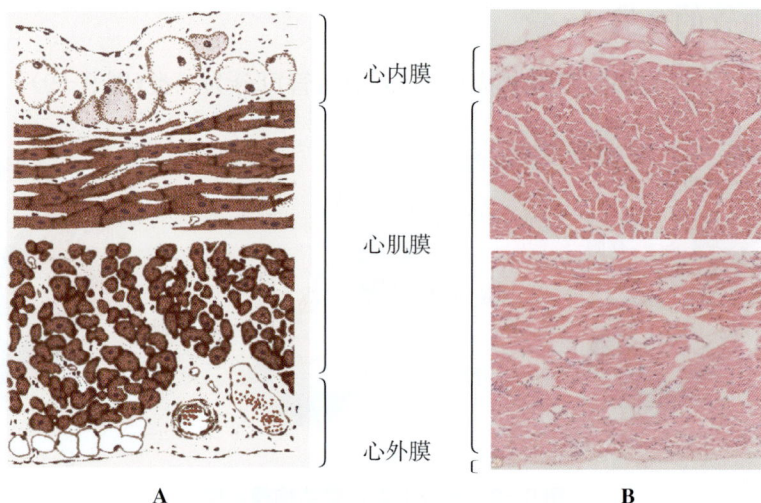

图 9-10　心脏壁的结构
A. 心脏壁结构模式图；B. 心脏壁结构光镜图(HE 染色,40×)

位于内皮下层和心肌膜之间,为疏松结缔组织,内有小血管和神经。在心室的心内膜下层,还有心脏传导系统的分支即浦肯野纤维。

2. 心肌膜

三层中最厚,由心肌纤维构成。①心肌纤维呈螺旋状排列,可分为内纵、中环和外斜三层。心肌纤维大多聚集成束,肌束间有少量结缔组织和丰富的毛细血管。②心肌膜在心房较薄,心室较厚,其中又以左心室最厚。心室肌内也有浦肯野纤维。心房肌纤维比心室肌纤维短而细。在电镜下,心房肌纤维含心房特殊颗粒,颗粒内含心房钠尿肽,具有很强的利尿、排钠、扩血管和降血压的作用。③在心房肌和心室肌之间,由致密结缔组织构成坚实的支架结构,称心骨骼。心房肌和心室肌分别附着于心骨骼,两部分心肌并不连续。

3. 心外膜

即心包的脏层,为浆膜,表面覆盖间皮,深层为薄层疏松结缔组织,内含血管、神经和脂肪组织。

二、心瓣膜

心瓣膜是心内膜向腔内凸起形成的薄片状结构,基部与心骨骼的纤维环相连。心瓣膜表面为内皮,内部为致密结缔组织,含有胶原纤维、弹性纤维及少量平滑肌纤维。心瓣膜位于房室孔和动脉口处,有房室瓣(二尖瓣、三尖瓣)和动脉瓣(主动脉瓣、肺动脉瓣)两种。心瓣膜的功能是阻止心房、心室和动脉之间的血液逆流。患风湿性心脏病时,心瓣膜内胶原纤维增生,使瓣膜变硬、变形,可导致瓣膜不能正常地关闭和开放。

三、心脏传导系统

心脏传导系统由心壁内特殊的心肌纤维组成。该系统包括窦房结、房室结、房室束、左右束支及其分支。窦房结为正常心跳的起搏点,位于右心房上腔静脉入口处的心外膜深部,其余分布在心内膜下层(图 9-11)。

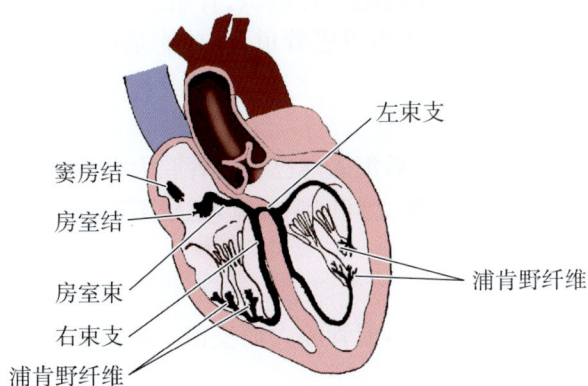

图 9-11 心脏传导系统模式图

组成心脏传导系统的特殊心肌纤维主要有 3 种类型,即起搏细胞、移行细胞和浦肯野纤维。这些细胞聚集成结或束,受交感、副交感和肽能神经纤维的调节。

1. 起搏细胞

简称 P 细胞,位于窦房结和房室结中央部位的结缔组织中,是心脏兴奋的起搏点。胞体较普通心肌纤维小,呈梭形或多边形,有分支连接成网,HE 染色浅,胞质中细胞器和肌原纤维少,糖原多。

2. 移行细胞

位于窦房结和房室结周边及房室束,具有传导冲动的作用。结构介于起搏细胞和普通心肌纤维之间,比普通心肌纤维细而短,胞质内含肌原纤维较起搏细胞略多。

3. 浦肯野纤维

又称束细胞,组成房室束及其分支,位于心室的心内膜下层和心肌膜。与普通心肌纤维相比,浦肯野纤维粗、短,形状不规则,有 1~2 个细胞核,胞质内含丰富的线粒体和糖原,肌原纤维较少,故 HE 染色浅(图 9-12)。细胞间有发达的闰盘,浦肯野纤维与心室肌纤维相连,可快速将冲动传导到心室各部,使心室肌同步收缩和舒张。

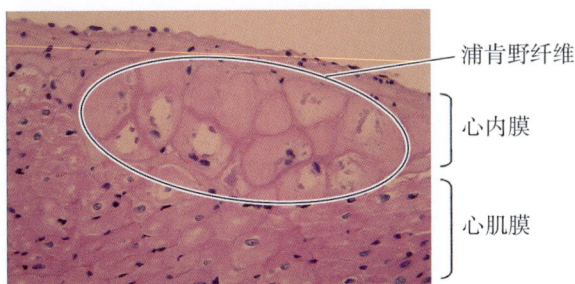

图 9-12 浦肯野纤维光镜图(HE 染色,400×)

第六节 淋巴管系统

淋巴管系统包括毛细淋巴管、淋巴管和淋巴导管。组织液回流到淋巴管内即称为淋巴,最后再通过淋巴导管回流至静脉。人体内除软骨组织、骨组织、骨髓、表皮、眼球、内耳及牙等处没有淋巴管道外,其余组织或器官大多有淋巴管道,其功能是将组织液中的水、电解质和大分子物质等输送入血液。

1. 毛细淋巴管

以盲端始于组织内,吻合成网,然后汇入淋巴管。管腔大而不规则,壁薄,仅由内皮和极薄的结缔组织构成,无周细胞。内皮细胞之间间隙较宽,基膜不连续,故通透性大,有利于大分子物质进出。

2. 淋巴管

结构与相应管径的中、小静脉相似,但管腔大而壁薄。由内皮、少量平滑肌和结缔组织构成,管腔内瓣膜较多。

3. 淋巴导管

包括胸导管和右淋巴导管。结构与大静脉相似,但管壁更薄,三层膜分界更不明显。

（傅　奕）

Chapter 10

Immune System

Immune system consists of groups of immune cells, lymphoid tissues and lymphoid organs, providing defense or immunity against invasion and damage by microorganisms and foreign substances. The immune cells comprise lymphocytes, antigen presenting cells (APC), granulocytes, mast cells and so on, which are present in the lymphoid tissues, or blood, lymph and other tissues. There are two types of lymphoid tissues: diffuse lymphoid tissue and lymphoid nodule. These tissues are the main components of peripheral lymphatic organs, and also widely distributed in the digestive and respiratory mucosae. Meanwhile, there are two categories of lymphoid organs: central lymphoid organs including thymus and bone marrow and peripheral lymphoid organs containing lymph nodes, spleen, tonsils, and so on.

The principle function of immune system includes: ①Immune defense: immune system protects the body against harmful effects of antigens, such as bacteria, viruses, abnormal cells and macromolecules. ② Immune surveillance: immune system recognizes and eliminates tumor-cells and virus-infected cells in the body. ③Immune homeostasis: immune system recognizes and removes senescent or dead cells in the body to maintain the homeostasis.

The immune system plays roles by immune reactions. There are two basic types: ①Cellular immunity: it is mediated mainly by T lymphocytes (T cells). In this process, T cells react against and kill microorganisms, foreign cells and virus-infected cells by releasing various immune effector molecules. ②Humoral immunity: it is mediated by B lymphocytes (B cells). Antigen stimulates B cells to proliferate and differentiate into plasma cells, which synthesize specific antibodies that inactivate foreign antigens. These two types of immune responses play an important role in coordination with each other.

The main function of the immune system is to distinguish "foreign" (i.e. non-self) from self, which is based on: ①major histocompatibility complex molecules (MHC), with species and individual specificity, are hallmarks of the body's own cells. That is, all the cells in the same individual have the same MHC molecules, but different individuals have different MHC molecules. MHC includes two key types called MHC class I and class II. All nucleated cells produce and expose on their surfaces MHC class I molecules presenting such "self-antigens", which T cells recognize as a signal to ignore those cells. MHC class II molecules are synthesized and transported to the cell surface similarly, but only in cells of the mononuclear phagocyte system and certain other cells, such as B cells and dendritic cells. ②There are more than one million types of specific antigen receptors on the surface of T and B cells, but each lymphocyte expresses only one type of antigen receptor. Therefore, each lymphocyte produces an immune reaction to only one antigen. But as an individual, lymphocytes can respond to a variety of antigens.

1 Main Immune Cells

1.1 Lymphocytes

Lymphocytes can be divided into three classes on the basis of their site of differentiation, function, and the presence of distinctive receptors in their membranes: T cells, B cells, and NK cells.

1.1.1　T cells

T cells constitute nearly 75% of blood lymphocytes. They originate in the bone-marrow, then migrate to the thymus, where they mature and are carried by the blood to other lymphoid tissues and lymphoid organs. Naive T cells are those that have not yet come into contact with antigens in the thymus. Once stimulated by an antigen, the naive T cells transform into metabolically active large lymphocytes, and proliferate and differentiate.

The mature T cells are small in size, most of them are effector T cells, the rest are memory T cells. Effector T cells exist only one week, whose function is to eliminate antigens quickly. Memory T cells, on the other hand, have a long lifespan, and can exist for years or even a lifetime. If the antigen appears again, memory T cells can rapidly react and stimulate the production of a large number of effector T cells, resulting in a stronger immune response, which makes the body maintain immunity to the antigen for a long time.

Important subpopulations of T cells include the following:

(1) Cytotoxic T cells (Tc, CTL, or Killer T cells): they act directly by producing perforin that opens holes in target cells (foreign cells, tumor cells or virus-infected cells), leading to cell lysis. Furthermore, Cytotoxic T cells also kill target cells by releasing granzymes, which trigger apoptosis of the target cells.

(2) Helper T cells (Th): they greatly assist immune responses by producing cytokines, that promote differentiation of B cells into plasma cells, activate cytotoxic T cells, and induce inflammatory reactions.

(3) Regulatory T cells (Tr or suppressor T cells): they are few in number, and serve to inhibit specific immune responses. As a result, the abnormalities in their number and function often lead to autoimmune diseases.

1.1.2　B cells

B cells represent 10%-15% of lymphocytes in the blood. B cells undergo maturation in the bone marrow, becoming naive B cells, then migrate to non-thymic lymphoid structures, where they reside, and proliferate when activated. Most of them differentiate into antibody-secreting plasma cells, which are responsible for humoral immunity. A few of them generate memory B cells, which react very rapidly to a second exposure to the same antigen.

1.1.3   NK cells

NK cells represent the remaining 10% of the circulating lymphocyte pool. NK cells are large granular lymphocytes derived from bone marrow. They can be activated and kill transformed or abnormal cells without antigen stimuli, or aid of antibodies and complement. NK cells are the first line of defense against tumor and virus infection.

1.1.4   Lymphocyte Recirculation

Lymphocytes leave lymph nodes by efferent lymphatic vessels and eventually enter the blood stream. Lymphocytes return to the lymph nodes by exiting the blood via the postcapillary venules (high endothelial venules) located in the diffuse lymphoid tissues. Briefly, the cycle of lymphocytes migrating between the blood and lymphoid organs (or lymphoid tissues), is called lymphocyte recirculation (Figure 10 - 1).

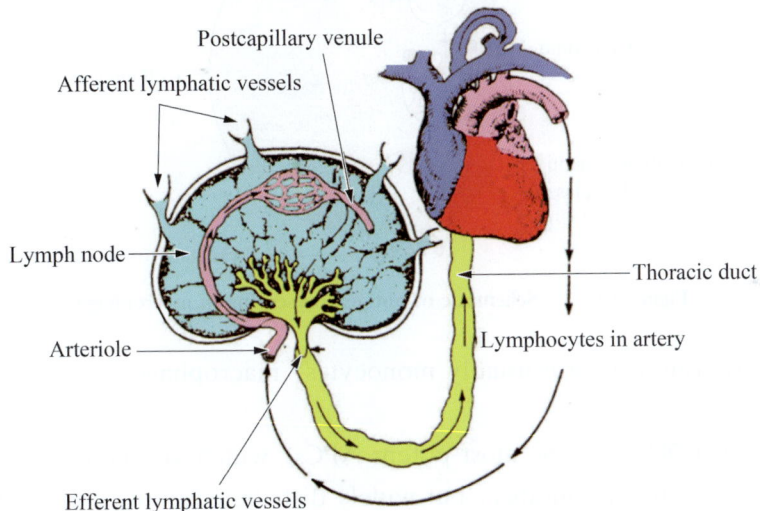

Figure 10 - 1   Schematic of lymphocyte recirculation

Recirculation enables lymphocytes to move from one part of the lymphoid system to another, and reach the sites within the body where they are needed. Moreover, the continuous recirculation of lymphocytes lead to a constant monitoring of all parts of the body by cells that alert the immune system of the presence of foreign antigens.

1.2 Macrophages and Mononuclear Phagocyte System (MPS)

Macrophages are derived from monocytes that circulate in the blood. Compared to monocytes, macrophages have undergone significant changes in morphology and function, exhibiting increased cell-size, more complex function and enhanced phagocytic activity.

Macrophages, which are distributed throughout the body, are present in most organs and constitute the mononuclear phagocyte system (MPS). MPS includes: macrophages, osteoclasts, microglia, Kupffer cells, pulmonary macrophages, and so on. To be classified as components of this system, all cells must be derived from monocytes, and exhibit intense phagocytic capacity. Furthermore, MPS cells also act as antigen presenting cells, and secrete several bioactive substances.

1.3 Antigen Presenting Cells

Antigen presenting cells (APCs) ingest antigens, partially digest them in lysosomes. Then small peptides from the antigens are combined with MHC class Ⅱ molecules, and return to the cell surface, which can be recognized by lymphocytes, then lymphocytes are activated (Figure 10 - 2).

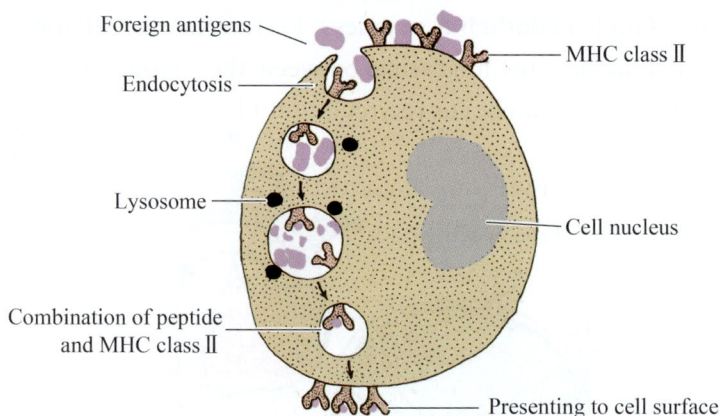

Figure 10 - 2   Schematic of antigen presenting in macrophage

Antigen presenting cells are usually monocytes, macrophages, dendritic cells, and B cells.

Dendritic cells (DCs) are the most potent APCs, which are named for their dendritic morphology. DCs are few in number, but widely distributed in different parts of the body with different names. They include epidermal Langerhans cells, DCs in interstitial tissues of the heart, liver, lung and kidney, veiled cells in lymph, interdigitating cells in peripheral lymphoid tissue and DCs in the blood. They are in different stages of development, belonging to different subtypes of DCs.

2 Lymphoid Tissues

Lymphoid tissue is the site where the immune response occurs. It consists of reticular tissues that form a meshwork to house other free cells. These cells include lymphocytes, macrophages, dendritic cells and plasma cells. Among them, lymphocytes are the major component. There are two types of lymphoid tissues: diffuse lymphoid tissue and lymphoid nodules.

2.1 Diffuse Lymphoid Tissue

Diffuse lymphoid tissue is composed mainly of T cells and is not sharply delineated from the surrounding connective tissue. A specific type of blood vessels, postcapillary venules, are common in diffuse lymphoid tissue. These venules have an unusual endothelial lining of tall cuboidal cells, so they are also called high endothelial venules (Figure 10 - 3), which are important channels for lymphocytes to travel between the blood and lymphoid tissues.

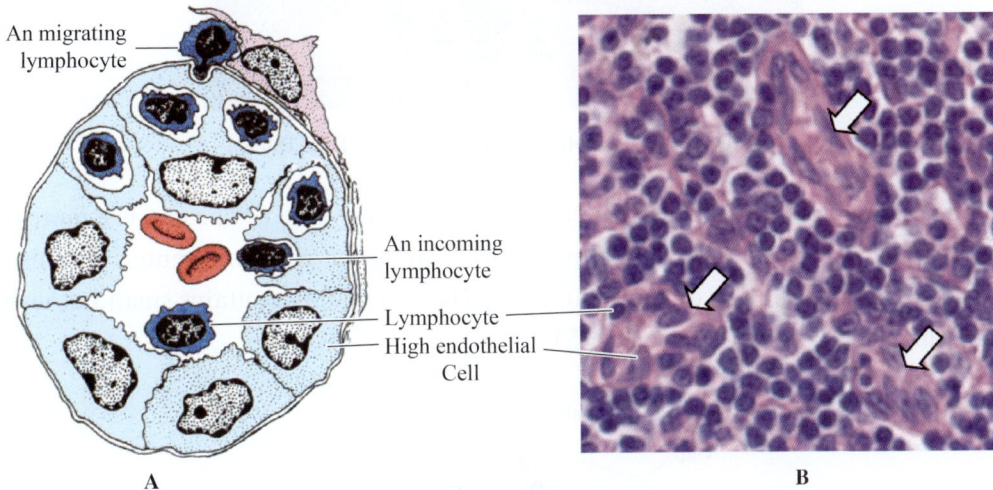

Figure 10 - 3 The structure of high endothelial venules
A. Schematic structure; B. Postcapillary venules (arrows, HE, 400×)

2.2 Lymphoid Nodules

Lymphoid nodules, also named as lymphatic follicles, are spherical with well-defined boundaries and are mainly composed of B cells, but also a certain amount of Th cells, follicular dendritic cells and macrophages (Figure 10 - 4). When stimulated by antigens, lymphoid nodules can develop an inner mass of pale staining cells, the germinal center, which is surrounded by a darkly stained mantle of small lymphocytes. Lymphoid nodules without germinal centers are called primary lymphoid nodules. Those with germinal centers are called secondary lymphoid nodules.

The germinal center is composed of the dark zone, the light zone and the cap. ①The dark zone is a small area, consisting mainly of large, naive B cells and Th cells. Due to the strong basophilia of the cells, this zone stains darkly. ②The light zone is larger than the dark zone, and is on the outer perimeter of the germinal center, staining lightly. It is

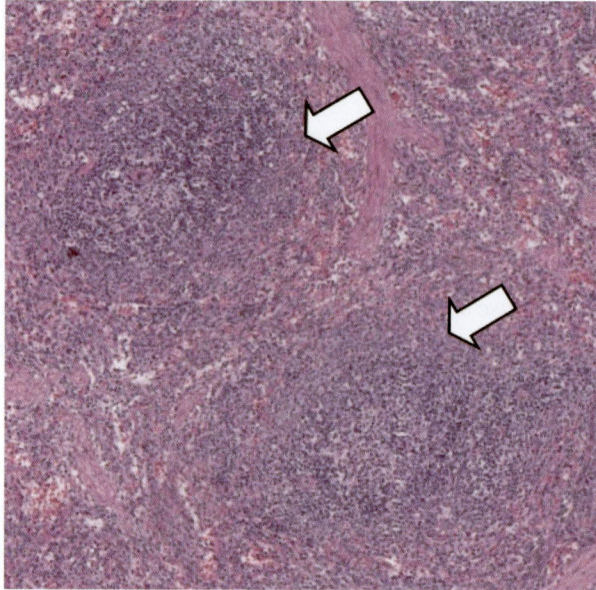

Figure 10 - 4   Lymphoid nodules (arrows, HE, 100×)

composed of medium-sized B cells, Th cells, macrophages, etc. ③The cap is a more darkly stained peripheral mantle, crescent-shaped, surrounding the germinal center. In this zone, the thickest part is at the top of the light zone. The cap mainly contains small but mature B cells, and memory B cells (Figure 10 - 5).

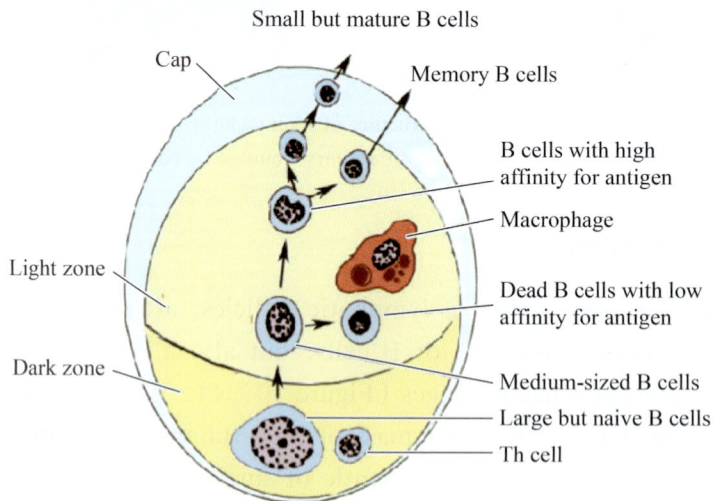

Figure 10 - 5   Schematic of the secondary lymphoid nodule and the distribution of B cells

The structure of lymphoid nodules is dynamic. After antigenic stimulation, primary lymphoid nodules form much larger and more prominent secondary lymphoid nodules. After 2 to 3 weeks of proliferation, most cells of the germinal center and mantle are dispersed and the structure of the secondary lymphoid nodule is gradually lost.

3   Lymphoid Organs

Lymphoid organs are composed of lymphoid tissues. There are two types: ①Central lymphoid organs: they include thymus and bone marrow, where T and B cells originate respectively. Lymphoid hematopoietic stem cells, that undergo different developmental pathways, form naive T cells in the thymus and naive B cells in the bone marrow. ② Peripheral lymphoid organs: they contain lymph nodes, spleen, tonsils, where immune reactions occur. Compared with the central lymphoid organs, the development of the peripheral lymphoid organs is later, and they are not fully developed until several months after birth.

3.1   Thymus

Fully formed and functional at birth, the thymus reaches maximal size at puberty. It then undergoes involution with slow replacement by adipose tissue, only a small amount of cortex and medulla remaining.

3.1.1   Structure of the Thymus

The thymus is a flat, bilobed structure. It has a connective tissue capsule that extends septa into the parenchyma, dividing the organ into many incompletely separated thymic lobules. Each lobule is composed of a peripheral dark zone known as the cortex and a central light zone, called the medulla, medullary areas of adjacent lobules may be confluent with each other (Figure 10 - 6).

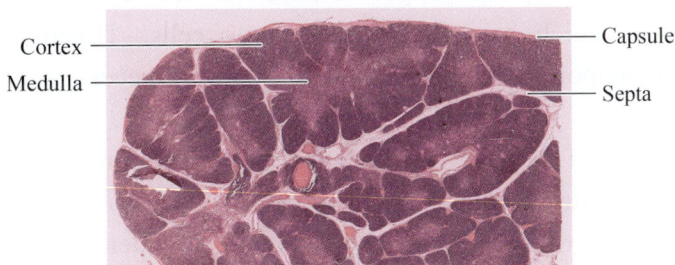

Figure 10 - 6   The thymus (HE, 40×)

The thymus provides a unique microenvironment for T cells development. The cells that make up this microenvironment are called thymic stromal cells, which mainly contain thymic epithelial cells, macrophages, interdigitating cells, mast cells, fibroblasts and so on. Thymic epithelial cells are the most important stromal cells. They not only form the scaffold of thymus microenvironment, but also secrete hormones, such as thymosin, thymopoietin, as well as some cytokines, which can regulate the differentiation and development of T cells.

3.1.1.1   Cortex

Cortex is located in the periphery of the lobules. The cortex contains an extensive population of dark-staining small lymphocytes (thymocytes), scattered thymic epithelial cells, and a few other stromal cells (Figure 10 – 7).

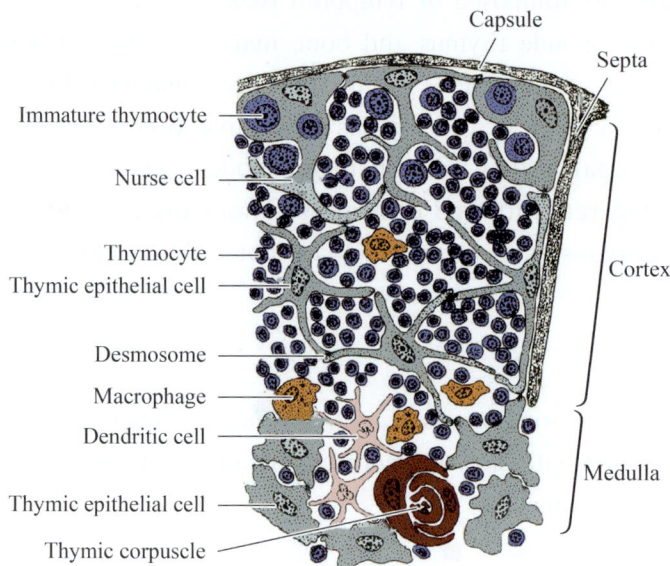

Figure 10 – 7　Schematic of the structure of thymus

(1) Thymic epithelial cells, also known as epithelial reticular cells, are primarily located beneath the capsule and interspersed among the thymocytes. They are stellate cells with long processes, and joined to similar adjacent cells by desmosomes. Some thymic epithelial cells under the capsule support clusters of maturing thymocytes with their cytoplasmic processes, which are called thymic nurse cells. Thymic epithelial cells can secrete thymosin, thymopoietin, and other factors that are necessary for the development of thymocytes.

(2) Thymocytes are T cells in different stages of differentiation and development, which are densely distributed in the cortex, accounting for 85%–90% of the total number of cortical cells. During the development, thymocytes undergo a stringent, two-stage selection process of quality control: positive selection and negative selection.

Positive selection occurs in the cortex, allowing only the survival of T cells that recognize MHC class I and class II molecules. Negative selection occurs in the deep cortex and medulla, allowing only the survival of T cells that do not react with self-antigens. Finally, only about 5% of all developing thymocytes pass both the positive and negative selection, becoming naive T cells. Most of thymocytes died by apoptosis and were removed by macrophages.

3.1.1.2　Medulla

Medulla is located in the center of each lobule, mainly consisting of a large number of more lightly stained thymic epithelial cells, as well as a few mature thymocytes, interdigitating cells, and macrophages.

(1) Thymic epithelial cells different from cortical epithelial cells in shape, they are spherical or polygonal with short processes, which are linked by desmosomes. These cells also secrete thymosin, thymopoietin, just as cortical epithelial cells do.

(2) Thymic corpuscles (Hassall's corpuscles) are unique to the medulla, and scattered in this region, increasing with age. These structures are concentrically arranged, consisting of flattened thymic epithelial cells. The outer cells of thymic corpuscles, with crescent-shaped nuclei, eosinophilic cytoplasm, are capable of division. The cells near the center of thymic corpuscles are degenerated and filled with keratohyalin granules and filaments. The cells in the core of thymic corpuscles are completely keratinized and strongly eosinophilic. Some have a central hyaline core (Figure 10-8). Their function is not well understood.

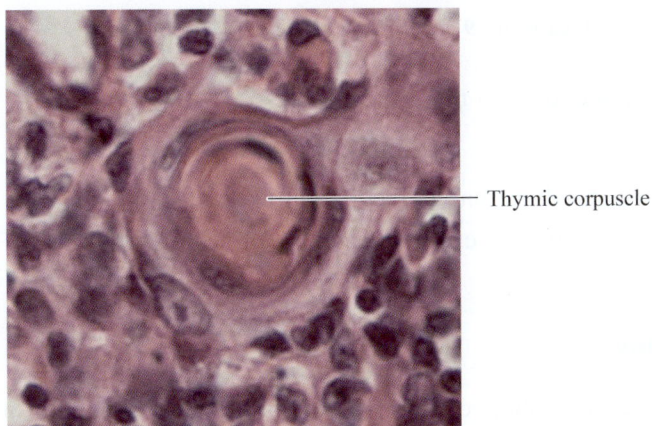

Figure 10 - 8   Thymic corpuscle (HE, 400×)

Blood supply to the thymus: the thymus is rich in blood supply. Arterioles enter the thymus through the capsule, and branch following the interlobular septa to the border between the cortical and medullary zones, finally reaching the cortex and medulla. The capillaries in the cortex converge at the cortex-medulla junction into high endothelial venules, from which naive T cells in the thymus enter the blood stream. Most of the capillaries in medulla are fenestrated and leave thymus through interlobular septa and capsule after merging into venules.

3.1.1.3   Blood-Thymus Barrier

Blood-thymus barrier is comprised as following (Figure 10-9):

continuous capillaries (endothelial cells are held together by zonulae occludens).
basal lamina of the capillaries.
thin perivascular space sheath containing macrophages.
basal lamina of thymic epithelial cells.
the processes of thymic epithelial cells.

This system prevents circulating antigens or some drugs from reaching the thymus

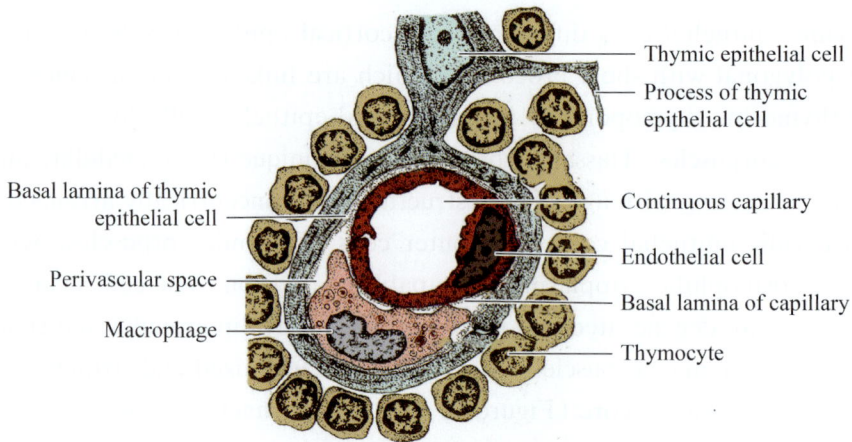

Figure 10 - 9　Schematic of the blood-thymus barrier

cortex, where T lymphocytes are being developed.

3.1.2　Function of the Thymus

Thymus is the organ where naive T cells mature.

Endocrine function: thymic epithelial cells can secrete thymosin, thymopoietin, and other hormones.

3.2　Lymph Nodes

Lymph nodes are bean-shaped, distributed throughout the body along the lymphatic vessels. A total of 500 to 600 lymph nodes are present, often in chains or groups, in strategic regions such as the hilus of the lung, groin, axillae, neck, mesenteries and so on. The size and structure of lymph nodes are closely related to the immune state of the body.

3.2.1　Structure of the Lymph Nodes

Each lymph node is covered by a thin layer of connective tissue, which is called capsule. Blood vessels enter (afferent) and leave (efferent) at the dent in the "bean", which is called the hilum. Efferent lymphatic vessels are also found at the hilum. Afferent lymphatic vessels penetrate the capsule and drain into the subcapsular sinus. The connective tissue capsule sends connected, radiating and stubby trabeculae into the interior of the node. Between trabeculae are lymphatic tissue and lymphatic sinuses. The parenchyma of each lymph node consists of an outer cortex and inner medulla (Figure 10 - 10,10 - 11).

3.2.1.1　Cortex

Cortex, just under the capsule consists of the superfacial cortex, paracortex zone and cortical sinuses.

(1) Superfacial cortex is adjacent to the subcapsular sinuses, and is composed of lymphoid nodules (with or without germinal centers), among which is diffuse lymphoid

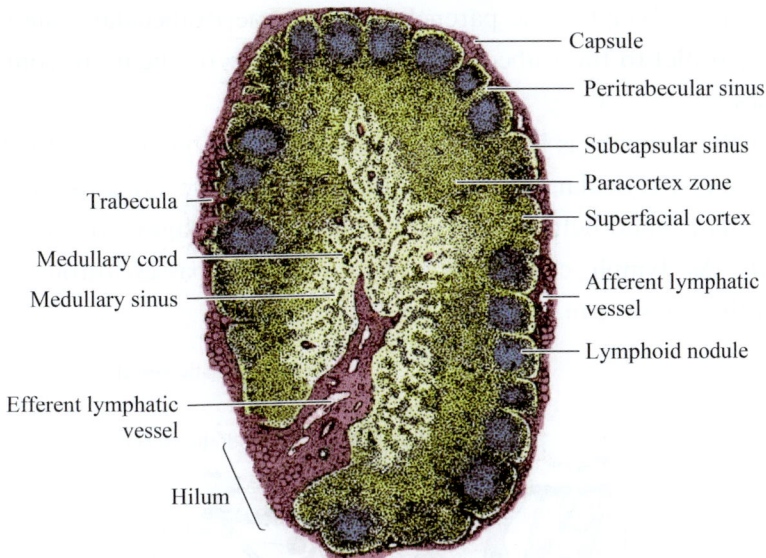

Figure 10 – 10   Schematic of the structure of a lymph node

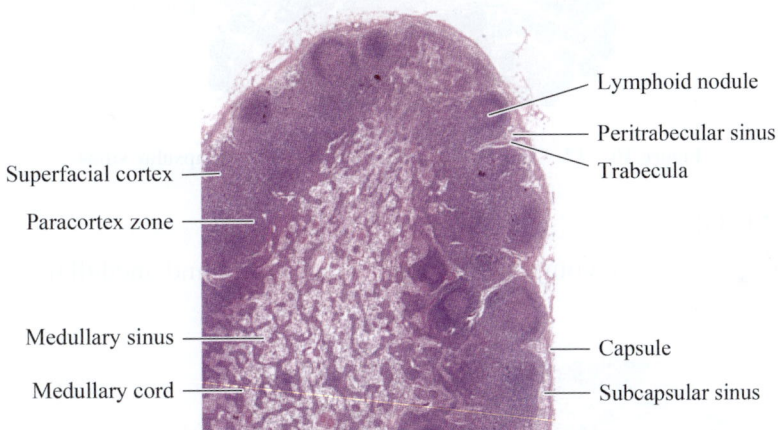

Figure 10 – 11   The lymph node (HE, 40×)

tissue. Superfacial cortex consists mostly of B lymphocytes, so it is B cell region of the cortex.

(2) Paracortex zone is located in the deep cortex, and is mainly the diffuse lymphoid tissue. This zone contains few, if any, nodules and many T lymphocytes, so it is the T cell region of the cortex. If the thymus of a newborn animal is removed, this area fails to develop, so it is also called thymus dependent area. Furthermore, there are many high endothelial venules in this area (Figure 10 – 3), which are important channels for lymphocytes in the blood to enter the paracortex zone.

(3) Cortical sinuses include the subcapsular sinuses and the peritrabecular sinuses, and

they are connected. The subcapsular sinuses are just under the capsule, forming a flat sac surrounding the entire lymph node parenchyma. The peritrabecular sinuses, usually with blind ends, run parallel to the trabeculae, and only a few of them are connected with the medullary sinuses.

The wall of these sinuses is lined by a flattened, discontinuous endothelium with a thin layer of stroma, a few reticular fibers and a flat layer of reticular cells. The sinus lumen is supported by stellate endothelial cells with many macrophages attached to the surface (Figure 10 - 12). As lymph containing antigens slowly passes through these sinuses, macrophages in the sinuses can clear antigens.

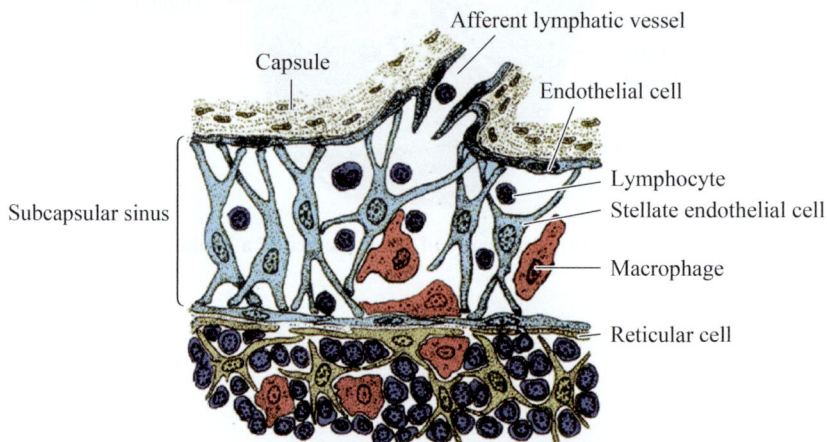

Figure 10 - 12　Schematic of the structure of subcapsular sinus

3.2.1.2　Medulla

Medulla has two major components: medullary cords and medullary sinuses (Figure 10 - 13).

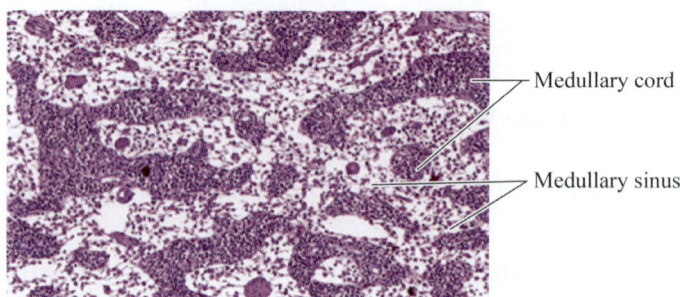

Figure 10 - 13　The lymph node medulla (HE, 100×)

(1) Medullary cords: they are branched cordlike masses of lymphoid tissue extending from the paracortex zone, also with high endothelial venules. They mainly contain B lymphocytes, macrophages and many plasma cells.

(2) Medullary sinuses: they are dilated spaces lined by discontinuous endothelium that

separate the medullary cords. They are continuous with the cortical sinuses, and have similar structure. However, the sinus lumen is wider, and with more macrophages than in cortical sinuses, which means a stronger lymph filtering function.

3.2.1.3   Pathway for Lymph Through a Lymph Node

Afferent lymph vessels cross the capsule of each node and pour lymph into the cortical sinuses (the subcapsular sinuses and the peritrabecular sinuses), then medullary sinuses, finally leave the node through efferent lymphatic vessels. The complex architecture of both the cortical and medullary sinuses slow the flow of lymph through the node, facilitating the uptake and removal of most of the bacteria and other antigens. Meanwhile, lymphocytes in the lymphoid tissue and the antibodies that they produce, are constantly converging into the lymph. As a result, the efferent lymph from nodes contains more lymphocytes and antibodies than the afferent lymph.

3.2.2   Function of the Lymph Nodes

(1) Lymph filtraion: lymph nodes are the body's filters. When lymph flows through lymph nodes, antigens (such as bacteria, viruses, toxins, etc.) can be removed by macrophages. The medullary sinuses are the main sites for lymph filtration.

(2) Immune response: lymph nodes are important sites for immune response. After antigens enter the lymph nodes, macrophages and other antigen presenting cells take up and process the antigens, then present them to the naive T cells or B cells, and activate them. The naive T and B cells then proliferate and differentiate to become a large number of effector lymphocytes and memory lymphocytes. Cellular and humoral immune responses often occur at the same time, but one or the other predominates depending on the nature of the antigen. When the cellular immune response is dominant, the paracortex zone is significantly enlarged and effector T cells increase. While the humoral immune response is dominant, both the number and the size of lymphoid nodules are increased, and the plasma cells in the medulla are also accumulated, accordingly producing more antibodies.

3.3 Spleen

During early fetal development, spleen is temporarily an organ of hematopoiesis, then this role is taken over by the bone marrow. In adults, the spleen is the largest lymphoid organ.

3.3.1   Structure of the Spleen

The spleen is surrounded by a thick capsule of dense connective tissue, which contains elastic fibers and smooth muscle fibers. The surface of the capsule is covered with mesothelium. At the hilum, on the medial surface of the spleen, the capsule gives rise to a number of trabeculae that extend into the splenic pulp. The spleen parenchyma consists of abundant red pulp and white pulp (Figure 10 - 14,10 - 15), without lymphatic sinuses.

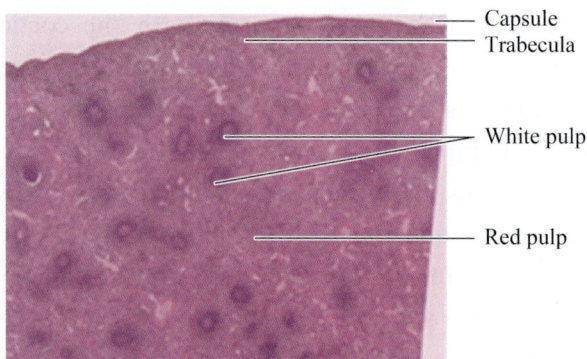

Figure 10 – 14   The spleen (HE, 40×)

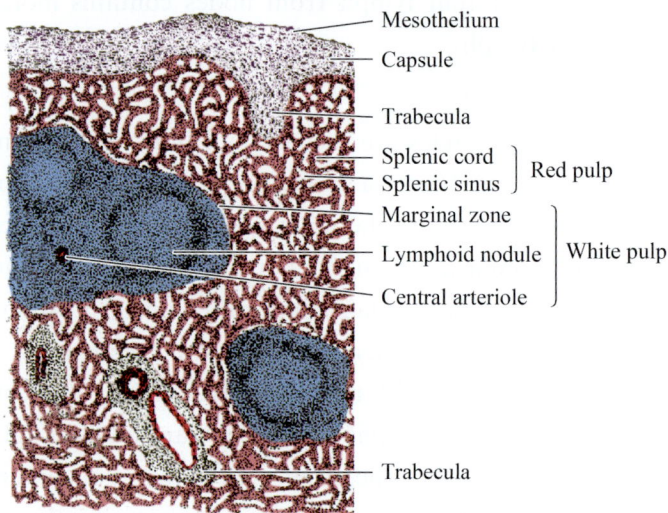

Figure 10 – 15   Schematic of the structure of spleen

3.3.1.1 White Pulp

On the surface of a cut through an unfixed spleen, there are scattered grayish-white spots, which are white pulp. In an HE stained section, the white pulp is a blue-purple mass structure. The small masses of white pulp consist of lymphoid nodules, the periarterial lymphatic sheath, and marginal zone (Figure 10 – 16), which correspond to the cortex of a lymph node.

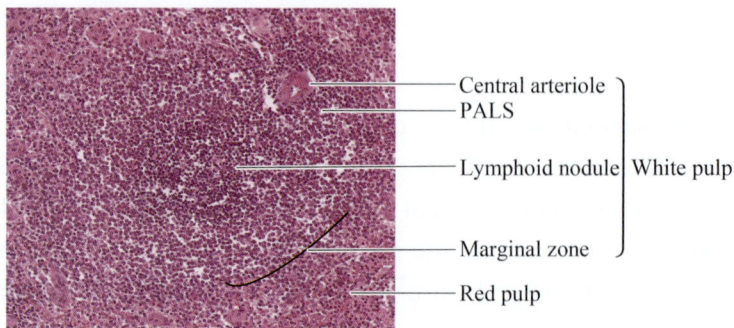

Figure 10 – 16   The white pulp (HE, 100×)

(1) Periarterial lymphatic sheath (PALS): small branches of the trabecular arteries are referred to as central arterioles. They are enveloped by a sheath of lymphocytes to form periarterial lymphatic sheath, which is primarily composed of T cells with some macrophages and interdigitating cells. Corresponding to the paracortex zone of lymph nodes, periarterial lymphatic sheath is also called thymus dependent area, but there are no high endothelial venules.

(2) Lymphoid nodules are located on one side of the periarterial lymphatic sheath, and are populated primarily by B cells. There are fewer lymphoid nodules in the spleen in healthy individuals. When stimulated by an antigen, the number of lymphoid nodules in the spleen increase significantly.

(3) Marginal zone is a narrow area located at the boundary between white pulp and red pulp. Some branches of the central arterioles terminate as marginal sinuses that are channels for antigens and lymphocytes in the blood to enter the white pulp. Conversely, lymphocytes in the white pulp can also participate in lymphocyte recirculation via marginal sinuses.

3.3.1.2 Red Pulp

A dark red tissue in the fresh state, comprises the majority of the spleen, accounting for 80% of spleen parenchyma. It consists of splenic cords and blood-filled splenic sinuses.

(1) Splenic cords are lymphoid tissues rich in blood cells and are irregular cords that are interconnected to form a meshwork. Separated by the splenic sinuses, splenic cords contain B cells, plasma cells, macrophages, and dendritic cells. To blood-borne antigens, macrophages and dendritic cells can stimulate the immune response through antigen presentation. Therefore, the splenic cords are the main sites for blood filtration.

(2) Splenic sinuses are venous sinuses with wide, irregular lumens and are interconnected. Unusual elongated endothelial cells line these sinuses, and sparsely wrapped in reticular fibers and highly discontinuous basal lamina. The spaces between endothelial cells are 0.2 to 0.5 μm, so that the blood cells in the splenic cords are able to pass easily from the spaces to the lumen of the sinuses (Figure 10 – 17). There are many macrophages outside the sinuses, and their processes can also penetrate into the sinus lumen through the space of the endothelial cells.

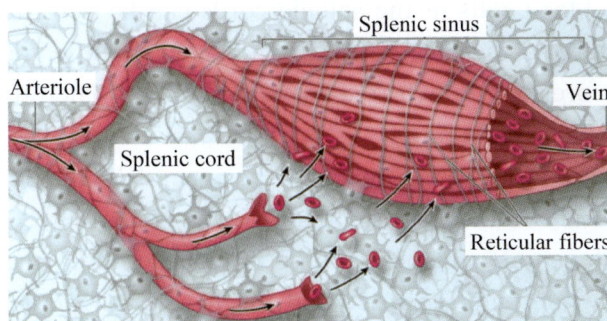

Figure 10 – 17　Schematic of the splenic sinus

3.3.1.3 Blood Supply to the Spleen

The splenic artery divides upon entering the hilum, branching into trabecular arteries. Then they leave the trabeculae to enter the white pulp, the arteries are known as central arterioles. Each central arteriole eventually leaves the white pulp and enters the red pulp, losing its sheath of lymphocytes and branching into several short straight penicillar arterioles that continue as capillaries. A few capillaries branching from the penicillar arterioles connect directly to the splenic sinuses. The other capillaries are uniquely open-ended, dumping blood into the splenic cords. From the sinuses, blood proceeds to small red pulp veins that converge to form trabecular veins, which in turn form the splenic vein in hilum, finally leave the spleen (Figure 10 – 18).

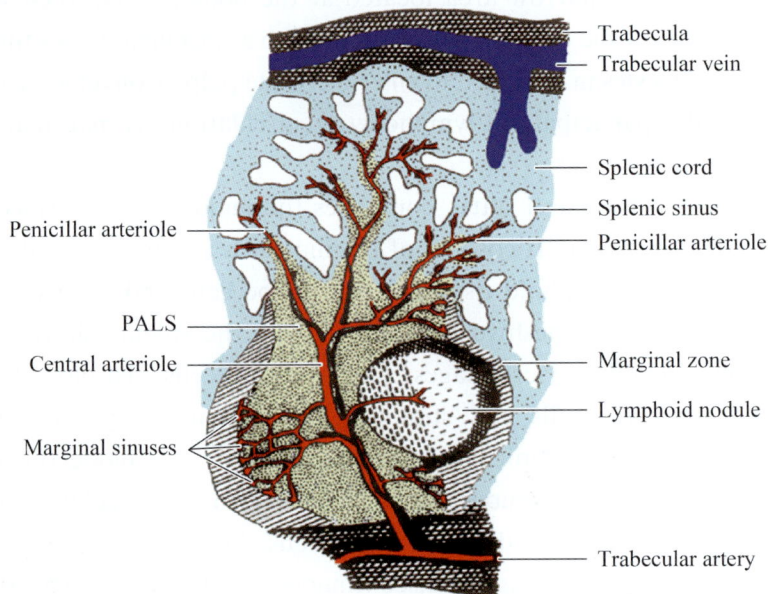

Figure 10 – 18 Schematic view of the blood circulation of the spleen

3.3.2 Function of the Spleen

(1) Blood filtration: the spleen is the major organ for clearing aged erythrocytes and platelets. Most of the blood cells in the splenic cords can be deformed, pass through the splenic sinuses and return to the blood circulation. Aged erythrocytes lose deformability, remain in the splenic cords and are cleared by macrophages. Therefore, the splenic cords are the main sites of blood filtration.

(2) Immune reaction: the spleen is also a peripheral lymphoid organ where blood-borne antigens (bacteria, viruses, plasmodium and schistosoma, etc.) trigger immune responses. When the humoral immune response is induced, both the number and size of lymph nodules in the white pulp increase, and the number of plasma cells in the splenic cord also increases. When the cellular immune response is induced, the periarterial lymphatic sheath becomes significantly thickened, and the spleen volume enlarges.

(3) Hematopoiesis: during the early fetal development, the spleen has a hematopoietic function. In adults, there are still a few hemopoietic stem cells in the spleen. When the body is under a severe blood loss state or some pathological conditions, the spleen can restore its hematopoietic function.

(4) Storage of blood: generally, there is about 40 ml blood stored in the splenic sinuses. This blood can enter the circulation when needed.

(Fu Yi)

第十章　免 疫 系 统

免疫系统由免疫细胞、淋巴组织和淋巴器官构成,执行机体的免疫防御功能。免疫细胞包括淋巴细胞、抗原呈递细胞、粒细胞、肥大细胞等,大多聚集于淋巴组织中,或散在于血液、淋巴及其他组织内。淋巴组织有弥散淋巴组织和淋巴小结两种,是周围淋巴器官的主要成分,也广泛分布于消化管和呼吸道等处。淋巴器官包括中枢淋巴器官(胸腺和骨髓)和周围淋巴器官(淋巴结、脾和扁桃体)。

免疫系统有三大主要功能:①免疫防御,可识别和清除侵入人体的抗原,包括病原微生物、异体细胞、异体大分子等。②免疫监视,可识别和清除体内突变的肿瘤细胞和被病毒感染的细胞。③免疫稳定,可识别和清除体内衰老或死亡的细胞,以维持内环境的稳定。

免疫系统通过免疫应答发挥功能。免疫应答有两类:①细胞免疫应答,指由T细胞对特异性抗原产生的免疫反应,然后通过特异致敏的T细胞释放多种免疫效应分子,从而清除靶细胞及抗原异物。②体液免疫应答,指由B细胞对特异性抗原所产生的免疫反应。B细胞在抗原刺激下,首先分化为浆细胞,然后浆细胞产生特异性的抗体,特异性的抗体与相应的抗原发生特异性结合,再通过中和解毒、凝集沉淀、调理吞噬等方式清除抗原。以上两类免疫应答相互协同、相互配合,共同发挥重要作用。

免疫系统发挥功能的本质特征是能辨别"自我"和"非我",其分子基础是:①主要组织相容性复合分子,简称MHC分子。MHC分子有种属特异性和个体特异性,是自身细胞的标志。即同一个体所有细胞的MHC分子都相同,而不同个体的MHC分子有区别。MHC分子主要包括MHC-Ⅰ类分子和MHC-Ⅱ类分子。所有有核细胞的表面都有MHC-Ⅰ类分子,而MHC-Ⅱ类分子仅分布于B细胞、树突状细胞和单核-吞噬细胞的表面。②T细胞和B细胞表面有特异性抗原受体,种类超过100万种,但每个淋巴细胞表面仅有一种抗原受体。因而每个淋巴细胞只针对一种抗原产生免疫应答;而作为一个个体,淋巴细胞可以针对多种抗原发生免疫应答。

第一节　主要的免疫细胞

一、淋巴细胞

根据来源、功能及表面标志,淋巴细胞可分为 T 细胞、B 细胞和 NK 细胞三类。

(一) T 细胞

占淋巴细胞总数的 75%,来源于骨髓,在胸腺中发育成熟,然后转移到周围淋巴器官或淋巴组织。在没有接触特异性抗原前,T 细胞保持相对静息的状态,称初始 T 细胞。一旦受抗原刺激后,初始 T 细胞便转化为代谢活跃的大淋巴细胞,并增殖分化。成熟的 T 细胞体积较小,大部分为效应性 T 细胞,少部分形成记忆性 T 细胞。效应性 T 细胞的寿命仅 1 周左右,能迅速清除抗原。而记忆性 T 细胞的寿命可长达数年,甚至终身。当记忆性 T 细胞再次遇到相同抗原时,能迅速转化增殖,形成大量效应性 T 细胞,产生更强大的免疫应答,从而使机体在较长时间内保持对该抗原的免疫力。

T 细胞可分为三个亚群:①细胞毒性 T 细胞,简称 Tc 细胞,能直接攻击病毒感染的细胞、异体细胞、肿瘤细胞等。当 Tc 细胞与靶细胞接触后,可通过释放穿孔素,使靶细胞溶解死亡。另外 Tc 细胞还可分泌颗粒酶,从小孔进入靶细胞,诱发靶细胞凋亡。②辅助性 T 细胞,简称 Th 细胞,可通过分泌多种细胞因子,辅助其他淋巴细胞发挥免疫应答。③调节性 T 细胞,简称 Tr 细胞,数量少,对机体免疫应答起负调控作用,因此其数量和功能异常往往可导致自身免疫性疾病。

(二) B 细胞

占淋巴细胞总数的 10%～15%,在骨髓成熟,成为初始 B 细胞,然后迁移到周围淋巴器官或组织。受抗原刺激后,初始 B 细胞可转化为大淋巴细胞,并增殖分化。大部分成为效应性 B 细胞,即浆细胞,可产生抗体,引发体液免疫应答。少部分成为记忆性 B 细胞,作用与记忆性 T 细胞相同。

(三) NK 细胞

约占淋巴细胞总数的 10%,来源于骨髓,为大颗粒淋巴细胞。其特点是不需要抗原刺激,也不需要借助抗体和补体便可活化,是机体抗肿瘤和抗感染免疫的第一道天然防线。

(四) 淋巴细胞再循环

周围淋巴器官和淋巴组织内的淋巴细胞可通过淋巴管进入血液循环,又可通过弥散淋巴组织内的毛细血管后微静脉返回淋巴组织或淋巴器官。这样周而复始,使淋巴细胞在血液循环和淋巴组织(器官)之间进行迁移和交换的现象,称淋巴细胞再循环(图 10-1)。通过淋巴细胞再循环,可以使分散于全身的免疫细胞成为一个相互关联的整体,同时也增加了淋巴细胞和抗原接触的机会,这样更有利于识别抗原,产生更有效的免疫应答。

二、巨噬细胞和单核吞噬细胞系统

巨噬细胞是由血液中的单核细胞穿出血管壁后分化而来的。与单核细胞相比,巨噬细胞在形态和功能上都发生了显著变化。体积增大,功能更为复杂,吞噬能力也增强。单核吞噬细

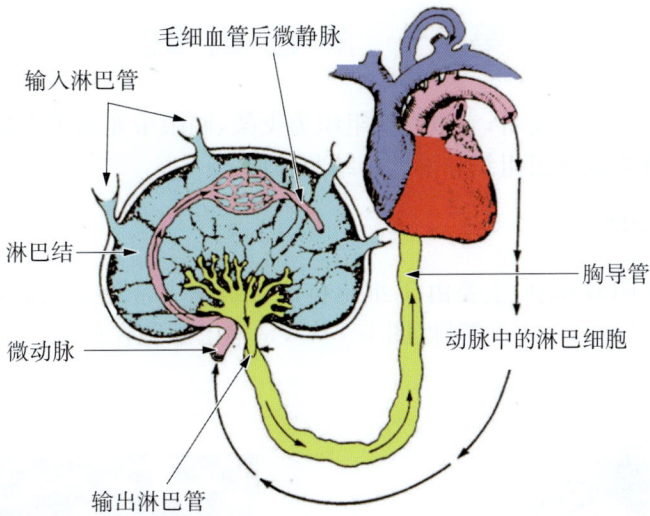

图 10-1 淋巴细胞再循环示意图

胞系统包括单核细胞和由其分化而来的、具有吞噬功能的细胞,如巨噬细胞、破骨细胞、小胶质细胞、肝巨噬细胞、肺巨噬细胞等。它们除了具有强大的吞噬能力外,也是主要的抗原呈递细胞,还能分泌多种生物活性物质。

三、抗原呈递细胞

抗原呈递细胞(antigen presenting cell,APC)是指能摄取和处理抗原,在细胞内形成抗原肽-MHC 分子复合物,然后将抗原肽呈递给 T 细胞,从而激发后者活化、增殖的一类免疫细胞(图 10-2)。主要有树突状细胞、单核-巨噬细胞和 B 淋巴细胞。

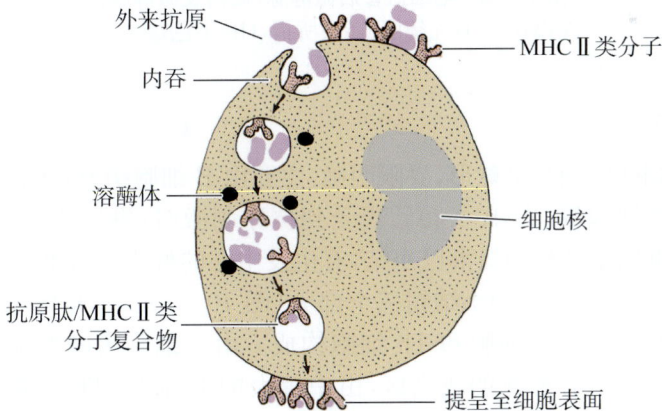

图 10-2 巨噬细胞抗原呈递示意图

树突状细胞(dendritic cell,DC)是目前发现的抗原呈递功能最强的 APC,因胞体有很多树枝状的突起而得名。DC 数量很少,但分布广泛,不同部位名称也不同,包括表皮的朗格汉斯细胞,心、肝、肺、肾的间质 DC,淋巴中的面纱细胞,外周淋巴组织中的交错突细胞及血液 DC 等,它们分别处于不同的发育成熟阶段,属于不同亚型的 DC。

第二节 淋巴组织

淋巴组织是免疫应答的场所,它以网状组织为支架,网眼中充满了大量淋巴细胞及其他免疫细胞。淋巴组织有弥散淋巴组织和淋巴小结两种形式。

一、弥散淋巴组织

弥散淋巴组织无明显界限,主要由 T 细胞构成。组织中常见毛细血管后微静脉,因其内皮细胞呈高柱状,故又称高内皮微静脉(图 10 - 3),是淋巴细胞在血液与淋巴组织之间进出的重要通道。

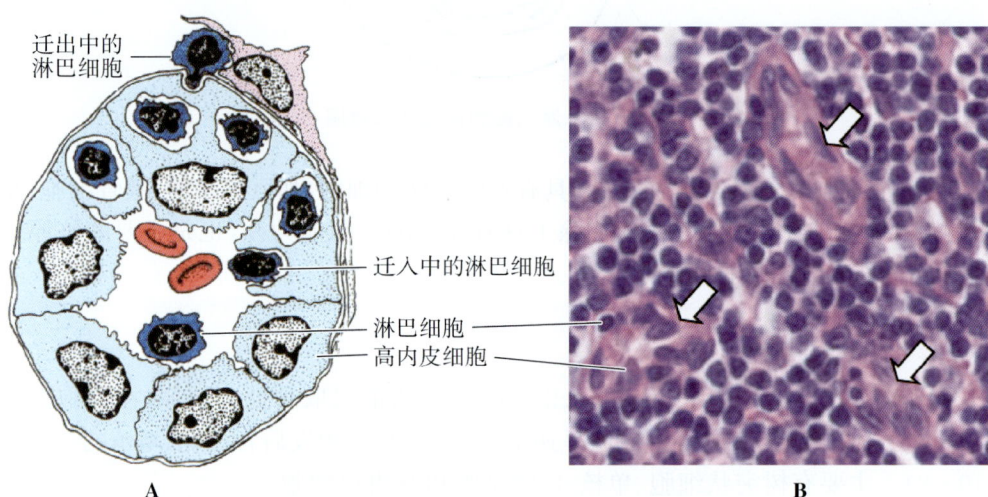

图 10 - 3 毛细血管后微静脉(高内皮微静脉)
A 模式图;B 光镜图(箭头所指,HE 染色,400×)

二、淋巴小结

淋巴小结,又称淋巴滤泡,呈球形,界限明确,主要由 B 细胞构成,还有一定量 Th 细胞、滤泡树突状细胞和巨噬细胞等(图 10 - 4)。当受到抗原刺激时,淋巴小结可增大,形成生发中心。无生发中心的淋巴小结称初级淋巴小结,有生发中心的称为次级淋巴小结。

生发中心可分为暗区、明区和小结帽三个部分(图 10 - 5)。①暗区,较小,位于生发中心的深部,主要由大而幼稚的 B 细胞和 Th 细胞构成。由于细胞嗜碱性强,故暗区着色较深。②明区,较大,位于生发中心外侧的浅染区,由中等大的 B 细胞、Th 细胞、巨噬细胞等构成。③小结帽,位于生发中心的周边,呈新月状,在明区顶部最厚,主要由小而成熟的 B 细胞和记忆性 B 细胞构成。

淋巴小结是个动态的结构。有抗原刺激时,淋巴小结增大、增多,通常在接触抗原后 2 周可达到高峰。当抗原被清除后,淋巴小结逐渐消失。

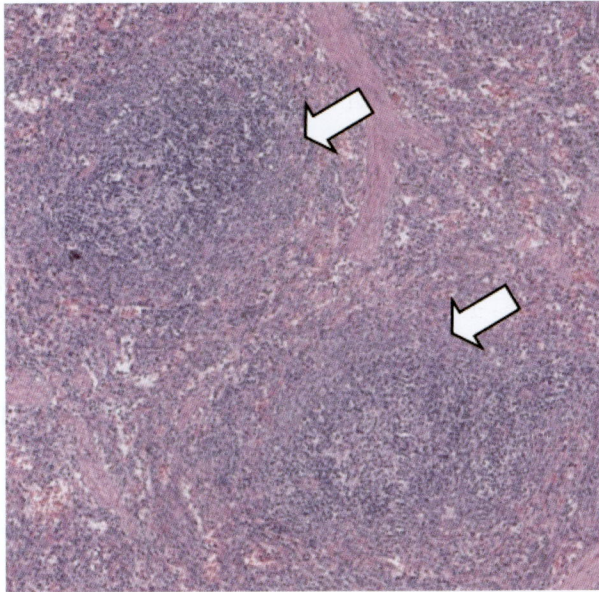

图 10-4 淋巴小结光镜图(HE 染色,100×)

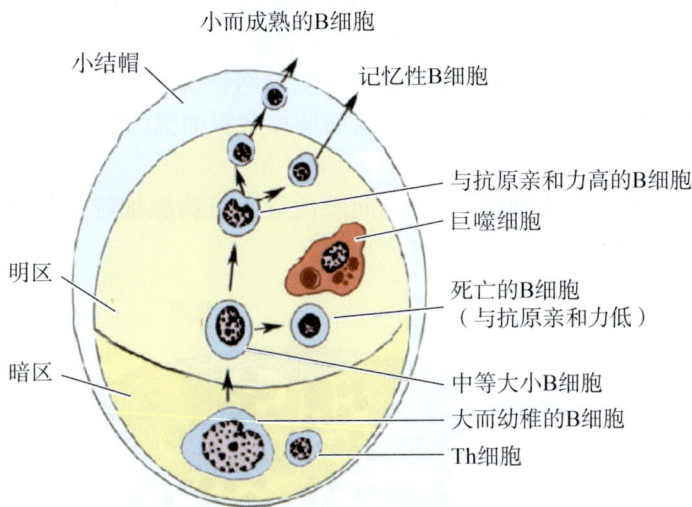

小而成熟的B细胞
小结帽
记忆性B细胞
与抗原亲和力高的B细胞
巨噬细胞
明区
死亡的B细胞
(与抗原亲和力低)
暗区
中等大小B细胞
大而幼稚的B细胞
Th细胞

图 10-5 次级淋巴小结结构示意图

第三节 淋巴器官

　　淋巴器官主要由淋巴组织构成,分中枢淋巴器官和周围淋巴器官。①中枢淋巴器官:包括胸腺和骨髓,是培育初始 T 细胞和初始 B 细胞的场所。淋巴性造血干细胞经历不同的分化发育途径,在胸腺形成初始 T 细胞,在骨髓形成初始 B 细胞。②周围淋巴器官:包括淋巴结、脾和扁桃体等,是机体发生免疫应答的场所。其发育较中枢淋巴器官晚,一般出生数月后才逐渐发育完善。

一、胸腺

胸腺在幼年时期体积较大,进入青春期后,逐渐开始退化。到老年时期,胸腺实质大部分被脂肪组织所替代,仅存少量的皮质和髓质。

(一)胸腺的结构

分左、右两叶,表面由薄层结缔组织构成被膜。被膜深入胸腺实质,形成小叶间隔,将实质分隔成许多胸腺小叶。每个小叶可分为皮质和髓质,相邻小叶间的髓质相互连续(图 10-6)。

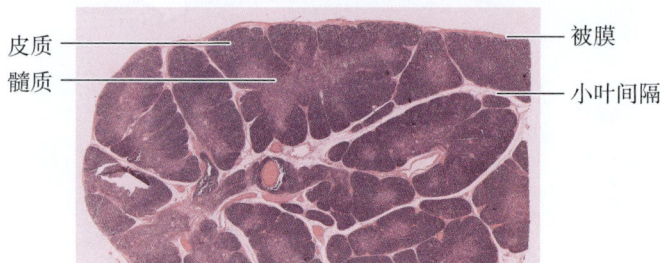

图 10-6 胸腺光镜图(HE 染色,40×)

胸腺为 T 细胞的发育提供了独特的微环境,构成这一微环境的细胞称为胸腺基质细胞,主要由胸腺上皮细胞、巨噬细胞、交错突细胞、肥大细胞、成纤维细胞等构成。其中,胸腺上皮细胞是最重要的基质细胞。它不仅构成胸腺微环境的网格状支架,还可分泌多种生物活性物质,如胸腺激素、神经肽类激素、细胞因子等,从而调控胸腺细胞的分化发育。

1. 皮质

位于小叶周边,以胸腺上皮细胞为支架,间隙内含大量胸腺细胞,故着色较深。此外还有少量基质细胞(图 10-7)。

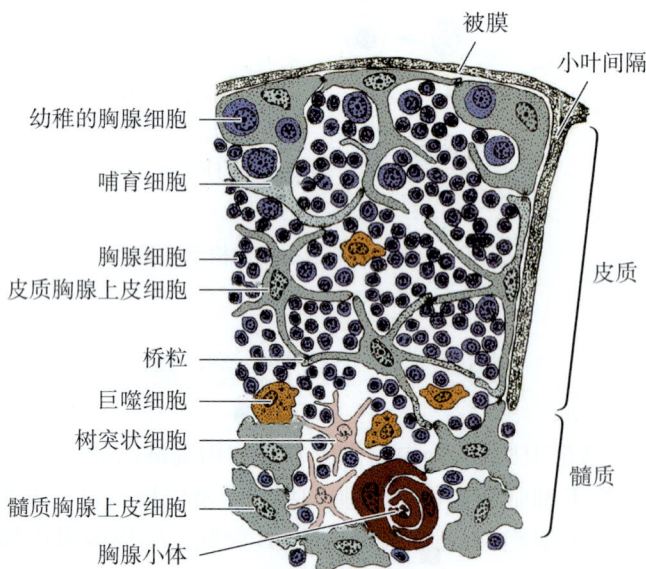

图 10-7 胸腺结构模式图

（1）胸腺上皮细胞：又称上皮性网状细胞，多分布于被膜下和胸腺细胞之间。星形，有突起，相邻细胞间以桥粒连接。有些被膜下的胸腺上皮细胞胞质丰富，可包绕胸腺细胞，称哺育细胞。胸腺上皮细胞能分泌胸腺素、胸腺生成素等，为胸腺细胞发育所必需。

（2）胸腺细胞：即处于不同分化发育阶段的 T 细胞，密集分布于皮质内，占皮质细胞总数的 85%～90%。在分化发育过程中，胸腺细胞要经历阳性选择和阴性选择。阳性选择发生在皮质外层，使 T 细胞具有 MHC 分子限制性识别能力；而阴性选择发生在皮质深层和髓质，淘汰能与机体自身抗原发生反应的 T 细胞，故最终只有不足 5% 的胸腺细胞能发育成熟，成为初始 T 细胞。而绝大部分的胸腺细胞凋亡，被巨噬细胞所吞噬。

2. 髓质

位于小叶中央，主要由大量胸腺上皮细胞构成，故着色浅。另外含少量成熟胸腺细胞（初始 T 细胞）、交错突细胞和巨噬细胞等。

（1）胸腺上皮细胞：形态与皮质上皮细胞不同，呈球形或多边形，胞体较大，突起较短，细胞之间也以桥粒相连。也能产生胸腺素和胸腺生成素。部分胸腺上皮细胞参与构成胸腺小体。

（2）胸腺小体：是胸腺髓质的特征性结构，随年龄增长而增加，散在分布，由胸腺上皮细胞呈同心圆状排列而成。胸腺小体外周的上皮细胞胞核呈新月状，胞质嗜酸性，可分裂；靠近小体中心的上皮细胞胞核逐渐退化，胞质含较多角蛋白；小体中心的上皮细胞则已完全角化，呈强嗜酸性，或已破碎，成均质透明状（图 10-8）。胸腺小体的功能目前尚不明确。

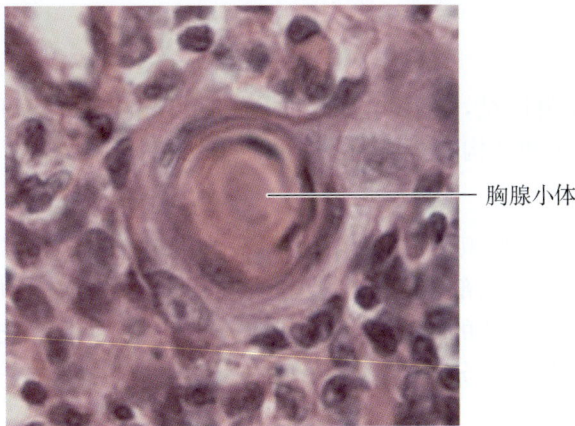

图 10-8　胸腺小体光镜图（HE 染色，400×）

3. 胸腺的血液供应

胸腺血供丰富，小动脉穿过胸腺被膜，沿小叶间隔至皮、髓交界处，形成微动脉，然后发出分支进入皮质和髓质。皮质内的毛细血管在皮、髓交界处汇合为高内皮微静脉，胸腺内成熟的初始 T 细胞由此进入血液。髓质的毛细血管多为有孔型，汇入微静脉后经小叶间隔及被膜离开胸腺。

4. 血-胸腺屏障

由胸腺皮质内的毛细血管及其周围的相关结构形成，包括：①连续毛细血管内皮，内皮细胞间有紧密连接。②内皮周围连续的基膜。③血管周隙，内含巨噬细胞。④上皮基膜。⑤一层连续的胸腺上皮细胞突起(图 10-9)。血-胸腺屏障可阻止血液中的抗原物质和某些药物等通过,从而维持内环境的稳定,保证胸腺细胞的正常发育。

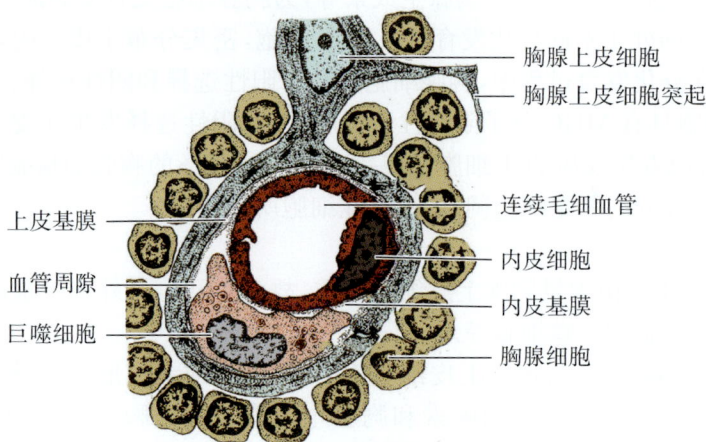

图 10-9 血-胸腺屏障结构模式图

(二)胸腺的功能

(1)培养初始 T 细胞的场所。

(2)内分泌功能。胸腺上皮细胞可分泌胸腺素、胸腺生成素、胸腺肽等。

二、淋巴结

人体有 500~600 个淋巴结,位于淋巴回流的通路上。淋巴结呈豆形,常成群分布于肺门、腹股沟、腋下等处,其大小和结构与机体的免疫状态密切相关。

(一)淋巴结的结构

淋巴结表面由薄层结缔组织构成被膜。数条输入淋巴管穿越被膜后与被膜下淋巴窦相通。淋巴结的一侧略凹陷,为门部,有血管、神经和输出淋巴管穿出。被膜和门部的结缔组织伸入淋巴结实质,形成相互连接的粗短支架,称为小梁。小梁之间为淋巴组织和淋巴窦。淋巴结的实质可分为皮质、髓质两部分,两者之间无明显分界(图 10-10、图 10-11)。

1. 皮质

位于被膜下方,由浅层皮质、副皮质区和皮质淋巴窦组成。

(1)浅层皮质:紧贴被膜下窦,由淋巴小结及小结之间的弥散淋巴组织构成,为皮质的 B 细胞区。

(2)副皮质区:位于皮质深层,为弥散淋巴组织。主要含 T 细胞,故为皮质的 T 细胞区。新生动物切除胸腺后,此区不发育,故又称胸腺依赖区。此区内有较多高内皮的毛细血管后微静脉,是血液中淋巴细胞进入副皮质区的重要通道。

(3)皮质淋巴窦:包括被膜下窦和小梁周窦,两者相互连通。被膜下窦位于被膜下方,成扁囊状包绕整个淋巴结实质。小梁周窦分布在小梁周围,末端常为盲端,仅少量与髓质淋巴窦连通。淋巴窦的窦壁为扁平的内皮细胞,外有薄层基质、少量网状纤维和一层扁平的网状细胞。窦腔由星状内皮细胞支撑,内皮细胞表面附着许多巨噬细胞(图 10-12)。当淋巴缓慢流

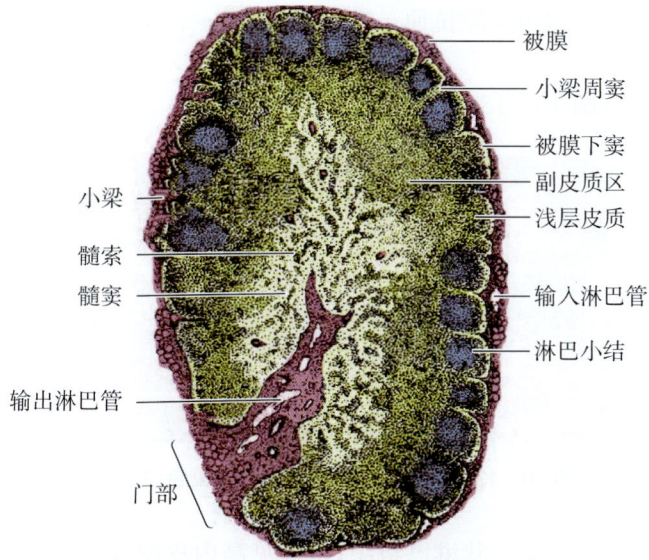

被膜
小梁周窦
被膜下窦
副皮质区
浅层皮质
输入淋巴管
淋巴小结
小梁
髓索
髓窦
输出淋巴管
门部

图 10-10 淋巴结结构模式图

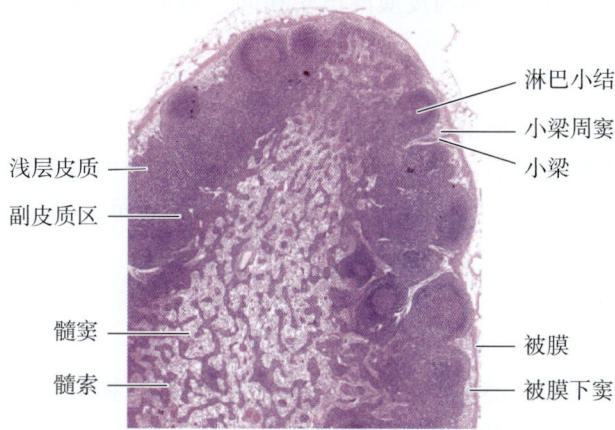

淋巴小结
小梁周窦
小梁
浅层皮质
副皮质区
髓窦
髓索
被膜
被膜下窦

图 10-11 淋巴结光镜图(HE 染色,40×)

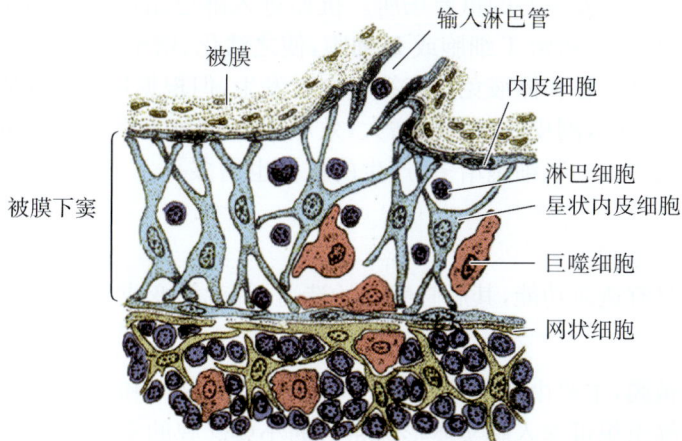

输入淋巴管
被膜
内皮细胞
淋巴细胞
星状内皮细胞
被膜下窦
巨噬细胞
网状细胞

图 10-12 淋巴结皮质被膜下窦结构模式图

经淋巴窦,窦腔内的巨噬细胞可清除抗原。

2. 髓质

由髓索和髓窦构成(图 10 - 13)。

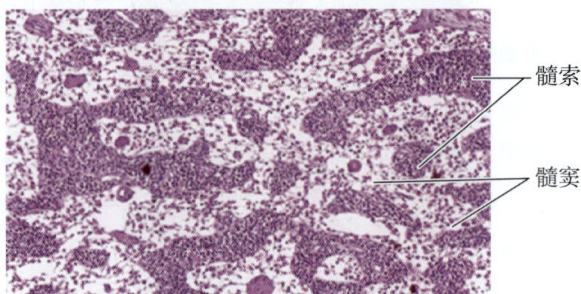

图 10 - 13　淋巴结髓质光镜图(HE 染色,100 ×)

(1)髓索:为相互连接的条索状淋巴组织,也可见高内皮微静脉。主要含 B 细胞、浆细胞、巨噬细胞等。

(2)髓窦:位于髓索之间,结构与皮质淋巴窦相同。但窦腔更宽大,腔内的巨噬细胞更多,故有较强的滤过功能。

3. 淋巴结内的淋巴通路

淋巴从输入淋巴管进入皮质淋巴窦(被膜下窦和小梁周窦),然后进入髓窦,继而从输出淋巴管流出。淋巴经淋巴窦滤过后,其中的细菌等抗原绝大部分可被清除。而淋巴组织中的淋巴细胞和产生的抗体,也会不断进入淋巴。因此,较输入淋巴而言,输出的淋巴中含更多的淋巴细胞和抗体。

(二)淋巴结的功能

1. 滤过淋巴

淋巴结是人体的过滤器。淋巴流经淋巴结时,其中的抗原物质(如细菌、病毒、毒素等)可被巨噬细胞吞噬。髓窦是滤过淋巴的主要部位。

2. 免疫应答

淋巴结是人体产生免疫应答的重要场所。抗原进入淋巴结后,巨噬细胞等抗原呈递细胞可摄取、处理抗原并呈递给初始 T 细胞或 B 细胞,使之活化、增殖、分化,产生大量的效应细胞和记忆细胞。细胞免疫应答和体液免疫应答常同时发生,但根据抗原的性质,会以其中一种为主。细胞免疫应答为主时,副皮质区明显增大,效应性 T 细胞增多。体液免疫应答为主时,淋巴小结增多、增大,髓质中的浆细胞增多,产生的抗体也增多。

三、脾

脾在胚胎时期具有造血功能,其后骨髓开始造血,脾就演变成人体最大的淋巴器官。

(一)脾的结构

脾表面有较厚被膜,主要由致密结缔组织构成,含弹性纤维和平滑肌纤维,表面覆有间皮。被膜和脾门部的结缔组织可深入脾实质形成粗大的小梁。脾的实质可分为白髓和红髓。脾内无淋巴窦(图 10 - 14、图 10 - 15)。

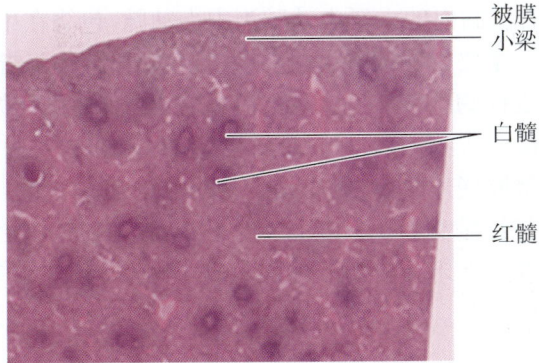

图 10 - 14　脾光镜图(HE 染色,40 ×)

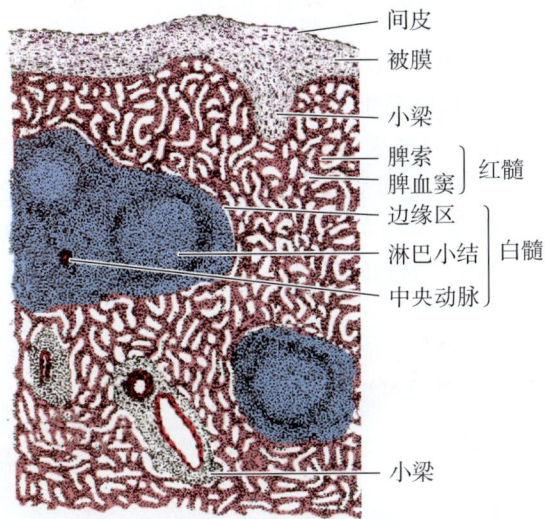

图 10 - 15　脾结构模式图

1. 白髓

在新鲜的脾切面上,可见散在分布的灰白色点状区域,即白髓。在 HE 染色的切片中,白髓为蓝紫色团块状结构。白髓相当于淋巴结的皮质,由动脉周围淋巴鞘、淋巴小结和边缘区构成(图 10 - 16)。

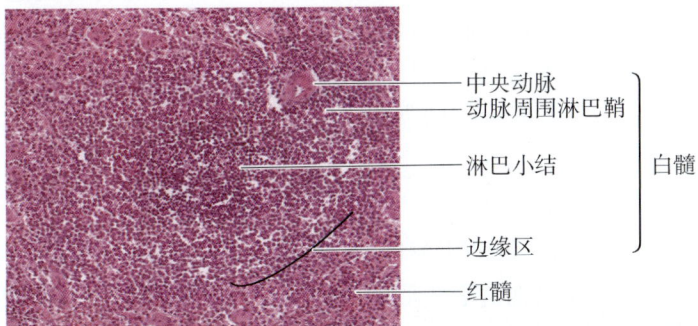

图 10 - 16　脾白髓光镜图(HE 染色,100 ×)

（1）动脉周围淋巴鞘：白髓内的主要小动脉为中央动脉,包绕在中央动脉周围的弥散淋巴组织,即动脉周围淋巴鞘。主要由大量 T 细胞、少量巨噬细胞及交错突细胞构成。此区相当于淋巴结的副皮质区,故也称胸腺依赖区,但无高内皮的毛细血管后微静脉。

（2）淋巴小结：又称脾小结,位于动脉周围淋巴鞘的一侧,主要由大量 B 细胞构成。健康人脾内淋巴小结较少,当抗原侵入时,淋巴小结数量明显增加。

（3）边缘区：即白髓与红髓交界的狭窄区域,是淋巴细胞首先接触抗原刺激而引起免疫应答的部位。中央动脉的侧支末端在此膨大,形成小血窦,称边缘窦。边缘窦是血液内抗原和淋巴细胞进入白髓的通道。反之,白髓内的淋巴细胞也可通过边缘窦参与淋巴细胞再循环。

2. 红髓

在新鲜的脾切面上,大部分组织呈深红色,即红髓。红髓约占脾实质的 80%,由脾索和脾血窦构成。

（1）脾索：为富含血细胞的淋巴组织,呈不规则索条状,相互连接成网,网孔即为脾血窦。脾索内含有较多 B 细胞、浆细胞、巨噬细胞和树突状细胞。

（2）脾血窦：为静脉性血窦,腔宽大、形态不规则、互连成网。窦壁由一层长杆状的内皮细胞平行排列而成,内皮外有不完整的基膜及网状纤维围绕,内皮细胞之间有 $0.2\sim0.5\,\mu\mathrm{m}$ 不等的间隙(图 10-17)。脾索内的血细胞可通过变形穿越内皮细胞间隙进入血窦。血窦外有较多巨噬细胞,其突起也可通过内皮细胞间隙伸入窦腔。

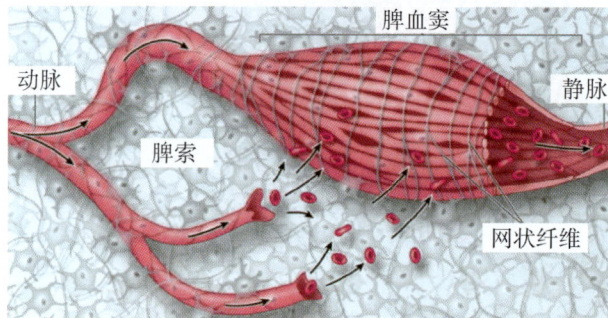

图 10-17 脾血窦结构模式图

3. 脾的血液供应

脾动脉从脾门入脾后,分支进入小梁,称小梁动脉。小梁动脉再分支进入白髓,称中央动脉。中央动脉主干穿出白髓后,进入脾索,形成直行的微动脉,形似笔毛,称笔毛微动脉。后者少数注入脾血窦,多数末端扩大,直接开口于脾索,因而大量血液直接进入脾索。脾血窦汇入小梁静脉,于脾门处汇合为脾静脉,离开脾(图 10-18)。

（二）脾的功能

1. 滤血

脾是清除衰老红细胞和血小板的主要器官。脾索中的血细胞大部分可经变形,穿过脾血窦,回到血循环。而衰老的红细胞由于变形能力降低,不能进入脾血窦,滞留在脾索中,被巨噬细胞清除。故脾索是滤血的主要部位。

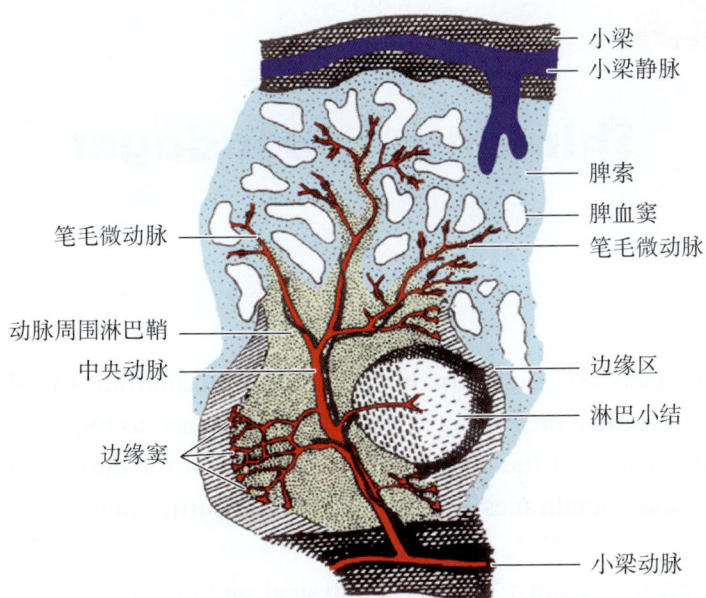

图 10-18　脾血液供应模式图

2. 免疫应答

脾是血源性抗原物质引发免疫应答的部位。血液中的病原体,如细菌、病毒、疟原虫、血吸虫等,都可引起脾发生免疫应答。当引发体液免疫应答时,脾内淋巴小结增多、增大,脾索内浆细胞增多;引发细胞免疫应答时,动脉周围淋巴鞘明显增厚,脾体积也显著增大。

3. 造血

在胚胎早期某一阶段,脾有造血功能。成年后,脾内仍有少量造血干细胞。当机体处在严重失血或病理状态下,脾仍可恢复造血功能。

4. 储血

正常情况下,脾血窦内储血约 40 ml。当机体需要时,这些血液可补充进入血循环。

（傅　奕）

Chapter 11

Skin and Appendages

The skin is the heaviest single organ of the body, accounting for about 16% of total body weight and, in adults, presenting $1.2-2.3\,\mathrm{m}^2$ of surface to the external environment. It covers the whole surface of the body and is continuous at the entry and exit points of the body with the mucous membranes lining the nose, mouth, anus, and reproductive and urinary openings.

The skin can protect against microbes, physical and chemical damage and ultraviolet radiation. Additionally, it plays an important role in regulating body temperature by secreting sweat from sweat glands. Moreover, the skin has a role as a sense organ detecting stimuli through specific sensory nerve receptors.

The skin is composed of 2 layers: the epidermis, an epithelial layer of ectodermal origin, and the dermis, a layer of connective tissue of mesodermal origin. The junction between epidermis and dermis is irregular, dermal projections are called papillae interdigitate, and epidermal protrusions are known as epidermis ridges. Beneath the dermis lies the hypodermis or subcutaneous tissue, which is a loose connective tissue. The hypodermis, which is not considered part of the skin, binds skin loosely to the subjacent tissues (Figure 11 - 1).

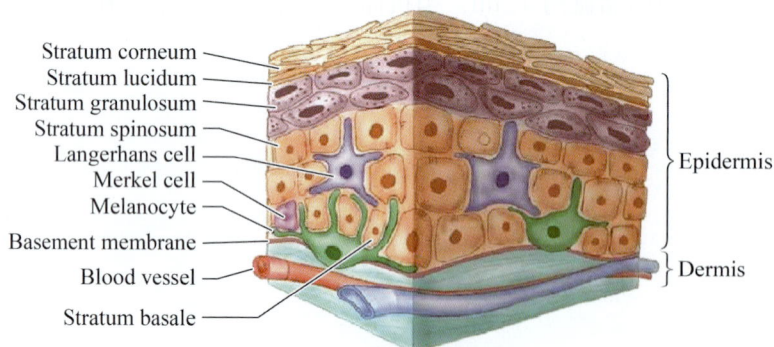

Figure 11 - 1   Diagram of skin

1   Epidermis

The epidermis is stratified squamous keratinized epithelium that can be divided into 5 layers, though these layers are only fully present in thick skin, such as on the palms of the hands and soles of the feet (Figure 11 – 2). It contains 2 cell types, keratinocytes and non-keratinocytes (melanocytes, Langerhans cells, and Merkel cells).

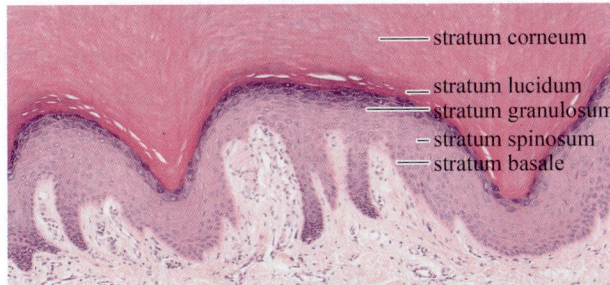

Figure 11 – 2   Layers of epidermis (Skin of human sole, HE, 100×)

1.1 Layers of Epidermis

1.1.1 Stratum Corneum

It is the outmost layer and consists of many horny cells, which are dead, plate-like enucleate keratinocytes with thickened plasma membranes. The cells in this layer are filled with mature keratin, which is a filamentous protein produced by keratinocytes in deeper layers of the epidermis. Keratin provides toughness and protection on the epidermis and helps to prevent water loss. The surface of the stratum corneum is constantly shedding, particularly when exposed to abrasion. However, this layer is constantly replenished as cells from deeper layers migrate towards the surface.

1.1.2 Stratum Lucidum

It is a thin, translucent layer visible only in the thickest skin, composed of extremely flattened eosinophilic cells. These cells are packed with keratin and do not possess nuclei or organelles.

1.1.3 Stratum Granulosum

This layer consists of 3 – 5 layers of flattened polygonal cells that are filled with coarse basophilic granules called keratohyalin granules. As the upper cells in this stratum die, they eventually become a part of the stratum lucidum.

1.1.4 Stratum Spinosum

It is the thickest layer of the epidermis. It is composed of several layers of polyhedral to flattened cells. In the cytoplasm, numerous bundles of keratin filaments are present, and there are also coarse basophilic granules called keratohyalin granules, which have no limiting membrane. Another type of granules, known as lamellated granules, contain lipids which can be discharged into intercellular spaces. The cells have numerous processes that give this layer a spine-studded appearance. Desmosomes are usually found between cells in this layer.

1.1.5 Stratum Basale

This layer consists of a single layer of basophilic cuboidal or columnar epithelial cells resting on the basement membrane separating the epidermis from the dermis. The cells in this layer undergo mitosis and are the stem cells of the epidermis. Some offspring cells of this layer begin to produce keratin filaments and migrate towards the upper layer.

1.2 Non-Keratinocytes

1.2.1 Merkel Cells

Merkel cells are distributed in the stratum basale. They resemble basal keratinocytes but have short processes and small dense granules (Figure 11 - 3). Free nerve endings form an expansion that is present at the base of Merkel cells. These cells may function as sensory mechanoreceptors, but other evidence suggests diffuse neuroendocrine system-related functions.

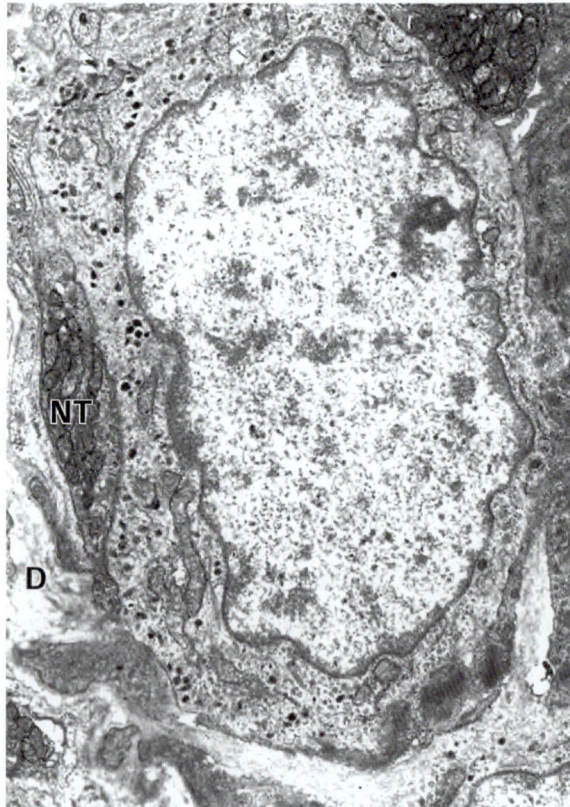

Figure 11 - 3   Electron micrograph of Merkel cell

1.2.2 Langerhans Cells

Langerhans cells are derived from bone marrow and mainly located in the stratum spinosum (Figure 11 - 4). They are star-shaped cells and contain many rod-like or racket-shaped cytoplasmic granules (Birbeck granules). In HE-stained sections, these cells are found to contain dark nuclei and light cytoplasm. They belong to the mononuclear phagocyte system and have a significant role in immunologic skin reactions. They are capable of binding, processing, and presenting antigens to T lymphocytes, thus participating in the stimulation of these cells.

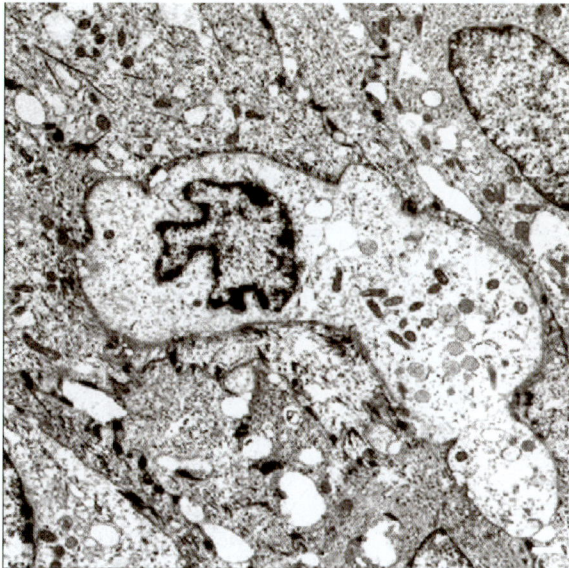

Figure 11 - 4   Diagram of Langerhans cell

1.2.3   Melanocytes

Melanocytes derive from the neural crest and migrate to the epidermis. They are scattered among the keratinocytes of the stratum basale but lack desmosomes. These cells have round cell bodies, central nuclei, and long cytoplasmic processes that pass between the cells of the stratum basale and spinosum to terminate in small indentations on the keratinocytes' surfaces. Their cytoplasm contains many mitochondria, a well-developed Golgi complex, short rough endoplasmic reticulum cisternae, and membrane bound melanosomes where melanin is synthesized. Melanin affects color of skin, eye, and hair. Once formed, melanin granules migrate within cytoplasmic extensions of the melanocyte and are transferred to cells of the stratum basale and spinosum, providing further protective action against the sun's ultraviolet light (Figure 11 - 5).

1.3   Dermis

The dermis is the connective tissue that supports the epidermis and connects it to the subcutaneous tissue (hypodermis). The surface of the dermis is very irregular and has many projections that interdigitate with projections of the epidermis. This layer has a rich

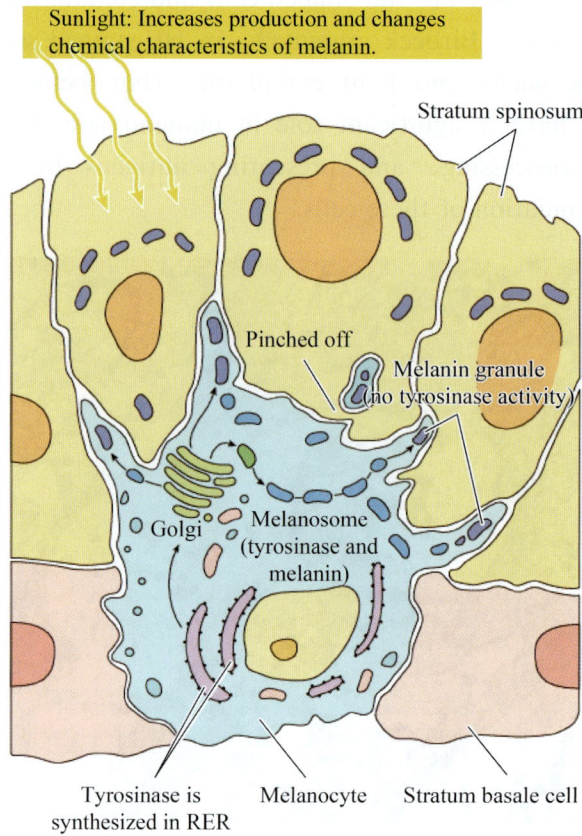

Figure 11 - 5   Diagram of Melanocyte

network of blood and lymph vessels, and contains epidermal derivatives including hair
follicles, sweat and sebaceous glands. The dermis is divided into 2 layers: the superficial
papillary layer and the deeper reticular layer (Figure 11 - 6).

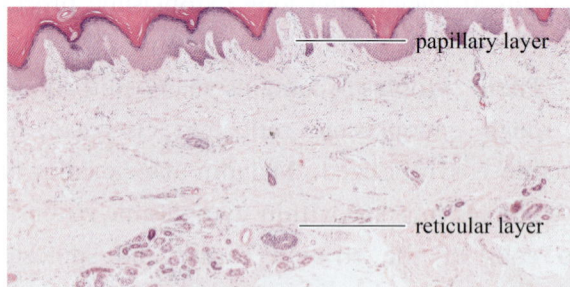

Figure 11 - 6   Layers of dermis (Skin of human sole, HE, 100×)

1.3.1   Papillary Layer

The papillary layer lies directly beneath the epidermal basement membrane and is
composed of loose connective tissue, rich in elastic fibers. Its projections, known as dermal
papillae interdigitate with the epidermal ridges, increasing the area of contact. The

papillary layer contains immune-protective cells, a rich capillary network, and abundant free nerve endings. Many dermal papillae contain encapsulated touch receptors called Meissner's corpuscles.

1.3.2 Reticular Layer

The reticular layer is a thicker layer composed of dense irregular connective tissue. This layer contains many arteriovenous anastomoses and a rich supply of nerves in both free nerve endings and encapsulated endings such as Pacinian corpuscles.

2 Subcutaneous Tissue

Beneath the dermis is subcutaneous tissue. The subcutaneous tissue layer consists of loose connective tissue that loosely connects the skin to the underlying organs, making it possible for the skin to slide over them. The hypodermis often contains fat cells that vary in number according to the area of the body and vary in size according to nutritional state.

3 Appendages of Skin

Epidermal derivatives or skin appendages include hairs, sweat glands, sebaceous glands, arrector pili muscles and nails (Figure 11 – 7).

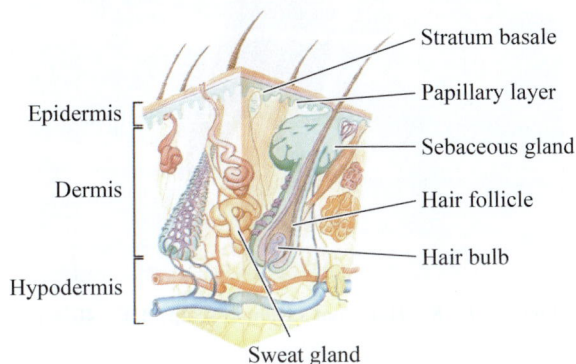

Figure 11 – 7 Diagram of the skin appendages

3.1 Hairs

Hairs are widespread over the body surface, although none is observed on palms, soles, parts of the genitalia, tips of fingers, toes and lips. The color, size, shape, and distribution of hairs vary according to race, age, sex, and body region.

3.1.1 Structure of Hair

The hair is divided into 3 parts: hair shaft, hair root and hair bulb (Figure 11 – 8). The hair shaft is exposed on the skin while the hair root is buried within; the hair shaft and hair root are composed of well-arranged keratinized epithelial cells, which are full of keratin and a varying number of melanin particles. The hair root is wrapped by the hair follicle that is divided into 2 layers. The inner layer is epithelial root sheath, which is continuous with the epidermis and wraps the hair root, and its structure is similar to that of the epidermis; The outer layer is a connective tissue sheath, which is continuous with the dermis and consists of a thin layer of densely connective tissue. The hair root and the lower end of the epithelial root sheath of the hair follicle are integrated and expand into a hair bulb. The epithelial cells of the hair bulb are called hair matrix cells, which are stem cells. They continue to proliferate, and some of the daughter cells differentiate to form hair roots and epithelial root sheath. These cells then migrate upwards. The melanocytes at the base of the hair bulb can transfer melanin particles to the epithelial cells. There is connective tissue on the bottom surface of the hair bulb, which is called hair papilla. it is rich in capillaries and nerve endings. Hair bulbs are the growth points of hair and hair follicles, and hair papilla can induce and nourish the growth of hair.

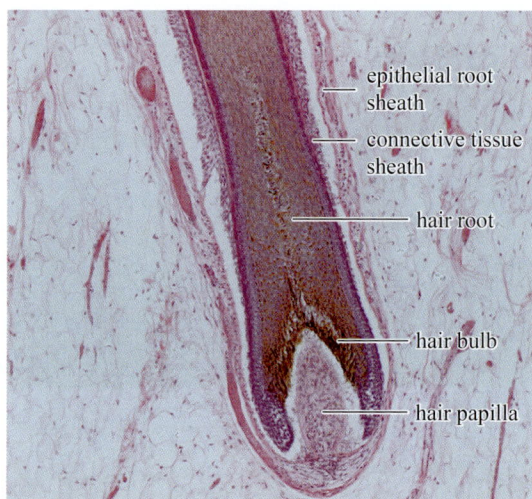

Figure 11 - 8   Hair root (Human scalp, HE, 40×)

The pigment of hair is produced by melanocytes that are distributed among the hair matrix cells. These pigments are then transferred into newly formed hair root epithelial cells. The color of the hair depends on the melanin content within the inner cortical cells of the hair shaft. When the melanin particles are scarce, the hair appears gray or brownish-yellow, and when it is completely deficient, the hair is white.

3.1.2   Growth and Renewal of Hair

The hair has a certain growth cycle. The growth cycle of hair on the head is usually 3 to 5 years, and the growth cycle of hair in other parts is only a few months.

During the growth phase, the hair bulbs are swollen, the hair papilla is rich in blood flow, and the hair matrix cells proliferate vigorously. During the resting phase, the hair bulbs and hair papilla become smaller and atrophic, and the hair matrix cells stop proliferating. Then the hair roots are not firmly connected to the hair bulbs and hair follicles. Before the old hair falls off, a new hair bulb and hair papilla are formed at the base of the hair follicle to form a new hair and push the old hair out.

Hormones, especially androgens, influence the pattern of terminal hair distribution and growth rate.

3.1.3   Sweat Glands

3.1.3.1   Eccrine Sweat Glands

Eccrine sweat glands are located in the skin throughout most of the body. Eccrine sweat glands are simple coiled tubular glands located deep in the dermis or in the underlying hypodermis. There is a slender, coiled duct passing from the secretory portion of each gland, which traverses the dermis and epidermis to open on the surface of the skin at a sweat pore (Figure 11 − 9).

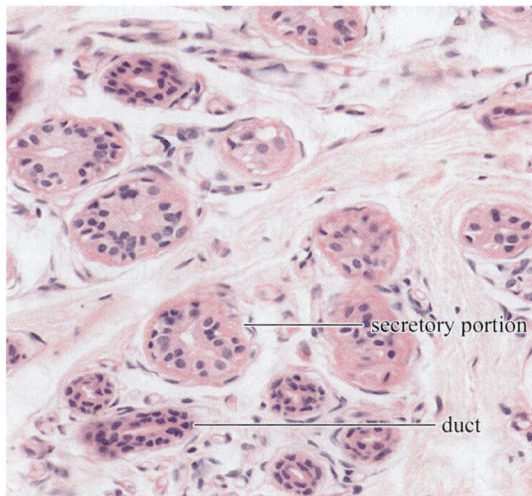

Figure 11 − 9   Eccrine sweat glands (Skin of human sole, HE, 200×)

The secretory portion of the gland consists of a simple cuboidal to low columnar epithelium surrounded by myoepithelial cells. Contractions of these myoepithelial cells assist in expelling fluid from the gland.

The duct of eccrine sweat glands is highly coiled and traverses the dermis and epidermis on its way to opening on the skin surface. The duct is composed of a stratified cuboidal epithelium made up of 2 layers.

Eccrine sweat glands play a major role in temperature regulation through the cooling that results from the evaporation of water from sweat on the body surface. The fluid secreted by the secretory portion of the gland is similar to blood plasma in regard to electrolyte balance, including potassium and sodium chloride as well as ammonia and urea.

3.1.3.2　Apocrine Sweat Glands

Apocrine sweat glands are found only in certain location: the axilla, the areola of nipple, and the anal region. Like eccrine glands, apocrine glands are coiled tubular glands. They are sometimes branched. The secretory portion of apocrine glands has a wider lumen than that of eccrine glands and is composed of cells of a single type. The cytoplasm of the glandular cell is eosinophilic. The apical cytoplasm contains numerous small granules containing the secretory material. These granules are subsequently released via exocytosis. Unlike eccrine glands, apocrine glands store their secretory product in the lumen.

The duct of the apocrine gland is similar to that of the eccrine gland. Meanwhile, it continues from the secretory portion of the gland in a relatively straight path to drain into the follicle canal. The duct epithelium is stratified cuboidal, usually 2-but sometimes 3-cell thick.

Apocrine glands produce a secretion that contains protein, carbohydrate, ammonia, lipid, and certain organic compounds that may color the secretion. In the axilla, the secretion is milky and slightly viscous. The secreted fluid is odorless, but bacterial action on the skin surface develops an acrid odor. Apocrine glands become functional at puberty; as with axillary and pubic hair, their development depends on sex hormones.

3.1.4　Sebaceous Glands

Sebaceous glands secrete sebum that coats the hair and skin surface. Except for the palms of the hands, soles of the feet, and the lateral sides of the fee, sebaceous glands are found throughout the body (Figure 11 - 10).

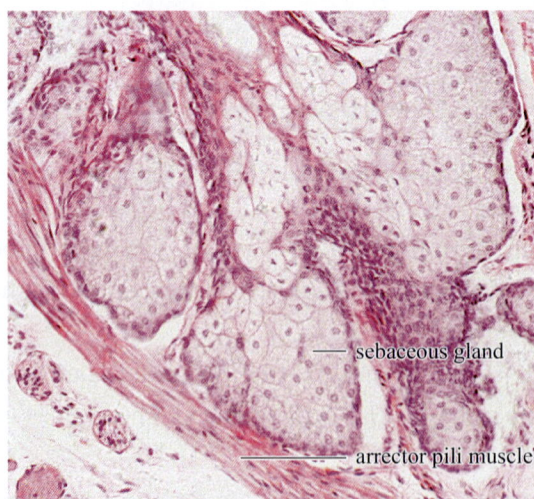

Figure 11 - 10　Sebaceous glands and arrector pili muscle (human scalp, HE, 100×)

Sebaceous glands develop as outgrowth of the external root sheath of the hair follicle, usually producing several glands per follicle. The ducts of the sebaceous glands open into the upper third of the follicular canal, where they discharge their secretory product to coat the hair shaft and eventually the skin surface. The oily substance produced in the gland is the product of holocrine secretion, which is named sebum. The entire cell produces the fatty product, fills with it, and undergoes programmed cell death as cellist is being filled. Ultimately, both the secretory product and cell debris are discharged from the gland as sebum into the infundibulum of a hair follicle, which forms the pilosebaceous canal with the short duct of the sebaceous gland. New cells are produced by mitosis of the basal cells at the periphery of the gland, and the cells of the gland remain linked to one another by desmosomes. The basal lamina of these cells is continuous with the basal lamina of both the epidermis and the hair follicle.

Sebaceous glands are under the influence of sex hormones and increase their activity greatly after puberty.

3.1.5   Arrector Pili Muscles

Hair and hair follicles grow obliquely in the skin. On the side of their blunt angle to the surface of the skin, there is a bunch of smooth muscles obliquely arranged, called arrector pili muscle (Figure 11 - 10). One end of it is attached to the hair follicle, while the other end is connected to the connective tissue of the dermal papillary layer. Contraction of arrector pili muscles result in the erection of the hair shaft to a more upright position and also cause a depression in the skin where the muscles attach to the dermis. This contraction produces the "gooseflesh" of common parlance.

3.1.6   Nails

Nails are plates of keratinized epithelial cells on the dorsal surface of each distal phalanx (Figure 11 - 11). The proximal part of the nail, hidden in the nail fold, is the nail root. The nail body, which corresponds to the stratum corneum of the skin, rests on a bed of epidermis called the nail bed. Only the stratum basale and the stratum spinosum are present in the nail bed. Nail body epithelium arises from the nail matrix. The proximal end of the matrix extends deep to the nail root. Cells of the matrix divide, move distally, and eventually cornify, forming the cells of the nail body.

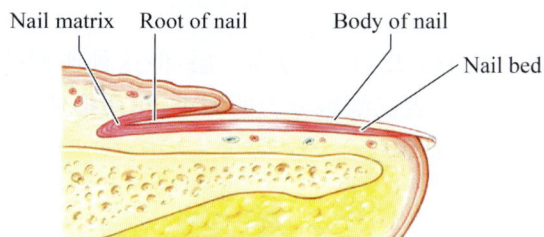

Figure 11 - 11   Diagram of the nail

(Zhang Jing)

第十一章 皮肤及其附属器官

皮肤是人体最重的器官,约占总体重的 16%。在成年人中,皮肤的表面积为 $1.2\sim2.3\,m^2$,面向外部环境。皮肤覆盖了身体的整个表面,并在身体出入口与口腔、鼻腔、肛门、生殖器和尿道开口处的黏膜相连续。皮肤能够抵御微生物、物理和化学损害及紫外线辐射,同时通过汗腺分泌汗液来调节体温。此外,皮肤还作为感觉器官,通过特定感觉神经感受外界刺激。

皮肤由两层组成:表皮(来自外胚层的上皮组织层)和真皮(来自中胚层的结缔组织层)。表皮与真皮的交界不规则,真皮的突起称为真皮乳头,与表皮的突起相互交错,被称为表皮嵴。真皮下方是皮下组织,也叫皮下脂肪组织,一般认为它不是皮肤的组成部分,只是将皮肤松散地连接到深部组织(图 11-1)。

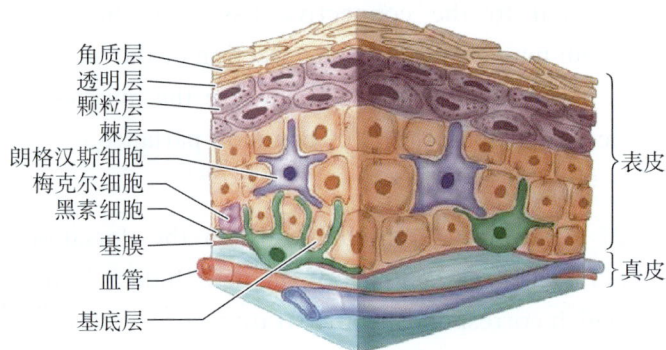

图 11-1 皮肤模式图

第一节 表 皮

表皮是一种角化的复层扁平上皮,可以分为 5 层,但这种典型的 5 层结构只存在于厚皮肤,例如手掌和脚底(图 11-2)。表皮细胞分为两大类,角质形成细胞和非角质形成细胞(黑素细胞、朗格汉斯细胞和梅克尔细胞)。

一、表皮的分层

1. 角质层

位于最表层,由多层角质细胞形成。角质细胞是已经死亡的细胞,细胞核消失且细胞膜增厚。该层细胞充满了由表皮深层的角质形成细胞产生的成熟角蛋白,它赋予表皮韧性和保护性,有助于防止水分散失。角质层的表面经常脱落,尤其在经受摩擦时。然而随着深层细胞不

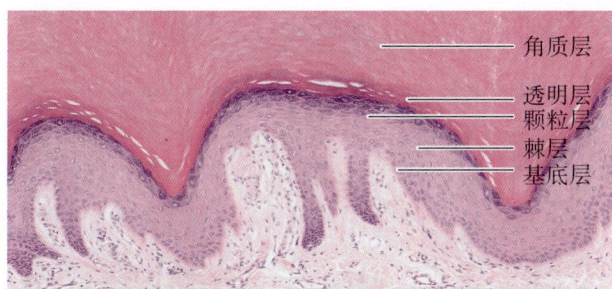

图 11-2 表皮的分层(人足底皮,HE 染色,100×)

断地向表层迁移,该层细胞得以更新和补充。

2. 透明层

该层较薄,且只在厚皮中出现。它是由非常扁平的嗜酸性细胞组成。这些细胞充满了角蛋白,没有细胞核或细胞器。

3. 颗粒层

该层包含 3~5 层扁平的多边形细胞,细胞内充满粗大的、嗜碱性的透明角质颗粒。该层上部的细胞死亡后即成为透明层的一部分。

4. 棘层

是表皮中最厚的一层,由数层多边形细胞和扁平细胞组成。在这些细胞的胞质中,存在着大量成束排列的角蛋白丝,从而形成了粗大的、嗜碱性的透明角质颗粒,且没有膜包被。细胞中还形成另一种膜被颗粒,为含有脂质成分的板层颗粒,可以将脂质排放到细胞间隙。该层细胞表面有较多短小的棘状突起,相邻细胞间的突起以桥粒相连。

5. 基底层

该层是由嗜碱性的单层立方上皮或柱状上皮细胞组成,位于表皮和真皮之间的基膜上。这层细胞具有增殖分化的潜能,是表皮的干细胞。基底层的细胞增殖形成的新细胞逐渐产生角蛋白丝并向表层迁移。

二、非角质细胞形成

1. 梅克尔细胞

梅克尔细胞分布在基底层中。它们类似于基底层角质形成细胞,但具有较短的突起和小而致密的颗粒(图 11-3)。常见感觉神经末梢末端膨大与该细胞底部紧密相接触。故梅克尔细胞可能作为感受器,但也有证据表明它们与弥散性神经内分泌系统相关。

2. 朗格汉斯细胞

朗格汉斯细胞来源于骨髓,主要位于棘层(图 11-4)。该细胞呈星形,细胞质内含有许多呈杆状或网球拍状的颗粒(伯贝克颗粒)。在 HE 染色的切片中,该细胞胞核深染而胞质清亮。朗格汉斯细胞属于单核吞噬细胞系统,在皮肤免疫反应中起着重要作用。该细胞能够捕获、处理抗原并将抗原呈递给 T 淋巴细胞,从而在 T 细胞的激活过程中发挥关键作用。

3. 黑素细胞

黑素细胞源自神经嵴并迁移到表皮。它们分散在基底层角质形成细胞中,但与角质形成细胞之间无桥粒连接。细胞呈圆形,核居中,向外伸出较长的突起,这些突起深入到基底层和

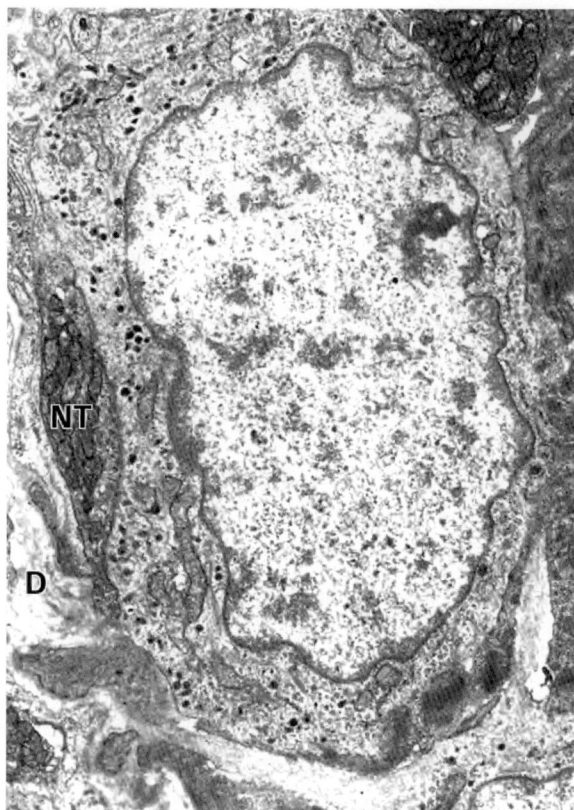

NT—神经末梢;D—真皮

图 11-3 梅克尔细胞电镜图

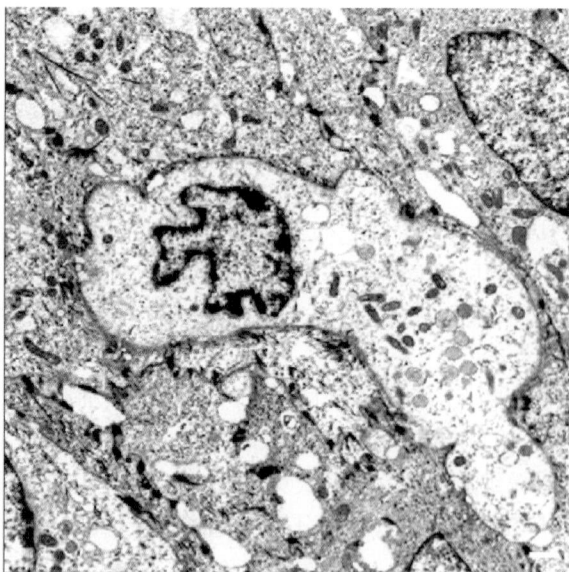

图 11-4 朗格汉斯细胞电镜图

棘层细胞之间,终止于角质形成细胞表面小的凹陷处。黑素细胞胞质中含有较多的线粒体、发达的高尔基复合体、粗面内质网及膜包被的黑色素体,其中含有合成的黑色素。黑色素决定了皮肤、眼睛和头发的颜色。一旦形成,黑色素颗粒会在黑色素细胞的胞质突起中迁移,并转移到基底层和棘层细胞中,从而进一步保护表皮深部细胞免受阳光中紫外线的辐射(图 11-5)。

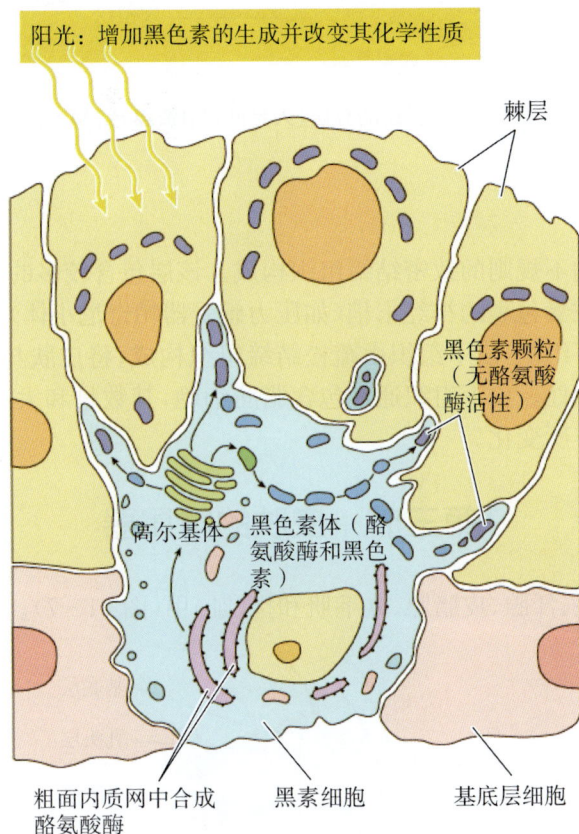

图 11-5 黑素细胞模式图

第二节 真 皮

真皮是由结缔组织组成,起到支持表皮并将其与皮下组织牢固连接的作用。真皮表面非常不规则,有许多突起,且与表皮的突起相互交错。该层具有丰富的血管和淋巴管,并包含毛囊、汗腺和皮脂腺等表皮衍生物。真皮分为两层:外侧的乳头层和深部的网织层(图 11-6)。

一、乳头层

乳头层紧靠表皮基膜的下方,由富含弹性纤维的疏松结缔组织构成。其向表皮突起形成真皮乳头,并与表皮相互交错,从而扩大了表皮和真皮的连接面。乳头层含有免疫细胞、丰富的毛细血管及游离神经末梢。许多真皮乳头内含有较多被囊包裹的触觉受体,称为迈斯纳小体(触觉小体)。

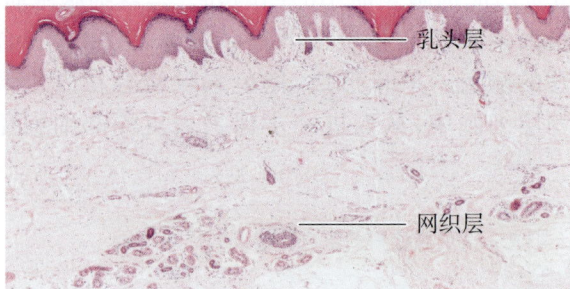

图 11-6　真皮的分层(人足底皮,HE 染色,40×)

二、网织层

网织层是由较厚的不规则的致密结缔组织构成。该层包含较多的血管、淋巴管和神经,包括游离神经末梢和有被囊包裹的神经末梢(如压力感受器帕奇尼小体)。

真皮的下方为皮下组织,皮下组织由疏松结缔组织构成,将皮肤与深部组织器官相连,并使皮肤具有一定的活动性。皮下组织通常包含脂肪细胞,其数量和大小依据身体部位的不同和营养状态的不同而有所变化。

第三节　皮肤的附属器

皮肤附属器包括毛、汗腺、皮脂腺、立毛肌和指(趾)甲(图 11-7)。

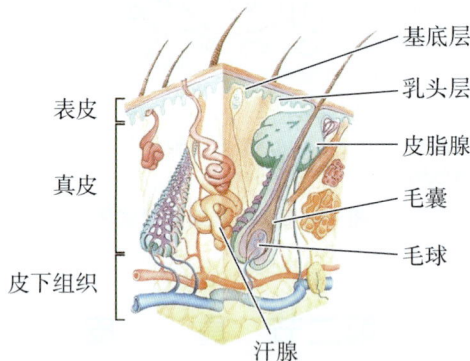

图 11-7　皮肤附属器模式图

一、毛

人体皮肤除手掌、脚掌、部分生殖器、指(趾)尖和嘴唇等部位以外,均有毛发分布。毛发的颜色、大小、形状及分布因人的种族、年龄、性别和身体部位不同而有所差异。

(一) 毛的结构

毛分为毛干、毛根和毛球三部分(图 11-8)。露在皮肤表面的为毛干,埋在皮肤内的为毛根;毛干和毛根由排列规则的角化上皮细胞组成,细胞内充满角蛋白并含有数量不等的黑素颗粒。包在毛根外面的毛囊分为两层,内层为上皮根鞘,与表皮相连续,包裹毛根,其结构也与表皮相似;外层为结缔组织鞘,与真皮相连续,由薄层致密结缔组织构成。毛根和毛囊上皮根鞘的下端合为一体,膨大为毛球。毛球的上皮细胞称毛母质细胞,为干细胞,它们不断增殖,部分干细胞分化形成毛根和上皮根鞘的细胞,并向上迁移。毛球基部的黑素细胞可将黑素颗粒转送到上皮细胞中。毛球底面有结缔组织突入其中形成毛乳头,内含丰富的毛细血管和神经末梢。毛球是毛和毛囊的生长点,毛乳头对毛的生长起诱导和营养作用。

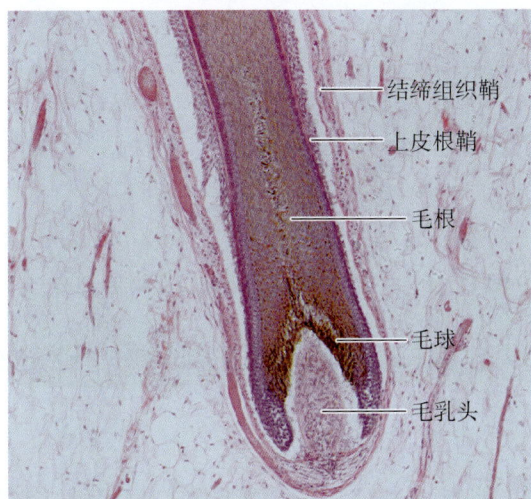

图 11-8 毛根(人头皮,HE 染色,40×)

毛的色素由分布在毛母质细胞间的黑素细胞生成,然后将色素输入新生的毛根上皮细胞中。毛发的颜色取决于毛干内角细胞中的黑色素含量。黑色素颗粒很少时毛发呈灰色或棕黄色,完全缺乏时呈白色。

(二) 毛的生长和更新

毛有一定的生长周期,头发的生长周期通常为3～5年,其他部位毛的生长周期只有数月。生长中的毛,其毛球膨大,毛乳头血流丰富,毛母质细胞增殖旺盛。转入静止期的毛球和毛乳头变小萎缩,毛母质细胞停止增殖,毛根与毛球、毛囊连接不牢。在旧毛脱落之前,于毛囊基部形成新的毛球和毛乳头,形成新毛,将旧毛推出。激素尤其是雄激素,会影响毛发的分布和生长速度。

二、汗腺

(一) 外泌汗腺

外泌汗腺分布在全身大部分的皮肤中。该汗腺是单曲管状腺,位于真皮深层或皮下组织中。每个腺体的分泌部分都连接一条细长的、高度盘曲的导管,穿过真皮层和表皮,开口于皮肤表面的汗孔(图 11-9)。

分泌部是由单层立方或矮柱状上皮组成,且被肌上皮细胞包绕。肌上皮细胞的收缩有助于腺液的分泌。

外泌汗腺的导管由两层立方上皮细胞组成。外泌汗腺在体温调节中起着重要作用,它通

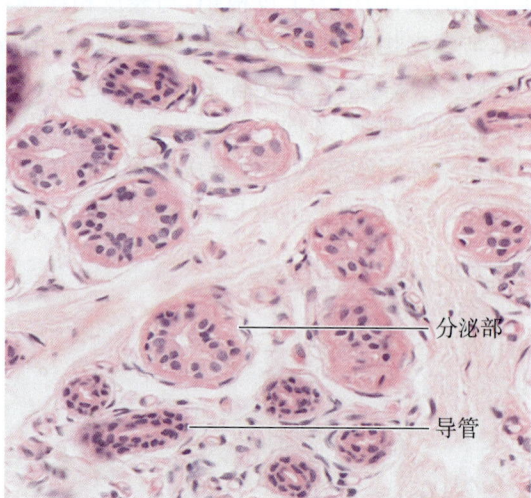

图 11-9 外泌汗腺(人足底皮,HE 染色,200×)

过体表汗液蒸发产生的冷却作用来调节体温。分泌部分泌的汗液成分与血浆相似,包括钾和氯化钠以及氨和尿素,从而维持电解质的平衡。

(二) 顶泌汗腺

顶泌汗腺主要分布在一些特定部位:腋下、乳晕和肛门区域。与外泌汗腺一样,顶泌汗腺也是弯曲管状腺体,有时有分支。该腺体分泌部的管腔比外泌汗腺的宽,由单层上皮细胞构成。腺细胞的胞质为嗜酸性。顶部胞质中含有较多颗粒,是细胞的分泌物,通过胞吐的形式分泌。与外泌汗腺不同,顶泌汗腺将其分泌物储存于导管中。

顶泌汗腺的导管与外泌汗腺的导管相似,然而,它从腺体分泌部发出后以相对笔直的路径开口于毛囊。导管上皮是复层立方上皮,通常为两层,有时三层。

顶泌汗腺分泌物含有蛋白质、碳水化合物、氨、脂质和某些可能使分泌物变色的有机化合物。腋窝的分泌物呈乳白色,微黏稠。分泌物在初分泌时是无味的,但通过细菌在皮肤表面的分解作用,它会产生刺鼻的气味。顶泌汗腺在青春期开始发挥功能,与腋毛和阴毛一样,它们的发育取决于性激素。

三、皮脂腺

皮脂腺分泌皮脂,覆盖于毛发和皮肤表面。除手掌、足底和足侧部外,皮脂腺分布在全身各处。

皮脂腺是由毛囊的外层根鞘发育而来,且每个毛囊通常可以形成几个腺体。皮脂腺的导管开口于毛囊的上三分之一段,并将其分泌物排入其中,覆盖于毛干表面,且最终分布于皮肤表面。腺体产生的油状物质,即皮脂,是全浆分泌的产物。即整个腺细胞逐渐产生并充满脂类物质,随即细胞凋亡、解体。最终,分泌物和细胞碎片以皮脂的形式从腺体排出,进入毛囊的漏斗部,并于皮脂腺的短导管之间形成了毛囊皮脂腺通道。腺体周边部的基底细胞通过有丝分裂不断产生新的腺细胞,且腺细胞之间通过桥粒相互连接。这些细胞的基膜与表皮和毛囊的基膜相延续(图 11-10)。

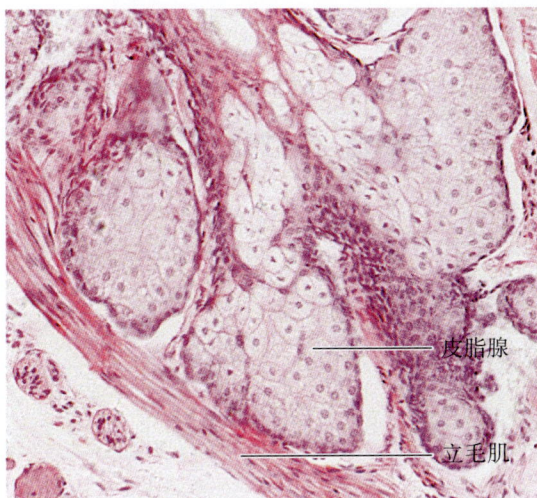

图 11-10 皮脂腺和立毛肌(人头皮,HE 染色,100×)

皮脂腺受性激素的影响,进入青春期分泌开始活跃。

四、立毛肌

毛和毛囊斜长在皮肤内,在它们与皮肤表面呈钝角的一侧,有一束斜行平滑肌,称立毛肌,其一端附着在毛囊上,另一端与真皮乳头层的结缔组织相连(图 11-10)。立毛肌的收缩会导致毛干竖立到更加直立的位置,也会导致与真皮层相连的皮肤凹陷。这种收缩产生了俗称"鸡皮疙瘩"的现象。

五、指(趾)甲

指(趾)甲为指(趾)端背面的呈层排列的角质形成细胞构成的硬角质板(图 11-11)。甲的近侧隐藏在甲沟中的部分称为甲根。甲体与皮肤角质层相对应,位于甲床的上方。甲床中只有基底层和棘层。甲体上皮来源于甲母质。甲母质近端延伸至甲根深处。甲母质细胞分裂增生,不断向指(趾)的远端移动,最终角化,形成甲体的细胞。

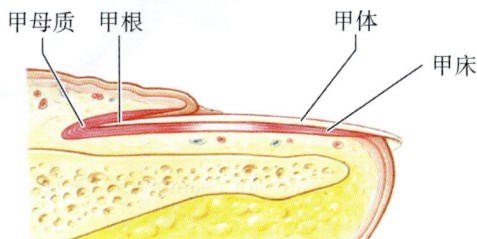

图 11-11 指甲模式图

(张 静)

Chapter 12

Eye and Ear

1 Eye

The eye is a photosensory organ consisting of the eyeball and accessory parts (conjunctiva, eyelids, lachrymal apparatus and extraocular muscles). The eyeball is a spherical structure and is mainly composed of eyeball wall and intraocular contents.

1.1 Eyeball Wall

The wall of eyeball consists of 3 concentric tunics, layers, or coats: the outer fibrous tunic (corneoscleral layer), the middle vascular tunic (uvea), and the inner neural tunic (retina) (Figure 12 – 1).

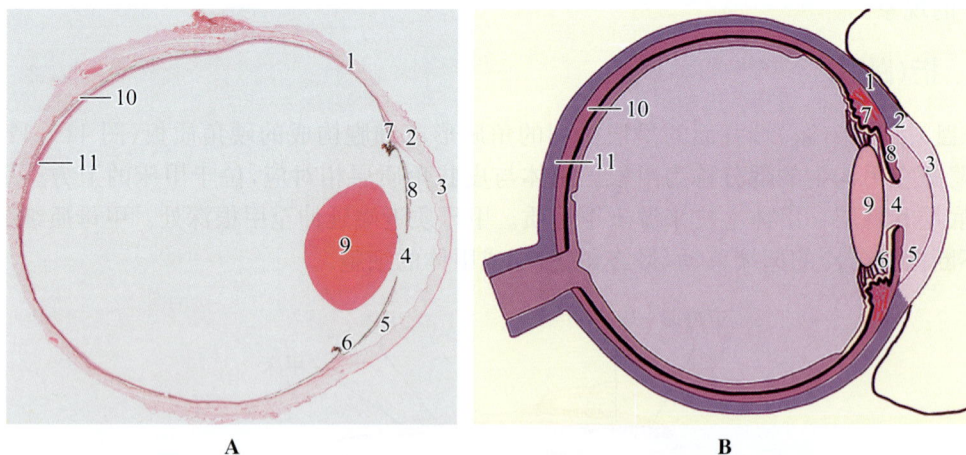

A   B

1. Sclera; 2. Limbus; 3. Cornea; 4. Pupil; 5. Anterior chamber; 6. Posterior chamber; 7. Ciliary body; 8. Iris; 9. Lens; 10. Choroid; 11. Retina

Figure 12 – 1   Structure of eyeball

A. Light microscopy image of the eyeball structure (3.5×); B. Schematic diagram of the eyeball structure

1.1.1   Tunica Fibrosa

The tunica fibrosa is composed of the sclera and the cornea. The white, opaque sclera covers the posterior 5/6 of the tunica fibrosa, whereas the colorless, transparent cornea covers the anterior 1/6 of the tunic. The junction between the sclera and the cornea is known as the limbus.

1.1.1.1　Sclera

The sclera, the white of the eye, is composed of dense connective tissue and nearly devoid of blood vessels. Sclera has a protective effect on the eyeball wall because of its tough texture. It also provides attachment for the extrinsic muscles of the eye.

1.1.1.2　Cornea

The cornea is a transparent disc-shaped structure that bulges out anteriorly from the eyeball. The cornea is thinner at its center, measuring around 0.5 mm, compared to the periphery which is approximately 1.0 mm thick. It can be divided into 5 distinct layers from anterior to posterior (Figure 12 – 2). The cornea is avascular, lacking blood vessels, but rich in free nerve endings. Additionally, it plays a crucial role in refracting light.

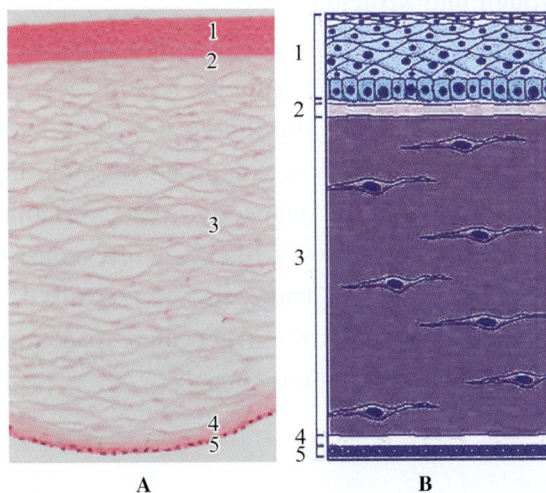

1. Corneal epithelium; 2. Anterior limiting lamina; 3. Corneal stroma; 4. Posterior limiting lamina; 5. Corneal endothelium

Figure 12 – 2　Structure of cornea
A. Light microscopy image of the cornea (100×); B. Structural schematic of the cornea

(1) Corneal Epithelium: It is a non-keratinized stratified squamous epithelium, with cells of 5 – 6 layers in a row, and there are no melanocytes. Both the basement membrane and the surface are smooth. The cells in the basal layer are columnar, in the middle layer they are polygonal, and in the superficial layer they are is flatten. The high mitotic rate of basal cells ensures the constant renewal of the corneal epithelium every 7 days on average. The corneal epithelium contains a rich supply of nerve endings, which contribute to the sensitivity and responsiveness of the cornea to external stimuli.

(2) Anterior limiting lamina: It's about 7 – 12 μm thick, transparent and homogeneous, containing stroma and collagen fibrils, but no cells.

(3) Corneal stroma: It accounts for approximately 9/10 of the total thickness of the cornea and is primarily composed of multiple layers of collagen lamellae. The collagen

fibrils within these lamellae are arranged in parallel, while the fibers between adjacent lamellae are perpendicular. Between the lamellae of the corneal stroma, there are scattered fibroblasts, also known as corneal cells. These cells are flat with multiple protrusions and produce fibers and stroma, participating in the repair of corneal injuries. The corneal stroma contains a significant amount of water.

（4）Posterior Limiting Lamina: Its structure is comparable to that of the anterior limiting lamina, being composed of stroma and collagen fibrils; however, it is thinner.

（5）Corneal Endothelium: It is a type of squamous epithelium that contributes to the renewal of the posterior limiting lamina.

The main reasons for corneal transparency are the regular arrangement of collagen fibrils, its high-water content, the absence of blood vessels, and the lack of melanocytes. These factors collectively contribute to the cornea's ability to maintain transparency, allowing light to pass through unobstructed.

1.1.1.3 Corneal Limbus

The corneal limbus is a 1 - 2 mm wide, annular region located at the junction of the cornea and sclera. Immediately inward of the limbus lies the scleral venous sinus, a large and irregularly shaped cavity whose wall is composed of endothelium, a discontinuous basement membrane, and a thin layer of connective tissue. Medial to the scleral venous sinus is the trabecular meshwork, a network-like structure consisting of trabeculae and trabecular spaces (Figure 12 - 3). The trabeculae are covered with endothelium and internally contain collagen fibers, while the trabecular spaces are filled with aqueous humor and are connected to the scleral venous sinus.

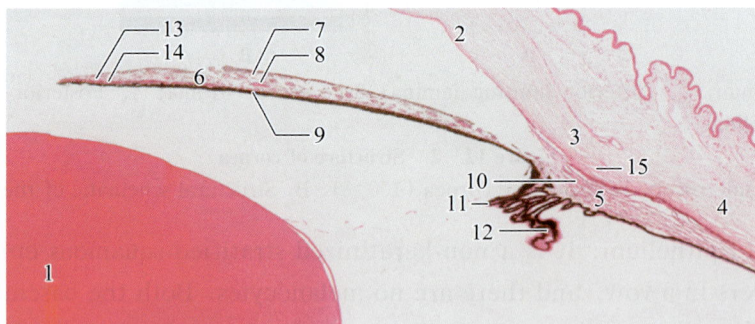

1. Lens; 2. Cornea; 3. Limbus; 4. Sclera; 5. Ciliary body; 6. Iris; 7. Anterior surface; 8. Iris stroma; 9. Iris epithelium; 10. Ciliary muscle; 11. Ciliary epithelium; 12. Ciliary processes; 13. Constrictor pupillary muscle; 14. Dilated pupillary muscle; 15. Canal of Schlemm & Trabecular meshwork

Figure 12 - 3　Light microscopy image of the anterior half of the eyeball (10×)

1.1.2　Vascular Tunic

The vascular tunic is composed of loose connective tissue rich in blood vessels and pigment cells. From front to back, it consists of 3 parts: the iris, the ciliary body, and the choroid.

1.1.2.1   Iris

The iris is a ring-shaped membrane situated between the cornea and the lens, measuring approximately 12 mm in diameter and 0.5 mm in thickness. It connects to the ciliary body at its periphery, while its center forms the pupil. The iris is structurally divided into 3 layers from anterior to posterior: the anterior border layer, iris stroma, and iris epithelium.

(1) Anterior Border Layer: It merges with the corneal epithelium and consists of discontinuous fibroblasts and pigment cells.

(2) Iris Stroma: It's thicker and composed of loose connective tissue rich in blood vessels and pigment cells. These pigment cells have irregular shapes with protrusions and are filled with melanin granules in their cytoplasm. Close to the pupillary margin, there is a circular arrangement of smooth muscle fibers, known as the sphincter pupillae, which contracts to narrow the pupil.

(3) Iris Epithelium: It comprises 2 layers of cells. The anterior layer, known as the dilator pupillae, consists of radially arranged myoepithelial cells centered around the pupil, which contract to dilate the pupil. The posterior layer is made up of cuboidal cells filled with melanin granules.

The color of the iris is influenced by the quantity and distribution of pigment cells within it.

1.1.2.2   Ciliary Body

The ciliary body is a ring-shaped structure located between the iris and choroid. It appears triangular in a sagittal section of the eyeball, wider at the front and narrower at the back. The anterior part of the ciliary body extends forward and inward with about 70 radially arranged ciliary processes, which emit radiating ciliary zonules connecting to the lens capsule. The posterior part of the ciliary body flattens gradually and terminates at the ora serrata.

The ciliary body consists of ciliary muscle, stroma, and epithelium (Figure 12 - 3). The ciliary muscle, composed of smooth muscle fibers, is the main component of the ciliary body. The muscle fibers have 3 orientations: longitudinal, radial, and circular. The stroma is connective tissue that is rich in blood vessels and pigment cells. The ciliary epithelium comprises 2 layers of cells: an outer layer of cuboidal pigmented epithelial cells and an inner layer of cuboidal or low columnar non-pigmented epithelial cells that secrete aqueous humor.

When the ciliary muscle contracts, the ciliary body protrudes forward, and the ciliary zonules relax. Conversely, when the muscle relaxes, the zonules tense, altering the position and curvature of the lens to adjust the focal length.

1.1.2.3   Choroid

The choroid (Figure 12 - 4), the posterior 2/3 of the vascular tunic, fills the space between the sclera and retina. It is loose connective tissue rich in blood vessels and pigment cells. Its innermost layer, adjacent to the retina, is a homogeneous and transparent membrane called the Bruch's membrane, composed of fibers and stroma.

1.1.3 Retina

The retina is divided into 2 parts: the blind portion and the visual portion. The blind portion, comprising the iris epithelium and ciliary epithelium, lacks photoreceptive capabilities. The visual portion, commonly referred to as the retina proper, lines the inner surface of the choroid and is a highly specialized layer of neural tissue responsible for photoreception. The junction between the blind and visual portions exhibits a serrated appearance, medically termed as the ora serrata.

1.1.3.1 Retina Layering

The retina (specifically referring to its visual portion) is mainly composed of 4 layers of cells, arranged from outer to inner as the pigment epithelium layer, photoreceptor layer, bipolar cell layer, and ganglion cell layer (Figure 12 - 4).

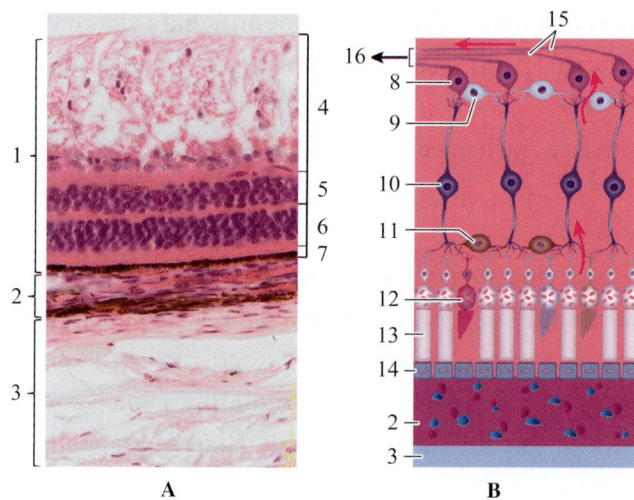

1. Retina; 2. Choroid; 3. Sclera; 4. Nuclei of ganglion cells; 5. Nuclei of bipolar cells; 6. Nuclei of rods and cones; 7. Pigmented layer of retina; 8. Ganglion cell; 9. Amacrine cell; 10. Bipolar cell; 11. Horizontal cell; 12. Cone; 13. Rod; 14. Pigment epithelium; 15. Nerve fibers; 16. optic nerve

Figure 12 - 4　Structure of retina

A. Light microscopy images (400×) of the retina, choroid and sclera; B. Schematic diagrams of retina

(1) Pigment Epithelial Layer: This layer is composed of a monolayer of cuboidal pigment epithelial cells. The basal surface of these cells tightly adheres to the Bruch's membrane, while their apical surface exhibit numerous protrusions that extend into the intercellular spaces of photoreceptor outer segments. Laterally, these cells are connected via tight junctions, intermediate junctions, and gap junctions. A prominent feature of these cells is the abundance of melanin granules and phagosomes within their cytoplasm. The melanin granules prevent photoreceptor cells from light-induced damage caused by

intense illumination. Phagosomes typically contain shed membrane disks from photoreceptor cells. Pigment epithelial cells perform numerous functions, such as storing vitamin A, participating in the formation of rhodopsin, and maintaining the stability of the retinal internal environment.

(2) Photoreceptor Layer: Photoreceptor cells, also known as visual cells, are sensory neurons that respond to light. These cells are divided into 3 parts: the cell body, the outer process (dendrite), and the inner process (axon). The cell body, which houses the nucleus, is slightly enlarged, and densely packed in multiple layers to form the photoreceptor layer. The outer process extends vertically towards the pigment epithelial layer and is divided into an inner segment and an outer segment, separated by a narrow, cilium-like structure called the connecting cilium. The inner segment, adjacent to the cell body, contains abundant mitochondria, rough endoplasmic reticulum, and Golgi complexes, and is the site of photoreceptor protein synthesis. The outer segment, which is the light-sensitive region, contains many parallel, stacked, flat membranous discs formed by the invagination of the plasma membrane on one side of the outer segment base (Figure 12 - 5). These membranous discs are equipped with photosensitive embedded proteins. The terminal end of the inner process primarily forms synaptic connections with bipolar cells.

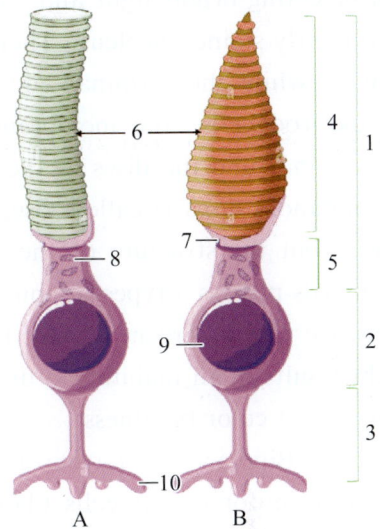

1. Outer process; 2. Cell body; 3. Inner process; 4. Outer segment; 5. Inner segment; 6. Membrane disks; 7. Connecting cilium; 8. Mitochondria; 9. Nucleus; 10. Synapses

Figure 12 - 5　Schematic diagram of rod cells and cone cells

A. Rod cell; B. Cone cell

Based on the shape of their outer processes and photoreceptive properties, photoreceptor cells are classified into 2 types: rods and cones. Cone cells are primarily distributed in the central retina, while rod cells are predominantly found in the peripheral region.

Rod Cell: Rod cells are much more numerous than cone cells and are primarily distributed in the peripheral retina, responsible for detecting dim light. These cells are slender in shape, with a small and densely stained nucleus. Their outer processes are rod-shaped (hence the name "rod cell"), while the terminal end of their inner processes is enlarged and globular. The membranous discs of rod cells are separated from the cell surface membrane, forming independent structures that continuously migrate towards the tip of the outer segment. As the discs at the tip age and detach, they are phagocytosed by pigment epithelial cells. The photosensitive protein on these membranous discs is called rhodopsin, which is sensitive to dim light. Rhodopsin consists of 11-cis-retinal and opsin.

Vitamin A is a crucial component for the synthesis of 11-cis-retinal. A deficiency in vitamin A can lead to a lack of rhodopsin, resulting in reduced vision in dim light, a condition known as night blindness.

Cone Cell: Cone cells are primarily distributed in the central retina and are responsible for detecting bright light and color. These cells are thicker than rod cells, with a larger and lightly stained nucleus. Their outer processes are cone-shaped (hence the name "cone cell"), while the terminal end of their inner processes is enlarged and pedunculated. Unlike rod cells, the membranous discs of cone cells are mostly attached to the cell membrane, and the discs at the tip do not detach. The photosensitive material on these membranous discs is called visual pigment, which is also composed of 11-cis-retinal and opsin, but the structure of the opsin differs from that of rhodopsin. Humans and most mammals possess 3 types of cone cells, each containing a different photosensitive pigment sensitive to red, green, or blue light. A deficiency in cone cells sensitive to red (or green) light results in an inability to distinguish red (or green) colors, a condition known as red (or green) color blindness.

(3) Bipolar Cell Layer: Bipolar cells are the vertically oriented interneurons that connect photoreceptor cells (both rods and cones) to ganglion cells in the retina. The dendrites of bipolar cells form synapses with the inner processes of photoreceptor cells, while their axons synapse with the dendrites of ganglion cells. Most bipolar cells connect multiple photoreceptor cells to multiple ganglion cells. However, a minority of these cells, known as midget bipolar cells, connect exclusively to a single cone cell and a single ganglion cell. These specialized cells are located at the edge of the fovea centralis in the retina.

This layer also contains other interneurons, such as horizontal cells and amacrine cells, which participate in the formation of local circuits within the retina for visual modulation.

Ganglion Cell Layer: Ganglion cells are multipolar neurons with long axons, mostly arranged in a single layer. Their dendrites primarily form synapses with bipolar cells, while their axons converge towards the posterior pole of the eyeball and exit the eyeball wall at the optic papilla to form the optic nerve. Most ganglion cells have larger cell bodies and form synaptic connections with multiple bipolar cells. However, a few ganglion cells located in the macular region have smaller cell bodies and form synapses with only one midget bipolar cell, known as midget ganglion cells.

Retinal Neuroglial Cells: These are mainly radial neuroglial cells, also known as Müller cells. They are elongated cells that span almost the entire thickness of the retina, except for the pigment epithelium. Their nuclei are located in the bipolar cell layer, and their processes extend between neurons, providing support, nutrition, insulation, and protection.

1.1.3.2 Macula Lutea

The macula lutea is located at the posterior pole of the retina, directly aligned with the optic axis. It has a transverse elliptical shape with a diameter of $1-3\,\text{mm}$ and a shallow depression at its center, known as the central fovea. The central fovea is the thinnest part of the retina, with a thickness of only $0.1\,\text{mm}$, consisting solely of pigment epithelium and cone cells. The bipolar cells and ganglion cells in this region are arranged obliquely towards the periphery, allowing light to directly fall on the cone cells. A one-to-one visual pathway is formed between the cone cells and the midget bipolar cells, as well as the midget ganglion cells, enabling precise signal transmission. Therefore, the central fovea is the most sensitive area of vision (Figure 12 – 6).

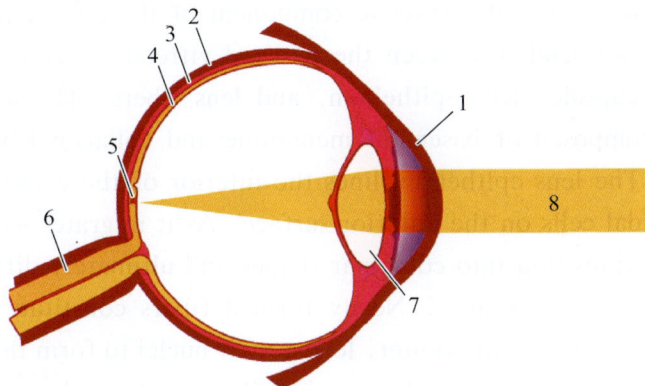

1. Cornea; 2. Sclera; 3. Choroid; 4. Retina; 5. Macula; 6. Optic nerve; 7. Lens; 8. Light

Figure 12 – 6   Schematic diagram of the macular lutea.

1.1.3.3   Optic Disc

The optic disc, also known as the papilla of the optic nerve, is located nasally to the macula. It appears as a circular, papilliform protrusion with a slightly concave center. It lacks photoreceptor cells, resulting in a physiological blind spot (Figure 12 – 6). This area serves as the convergence point for the axons of all retinal ganglion cells, which then exit the eyeball to form the optic nerve. Additionally, the central retinal artery and vein traverse through the optic disc.

1.2   Contents of the Eyeball

The contents of the eyeball include the aqueous humor, lens, and vitreous humor, all of which are colorless and transparent. Together with the cornea, they constitute the refractive system of the eye.

1.2.1   aqueous humor

Aqueous humor is the clear fluid that fills the anterior and posterior chambers of the eye. It is produced by the ciliary body through a combination of blood filtration and secretion from non-pigmented epithelial cells. Formed in the posterior chamber, it flows through the pupil into the anterior chamber and then exits via the trabecular meshwork at the angle of the anterior chamber, draining into the scleral venous sinus. From there, it enters the blood circulation through the anterior ciliary veins (Figure 12 - 3). Aqueous humor not only contributes to the refractive process but also provides nourishment to the lens and cornea, simultaneously helping maintain intraocular pressure. Under physiological conditions, there is a dynamic balance between the production and drainage of aqueous humor. An imbalance, such as excessive production or impaired drainage, can lead to increased intraocular pressure and subsequent damage to vision, a condition known as glaucoma.

1.2.2　Lens

The lens is the most crucial refractive component of the eye, a resilient, biconvex, transparent structure suspended between the iris and vitreous body by zonular fibers. It consists of the lens capsule, lens epithelium, and lens fibers. The lens capsule, a thin membranous layer composed of basement membrane and collagen fibrils, surrounds the entire lens surface. The lens epithelium lines the interior of the capsule, presenting as a single layer of cuboidal cells on the anterior surface. As it migrates towards the equator, these cells gradually transition into columnar shapes and ultimately differentiate into lens fibers, forming the lens's substance. Newly formed fibers constitute the cortex, while older fibers are pushed towards the center, losing their nuclei to form the lens nucleus. The lens lacks blood vessels and nerves, relying primarily on aqueous humor for nourishment. Visual impairment resulting from lens opacity is known as cataract.

1.2.3　Vitreous Body

The vitreous body is one of the refractive media located between the lens and the retina. It is enclosed by a transparent membrane called the hyaloid membrane and consists of a colorless, transparent gel-like substance. This substance is composed of 99% water, and also contains collagen fibrils, vitreous proteins, hyaluronic acid, and a small number of cells.

1.3　Accessory Organs of the Eye

The accessory organs of the eye, like the eyelids, lacrimal apparatus, and extraocular muscles, protect and move the eyeball.

1.3.1　Eyelid

The eyelid is a thin, plate-like structure consisting of 5 layers, arranged from anterior to posterior as skin, subcutaneous tissue, muscular layer, tarsus, and palpebral conjunctiva (Figure 12 - 7).

1.3.1.1　Skin

The skin of the eyelid is thin and soft. At the margin of the eyelid, there are eyelashes. The roots of the eyelashes are accompanied by small sebaceous glands, known as the tarsal glands or glands of Zeis. Near the eyelashes, there are coiled sweat glands called the glands of Moll.

1.3.1.2 Subcutaneous Tissue

This layer consists of loose connective tissue, which is prone to edema or congestion.

1.3.1.3 Muscular Layer

The muscular layer of the eyelid predominantly comprises skeletal muscle fibers.

1.3.1.4 Tarsus

Composed of dense connective tissue, the tarsus is hard like cartilage and serves as the support structure for the eyelid. Within the tarsus are parallel-arranged sebaceous glands that open at the eyelid margin, known as the tarsal glands. Their secretions lubricate the eyelid margin and protect the cornea. Obstruction and infection of the tarsal gland ducts can lead to the formation of a tarsal gland cyst (chalazion).

1.3.1.5 Palpebral Conjunctiva

This is a thin layer of mucosa with stratified columnar epithelium containing goblet cells. Its lamina propria

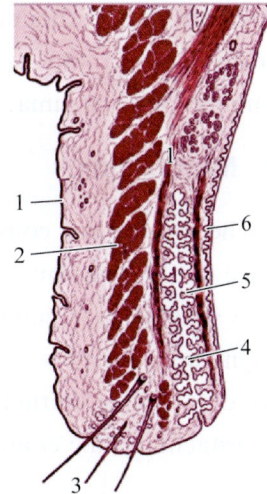

1. Skin; 2. Orbicularis oculi muscle; 3. Eyelashes; 4. Meibomian; 5. Tarsal plate; 6. Conjunctiva

Figure 12 – 7   Schematic diagram of the eyelid structure

consists of a thin layer of connective tissue. The palpebral conjunctiva transitions into the bulbar conjunctiva at the conjunctival fornix.

1.3.2 Lacrinal Gland

The lacrimal gland is a serous compound tubular acinar gland. It secretes tears that are drained via ducts into the conjunctival fornix, serving to lubricate and cleanse the cornea and conjunctiva.

2   Ear

The ear, consisting of the outer, middle, and inner ear, functions as the organ of hearing and balance. While the outer and middle ear receive and conduct sound waves, the inner ear is responsible for perceiving auditory and vestibular sensations. This textbook primarily focuses on the inner ear.

2.1 Outer Ear

The outer ear comprises the auricle, external auditory canal, and tympanic membrane. The auricle, supported by elastic cartilage, is covered by a thin layer of skin. The skin of the external auditory canal contains ceruminous glands, structurally similar to apocrine sweat glands, which secrete cerumen. The tympanic membrane, an oval-shaped translucent thin film, separates the external auditory canal from the middle ear. Its outer surface is covered by stratified squamous epithelium, while its inner surface is lined with simple cuboidal epithelium, with a thin layer of connective tissue in between. Due to its delicate nature, the tympanic membrane is prone to perforation or rupture from inflammation or trauma.

2.2 Middle Ear

The middle ear comprises the tympanic cavity and the Eustachian tube. The inner surface of the tympanic cavity and the 3 ossicles are covered by a mucosa, lined by either simple squamous or cuboidal epithelium. The mucosal lining of the Eustachian tube near the tympanic cavity is simple columnar epithelium, while it transitions to pseudostratified ciliated columnar epithelium near the nasopharynx. Additionally, the lamina propria of the Eustachian tube contains mixed glands.

2.3 Inner Ear

The inner ear, located within the petrous part of the temporal bone, consists of a series of curved canals with a complex structure resembling a "maze", hence also known as the labyrinth. It comprises the bony labyrinth (osseous labyrinth) and the membranous labyrinth. The membranous labyrinth is suspended within the bony labyrinth.

The bony labyrinth is a complex space divided into 3 main parts: the cochlea, vestibule, and semicircular canals (Figure 12 – 8), which are interconnected. The inner walls of these structures are lined with periosteum, and the labyrinth is filled with perilymph.

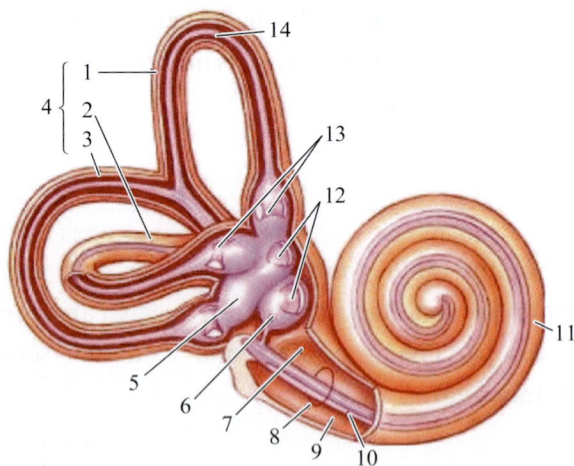

1. Anterior; 2. Lateral; 3. Posterior; 4. Semicircular canals; 5. Utricle; 6. Saccule; 7. Vestibular duct; 8. Cochlear duct; 9. Tympanic duct; 10. Organ of Corti; 11. Bony labyrinth of cochlea; 12. Maculae; 13. Cristae ampullaris; 14. Membranous semicircular canals

Figure 12 – 8   Structural schematic diagram of bony labyrinth, membranous labyrinth and receptors

The membranous labyrinth is a membranous structure suspended within the bony labyrinth, resembling its shape, and similarly divided into 3 parts: the cochlear duct, the vestibular membrane (comprising the utricle and saccule), and the membranous semicircular canals. These 3 components are interconnected. The wall of the membranous labyrinth is composed of simple squamous epithelium and lamina propria, where specialized sensory receptors for hearing and equilibrioception are formed by thickening of the mucosa and specialization of the epithelial cells.

The membranous labyrinth cavity is filled with endolymph, which is separated from the perilymph outside. The lymph serves various functions, including nourishing the inner ear and transmitting sound waves.

2.3.1   Cochlea, Cochlear Duct, and Spiral Organ

2.3.1.1   Cochlea

The cochlea, resembling a snail shell in appearance, is a complex structure formed by the winding of both a bony and a membranous cochlear duct (also referred to as the scale media) around a central axis for approximately 2 and 1/2 turns. The membranous duct divides the bony cochlear duct into 2 compartments: the upper scale vestibuli and the lower scale tympani (Figure 12 – 9). Both of these compartments are filled with perilymph and are connected at the cochlea's apex via the cochlear aperture. The cochlear axis, conical in shape and composed of spongy bone, harbors the spiral ganglion within its interior.

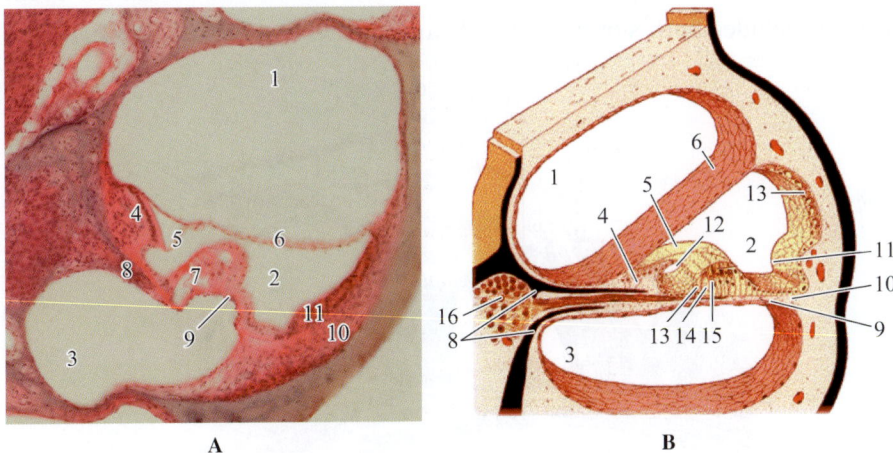

A   B

1. Scala vestibuli; 2. Scala media; 3. Scala tympani; 4. Spiral limbus; 5. Tectorial membrane; 6. Vestibular membrane; 7. Spiral organ; 8. Osseous spiral lamina; 9. Basilar membrane; 10. Spiral ligament; 11. Stria vascularis; 12. Internal spiral tunnel; 13. Inner hair cells; 14. Inner tunnel; 15. Pillar cells; 16. Spiral ganglion

Figure 12 – 9   Structure of cochlea duct and spiral organ
A. Photomicrograph (66×) of cochlear duct and spiral organ; B. Schematic diagram

2.3.1.2   Cochlear Duct

The cochlear duct is a spiral-shaped membranous canal that contains endolymph. When viewed in cross-section, it exhibits a triangular shape and is composed of 3 distinct walls.

Superior Wall: Also referred to as the vestibular membrane, it is covered by simple squamous epithelium on both sides, with a very thin layer of connective tissue in between.

Lateral Wall: It consists of the spiral ligament and its overlying epithelium. The spiral ligament is formed by the thickening of the periosteum on the lateral wall of the cochlea. Notably, the overlying epithelium, which contains capillaries extending from the lamina propria, is known as the stria vascularis and is intimately involved in the production of endolymph.

Inferior Wall: This is comprised of the osseous spiral lamina on the medial side and the membranous spiral lamina (also known as the basilar membrane) on the lateral side. The osseous spiral lamina is a thin, spiral-shaped structure formed by the extension of bony tissue outwards from the modiolus. The periosteum thickens and protrudes into the membranous cochlear duct to form the spiral limbus. Cells on its surface secrete glycoproteins, resulting in the formation of the tectorial membrane that is suspended above the spiral organ. The basilar membrane consists of 2 layers of epithelium sandwiching a basal lamina, connecting medially to the osseous spiral lamina and laterally to the spiral ligament. The epithelial thickening of the basilar membrane forms the organ of Corti.

2.3.1.3 Spiral Organ

The spiral organ, alternatively referred to as the organ of Corti, is a distinctively spiral-shaped structure that is positioned on the basilar membrane within the cochlear duct. Its composition includes both supporting cells and hair cells (Figure 12 - 10).

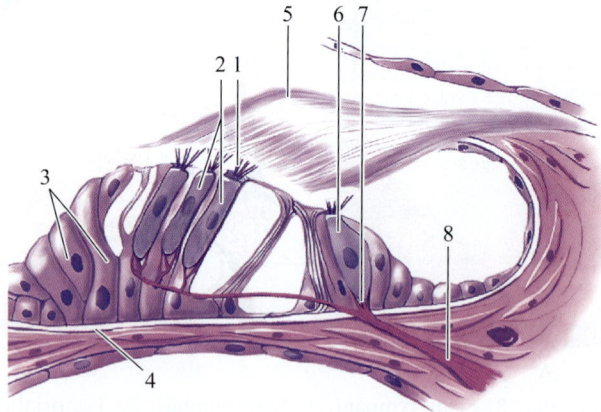

1. Hairs (Stereocilia); 2. Outer hair cells; 3. Supporting cells;
4. Basilar membrane; 5. Tectorial membrane; 6. Inner hair cells; 7. Afferent nerve fibers; 8. Fibers of cochlear nerve
Figure 12 - 10　Structural schematic diagram of spiral organ

Supporting Cells: Mainly pillar cells and phalangeal cells.

Pillar cells: There are 2 rows, inner and outer, which are referred to as inner and outer pillar cells respectively. They feature a broad base and a slender middle section. The bases and apices of these cells are connected on each side, respectively, while their middle portions are separated, forming a triangular inner tunnel. The cytoplasm of pillar cells is rich in tonofilaments, providing support.

Phalangeal Cells: There is 1 row of inner phalangeal cells on the inner side of the inner hair cells and 3 – 5 rows of outer phalangeal cells on the outer side of the outer pillar cells. The phalangeal cell is tall and columnar, with a concave top supporting a hair cell and a finger-like projection extending to the free surface of the spiral organ.

Hair Cells: These are sensory epithelial cells. There is 1 row of inner hair cells on top of the inner phalangeal cells and 3 – 5 rows of outer hair cells on top of the outer phalangeal cells. Inner hair cells are flask-shaped, while outer hair cells are tall and columnar. The apex of each hair cell bears 30 – 60 stereocilia, arranged in 3 – 4 rows in a "U" shape on inner hair cells and 3 – 5 rows in a "U" or "W" shape on outer hair cells. The stereocilia on the outer side gradually increase in height compared to those on the inner side, with the tallest ones found on the outermost hair cells being inserted into the gelatinous tectorial membrane. The base of the hair cells forms synapses with the dendritic endings of bipolar cells from the cochlear ganglion.

The basilar membrane of the spiral organ contains numerous collagen-like filaments called auditory strings, which radiate from the inner to the outer side. From the base to the apex of the cochlea, the basilar membrane widens gradually while the auditory fibers lengthen, resulting in a transition of resonant sound waves from higher frequencies at the base to lower frequencies at the apex.

The spiral organ is the auditory receptor. Sound waves enter through the external auditory canal, causing the tympanic membrane to vibrate. These vibrations are transmitted via the ossicular chain to the oval window, initiating vibrations in the perilymph of the scala vestibuli. Subsequently, these vibrations either cause the endolymph in the membranous cochlear duct to vibrate via the vestibular membrane or are transmitted through the helicotrema to the scala tympani, inducing resonance in the basilar membrane and spiral organ. Depending on the frequency of the vibrations, corresponding auditory strings resonate, causing the stereocilia of the hair cells in contact with the tectorial membrane to bend. This stimulates the hair cells, and the resulting excitation is transmitted via the cochlear nerve to the central nervous system, generating the sensation of hearing. Any disruption in this process can lead to hearing loss.

2.3.2　Semicircular Canals, Semicircular Ducts, and Crista Ampullaris

2.3.2.1　Semicircular Canals

The semicircular canals, situated in the posterolateral region of the inner ear, are comprised of 3 mutually perpendicular half-ring-shaped bony canals. These canals connect to the vestibule via dilated areas known as ampullae.

2.3.2.2　Semicircular Ducts

The semicircular ducts are nested within the bony semicircular canals, and at the ampulla, a ridge-like elevation called the crista ampullaris is formed by the thickening of one side of the membrane.

2.3.2.3 Crista Ampullaris

The crista ampullaris is composed of an epithelium that includes supporting cells and hair cells, which are overlaid by a conical, gelatinous structure known as the cupula (Figure 12 – 11).

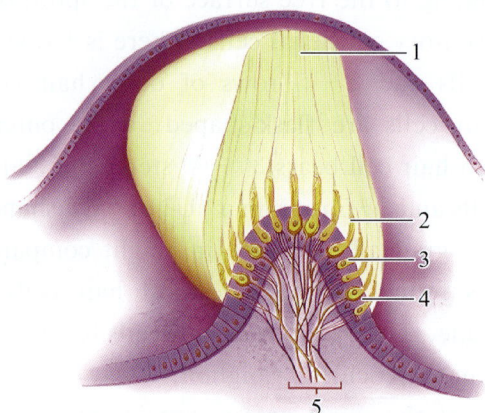

1. Cupula; 2. Hair; 3. Hair cell; 4. Supporting cell; 5. Nerves

Figure 12 – 11 Structural schematic diagram of crista ampullaris

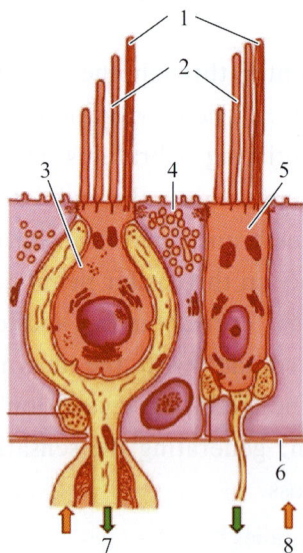

1. Kinocilia; 2. Stereocilia; 3. Type Ⅰ hair cell; 4. Supporting cell; 5. Type Ⅱ hair cell; 6. Basal lamina; 7. Efferent nerve endings; 8. Afferent nerve endings

Figure 12 – 12 Schematic diagram of hair cells in crista ampullaris

The supporting cells are tall and columnar, with secretory granules at their apical cytoplasm that secrete glycoproteins to form the cupula. These supporting cells provide support and nourishment to the hair cells.

There are two types of hair cells (Figure 12 – 12): type Ⅰ and type Ⅱ. Type Ⅰ cells are flask-shaped, while type Ⅱ cells are long and cylindrical. The free surface of the hair cells bears 50 – 100 stereocilia arranged in a staircase pattern. The longest stereocilium is accompanied by a longer kinocilium on one side, and both the stereocilium and kinocilium extend into the cupula. The cupula is formed by glycoproteins secreted by the supporting cells. Afferent nerve fibers from the vestibular nerve terminate at the base of the hair cells.

The crista ampullaris is a vestibular receptor. During rotational or accelerating head movements, the endolymph in the semicircular duct flows, causing the cupula to deflect. This deflection stimulates the hair cells, generating excitation that is transmitted to the central nervous system via the vestibular nerve.

2.3.3   Vestibule, Utricle / Saccule, and Maculae

2.3.3.1   Vestibule

The vestibule is a dilated bony cavity that connects the semicircular canals and cochlea.

2.3.3.2   Utricle/Saccule

The membranous vestibule is nested within the bony vestibule and consists of the utricle and saccule. Localized thickenings of the mucosa on the lateral wall of the utricle and the anterior wall of the saccule form patch-like structures called the macula utriculi and macula sacculi, respectively. Both the macula utriculi and macula sacculi are vestibular receptors, collectively referred to as the maculae acustica.

2.3.3.3   Maculae

The basic structure of the maculae is similar to that of the crista ampullaris, consisting of supporting cells and hair cells (Figure 12 − 13), but the surface is flat. The secretions of the supporting cells form a gelatinous membrane called the otolithic membrane on the surface of the maculae. This membrane contains tiny calcium carbonate crystals called otoliths. The kinocilium and stereocilia of the hair cells also extend into the otolithic membrane.

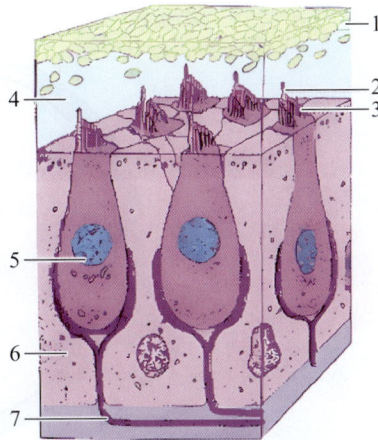

1. Otoliths; 2. Kinocilia; 3. Stereocilia; 4. Gelatinous layer; 5. Hair cell; 6. Supporting cell; 7. Nerves

Figure 12 − 13   Structural schematic diagram of the maculae acustica

The maculae senses linear acceleration and the static position of the head. Due to the perpendicular arrangement of the saccular and utricular maculae, and the much higher density of otoliths compared to endolymph, the otolithic membrane experiences a constant gravitational pull, stimulating hair cells regardless of head position. This excitation is then transmitted to the central nervous system via the vestibular nerve.

(*Sun Shen*)

第十二章 眼 和 耳

第一节 眼

眼是感光器官,主要由眼球及其附属结构(结膜、眼睑、泪器和眼外肌)组成。眼球近似球形,由眼球壁和眼内容物组成。

一、眼球壁

眼球壁由 3 个同心的层组成:外层纤维膜(角巩膜层)、中层血管膜(葡萄膜)和内层神经层(视网膜)(图 12-1)。

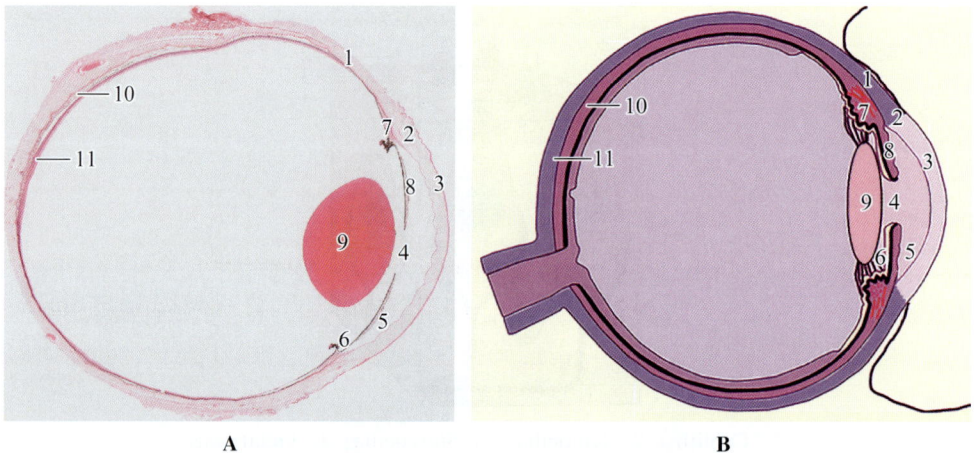

A   B

1—巩膜;2—角膜缘;3—角膜;4—瞳孔;5—前房角;6—后房角;7—睫状体;8—虹膜;9—晶状体;10—脉络膜;11—视网膜

图 12-1 眼球结构
A.眼球的光镜图(HE 染色,3.5×);B.眼球的结构模式图

(一) 纤维膜

纤维膜由巩膜和角膜组成。白色不透明的巩膜覆盖纤维膜的后面约 5/6,而无色透明的角膜覆盖前 1/6。巩膜和角膜之间的连接称为角膜缘。

1. 巩膜

巩膜(sclera)是眼睛的白色部分,由致密结缔组织组成,几乎没有血管。因巩膜质地坚硬,对眼球壁具有保护作用。另外,巩膜还为眼外肌提供附着点。

2. 角膜

角膜是眼球前部向外凸出的透明圆盘状结构。中央薄,平均 0.5 mm,而周边较厚,平均 1.0 mm。角膜从前至后分为 5 层(图 12-2),没有血管,含有丰富游离神经末梢。角膜具有屈光作用。

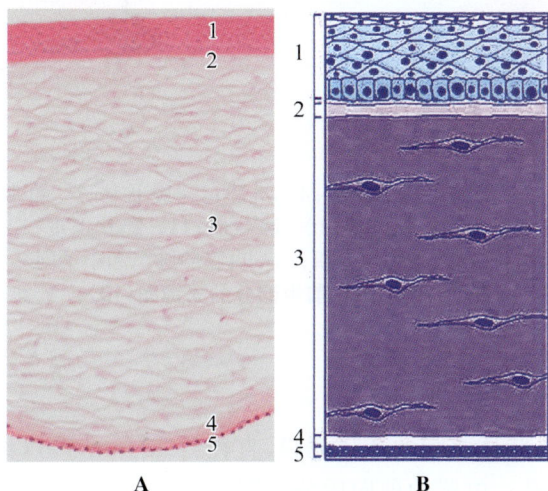

1—角膜上皮;2—前界层;3—角膜基质;4—后界层;5—角膜内皮

图 12-2　角膜结构

A. 角膜的光镜图(100×);B. 角膜结构模式图

(1) 角膜上皮:是未角化的复层扁平上皮,有 5~6 层细胞,排列整齐,其中无黑素细胞。基底面和表面均平坦。基底层为一层矮柱状细胞,具有增殖能力,中间层为多边形细胞,表层则是扁平细胞。角膜上皮平均 7 天更新一次。角膜上皮内含丰富的游离神经末梢,所以感觉敏锐。

(2) 前界层:厚 7~12 μm,透明均质状,含基质和胶原原纤维,不含细胞。

(3) 角膜基质:约占角膜全厚的 9/10,主要由多层胶原板层组成,板层内胶原原纤维的排列方向互相平行,相邻板层间纤维则互相垂直。板层之间有散在分布的成纤维细胞,又称为角膜细胞,扁平多突起,产生纤维和基质,参与角膜损伤的修复。角膜基质内含较多水分。

(4) 后界层:结构与前界层类似,由基质和胶原原纤维组成,但更薄。

(5) 角膜内皮:为单层扁平上皮。参与后界层的更新。

角膜透明的主要原因是胶原原纤维规则排列、富含水分、无血管、无黑素细胞。

3. 角膜缘

角膜缘为角膜和巩膜交界处的环形带状区域,宽 1~2 mm。角膜缘内侧有环行的巩膜静脉窦,窦腔较大而不规则,窦壁由内皮、不连续的基膜和薄层结缔组织构成。巩膜静脉窦内侧为小梁网,呈网络状,由小梁和小梁间隙构成(图 12-3)。小梁表面覆盖内皮,内部为胶原纤维。小梁间隙内含房水,与巩膜静脉窦相通。

(二) 血管膜

血管膜由富含血管和色素细胞的疏松结缔组织构成。从前向后依次为虹膜、睫状体和脉

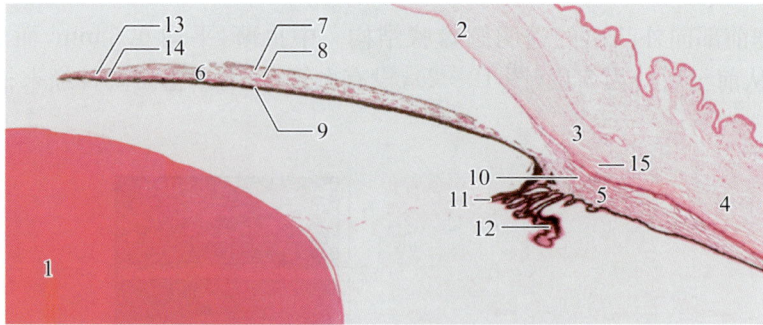

1—晶状体;2—角膜;3—角膜缘;4—巩膜;5—睫状体;6—虹膜;7—前缘层;8—虹膜基质;9—虹膜上皮;10—睫状肌;11—睫状上皮;12—睫状突;13—瞳孔括约肌;14—瞳孔开大肌;15—巩膜静脉窦和小梁网

图12-3　眼球前半部分的光镜图(10×)

络膜三部分。

1. 虹膜

虹膜是位于角膜和晶状体之间的环状薄膜,直径约12 mm,厚度约0.5 mm。虹膜外周与睫状体相连,而中央为瞳孔。虹膜由前向后分三层。

(1)前缘层与角膜上皮相延续,为一层不连续的成纤维细胞和色素细胞。

(2)虹膜基质较厚,为富含血管和黑素细胞的疏松结缔组织。黑素细胞的形态不规则,有突起,胞质内充满黑素颗粒。近瞳孔缘处有围绕瞳孔环行排列的平滑肌,称瞳孔括约肌,收缩时使瞳孔缩小。

(3)虹膜上皮由前后两层细胞组成。前层为肌上皮细胞,以瞳孔为中心呈放射状排列,称为瞳孔开大肌,收缩时使瞳孔开大。后层细胞呈立方形。胞质内充满黑素颗粒。黑素细胞的数量和分布影响虹膜的颜色。

2. 睫状体

睫状体是位于虹膜与脉络膜之间的环状结构。在眼球矢状切面上呈三角形,前宽后窄。睫状体前部向前内方伸出约70个呈放射状排列的睫状突,而睫状突表面则发出辐射状的睫状小带连至晶状体囊内。睫状体后部渐平坦,终止于锯齿缘。

睫状体由睫状肌、基质和上皮组成(图12-3)。睫状肌为平滑肌,是睫状体的主要组成成分。肌纤维有纵行、放射状和环行三种走向。基质为富含血管和色素细胞的结缔组织。睫状体上皮由两层细胞组成,外层为立方形的色素上皮细胞,内层为立方形或矮柱状的非色素上皮细胞,可分泌房水。

睫状肌收缩时,睫状体前突,睫状小带松弛;反之,则紧张,借此改变晶状体的位置和曲度,从而调节焦距。

3. 脉络膜

脉络膜为血管膜的后2/3部分,充填于巩膜和视网膜之间,是富含血管和色素细胞的疏松结缔组织。最内层与视网膜相贴,为一均质透明的薄膜,称玻璃膜(Bruch's membrane),由纤维和基质组成(图12-4)。

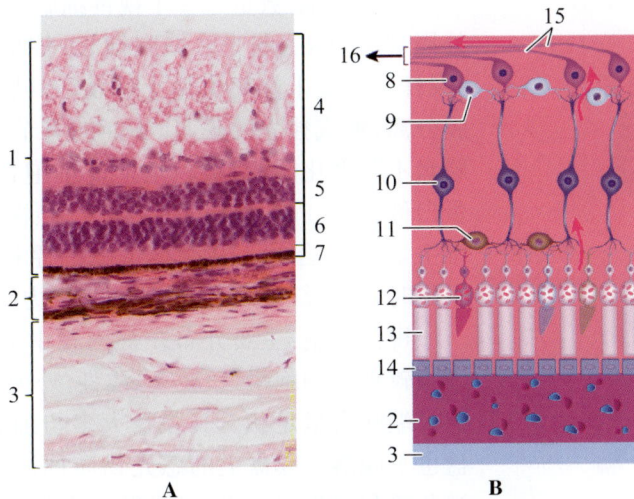

1—视网膜;2—脉络膜;3—巩膜;4—节细胞层;5—双极细胞层;6—视细胞层;7—色素上皮层;8—节细胞;9—无长突细胞;10—双极细胞;11—水平细胞;12—视锥细胞;13—视杆细胞;14—色素上皮;15—神经纤维;16—视神经

图 12-4 视网膜结构
A.视网膜、脉络膜和巩膜的光镜图(400×);B.视网膜的模式图

(三) 视网膜

视网膜分为盲部与视部。盲部包括虹膜上皮和睫状体上皮,不能感光。视部衬于脉络膜内侧,为高度特化的神经组织,是感光部位,即通常所称的视网膜。盲部与视部交界处呈锯齿状,称锯齿缘(ora serrata)。

1. 视网膜分层

视网膜(以下所述视网膜指视网膜视部)主要由 4 层细胞构成,由外向内依次为色素上皮层、视细胞层、双极细胞层和节细胞层(图 12-4)。

(1) 色素上皮层:由色素上皮细胞构成的单层立方上皮。细胞基底面紧贴玻璃膜,顶部有大量突起伸入视细胞的外节之间,侧面有紧密连接、中间连接、缝隙连接。色素上皮细胞的主要特点是胞质内含许多粗大的黑素颗粒和吞噬体。黑素颗粒可防止强光对视细胞的损害。吞噬体内通常为视细胞脱落的膜盘。色素上皮细胞功能较多,如储存维生素 A、参与视紫红质形成及稳定视网膜的内环境等。

(2) 视细胞层:视细胞是感受光线的感觉神经元,又称感光细胞。细胞分为胞体、外突(即树突)和内突(即轴突)三部分。胞体是细胞核所在部位,略微膨大。胞体紧密排列成多层,构成视细胞层。外突垂直伸向色素上皮细胞层,分为内节和外节,二者之间有一缩窄处为纤毛性结构,称连接纤毛。内节邻接胞体,含丰富的线粒体、粗面内质网和高尔基复合体,是合成感光蛋白的部位。外节为感光部位,含有大量平行层叠的扁平状膜盘。膜盘是由外节基部一侧的胞膜向胞质内陷形成的(图 12-5),其上有能感光的镶嵌蛋白。内突末端主要与双极细胞形成突触联系。

根据外突形状和感光性质不同,视细胞分为视杆细胞和视锥细胞两种。视锥细胞主要分布在视网膜中部,视杆细胞主要分布在周围。

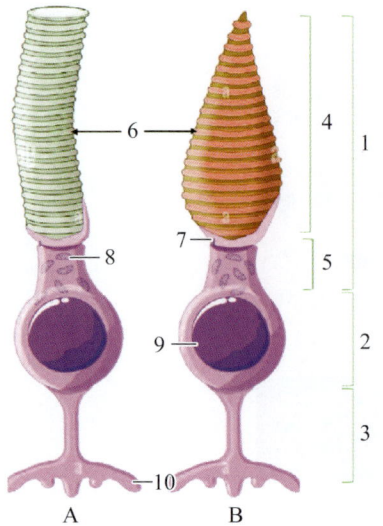

1—外突；2—胞体；3—内突；4—外节；5—内节；6—膜盘；7—连接纤毛；8—线粒体；9—细胞核；10—突触

图 12 - 5　视杆细胞和视锥细胞的模式图

A. 视杆细胞；B. 视锥细胞

视杆细胞：数量远多于视锥细胞，主要分布在视网膜的外周部分，感受弱光。细胞细长，核小、深染，外突呈杆状(视杆)，内突末端膨大呈小球状。其膜盘与细胞表面细胞膜分离，形成独立的膜盘，不断向外节顶端推移，而顶端的膜盘不断老化脱落，被色素上皮细胞吞噬。膜盘上的感光蛋白称视紫红质，感弱光。由 11 -顺视黄醛和视蛋白组成。维生素 A 是合成 11 -顺视黄醛的原料。当人体维生素 A 不足时，视紫红质缺乏，导致弱光视力减退，即为夜盲症。

视锥细胞：主要分布在视网膜中部，感受强光和颜色。细胞较视杆细胞粗，核较大，浅染，外突呈圆锥形(视锥)，内突末端膨大呈足状。其膜盘大多与细胞膜不分离，顶端膜盘也不脱落。膜盘上的感光物质称视色素，也是由 11 -顺视黄醛和视蛋白组成，但视蛋白的结构与视紫红质的不同。人和绝大多数哺乳动物有三种视锥细胞，分别含有红敏色素、绿敏色素和蓝敏色素。如缺少感红光(或绿光)的视锥细胞，则不能分辨红(或绿)色，为红(或绿)色盲。

（3）双极细胞层：双极细胞是连接视细胞和节细胞的纵向中间神经元。其树突与视神经的内突形成突触，轴突与节细胞的树突形成突触。大多数双极细胞可连接多个视细胞和节细胞，然而也有少数细胞只与一个视锥细胞和一个节细胞联系，称侏儒双极细胞，其位置在视网膜中央凹边缘。

此层还有其他中间神经元，如水平细胞、无长突细胞等，参与构成视网膜内的局部环路，进行视觉调节。

（4）节细胞层：节细胞是具有长轴突的多极神经元，大多排列成单层，其树突主要与双极细胞形成突触，轴突向眼球后极汇聚，在视神经乳头处穿出眼球壁，形成视神经。节细胞大多数胞体较大，与多个双极细胞形成突触联系；少数位于黄斑处的节细胞胞体较小，只与一个侏儒双极细胞形成突触，称侏儒节细胞。

视网膜神经胶质细胞：主要是放射状胶质细胞，又称米勒细胞(Müller cell)。细胞狭长，几乎贯穿除色素上皮外的视网膜全层，其胞核位于双极细胞层，突起伸展于神经元之间，具有支持、营养、绝缘和保护作用。

2. 黄斑

黄斑是视网膜后极正对视轴的一个浅黄色区域，呈横向椭圆形，直径 1～3 mm，其中央有一浅凹，称中央凹。中央凹是视网膜最薄的部分，厚度仅 0.1 mm，只有色素上皮和视锥细胞。此处的双极细胞和节细胞均斜向外周排列，故光线可直接落在视锥细胞上。其视锥细胞与侏儒双极细胞、侏儒节细胞之间构成一对一的视觉通路，从而实现精确的信号传导。因此，中央凹是视觉最敏锐的部位(图 12 - 6)。

3. 视盘

视盘又称视神经乳头，位于黄斑鼻侧，圆盘状，呈乳头状隆起，中央略凹。此处无感光细胞，为生理盲点。所有节细胞的轴突在此汇集，穿出眼球壁形成视神经；视网膜中央动、静脉也在此穿过。

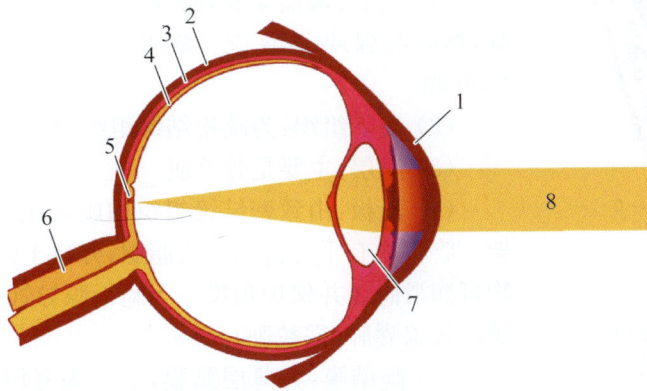

1—角膜；2—巩膜；3—脉络膜；4—视网膜；5—黄斑；6—视神经；7—晶状体；8—光线
图 12－6　黄斑模式图

二、眼内容物

包括房水、晶状体和玻璃体，均无色透明，与角膜共同组成眼的屈光系统。

1. 房水

房水为充满于眼房的透明液体。房水来自睫状体的血液渗出和非色素上皮细胞分泌，形成于后房，再经瞳孔至前房，继而在前房角经小梁间隙进入巩膜静脉窦，最终由睫状前静脉导入血循环（图 12－3）。房水具有屈光作用，还可营养晶状体和角膜，以及维持眼压。生理状况下，房水的产生和回流动态平衡。房水产生过多或回流受阻时，会增高眼压，使视力受损，称青光眼。

2. 晶状体

晶状体是眼球中最重要的屈光装置，为具有弹性的扁圆形双凸透明体，借睫状小带悬挂于虹膜和玻璃体之间。晶状体由晶状体囊、晶状体上皮和晶状体纤维组成。晶状体囊包绕整个晶状体表面，为一薄层囊状结构，由基膜和胶原原纤维组成。晶状体上皮在晶状体囊内，在前表面时为单层立方上皮，而在向赤道移行过程中渐渐变为柱状，并最终分化为晶状体纤维，构成晶状体实质。新形成的纤维构成皮质，老的纤维被推向中心，胞核逐渐消失，构成晶状体核。晶状体内无血管和神经，主要靠房水供给营养。晶状体混浊导致的视觉障碍，称白内障。

3. 玻璃体

玻璃体为屈光介质之一，位于晶状体与视网膜之间。外包透明的薄膜称玻璃体膜，其内为无色透明的胶状体，其中水分占 99%，还含有胶原原纤维、玻璃体蛋白、透明质酸和少量细胞。

三、眼附属器官

包括眼睑、泪器和眼外肌等，对眼球起保护、运动等作用。

1. 眼睑

为薄板状结构，有 5 层结构，由前至后依次为皮肤、皮下组织、肌层、睑板和睑结膜（图 12－7）。

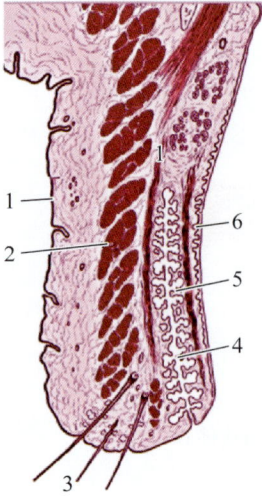

1—皮肤；2—眼轮匝肌；3—睫毛；
4—睑板腺；5—睑板；6—结膜

图 12-7　眼睑结构的模式图

（1）皮肤：薄而柔软，睑缘处有睫毛，睫毛根部有小的皮脂腺，称睑缘腺或 Zeis 腺。睫毛附近有螺旋状汗腺，称睫腺或 Moll 腺。

（2）皮下组织：为疏松结缔组织，易水肿或淤血。

（3）肌层：主要是骨骼肌。

（4）睑板：由致密结缔组织构成，坚硬如软骨，是眼睑的支架。睑板内有平行排列的皮脂腺，开口于睑缘，称睑板腺，分泌物可润滑睑缘并保护角膜。当睑板腺导管阻塞和感染时，会形成睑板腺囊肿(霰粒肿)。

（5）睑结膜：为薄层黏膜，上皮为复层柱状，有杯状细胞，固有层为薄层结缔组织。睑结膜在结膜穹窿处移行为球结膜。

2. 泪腺

为浆液性复管泡状腺。分泌的泪液经导管排至结膜穹窿部，具有润滑、清洁角膜和结膜的作用。

第二节　耳

耳是听觉和位觉器官，由外耳、中耳和内耳组成。外耳和中耳接收和传导声波，内耳感受听觉和位置觉。本书主要介绍内耳。

一、外耳

外耳由耳廓、外耳道和鼓膜构成。耳廓以弹性软骨为支架，外包薄层皮肤。外耳道的皮肤内有耵聍腺，结构类似大汗腺，分泌耵聍。**鼓膜**为椭圆形的半透明薄膜，分隔外耳道与中耳。鼓膜外表面为复层扁平上皮，内表面为单层立方上皮，中间为薄层结缔组织。鼓膜很薄，炎症或外伤都能导致穿孔或破裂。

二、中耳

中耳包括鼓室和咽鼓管。鼓室内表面和三块听小骨表面覆有黏膜，上皮为单层扁平或立方。咽鼓管近鼓室段的黏膜上皮为单层柱状，近鼻咽段为假复层纤毛柱状，固有层内有混合腺。

三、内耳

内耳位于颞骨岩部中，为一系列弯曲管道，结构复杂，形同"迷宫"，故又称迷路。它由骨迷路和膜迷路组成。膜迷路悬于骨迷路内。

骨迷路是一个由三部分组成的复杂空间，由前至后依次为耳蜗、前庭和半规管(图 12-8)，它们互相通连，内壁上都衬以骨膜，迷路内充满外淋巴。

膜迷路是悬于骨迷路内的膜性结构，形态与骨迷路相似，也相应地分为三部分，即膜蜗管、膜前庭(椭圆囊和球囊)和膜半规管，三者也互相通连。管壁的黏膜由单层扁平上皮和固有层构成，其上可见由黏膜增厚、上皮细胞特化形成的听觉或位觉感受器。

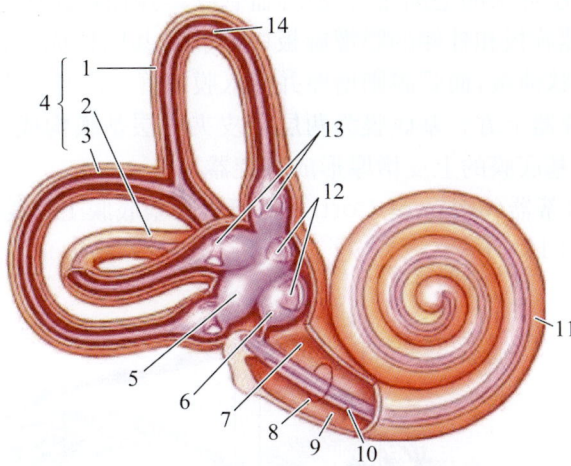

1—前；2—水平；3—后；4—半规管；5—椭圆囊；6—球囊；7—前庭；8—膜蜗管；9—鼓室导管；10—螺旋器；11—耳蜗；12—位觉斑；13—壶腹嵴；14—膜半规管

图 12-8　骨迷路、膜迷路及感受器结构模式图

膜迷路腔内充满内淋巴,内、外淋巴互不相通。淋巴有营养内耳和传递声波等作用。

1. 耳蜗、膜蜗管和螺旋器

(1)耳蜗:形如蜗牛壳,是由骨蜗管和其内嵌套的膜蜗管围绕中央的蜗轴旋绕两周半而成。骨蜗管被膜蜗管(又称中阶)分隔为上、下两部分,上方为前庭阶,下方为鼓室阶(图 12-9),两者均含外淋巴,在蜗顶处经蜗孔相通。蜗轴圆锥形、由松质骨构成,内有耳蜗神经节。

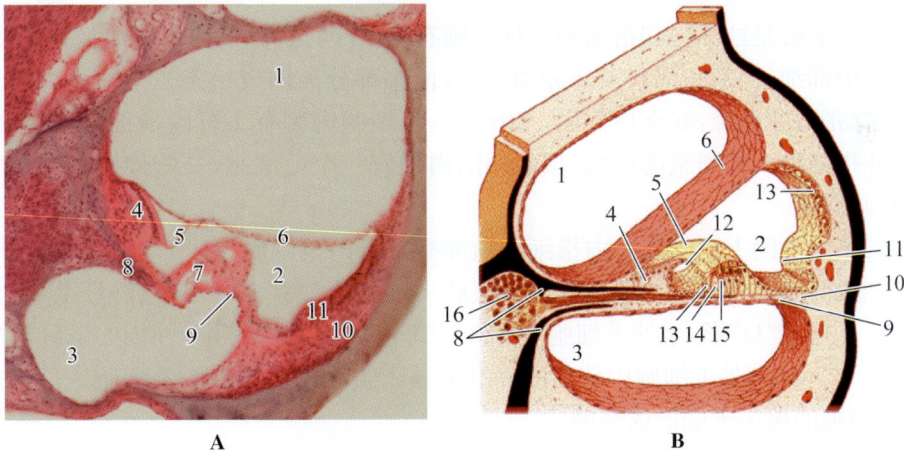

1—前庭阶；2—中阶；3—鼓室阶；4—螺旋缘；5—盖膜；6—前庭膜；7—螺旋器；8—骨螺旋板；9—基底膜；10—螺旋韧带；11—血管纹；12—内螺旋隧道；13—内毛细胞；14—内隧道；15—柱状细胞；16—螺旋神经节

图 12-9　耳蜗管及螺旋器结构
A 耳蜗管及螺旋器光镜图(66×);B.耳蜗管基螺旋器模式图

(2)膜蜗管:为螺旋形、膜性管道,内含内淋巴。横切面呈三角形,由 3 个壁组成。

上壁:为前庭膜,膜的两面覆盖单层扁平上皮,中间为极薄的结缔组织。

外侧壁:由螺旋韧带和其表面的上皮构成。螺旋韧带由耳蜗外侧壁的骨膜增厚形成;而表面上皮因其内含有固有层伸入的毛细血管,故称血管纹,与内淋巴的产生有关。

下壁:由内侧的骨螺旋板和外侧的膜螺旋板(基底膜)共同构成。骨螺旋板是蜗轴的骨组织向外伸出形成的螺旋状薄板,而骨膜则增厚并突入膜蜗管形成螺旋缘,其表面的细胞分泌糖蛋白形成盖膜,悬于螺旋器上方。基底膜为两层上皮夹一层基膜构成,内侧与骨螺旋板相连,外侧与螺旋韧带相连。基底膜的上皮增厚形成螺旋器。

(3)螺旋器:又称科蒂器(organ of Corti),是膜蜗管基底膜上呈螺旋状的膨隆结构,由支持细胞和毛细胞组成(图12-10)。

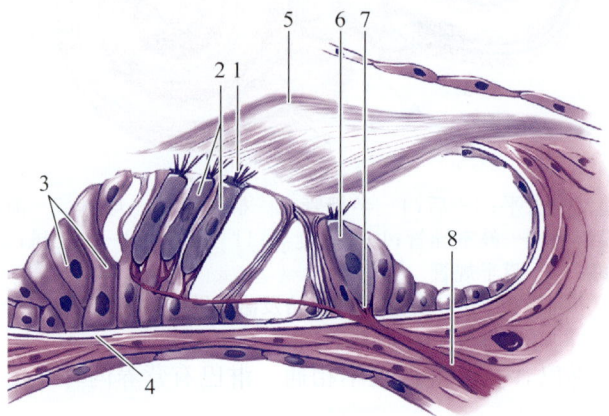

1—听毛(静纤毛);2—外毛细胞;3—支持细胞;4—基底膜;5—盖膜;6—内毛细胞;7—传入神经纤维;8—耳蜗神经纤维

图12-10 螺旋器结构的模式图

支持细胞:主要是柱细胞和指细胞。柱细胞有内、外两行,分别称内柱细胞和外柱细胞,它们底部宽大、中部细长,基底部和顶部分别相连,而中部分离围成一条三角形的内隧道。柱细胞的胞质富含张力原纤维,起支持作用。指细胞,内细胞内侧有1行内指细胞,外柱细胞外侧有3～5行外指细胞。指细胞高柱状,顶部凹陷内托着一个毛细胞,一侧伸出一个指状突起抵达螺旋器的游离面。

毛细胞:感觉性的上皮细胞。内指细胞顶部有1行内毛细胞,外指细胞顶部有3～5行外毛细胞。内毛细胞呈烧瓶形,外毛细胞呈高柱状。细胞顶部有30～60根静纤毛,它们于内毛细胞上有3～4行呈"U"形,于外毛细胞上有3～5行呈"U"或"W"形;外侧的静纤毛较内侧的逐排增高(图12-10),外毛细胞中较高的静纤毛插入盖膜的胶质中。毛细胞底部与来自耳蜗神经节双极细胞的树突末端形成突触。

螺旋器基底膜中含有大量的胶原样细丝,称听弦,听弦从内向外呈放射状排列。从蜗轴底部至顶部,基底膜由窄变宽、听弦由短变长,使得声波共振从底部的高频率过渡到顶部的低频率。

螺旋器是听觉感受器。声波由外耳道传入,使鼓膜振动,经听骨链传至卵圆窗,引起前庭阶外淋巴振动;继而经前庭膜使膜蜗管的内淋巴振动,或者经蜗孔传到鼓室阶,引起基底膜及螺旋器共振。依照振动频率的高低,相应的听弦发生共振,与盖膜接触的毛细胞的静纤毛因此受力弯曲,毛细胞受刺激,兴奋经耳蜗神经传至中枢,产生听觉。以上任何环节的异常都可导致耳聋。

2. 半规管、膜半规管及壶腹嵴

（1）半规管：位于内耳的后外侧，为 3 个相互垂直的半环形骨管，与前庭相连处分别形成一个膨大称壶腹。

（2）膜半规管：嵌套于骨半规管内；在壶腹部其一侧黏膜增厚形成嵴状隆起，称壶腹嵴。

（3）壶腹嵴：其上皮由支持细胞和毛细胞组成，其上覆盖圆锥形的胶质壶腹帽（图 12 - 11）。

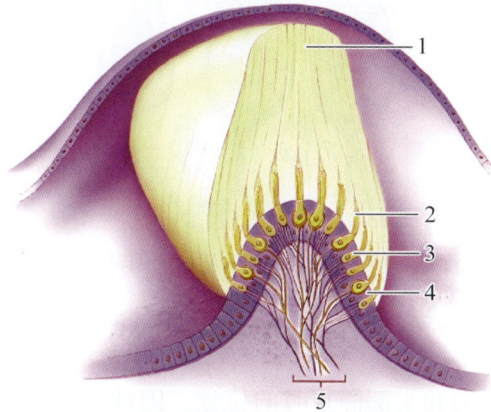

1—壶腹帽；2—毛；3—毛细胞；4—支持细胞；5—神经纤维

图 12 - 11　壶腹嵴结构的模式图

支持细胞呈高桩状，顶部胞质有分泌颗粒，分泌糖蛋白形成壶腹帽。支持细胞对毛细胞有支持和营养作用。

毛细胞分 I 型和 II 型两种（图 12 - 12）。I 型细胞呈烧瓶状，II 型细胞呈长圆柱状。毛细胞游离面有 50～100 根静纤毛阶梯状排列，最长的静纤毛一侧有一根较长的动纤毛。两种纤毛均伸入壶腹帽内。壶腹帽由支持细胞分泌的糖蛋白形成。前庭神经中的传入纤维末梢分布于毛细胞的基部。

壶腹嵴是位觉感受器。当身体或头部进行旋转变速运动时，膜半规管的内淋巴流动使壶腹帽偏斜，进而刺激毛细胞产生兴奋，经前庭神经传入中枢。

3. 前庭、膜前庭及位觉斑

（1）前庭：为一膨大的骨性腔隙，连接半规管和耳蜗。

（2）膜前庭：嵌套于前庭内，由椭圆囊和球囊组成。椭圆囊外侧壁和球囊前壁的黏膜局部增厚，呈斑块状，分别称椭圆囊斑和球囊斑。椭圆囊斑和球囊斑均为位觉感受器，故合称位觉斑。

（3）位觉斑：基本结构类似壶腹嵴，也由支持细胞和毛细胞组成（图 12 - 13），但表面平坦。支持细胞的分泌物在位觉斑表面形成一层胶质膜，称耳石膜或位砂膜，内有细小

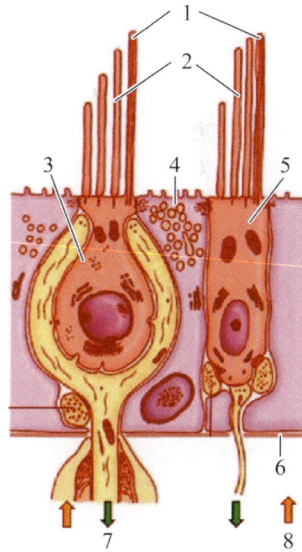

1—动纤毛；2—静纤毛；3—I 型毛细胞；4—支持细胞元；5—II 型毛细胞；6—基膜；7—传出神经末梢；8—传入神经末梢

图 12 - 12　壶腹嵴毛细胞的模式图

的碳酸钙结晶,即位砂。毛细胞顶部的动纤毛和静纤毛也伸入耳石膜内。

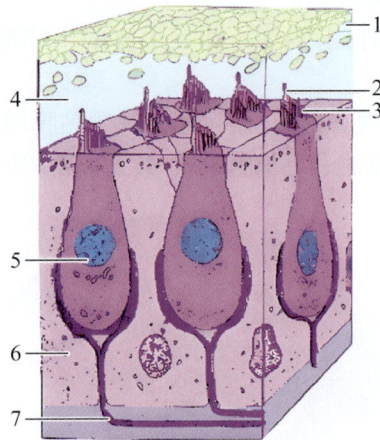

1—耳石;2—动纤毛;3—静纤毛;4—耳石膜;5—毛细
胞;6—支持细胞;7—神经纤维

图 12-13 位觉斑结构的模式图

位觉斑感受直线变速运动和头部静止时的位觉。因球囊斑和椭圆囊斑互成直角,而位砂的比重远大于内淋巴以至于惯性大,故无论头处在何种位置,耳石膜都能受到重力的作用而刺激毛细胞,产生的兴奋经前庭神经传入中枢。

(孙 申)

Chapter 13

Endocrine System

The endocrine system is made up of individual endocrine glands and endocrine cells that present in other organs. Together with the nerve system, it has evolved for controlling and coordinating the function of the various organs of the body. The main function of endocrine cells is to produce hormones. Hormones are molecules that function in the body as chemical signals. Hormones are usually carried by the vascular circulation around the body where they interact with target cells. They achieve their specific action by interacting with receptor molecules expressed by the target cells in various tissues and organs. In general, hormones are involved in regulating metabolic activities in cells in many organs and tissues of the body, many of which are important in controlling homeostasis.

According to biochemical structure, hormones can be divided into 2 types: nitrogen-containing hormones and steroid hormones. Accordingly, endocrine cells are classified into 2 types according to chemical nature of hormones released. Nitrogen-containing hormone-secreting cells: these cells contain rough endoplasmic reticulum, Golgi complex and membrane bound secretory granules. They are usually found in thyroid, parathyroid, adrenal medulla, pituitary and pineal glands, etc. Steroid hormones-secreting cells: these cells contain abundant smooth endoplasmic reticulum, mitochondria with tubular cristae and lipid droplets. They are found only in adrenal cortex and gonads.

Endocrine cells usually aggregate as endocrine glands, they are arranged in glomerulus, cords, reticulum or in follicles. Endocrine glands are ductless and rich in capillaries between cells. They can release hormones either into the vascular system (endocrine) or to their surroundings (paracrine), and bind to specific receptors of target cells.

The endocrine glands include the thyroid, parathyroid glands, adrenal glands, hypophysis and pineal gland.

1　Thyroid

The thyroid gland consists of 2 lobes united by an isthmus. It is covered by thin capsule of loose connective tissue. The parenchyma of thyroid is composed of spherical follicles of various sizes and parafollicular cells. Between follicles is delicate connective tissue containing fenestrated capillaries (Figure 13 - 1,13 - 2).

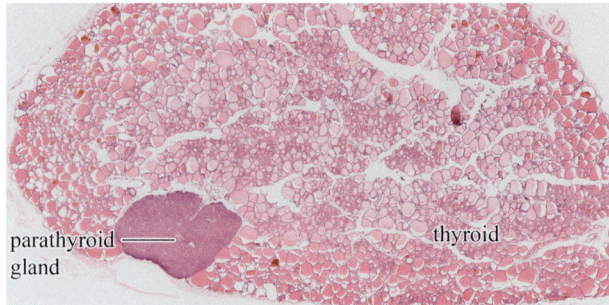

Figure 13 - 1   Thyroid gland and parathyroid gland (HE, 12×)

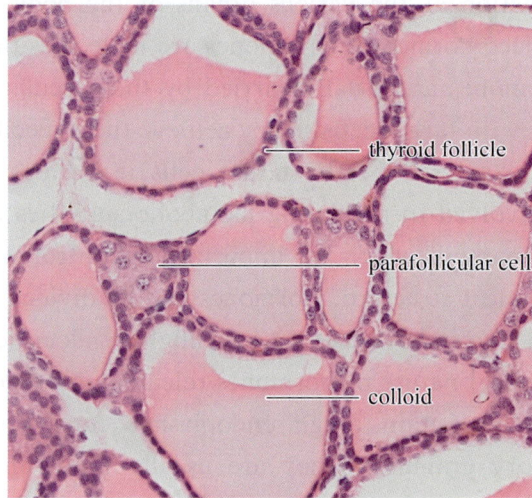

Figure 13 - 2   Thyroid follicle (HE, 200×)

1.1 Thyroid Follicles

Thyroid is composed of thousands of follicles formed by simple cuboidal epithelium. The height of the epithelium varies with function: usually low cuboidal in an underactive gland and high in an overactive one. In the cavity of thyroid follicles, present the homogeneous, acidophilic, gelatinous substance, known as colloid, whose chemical composition is iodinated thyroglobulin.

The follicular epithelial cells are cuboidal cells with a round nucleus in the center of the cell and a weakly basophilic cytoplasm. Electron microscopy shows that these cells contain rich rough endoplasmic reticulum and abundant lysosomes, well-developed Golgi complex in supra-nuclear area, secretory granules and pinocytotic colloid vesicles in apical part.

The follicular epithelial cells could synthesize and release thyroid hormones, triiodothyronine (T_3) and thyroxine (T_4). The process is as following: amino acids are taken up from the bloodstream at the base of follicular epithelial cells. The pre-thyroglobulin is synthesized on the rough endoplasmic reticulum, followed by glycosylation in the Golgi apparatus, and packaging in vesicles. Fusion of vesicles with apical plasma membrane leads to exocytosis of thyroglobulin into follicle cavity. Meanwhile, uptake of circulating iodide at the basal cell membrane is followed by oxidation by peroxidase and transfer to cell apices. Enzymes in apical microvilli that project into colloid catalyze iodination of tyrosine residues in thyroglobulin. Iodinated thyroglobulin is formed and stored in the follicular cavity (Figure 13-3).

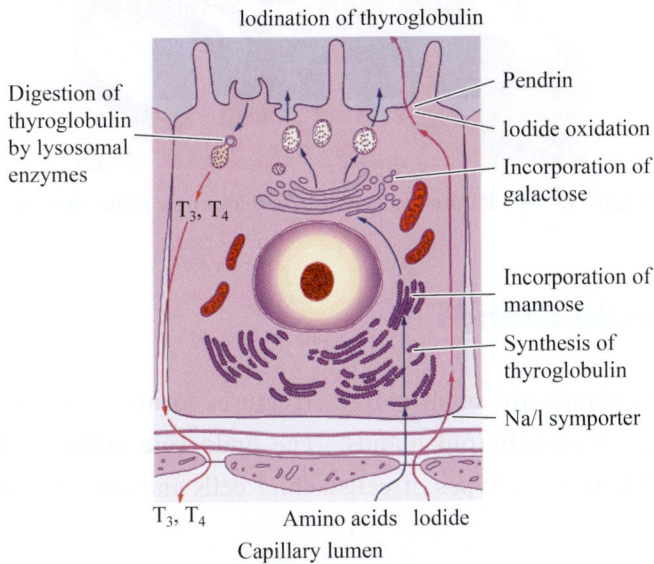

Figure 13-3 Diagram of steps in thyroid hormone synthesis

Stimulation by thyroid stimulating hormone (TSH) causes follicular epithelial cells to endocytose portions of colloid and form vesicles containing iodinated thyroglobulin. They fuse with lysosomes that cleave thyroglobulin. Resultant T_3 and T_4 are released into the bloodstream.

T_3 and T_4 could increase metabolic rates of most body tissues and are essential for normal growth, maturation, and mental activity. They also influence development of central nerve system during fetal and neonatal life.

1.2 Parafollicular cells

The parafollicular cells, or C cells, are found as part of the follicular epithelium or as isolated clusters between thyroid follicles. They are large and pale stained with HE, argyrophilic with silver staining. Electron microscopy shows many small secretory granules in cytoplasm. These cells are responsible for the synthesis and secretion of calcitonin, which decreases blood calcium level by inhibiting bone resorption of osteoclasts (Figure 13-4).

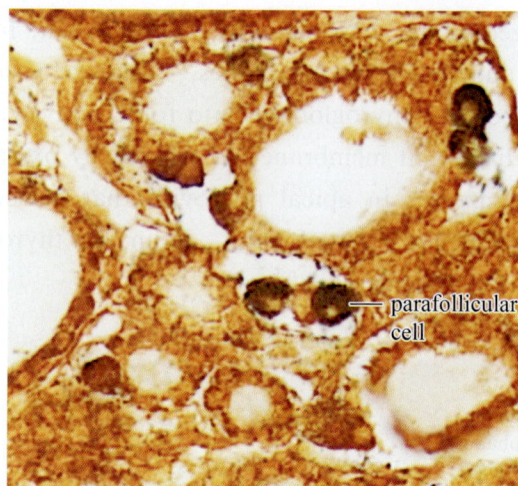

Figure 13 - 4   Parafollicular cell (Thyroid, silver stain, 400×)

2   Parathyroid Glands

The parathyroid glands are small paired structures located behind the thyroid gland. Humans usually have 4 parathyroid glands. The endocrine cells of the parathyroid are arranged in cords. There are 2 types of cells: chief cells and oxyphil cells.

2.1   Chief Cells

Chief cells are small polygonal cells with pale-staining cytoplasm. These cells secrete parathyroid hormone (PTH) which elevates blood calcium by increasing activity of osteoclasts. Under the co-regulation of parathyroid hormone and calcitonin, the body maintains the stability of blood calcium.

2.2   Oxyphil Cells

Oxyphil cells are generally found in groups between chief cells. They are larger polygonal cells, and their cytoplasm appears acidophilic because of many mitochondria. The function of oxyphil cells is not known.

3   Adrenal Glands

Adrenal glands are covered by a capsule of dense connective tissue, which with abundant sinusoids, extends into the interior glands. The parenchyma of the gland is divided into 2 regions: an outer portion known as cortex and an inner portion called medulla (Figure 13 - 5).

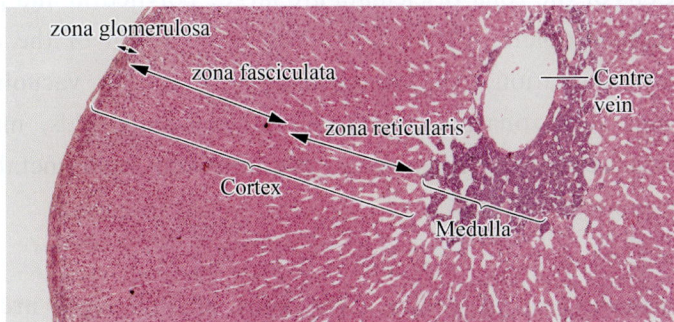

Figure 13 - 5　Structure of Adrenal gland (Adrenal gland, HE, 40×)

3.1　Cortex

The adrenal cortex occupies about 80% of the total volume of the adrenal glands. According to the arrangement of the gland cells, cortex can be subdivided into 3 concentric layers whose limits are usually not sharply defined: the zona glomerulosa, the zona fasciculata, and the zona reticularis (Figure 13 - 6, Figure 13 - 7).

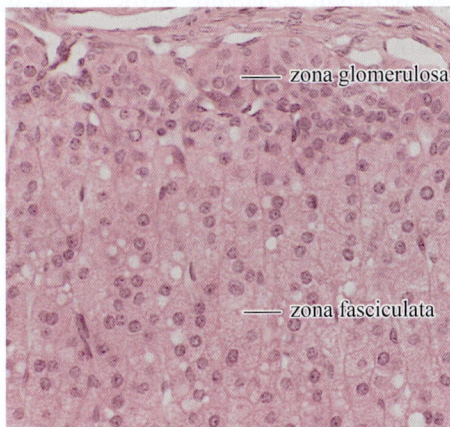

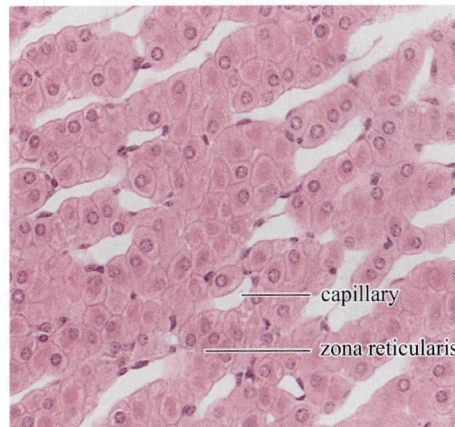

Figure 13 - 6　Zona glomerulosa and zona fasciculata (Adrenal gland, HE, 200×)

Figure 13 - 7　Zona reticularis (Adrenal gland, HE, 200×)

3.1.1　Zona Glomerulosa

This layer, immediately beneath the connective tissue capsule, represents 10% - 15% of the cortex. The small columnar or pyramidal cells of this zone are arranged in clusters. The zona glomerulosa secretes mineralocorticoids, primarily aldosterone, that act mainly on the distal renal tubules as well as on the gastric mucosa, stimulating the absorption of sodium.

3.1.2　Zona Fasciculata

It is the thickest layer of cortex. The cells of this layer are arranged in straight cords,

1 or 2 cells thick. Cells of the zona fasciculata are large, polyhedral and pale stained, with a great number of lipid droplets in their cytoplasm. As a result of the dissolution of the lipids during tissue preparation, the fasciculata cells appear vacuolated in common histologic preparations. The zona fasciculata secretes glucocorticoids, mainly cortisol and corticosterone, which regulate carbohydrate, protein and lipid metabolism, and also suppress immune responses.

3.1.3 Zona Reticularis

It is the innermost layer of cortex. The cells of this layer are arranged as an anastomosing network of short cords. These cells are small, acidophilic and dark stained, with many lipofuscin pigment granules in cytoplasm. The zona reticularis produces sex hormones, mainly androgens and cortisol in small amounts.

3.2 Medulla

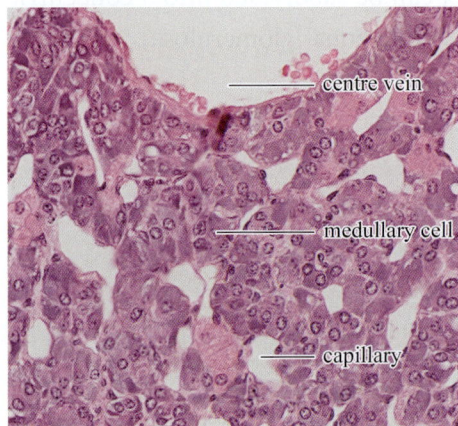

Figure 13 - 8   Medulla (adrenal gland, HE, 200×)

The adrenal medulla is composed of polyhedral cells arranged in cords or clumps (Figure 13 - 8). A profuse capillary supply intervenes between adjacent cords. The medulla cells contain chromaffin granules which can be stained deep brown when exposed to chromaffin salts, so they are also called chromaffin cells.

Electron microscopy shows that medullary parenchymal cells have abundant membrane-limited electron-dense secretory granules. According to the content of these granules, the chromaffin cells can be divided into 2 types: epinephrine-secreting cells, have smaller and less electron-dense granules containing epinephrine; norepinephrine-secreting cells, have larger and more electron-dense granules containing norepinephrine. Chromaffin cells produce the catecholamines (epinephrine and norepinephrine) which cause general physiological changes that prepare the body for physical activity. For example, epinephrine increases the heart rate and norepinephrine increases the blood pressure and blood flow to the heart, brain, and skeletal muscle.

4 Hypophysis

The hypophysis, or pituitary gland, weighs about 0.5 g, and lies in a cavity of the sphenoid bone. It actually consists of the neurohypophysis and the adenohypophysis. The neurohypophysis consists of the pars nervosa and the smaller infundibulum, or neural stalk. The neural stalk is composed of the stem and median eminence. The adenohypophysis is subdivided into 3 portions: pars distalis, pars intermedia and pars tuberalis (Figure 13 – 9).

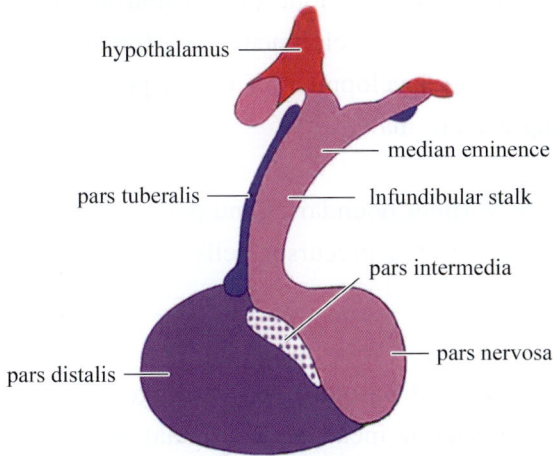

Figure 13 – 9   Diagram of hypophysis

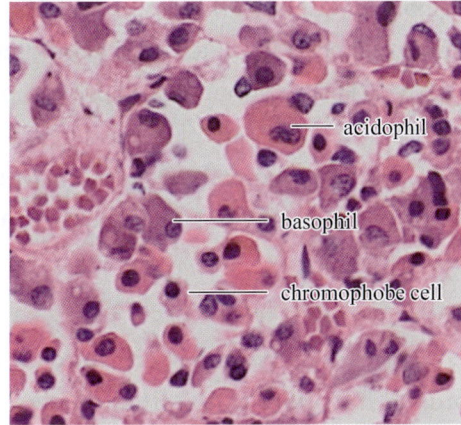

Figure 13 – 10   Three types of cells in pars distalis (hypophysis, HE, 400×)

4.1 Adenohypophysis

4.1.1   Pars Distalis

The glandular cells of the pars distalis are arranged into cords interspersed with sinusoids and few connective tissues. In routine HE preparations, these cells are of 2 types: chromophobes and chromophils. Chromophils are also divided into basophils and acidophils according to their affinity for basic and acid dyes. The subtypes of basophil and acidophil cells are named for the hormones they produce (Figure 13 – 10).

4.1.1.1   Acidophils

Acidophils take up about 40% cells in pars distalis. Cells are round or ovoid with acidophilic granules in cytoplasm. There are 2 varieties of the acidophils: somatotrophs and mammotrophs.

Somatotroph: these cells synthesize and release growth hormone, which stimulates body growth, particularly growth of long bones.

Mammotroph: these cells secret prolactin, which promotes milk secretion.

4.1.1.2   Basophil

Basophils account for 10% of cells in pars distalis. These cells are oval or polyhedral with basophilic granules in cytoplasm. There are 3 types of basophils: thyrotrophs, corticotrophs and gonadotrophs.

Thyrotrophs: these cells produce TSH, which stimulates growth of thyroid follicle, and synthesis and release of thyroid hormones.

Corticotrophs: these cells secrete adrenocorticotrophic hormone (ACTH), which stimulates secretion of glucocorticoids from zona fasciculata and reticularis of adrenal cortex.

Gonadotrophs: these cells secrete follicle-stimulating hormone (FSH) and luteinizing hormone (LH). FSH promotes ovarian follicle development in females and spermatogenesis in males. LH promotes ovulation and development of the corpus luteum in female. LH also stimulates androgen by Leydig cells in male.

4.1.1.3 Chromophobe Cell

Chromophobe cells are clusters of small cells without boundaries and pale stained. Few secretory granules indicate that they are undifferentiated precursor cells or degranulated chromophils.

4.1.2 Pars Intermedia

The pars intermedia is composed of chromophobes and basophil cells arranged either in cords or in colloid-containing follicles. These cells secrete melanocyte stimulating hormone (MSH) which promotes the production of melanin in melanocytes (Figure 13 - 11).

4.1.3 Pars Tuberalis

The pars tuberalis is a funnel-shaped region surrounding the infundibulum of the neurohypophysis. most of the cells of this portion secrete FSH and LH, and are arranged in cords alongside the blood vessels.

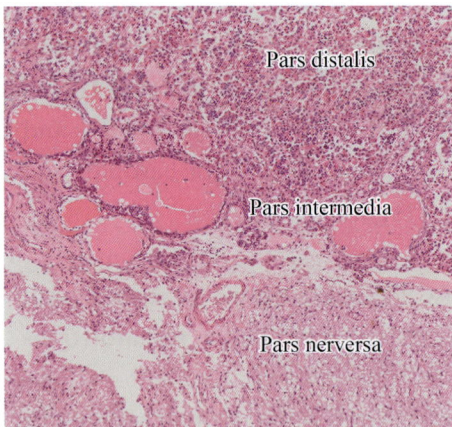

Figure 13 - 11　Pars intermedia (Hypophysis, HE, 40×)

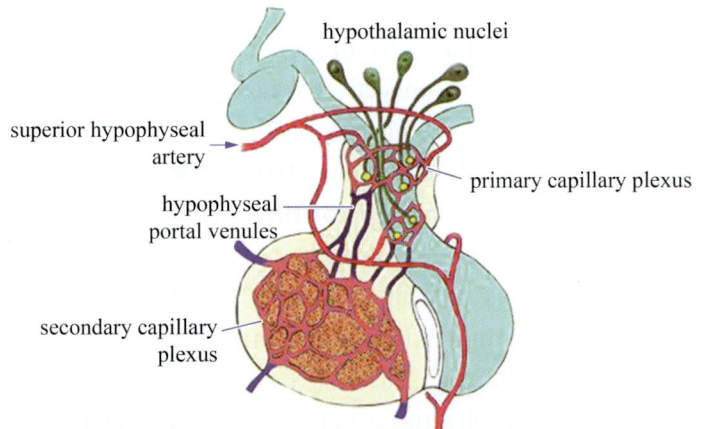

Figure 13 - 12　Diagram of hypophyseal portal system

4.1.4 Hypophyseal Portal System

Hypophyseal portal system includes (Figure 13 - 12):

(1) The primary capillary plexus in the stalk and median eminence, formed by superior hypophyseal arteries.

(2) The hypophyseal portal venules from the primary plexus in pars tuberalis.

(3) The secondary capillary plexus in pars distalis, formed from the portal venules.

4.1.5   Relationship Between Pars Distalis and Hypothalamus

Various hormones secreted by neuroendocrine cells in the arcuate nucleus and other nuclei of the hypothalamus are transported and released through the axons of nerve cells to the first level capillary network at Fenderson's funnel, and then transported through the pituitary portal vein to the second level capillary network in the distal part, regulating the secretion activity of various glandular cells in the distal part. These hormones can be divided into 2 categories: one promotes the secretion of glandular cells, called releasing hormones, and the other inhibits the secretion of glandular cells, called releasing inhibitory hormones. At present, the known release hormones include growth hormone releasing hormone, prolactin releasing hormone, gonadotropin-releasing hormone, thyrotropin releasing hormone, adrenocorticotropin-releasing hormone, and melanocyte stimulating hormone releasing stimulation. Releasing inhibitory hormones include: somatostatin, prolactin releasing inhibitory hormones, etc.

From this, it can be seen that the hypothalamus enters the pituitary gland through the pituitary portal system through the secretion of releasing hormones and releasing inhibitory hormones, in order to promote or inhibit the secretion activity of various cells in the pituitary gland, forming the hypothalamic pituitary system. The various hormones secreted by pituitary cells can also regulate the secretion activity of these neuroendocrine cells in the hypothalamus through a short feedback mechanism (Figure 13 - 13).

4.2 Neurohypophysis

The neurohypophysis develops from a downgrowth of the hypothalamus. It is divided into the pars nervosa and the infundibulum.

The pars nervosa is composed of large numbers of unmyelinated nerve fibers, sinusoids, and pituicytes. The unmyelinated nerve fibers originate from the secretory neurons of hypothalamic supraoptic and paraventricular nuclei. The neurosecretions are transported along the axons and accumulate at their endings in the pars nervosa. These dilated expansions of the axons contain aggregates of neurosecretory material, which form Herring bodies. Under light microscopy, these bodies appear as amorphous, lightly eosinophilic amorphous areas in close contact with capillaries.

Two hormones are stored and released in pars nervosa.

Vasopressin: it stimulates water resorption in kidneys and contraction of vascular smooth muscle.

Oxytocin: it promotes contraction of uterine smooth muscle during parturition and contraction of myoepithelial cells in mammary glands during lactation.

Pituicytes are neuroglial cells with irregular shape and short processes containing lipid droplets and pigment granules in their cytoplasm.

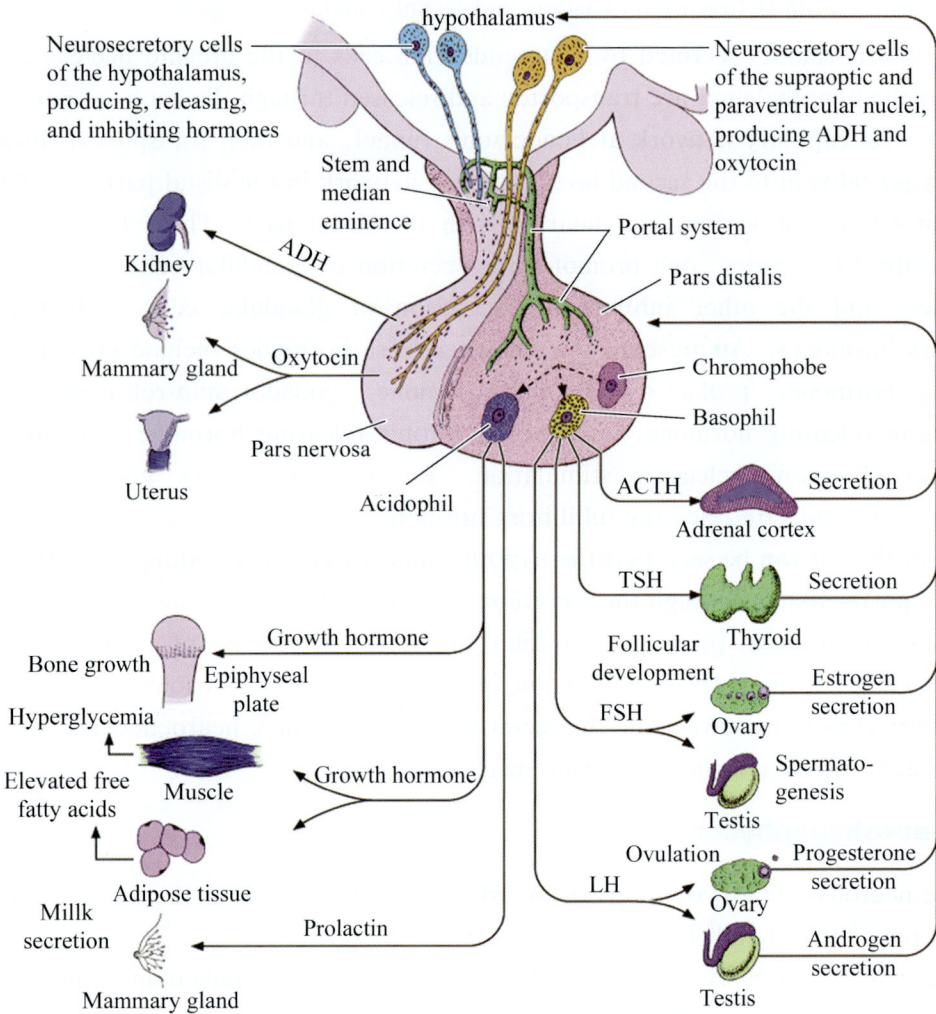

Figure 13 - 13 Schematic diagram showing effects of hypothalamic and hypophyseal hormones on target organs and the feedback mechanisms that control their secretion

5 Pineal Gland

The pineal gland is a flattened conical organ. It is found in the posterior extremity of the third ventricle, above the roof of the diencephalon, to which it is connected by a short stalk. The pineal gland is covered by pia mater. Connective tissue, which originate from pia mater, penetrate the pineal tissue into many irregular lobules. Each lobule consists of several types of cells, principally pinealocytes and astrocytes.

Pinealocytes have a slight basophilic cytoplasm with large irregular nuclei and sharply defined nucleoli. When impregnated with silver salts, the pinealocytes appear to have long and tortuous branches reaching out to the vascular connective tissue septa, where they end as flattened dilatations. Pinealocytes produce, mainly at night, melatonin that regulates circadian rhythm.

(Zhang Jing)

第十三章　内分泌系统

内分泌系统由独立的内分泌腺和分布于其他器官内的内分泌细胞组成。它和神经系统共同控制和协调机体各个器官的功能。

内分泌细胞的主要功能是分泌激素。激素是作为化学信号在体内发挥作用的分子。激素主要通过血液循环作用于机体特定的靶细胞,与靶细胞中的受体相结合发挥其特定作用。一般来说,激素参与调节机体多种器官和组织中的细胞代谢活动,尤其是调控机体内环境的稳定。根据生物化学结构,激素可分为两大类:含氮激素和类固醇激素。因此,内分泌细胞被分为含氮激素分泌细胞和类固醇激素分泌细胞。前者含有粗面内质网、高尔基复合体和膜包被的分泌颗粒,见于甲状腺、甲状旁腺、肾上腺髓质、垂体和松果体等;后者含有丰富的滑面内质网、管状嵴线粒体和脂滴,存在于肾上腺皮质和性腺。

内分泌细胞通常聚集成为内分泌腺,腺细胞通常排列成团状、索状、网状或围成滤泡状。内分泌腺是无导管的,腺细胞之间有丰富的毛细血管。它们向循环系统(内分泌)或其周围(旁分泌)释放激素,并与靶细胞上特定受体相结合。

内分泌腺包括甲状腺、甲状旁腺、肾上腺、垂体和松果体。

第一节　甲　状　腺

甲状腺分为两叶,中间由峡部相连。表面包裹有薄层结缔组织被膜。甲状腺实质由大小不等的球形滤泡和滤泡旁细胞组成。滤泡之间有少量的结缔组织和丰富的有孔毛细血管和毛细淋巴管(图 13-1、图 13-2)。

一、甲状腺滤泡

甲状腺由数千个滤泡组成,这些滤泡是由单层立方上皮围成,但上皮细胞的高度可随功能状态不同而变化:在功能不活跃时通常呈矮立方形,在功能活跃时上皮细胞则增高。甲状腺滤泡腔中充满均质嗜酸性的凝胶状物质,称为胶质,其化学成分为碘化的甲状腺球蛋白。

滤泡上皮细胞为立方形,核圆居中,胞质弱嗜碱性。电镜显示该细胞含有丰富的粗面内质网、溶酶体、位于核上区发达的高尔基复合体及分布于顶部胞质的分泌颗粒和胶质小泡。

滤泡上皮细胞能够合成并释放甲状腺激素:三碘甲状腺原氨酸(T_3)和甲状腺素(T_4)。其

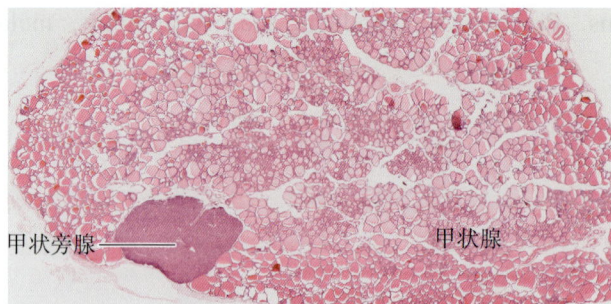

图 13-1 甲状腺和甲状旁腺(HE 染色,12×)

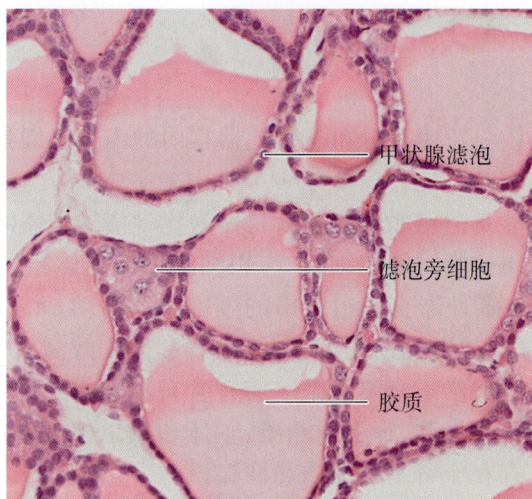

图 13-2 甲状腺滤泡(甲状腺染色,HE,200×)

过程如下:滤泡上皮细胞从基底部的血液中摄取氨基酸,在粗面内质网合成甲状腺球蛋白前体,继而在高尔基复合体中进行糖基化,并浓缩形成分泌颗粒。分泌颗粒与细胞顶部胞膜融合,以胞吐的方式将甲状腺球蛋白排放到滤泡腔中。同时,滤泡上皮细胞通过基底部胞膜摄取血液中的碘离子,经过氧化物酶氧化并转移到细胞顶部。顶部微绒毛伸入胶质中,其上的酶催化甲状腺球蛋白中酪氨酸残基的碘化,形成了碘化的甲状腺球蛋白,储存在滤泡腔中(图 13-3)。

在促甲状腺激素(thyroid-stimulating hormone,TSH)的作用下,滤泡上皮细胞以胞吞的方式将滤泡腔内碘化的甲状腺球蛋白吸收入胞质,并形成胶质小泡。胶质小泡与溶酶体融合,其中的碘化的甲状腺球蛋白被分解,生成的 T_3 和 T_4 被释放到血液中。

T_3 和 T_4 能够增进机体的新陈代谢,对机体的正常生长、成熟和智力活动至关重要。同时也会影响胎儿和婴幼儿中枢神经系统的发育。

二、滤泡旁细胞

滤泡旁细胞,又称 C 细胞,位于滤泡上皮细胞之间,或成群分布于甲状腺滤泡之间。HE 染色胞体较大、胞质浅染,镀银染色呈现嗜银性。电镜下显示细胞质中有较多小的分泌颗粒。该细胞可合成分泌降钙素,降钙素通过抑制破骨细胞对骨的重吸收来降低血钙水平(图 13-4)。

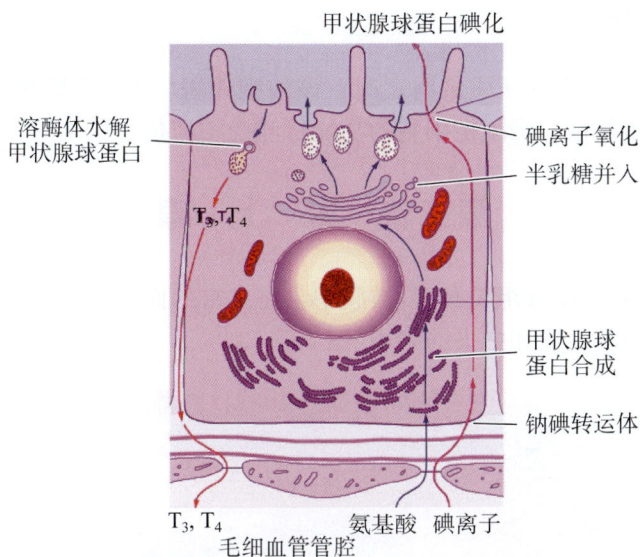

甲状腺球蛋白碘化

溶酶体水解
甲状腺球蛋白

碘离子氧化

半乳糖并入

T_3,T_4

甲状腺球
蛋白合成

钠碘转运体

T_3, T_4　　　氨基酸　碘离子
毛细血管管腔

图 13-3　甲状腺激素合成过程示意图

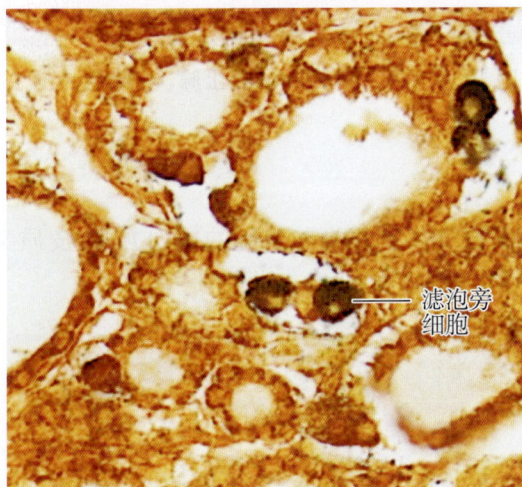

滤泡旁
细胞

图 13-4　滤泡旁细胞(甲状腺,银染,400×)

第二节　甲状旁腺

甲状旁腺位于甲状腺的背面,成对分布。人类通常有 4 个甲状旁腺。
甲状旁腺的内分泌细胞通常排列成索状,分为两种类型:主细胞和嗜酸性细胞。

一、主细胞

主细胞体积较小,呈多边形,胞质浅染。该细胞分泌甲状旁腺激素(PTH),通过增强破骨
细胞的活性来提高血钙水平。在甲状旁腺激素和降钙素的共同调节下,机体维持血钙的稳定。

二、嗜酸性细胞

嗜酸性细胞一般成群存在于主细胞之间。该细胞体积较大,呈多边形。由于胞体含有较多线粒体,细胞质呈嗜酸性。嗜酸性细胞的功能目前尚不清楚。

第三节 肾 上 腺

肾上腺表面包裹致密结缔组织被膜,被膜中含有丰富的血窦,并伸入腺体内部。肾上腺实质分为两个部分:周边的皮质和中央的髓质(图13-5)。

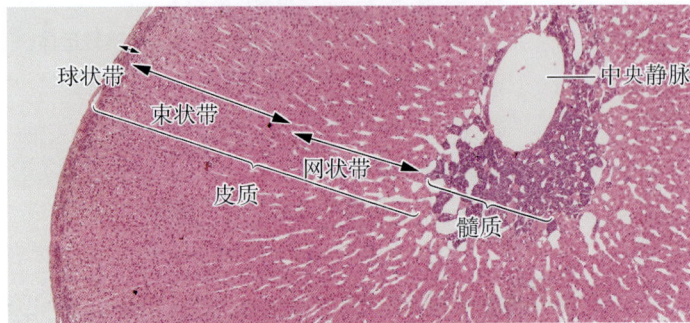

图13-5 肾上腺的结构(肾上腺,HE染色,40×)

一、皮质

皮质约占肾上腺总体积的80%。根据腺细胞的排列方式,皮质又可分为三个带:球状带、束状带和网状带,其间并无明确界限(图13-6、图13-7)。

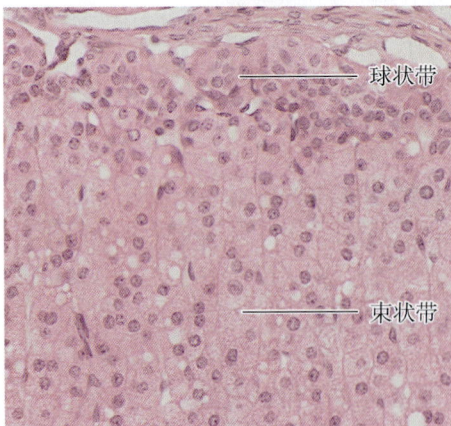

图13-6 球状带和束状带(肾上腺,HE染色,200×)

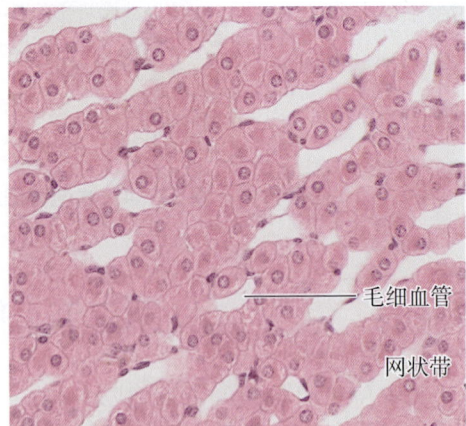

图13-7 网状带(肾上腺,HE染色,200×)

1. 球状带

球状带位于被膜下方,占皮质总体积的10%～15%。细胞较小,呈矮柱状或锥体形,排列成球团状。球状带分泌盐皮质激素,主要是醛固酮,作用于肾远端小管和胃黏膜,促进钠离子的吸收。

2. 束状带

束状带是皮质中最厚的部分。细胞排列成单行或双行的细胞索。束状带细胞体积较大,呈多边形,染色浅,胞质内含有大量脂滴。在组织切片制备过程中,脂滴被溶解,故胞质呈泡沫状。束状带分泌糖皮质激素,主要是皮质醇和皮质酮,调节糖、蛋白质和脂类代谢,也有抑制免疫应答的作用。

3. 网状带

网状带位于皮质的最内层。细胞排列成索并相互吻合成网。网状带细胞较小,嗜酸性,染色较深,胞质中含有较多脂褐素。网状带分泌性激素,主要是雄激素和少量的皮质醇。

二、髓质

肾上腺髓质由多边形的髓质细胞组成,排列成索状或团状(图 13-8)。细胞团或索之间有大量的毛细血管。髓质细胞含有嗜铬颗粒,当其接触到铬盐时,颗粒可被染成深棕色,故髓质细胞又称为嗜铬细胞。

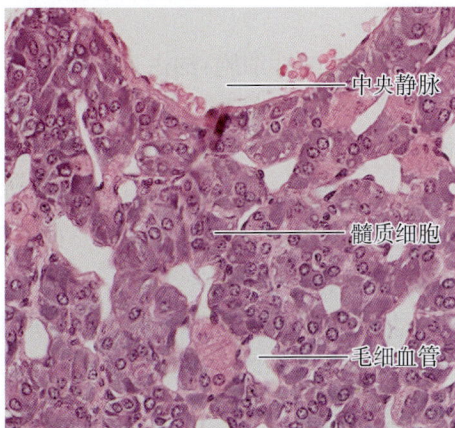

图 13-8 髓质(肾上腺,HE 染色,200×)

电镜显示髓质细胞含有许多电子密度高的膜包被的分泌颗粒。根据这些颗粒的内含物质不同,嗜铬细胞可分为两种类型:一种为肾上腺素细胞,其颗粒较小且电子密度低,颗粒内含肾上腺素;另一种为去甲肾上腺素细胞,其颗粒较大且电子密度高,颗粒内含去甲肾上腺素。嗜铬细胞分泌儿茶酚胺类物质(肾上腺素和去甲肾上腺素),能够引起全身生理变化,为身体活动做准备。例如,肾上腺素可以提高心率,去甲肾上腺素使得血压增高,心脏、脑和骨骼肌的血流加速。

第四节 垂 体

垂体重约 0.5 g,位于颅底蝶鞍垂体窝内,由神经垂体和腺垂体两部分组成。神经垂体分为神经部和较小的漏斗。漏斗包括漏斗柄和正中隆起。腺垂体分为 3 个部分:远侧部、中间部和结节部(图 13-9)。

一、腺垂体

1. 远侧部

腺细胞排列成索状,其间有丰富的窦状毛细血管和少量结缔组织。在常规 HE 染色标本中,这些细胞分为两种类型:嗜色细胞和嫌色细胞。嗜色细胞根据其对碱性和酸性染料亲和力不同,又分为嗜碱性细胞和嗜酸性细胞。而嗜碱性细胞和嗜酸性细胞的亚型则是以它们分泌的激素来命名的(图 13-10)。

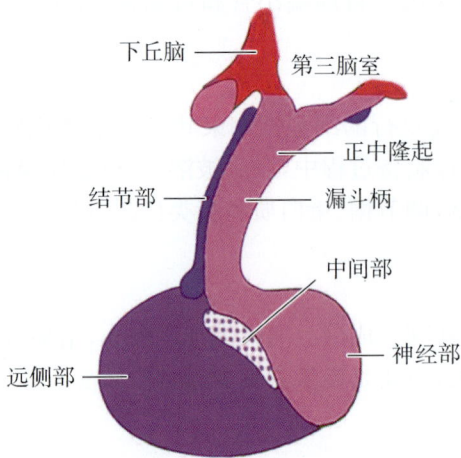

图 13-9 垂体的模式图

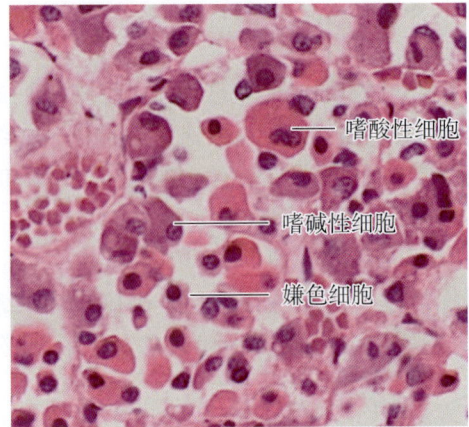

图 13-10 远侧部的三种细胞(垂体,HE 染色,400×)

（1）嗜酸性细胞：约占远侧部腺细胞总数的40%。细胞呈圆形或卵圆形，胞质中含有嗜酸性颗粒。嗜酸性细胞分为两种：生长激素细胞和催乳激素细胞。前者合成并释放生长激素，促进身体生长，尤其是长骨的生长；后者分泌催乳激素，促进乳汁分泌。

（2）嗜碱性细胞：约占远侧部腺细胞总数的10%。细胞呈椭圆形或多边形，胞质中含有嗜碱性颗粒。嗜碱性粒细胞分为三种类型：促甲状腺激素细胞、促肾上腺皮质激素细胞和促性腺激素细胞。

促甲状腺激素细胞分泌 TSH，刺激甲状腺滤泡的生长及甲状腺激素的合成和释放；促肾上腺皮质激素细胞分泌促肾上腺皮质激素(adrenocorticotropic hormone，ACTH)，刺激肾上腺皮质束状带和网状带分泌糖皮质激素；促性腺激素细胞分泌卵泡刺激素(follicle stimulating hormone，FSH)和黄体生成素(luteinizing hormone，LH)。FSH 促进女性卵泡发育和男性精子发生。LH 促进女性排卵、黄体发育和刺激男性睾丸间质细胞分泌雄激素。

（3）嫌色细胞：体积小，成群分布，细胞界限不清，着色浅。胞质内含少量分泌颗粒，表明该细胞是未分化的前体细胞，又或者是脱颗粒的嗜色细胞。

2. 中间部

中间部由嫌色细胞和嗜碱性细胞组成，排列成索状或围成含有胶体的滤泡。该细胞可分泌黑素细胞刺激素(melanocyte stimulating hormone，MSH)，促进黑素细胞中黑色素的形成（图 13-11）。

3. 结节部

结节部是围绕神经垂体的漏斗柄形成的一个漏斗状区域。该部大多数细胞分泌 FSH 和 LH，细胞排列成纵行条索且随血管分布。

4. 垂体门脉系统

垂体门脉系统包括（图 13-12）：

（1）垂体上动脉在垂体柄和正中隆起处形成第一级毛细血管网。

（2）第一级毛细血管网在结节部汇聚形成垂体门微静脉。

（3）垂体门微静脉下行至远侧部再次分支吻合，形成第二级毛细血管网。

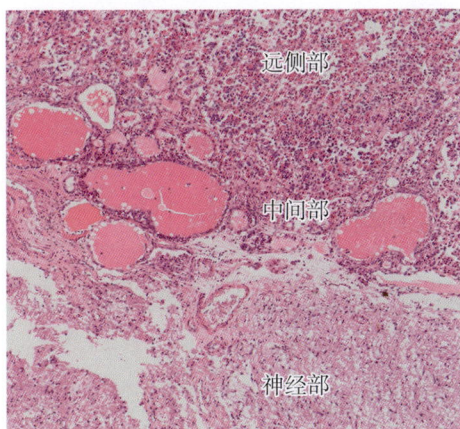

图 13-11 中间部(垂体,HE 染色,40×)

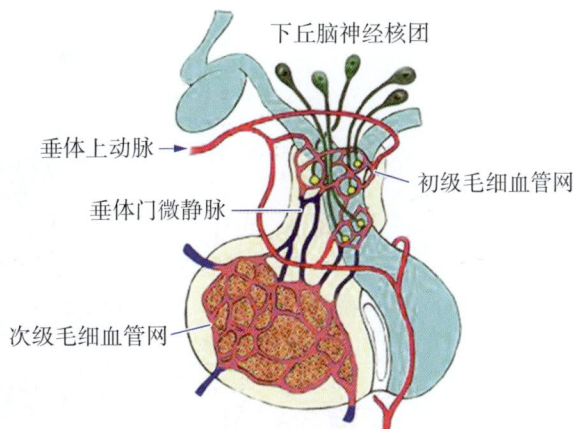

图 13-12 垂体门脉系统模式图

5. 下丘脑与腺垂体的关系

下丘脑的弓状核等核团内的神经内分泌细胞所分泌的各种激素,经神经细胞的轴突运输、释放入漏斗处的第一级毛细血管网,继而经垂体门微静脉输送至远侧部的第二级毛细血管网,分别调节远侧部各种腺细胞的分泌活动。这些激素可分为两类:一类促进腺细胞的分泌,称释放激素;另一类抑制腺细胞的分泌,称释放抑制激素。目前已知的释放激素有:生长激素释放激素、催乳激素释放激素、促性腺激素释放激素、促甲状腺激素释放激素、促肾上腺皮质激素释放激素、黑素细胞刺激素释放激素等。释放抑制激素有:生长抑素、催乳激素释放抑制激素等。

由此可见,下丘脑通过所分泌的释放激素和释放抑制激素,经垂体门脉系统进入腺垂体,以促进或抑制腺垂体内各种细胞的分泌活动,形成下丘脑-腺垂体系。腺垂体细胞分泌的各种激素,又可通过短反馈机制调节下丘脑中这些神经内分泌细胞的分泌活动(图 13-13)。

二、神经垂体

神经垂体是由下丘脑向下生长发育而来的,分为神经部和漏斗部图。

神经部由大量无髓神经纤维、血窦和垂体细胞组成。无髓神经纤维来源于下丘脑视上核和室旁核的神经内分泌细胞。分泌颗粒沿轴突被运输至神经部,并在轴突终末聚集成团。这些神经分泌物质的聚集体使得轴突局部膨大,形成赫林体。在光学显微镜下,呈现为靠近毛细血管分布的均质状、弱嗜酸性团块。

神经部储存和释放两种激素:加压素和催产素。前者刺激肾脏的水分吸收和血管平滑肌的收缩;后者在分娩时促进子宫平滑肌收缩,哺乳时促进乳腺肌上皮细胞收缩。

垂体细胞是一种形状不规则、突起较短的神经胶质细胞,胞质中含有脂滴和色素颗粒。

第五节 松 果 体

松果体呈扁圆锥形,位于第三脑室的后端,间脑顶部上方,通过细柄与间脑相连。松果体表面包以软脑膜。软脑膜结缔组织深入松果体实质,将其分成若干不规则的小叶。每个小叶由几种不同类型的细胞组成,主要是松果体细胞和星形胶质细胞。

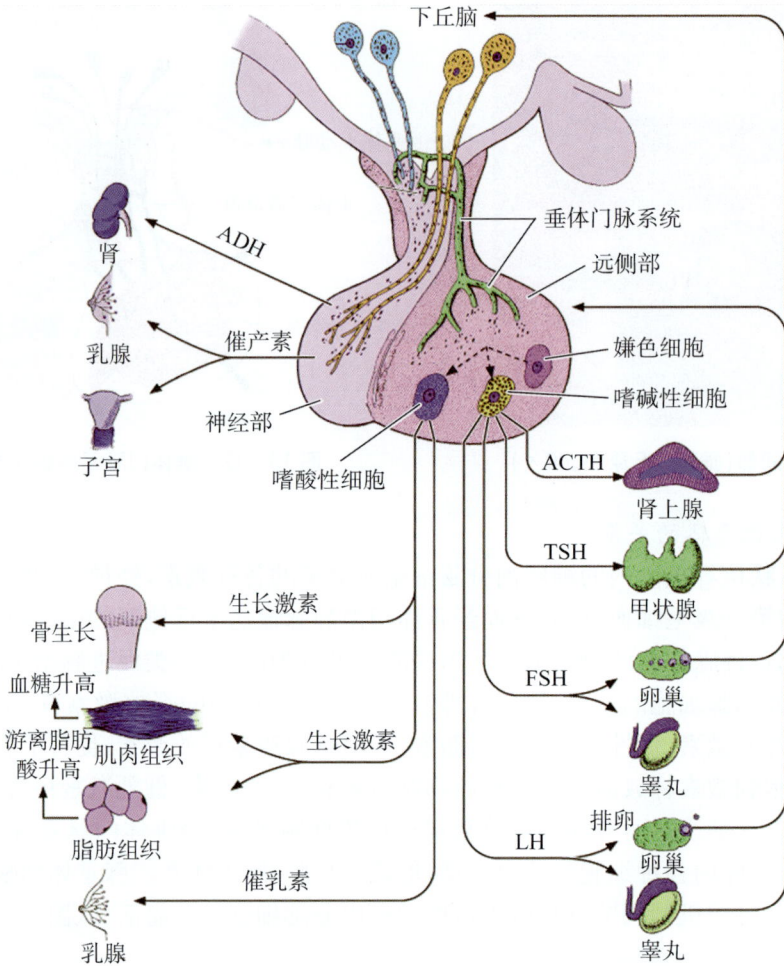

图 13 - 13　下丘脑、垂体激素对靶器官的作用示意图

松果体细胞胞质弱嗜碱性,核大而不规则,核仁清晰。在银染标本中,松果体细胞显示出长而弯曲的分支,延伸到血管周围的结缔组织,在血管附近形成膨大的终末。松果体细胞主要在夜间产生调节昼夜节律的褪黑激素。

（张　静）

Chapter 14

Digestive Tract

The digestive tract is a hollow tube of varying diameters whose length is approximately 9 meters. This tube includes the oral cavity, pharynx, esophagus, stomach, small and large intestines. The wall of these organs has the same basic structural organization, and each has its own characteristics corresponding to its function.

1 General Features of the Digestive Tract

From the esophagus to the large intestine, the wall of each organ is formed by 4 distinct layers. From the lumen outward, they are as follows: mucosa, submucosa, muscularis externa and adventitia (Figure 14 – 1).

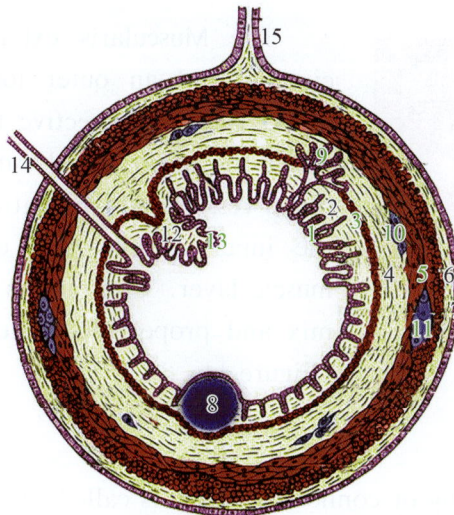

1. Epithelium; 2. Lamina propria; 3. Muscularis mucosae; 4. Submucosa; 5. Muscularis; 6. Adventitia; 7. Serosa; 8. Lymph nodes; 9. Submucosal gland; 10. Submucosal plexus; 11. Myenteric plexus; 12. Plica; 13. Villus; 14. Duct of associated gland; 15. Mesothelium

Figure 14 – 1   Schematic structure of a portion of the digestive tract

1.1 Mucosa

The mucosa comprises an epithelial lining, a lamina propria and the muscularis mucosae. The mucosa has 3 principal functions: protection, absorption and secretion. The epithelium is stratified squamous in the oral cavity, pharynx, esophagus and anal canal with protective function; it is simple columnar in the stomach and intestines, mainly for digestion and absorption. The lamina propria is the loose connective tissue layer that is rich in blood, lymph vessels and smooth muscle fibers, the lamina propria of stomach and intestine also contain glands and lymphoid tissue. The muscularis mucosae consists of a thin inner circular layer and an outer longitudinal layer of smooth muscle fibers is responsible for the mobility of the mucosa. This layer forms the boundary between mucosa and submucosa.

1.2 Submucosa

The submucosa consists of a dense irregular connective tissue layer containing blood vessels, lymphatic vessels, and a submucosal (Meissner's) nerve plexus. It may also contain glands and lymphoid tissue. For example, they are present in the esophagus and the duodenum.

1.3 Muscularis Externa

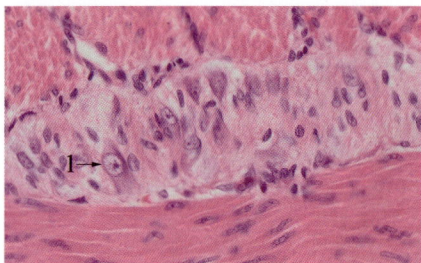

1. Neuron
Figure 14 - 2　Myenteric plexus (HE)

The Muscularis externa consists of an inner circular and an outer longitudinal smooth muscle layer. A thin connective tissue layer containing the myenteric (also called Auerbach's) nerve plexuses, blood vessels and lymphatic vessels is located between the inner circular and outer longitudinal smooth muscle layer. Contraction of the muscularis externa mix and propel the contents of the digestive tract (Figure 14 - 2).

1.4 Adventitia

The adventitia consisting of connective tissue is called fibrosa, which is found where the wall of the tube is directly attached or fixed to adjoining structures (the esophagus, duodenum and ascending and descending colon). The adventitia consisting of a serous membrane containing mesothelium (a simple squamous epithelium) and small amount of underlying connective tissue is called Serosa. The digestive canal with serosa (the stomach, jejunum, ileum, transverse colon and sigmoid colon) is suspended in the shallowest layer of peritoneal cavity, with smooth surface, which facilitates the organ movement.

2   Oral Cavity and Pharynx

The epithelium and underlining connective tissue constitute the oral mucosa. Most oral cavity (the soft palate, lips, cheeks, etc.) possesses the nonkeratinized squamous epithelium and the lamina propria is vascular connective tissue. The gingiva, hard palate and dorsal surface of the tongue are covered by the keratinized stratified squamous epithelium, and the lamina propria in these regions rests directly on bony tissue. Skeletal muscle underlies the mucosa in the lips, cheeks, tongue, floor of the mouth, and soft palate.

2.1   Tongue

The tongue is composed of superficial mucosa and deep lingual muscle. The lingual muscle is composed of longitudinal, transverse and vertical skeletal muscle fiber bundles. The mucosa comprises a stratified squamous epithelium and a lamina propria.

The root anchors the tongue into the hyoid bone. Dorsal surface of the tongue body is divided into an anterior 2/3 and a posterior 1/3 by a V-shaped groove. Behind this boundary, the posterior 1/3 of the surface shows small bulges composed of lymphoid nodules and the lingual tonsils. The anterior 2/3 of the dorsal surface have many papillae, which are elevations of the oral epithelium and lamina propria. There are mainly 3 types of papillae (Figure 14 – 3).

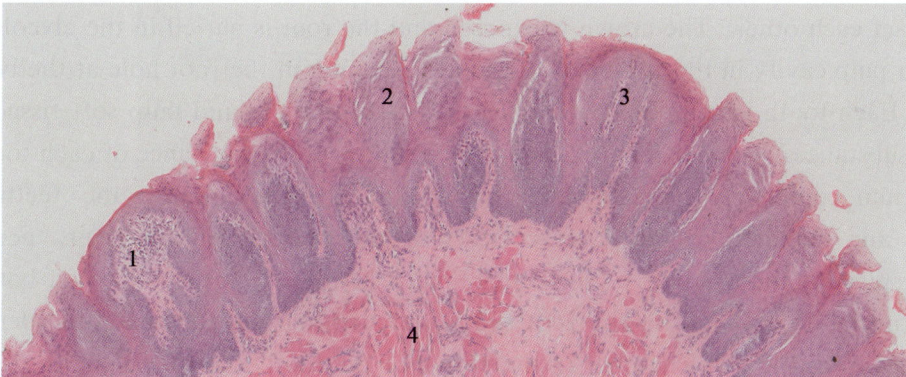

1. Circumvallate papillae; 2. Filiform papillae; 3. Fungiform papillae; 4. Skeletal muscle fibers
Figure 14 – 3   Papillae (HE)

2.1.1   Filiform Papillae

The filiform papillae are quite numerous and are present over the entire surface of the tongue. They are conical shape with no taste buds, and their stratified squamous epithelium is highly keratinized.

2.1.2 Fungiform Papillae

The fungiform papillae are mushroom-shaped and possess a few taste buds on their upper surface. The epithelium of fungiform papillae is stratified squamous nonkeratinized.

2.1.3 Circumvallate Papillae

The circumvallate papillae are 7 – 12 extremely large circular papillae, which are located in front of the V-shaped groove. Numerous serous glands (taste gland) are located in the lamina propria, which drain their contents into the deep groove that encircles the periphery of each papilla. The great number of taste buds present along the sides of these papillae. The secretion removes food particles from the vicinity of the taste buds so that they can receive and process new gustatory stimuli.

Each taste bud is onion-shaped, is completely intraepithelial, and is composed of 60 – 80 spindle-shaped neuroepithelial taste cells (Figure 14 – 4). The cells are compacted together and form an opening known as a taste pore at the epithelial surface. Apically, they possess long microvilli known as taste hairs, which pass through the taste pore and are exposed to the moist environment of the oral cavity. Synaptic vesicles were found in the basal part of the cytoplasm, and synapses were formed between the basal surface and taste nerve terminals. There are pyramidal basal cells in the deep part of taste buds, which are differentiated cells and can differentiate into taste cell. Taste buds are taste receptors.

2.2 Tooth

Each tooth is composed of a crown and a root and the cervix, where the crown and root contact each other. The crown is exposed and the root is buried in the alveolar bone. There is a pulp cavity in the center of the tooth, opening in the root hole at the bottom of the root. Each tooth is composed of calcified hard substances and pulp soft tissue. Three calcified substances, enamel, dentin, and cementum form the substance of each tooth. The periodontium comprises the structures responsible for maintaining the teeth in the maxillary and mandibular bones. It consists of the periodontal ligament, periodontal ligament, gingiva and alveolar periosteum (Figure 14 – 5). Dentin is located both in the crown (coronal dentin) and in the root (radicular dentin) and surrounds the dental pulp cavity, known as the pulp chamber in the crown of the tooth and root canal in the root of the tooth. A very vascularized and highly ordered connective tissue is called the dental pulp, that fills the pulp cavity. Dental pulp has nutritional effect on dentin and enamel.

Dentin is the bulk of a tooth. It is 65% – 70% calcium salts and 30% – 35% type I collagen fibers. Odontoblasts are arranged between dentin and medulla; they continue to form organic matrix of dentin throughout the tooth's life.

2.2.1 Enamel

Enamel covers coronal dentin. It is the hardest tissue in the body; it is 96% calcium salts and 4% organic matrix consisting mostly of the protein enamelin.

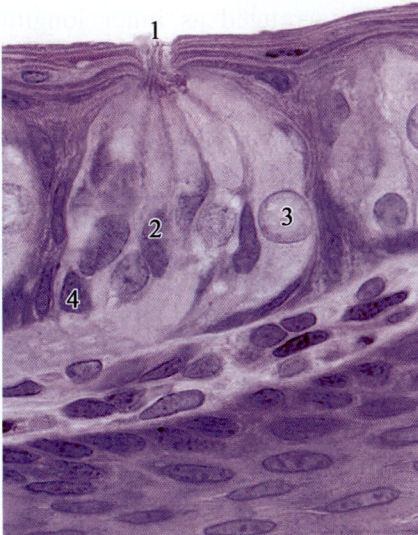

1. Taste pore; 2. Support cell; 3. Taste cell; 4. Basal cells

Figure 14 – 4   Taste buds (HE)

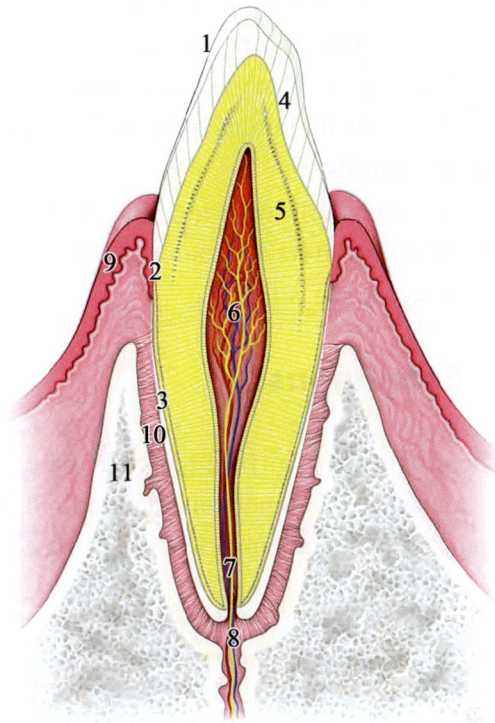

1. Dental crown; 2. Cervix of the tooth; 3. Root of the tooth; 4. Enamel; 5. Dentin; 6. Dental pulp; 7. Root canal; 8. Apical foramen; 9. Gingiva; 10. Periodontal ligament; 11. Alveolar bone

Figure 14 – 5   Diagram of a sagittal section from an incisor tooth in position in the mandibular bone

2.2.2   Cementum

Cementum covers radicular dentin surface, and meet the cervical end of enamel. Its composition and structure are similar to that of bone tissue.

2.2.3   Periodontal Ligament

The periodontal ligament is a connective tissue with bundles of collagen fibers inserted into the cementum and alveolar bone, fixing the tooth firmly in its bony socket.

2.2.4   Gingiva

Gingiva comprises a stratified squamous epithelium and a lamina propria. The cervix of each tooth is surrounded by the gingiva.

2.3   Pharynx

Pharynx is the crossing area of digestive tract and respiratory tract, being divided into 3 parts: oral pharynx, nasal pharynx and laryngeal pharynx.

The mucosa consists of epithelium and lamina propria. Its mucosa is lined by stratified squamous epithelium in oral pharynx, but pseudostratified ciliated columnar epithelium in nasal and laryngeal pharynx. The mucosa of the pharynx also has many small mucous salivary glands in its lamina propria, composed of dense connective tissue. The pharynx contains the tonsils.

In the muscularis externa, the skeletal muscles are arranged as inner longitudinal pharyngeal constrictors and outer circular or diagonal pharyngeal muscles.

The outer layer is fibrosa.

3 Esophagus

The esophagus is a fixed muscular tube that delivers food and liquid from the pharynx to the stomach. The lumen has longitudinal folds. When a bolus of food passes through the esophagus, the lumen expands without mucosal injury (Figure 14 - 6).

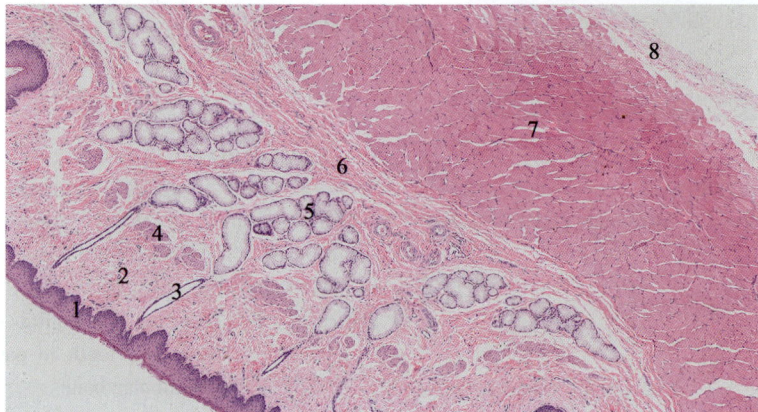

1. Epithelium; 2. Lamina propria; 3. Duct of Esophageal gland; 4. Muscularis mucosae; 5. Esophageal glands; 6. Submucosa; 7. Muscularis; 8. Fibrosa
Figure 14 - 6   Photomicrograph of a section of the upper region of the esophagus (HE)

3.1 Mucosa

It is composed of a stratified squamous nonkeratinized epithelium, a lamina propria and only longitudinal smooth muscle fibers of the muscularis mucosae.

3.2 Submucosa

The submucosa is composed of dense irregular connective tissue that contains larger blood and lymphatic vessels, diffuse lymphatic tissue and lymphatic nodules nerve fibers, and ganglion cells. There are groups of mucus-secreting glands, the esophageal glands, whose ducks passed through the mucosa and opened into the esophageal lumen.

3.3   Muscularis Externa

The muscularis externa consists of 2 muscle layers: an inner circular layer and an outer longitudinal layer. The upper 1/3 is skeletal, the middle 1/3 is skeletal and smooth, whereas the lower 1/3 is smooth muscle.

3.4   Adventitia

The adventitia is only covered by fibrosa where it is attached to adjacent structures by connective tissue.

4   Stomach

The stomach is an expand segment of the digestive tube. It receives food from the esophagus, and produce mixture called chyme with addition of gastric secretions. The stomach has the same general structural characteristics throughout, consisting of a mucosa, submucosa, muscularis externa and serosa. The mucosa and submucosa of the non-distended stomach lie in longitudinal folds known as rugae. When the stomach is filled with food, these folds flatten out.

4.1   Mucosa

The stomach's surface is divided into bulging irregular areas called gastric areas by grooves. The mucosa epithelium invaginates into the lamina propria forming gastric pits. The gastric glands open into the bottom of the gastric pits (Figure 14 – 7, 14 – 8, 14 – 9).

4.1.1   Epithelium

The epithelium that lines the surface and the gastric pits of the stomach is simple columnar. The columnar cells are surface mucous cells. Each cell possesses an oval nucleus near the bases of the cells, a large apical cup of mucinogen granules which typically appear empty in H&E sections because the mucinogen is lost in fixation and dehydration; there are intracellular tight junctions. These cells secrete an alkaline mucus containing high bicarbonate concentration. The mucous secretion forms a thick, viscous, gel-like coat that adheres to the epithelial surface, and it protects the epithelium from the acidic content of the gastric juice. The surface mucous cells continuously shed and are replaced by the stem cells found in the bottom of the gastric pits, which have a turnover time of 3 – 5 days. Normal gastric epithelium has no goblet cells. If Goblet cells appear in gastric mucosa, it is pathologically defined as the intestinal metaplasia of stomach, which may be the prophase of gastric cancer.

4.1.2   Lamina Propria

The lamina propria of the stomach houses gastric glands; depending on the region of

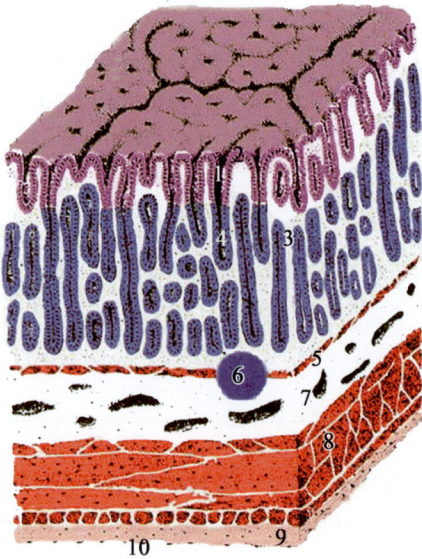

1. Gastric pit; 2. Simple columnar epithelium; 3. Lamina propria; 4. Fundic gland; 5. Muscularis mucosae; 6. Lymph nodes; 7. Submucosa; 8. Muscularis; 9. serosa; 10. Mesothelium

Figure 14 - 7   Diagram of stomach

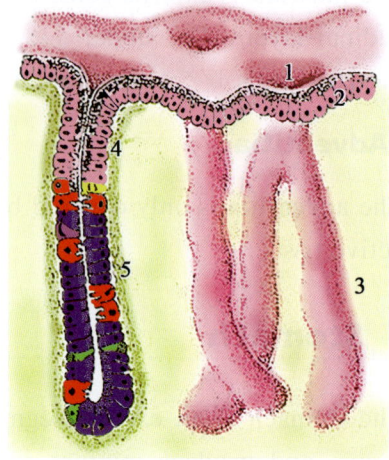

1. Gastric pit; 2. Simple columnar epithelium; 3. Lamina propria; 4. Gastric pit; 5. Fundic gland; Yellow: Stem cells; Rose red: mucous neck cells; Red: parietal cells; Blue: chief cell; Green: Endocrine cells

Figure 14 - 8   Diagram of fundic glands

the stomach, these are cardiac, fundic, or pyloric. There is a small amount of connective tissue between the glands and between the gastric pits. Besides fibroblasts, there are also many lymphocytes, plasma cells, mast cells, eosinophils and scattered smooth muscle fibers.

4.1.2.1   Fundic Glands

The lamina propria of the fundus and body is filled with fundic glands. They are brancher, tubular glands, 3 - 7 of which open into the bottom of each gastric pit. Each fundic glands has 3 regions: the isthmus, neck, and base. All gastric glands are composed of parietal cells, chief cells, mucous neck cells, endocrine cells, and stem cells (Figure 14 - 9, 14 - 10).

Parietal Cells/Oxyntic Cells: They are present in the upper half (the isthmus regions and the neck regions) of gastric glands. They are rounded or pyramidal cells, with one centrally spherical nucleus and intensely eosinophilic cytoplasm (Figure 14 - 10). When examined with the transmission electron microscope (Figure 14 - 11), the parietal cells are seen to have an extensive intracellular secretory canaliculus that communicates with the lumen of the gland. Numerous microvilli project from the surface of the canaliculi, and many smooth tubules or vesicles are present in the cytoplasm adjacent to the canaliculi is called tubulovesicular membrane system.

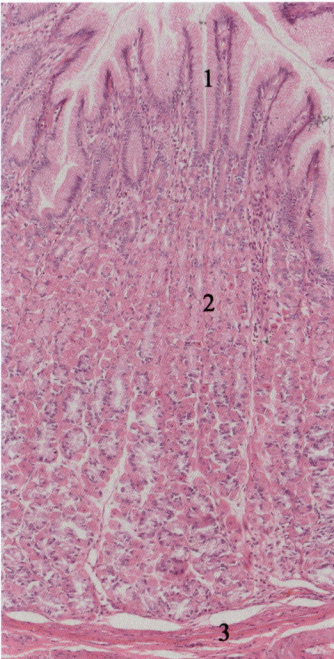

1. Gastric pit; 2. Fundic gland;
3. Muscularis mucosae
Figure 14 − 9   Photomicrograph of a
section of the fundic
gastric mucosa (HE)

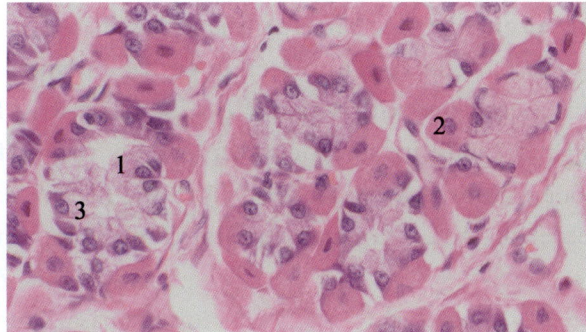

1. Fundic gland; 2. Parietal cells; 3. Chief cells
Figure 14 − 10   Photomicrograph of fundic glands (HE)

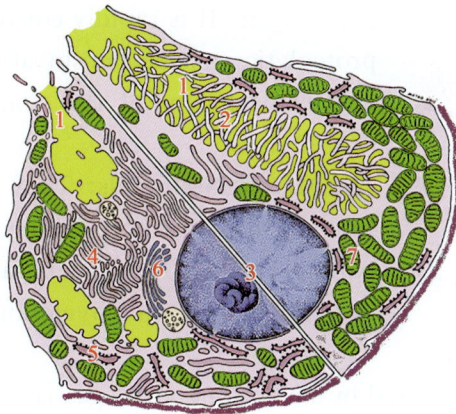

1. intracellular canaliculi; 2. microvilli; 3. Nucleus; 4. Tubulovesicles;
5. Rough endoplasmic reticulum; 6. Golgi complex; 7. Mitochondria
Figure 14 − 11   Composite diagram of a parietal cell, showing the
ultrastructural differences between a resting cell (left)
and an active cell (right)

These cells alter their morphology during HCl secretion. In the resting cells, few microvilli and a number of tubulovesicular structures can be seen. In an actively secreting cell, the canaliculi communicate with the lumen of the gland, the number of microvilli in the canaliculi increases and the tubulovesicular system is reduced significantly or disappears. It is believed that the membranes of the tubulovesicular system serve as a reservoir of intracellular canaliculi. Numerous mitochondria also found in cytoplasm. The parietal cells live for approximately 200 days before being replaced by stem cells.

They secrete hydrochloric acid (HCl). The membranes of the intracellular secretory canaliculus contain active proton pumps ($H^+/K^+ - ATPase$) and Cl^- channels. They can import H^+ formed in parietal cells and Cl^- absorbed from blood into tubules respectively to form hydrochloric acid that is secreted into gland cavity. Mitochondria supply the high levels of energy necessary for this process.

The parietal cells also secrete gastric intrinsic factor, a glycoprotein that binds to and forms a complex with vitamin B_{12} in the gastric lumen. When this complex reaches the ileum, it binds to specific receptors on the surface absorptive cells, and the vitamin becomes absorbed. A lack of intrinsic factor leads to B_{12} deficiency that results in a disorder of the erythrocyte-forming known as pernicious anemia.

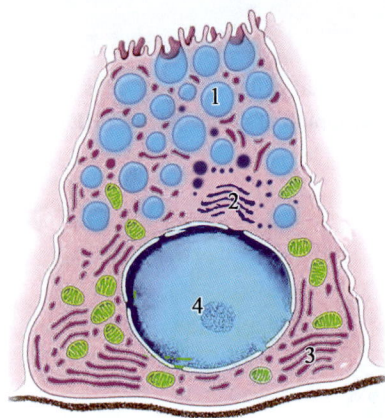

1. Zymogen granules; 2. Golgi complex; 3. Rough endoplasmic reticulum; 4. Nucleus

Figure 14 – 12　Diagram of a chief cell

Chief Cells/Zymogenic Cells: They are located in the lower (basal) region of the fundic glands. Chief cells are typical protein-secreting cells (Figure 14 – 12). They are columnar shaped with a round nucleus near to the bases of the cells. The cytoplasm around nucleus is strongly basophilic (Figure 14 – 10). Zymogen granules in their apical cytoplasm contain the inactive enzyme pepsinogen. It is rapidly converted into the highly active proteolytic enzyme pepsin after being released into the acid environment of the stomach. They live for about 60 – 90 days.

Mucous Neck Cells: They are located in the neck of fundic glands and occur singly or in clusters between the parietal cells. They manufacture soluble mucus that becomes part of the chyme and lubricates it. These cells live for approximately 6 days.

Stem Cells: They are scattered in the bottom of the gastric pits and upper region fundic glands but few in number. they are low columnar cells with oval nuclei near the bases of the cells. they replace the epithelial lining of the stomach and the cells of the glands by mitosis.

Endocrine Cells: Enteroendocrine cells secrete their products into either the lamina propria or underlying blood vessels. They are found in the neck and bases of gastric glands. They live for about 60 to 90 days. They produce hormones such as histamine, gastrin, somatostatin, secretin and cholecystokinin (Table 14 – 1, 14 – 2).

Table 14 - 1   Physiologic Actions of Gastrointestinal Hormones

Hormone	Site of Synthesis	Major Action	
		Stimulates	Inhibits
Gastrin	G cells in stomach	Gastric acid secretion	
Ghrelin	Gr cells in stomach	GH secretion Appetite and perception of hunger	Lipid metabolism Fat utilization in adipose tissue
Cholecystokinin (CCK)	I cells in duodenum and jejunum	Gallbladder contraction Pancreatic enzyme secretion Pancreatic bicarbonate ion secretion Pancreatic growth	Gastric emptying
Secretin	Scells in duodenum	Pancreatic enzyme secretion Pancreatic bicarbonate ion secretion Pancreatic growth	Gastric acid secretion
Gastric inhibitory peptide (GIP)	K cells in duodenum and jejunum	Insulin release	Gastric acid secretion
Motilin	Mo cells in duodenum and jejunum	Gastric motility Intestinal motility	

Table 14 - 2   Physiologic Actions of Gastrointestinal Hormones

Hormone	Site of Synthesis	Major Action	
		Stimulates	Inhibits
Candidate hormones			
Pancreatic polypeptide	PP cells in pancreas	Gastric emptying and gut motility	Pancreatic enzyme secretion Pancreatic bicarbonate secretion
Peptide YY	L cells in ileum and colon	Electrolyte and water absorption in the colon	Gastric acid secretion Gastric emptying Food intake
Glucagon-like peptide-1 (GLP - 1)	L cells in ileum and colon	Insulin release	Gastric acid secretion Gastric emptying
Paracrine hormones			
Somatostatin	D cells in mucosa throughout GI tract		Gastrin release Gastric acid secretion Release of other GI hormones
Histamine	Mucosa throughout GI tract	Gastric acid secretion	
Neurocrine hormones			
Bombesin	Stomach	Gastrin release	

(续表)

Hormone	Site of Synthesis	Major Action	
		Stimulates	Inhibits
Enkephalins	Mucosa and smooth muscle throughout GI tract	Smooth muscle contraction	Intestinal secretion
Vasoactive inhibitorypeptide (VIP)	Mucosa and smooth muscle throughout GI tract	Pancreatic enzyme secretion Intestinal secretion	Smooth muscle contraction Sphincter contraction

4.1.2.2 Cardiac Glands

They are distributed in the area $1-3$ cm wide near the cardia. Cardiac glands are composed of mucus-secreting cells.

4.1.2.3 Pyloric Glands

They are distributed in the area about $4-5$ cm wide near the pylorus. Pyloric glands have longer pits and shorter branched, coiled, tubular secretory portions. Parietal cells are scarce here. Gastrin (G) cells (which release gastrin) intercalated among the mucous cells of pyloric glands. Gastrin stimulates the parietal cells to release acid, and promote the proliferation of gastrointestinal mucosa cells.

Gastric juice is a mixture of three kinds of glandular secretions.

Mucous-HCO$_3^-$ Barrier/Stomach Mucous Barrier: Gastric juice contains high concentration of hydrochloric acid, which is highly corrosive. Pepsin can decompose protein, but gastric mucosa is as corrosion-resistant as ceramics, which is mainly due to the presence of stomach mucous barrier. It resides in the surface layer of the mucosa and is believed to be formed from the surface mucus and the tight junction, which fuse the surface mucous cells together. The mucous layer is $0.25-0.5$ cm thick, mainly composed of visible, gel-like mucus containing high bicarbonate and potassium concentration. The mucus layer separates the epithelium from pepsin, and the high concentration of HCO$_3^-$ makes local pH of 7. It does not only inhibit the enzyme activity, but also neutralize the infiltrated H^+ to form H_2CO_3, which is rapidly decomposed into H_2O and CO_2 by carbonic anhydrase of gastric epithelial cells. In addition, the rapid renewal of gastric epithelial cells also enables the stomach to repair the damage timely. Stomach Mucous Barrier protecting stomach mucosa from auto digestion. If the barrier is destroyed, it will cause self-digestion of gastric tissue, forming gastritis or gastric ulcer.

4.1.3 Muscularis Mucosae

The muscularis mucosae is composed of 2 relatively thin layers of smooth muscle fibers, usually arranged as an inner circular and outer longitudinal layer.

4.2 Gastric Submucosa

The submucosa is composed of a dense connective tissue containing variable amounts of adipose tissue and blood vessels, as well as the nerve fibers and the submucosal (Meissner's) plexus.

4.3 Gastric Muscularis Externa and Adventitia

The muscularis of the stomach is traditionally described as consisting of an outer longitudinal layer, a middle circular layer, and an inner oblique layer. At the pylorus and cardia, the middle layer is greatly thickened to form the pyloric sphincter and cardiac sphincter. The stomach is covered by a thin serosa.

5 Small Intestine

The small intestine is divided into 3 portions: duodenum, jejunum and ileum. It is the principal site for digestion and absorption.

5.1 Mucosa

The mucosa of all 3 regions displays intestinal villi, extensions of the lamina propria, covered by a simple columnar type of, are 0.5 – 1.5 mm long. In the duodenum they are leaf shaped, gradually assuming fingerlike shape as they reach the ileum and are short conical shaped in the ileum. Additionally, a series of permanent folds the plicae circulares, consisting of submucosa and mucosa extend into the lumen (Figure 14 – 13, 14 – 14).

The small intestinal glands housed in the lamina propria, which are formed by the epithelium of villus root invading into the lamina propria. They are single tubular glands, also known as crypts of Lieberkühn. They open onto the luminal surface of the intestine at the base of the villi. The epithelium of the glands is continuous with that of the villi.

5.1.1 Epithelium

The epithelium of the villi is composed of goblet, surface absorptive, and endocrine cells. The intestinal glands contain absorptive cells, goblet cells, endocrine cells, regenerative cells, as well as Paneth's cells.

Absorptive cells: The absorptive cells are the predominant cells covering the villi and they occur in small numbers in the crypts. They are tall columnar cells, each with an oval nucleus in the basal of the cell. At the apex of each cell possess 2 000 – 3 000 microvilli, forming the striated (brush) border under light microscope. Their tips have a thick cell coat of glycocalyx, rich in disaccharidases and peptidases and other digestive enzymes. The main function of these cells is to digest and absorb sugar, protein, fat and other nutrients substances. It has been calculated that plicae increase the intestinal surface 3 times, the villi increase it 10 times, and the microvilli increase it 20 times, for a total increase of approximately 400 – 600 times.

Their plasma rich in smooth endoplasmic reticulum and Golgi Complex, which manufacture chylomicron (triglyceride and lipoprotein cover), move to the basolateral

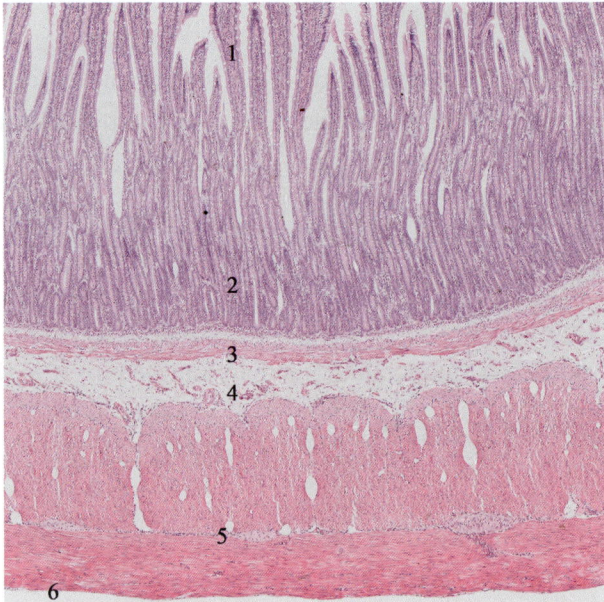

1. Small intestinal villi; 2. Small intestinal gland;
3. Muscularis mucosae; 4. Submucosa; 5. Muscularis;
6. Adventitia

Figure 14 - 13   Photomicrograph of a section of the jejunum (HE)

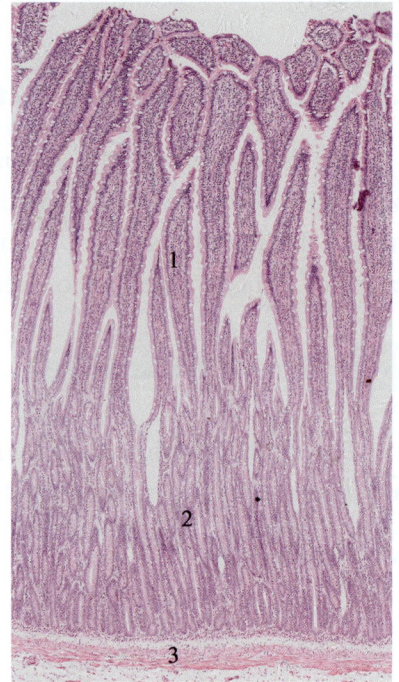

1. Small intestinal villi; 2. Small intestinal gland; 3. Muscularis mucosae

Figure 14 - 14   Photomicrograph of a section of the jejunum (HE)

plasma membrane and flow into extracellular space chylomicrons that pass through the basement membrane and enter the central lacteal. Absorptive cells attach to neighboring cells by tight junctions near the free surface of cells, prevent the material in the intestinal lumen from entering the tissue from the intercellular space.

Additionally, absorptive cells participate in secretion of secretory IgA; absorptive cells located in the duodenum and upper jejunum release enterokinase which convert inactive trypsinogen into active trypsin.

Goblet Cells: Goblet cells are interspersed between the absorptive cells. They increase in number from the duodenum to the terminal part of the ileum. Goblet cells produce mucus, whose function is to protect and lubricate the lining of the intestine.

Paneth's Cells: Paneth's cells are located in the bases of the small intestinal glands.

They are pyramidal-shaped with basal nucleus whose apical region contain numerous large acidophilic secretory granules. These cells manufacture the enzyme lysozyme as well as defensins (cryptids), both displaying the antibacterial effects.

Enteroendocrine Cells: Many kinds of enteroendocrine cells scattered in the small intestine epithelium (Table 14 - 1, Table 14 - 2). they produce hormones such as cholecystokinin (CKK), secretin, which increase pancreatic and gallbladder activity and inhibit gastric secretory function and motility.

Stem Cells: Stem cells are located in the basal half of the crypts of Lieberkühn. They are columned and small. The cells proliferate in the way of mitosis, differentiation and migration to replace all of the cell types described above; they move toward the crypt base or toward the tips of the villi, from which they are finally sloughed into the lumen. Stem cells function as a population of cells that replace the entire intestinal epithelium every 4 – 7 days.

5.1.2   Lamina Propria

The lamina propria of small intestine is composed of loose connective tissue with blood and lymph vessels nerve fibers, and smooth muscle fibers.

In addition, the lamina propria core of each villus contains 1 – 2 central lacteals, which is a blind-ending lymphatic capillary (Figure 14 – 15). The central lacteals run to the region of lamina propria above the muscularis mucosae, where they form a plexus. They are larger than the blood capillaries, but their wall is so close together that appear to collapsed. They are important for the absorption of lipids. Individual amino acids, sugars and other hydrolyze substance enter the surface absorptive cells transferred into the lamina propria where they enter the blood capillaries.

Smooth muscle cells derived from the muscularis mucosae extend into the core of villus and accompany the central lacteal and blood capillaries. These smooth muscle fibers may account for shorten of the villi, speed up during digestion and help propel nutrients in the blood and lymphatic capillaries to the general circulation.

The lamina propria contains scattered lymphocytes and lymphatic nodules. The duodenum and the jejunum have individual lymphatic nodule and the ileum houses large accumulations of lymphatic nodules as known Peyer's patches, which may reach submucosa.

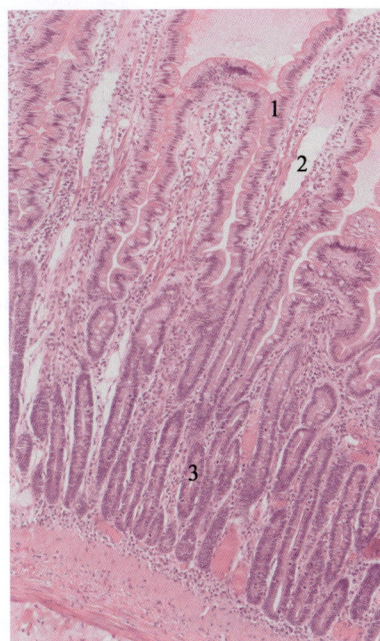

1. Epithelium; 2. The lumen of central lacteal; 3. Small intestine gland

Figure 14 – 15   Photomicrograph of central lacteals (HE)

5.1.3   Muscularis Mucosae

The muscularis mucosae consists of a thin inner circular layer and an outer longitudinal layer of smooth muscle fibers.

5.2   Submucosa

The submucosa consists of dense connective tissue that is rich in blood and lymphatic vessels.

The submucosa of the duodenum contains the submucosal glands and the duodenal glands (Brunner's glands). They are coiled tubular glands opening into the intestinal glands. The mucous cells of these glands produce an alkaline mucus (pH $8.1 - 9.3$), which protects the duodenal lining from Gastric Acid erosion (Figure $14 - 16$).

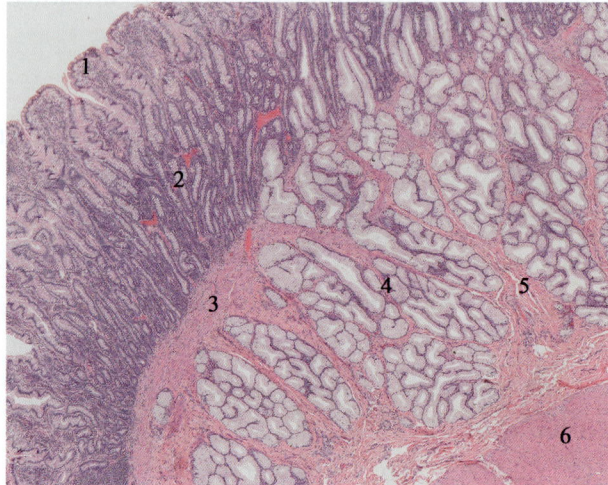

1. Small intestinal villi; 2. Small intestinal gland; 3 Muscularis mucosae; 4. Duodenal gland; 5 Submucosa; 6. Muscularis

Figure $14 - 16$ Photomicrograph of a section of duodenum (HE)

The secretion of small intestinal epithelium and glands is called small intestinal fluid. The daily secretion of adults is $1 - 3$ L, and it also contains a lot of water, NaCl, KCl and so on.

5.3 Muscularis Externa and Advetitia

The Muscularis externa consists of an inner layer of circularly arranged smooth muscle cells and an outer layer of longitudinally arranged smooth muscle cells.

Most small intestine is covered by the serosa, except that part of duodenum is fibrous membrane.

6   Large Intestine

The large intestine is subdivided into the cecum, the colons, the rectum, the anal canal, and the appendix. The principal functions of the large intestine are reabsorption of water and electrolytes, formation and storage of faeces and fermentation of some of the indigestible food matter by bacteria. The Cecum, the Colons, and the Rectum own the same structural features (Figure $14 - 17, 14 - 18$).

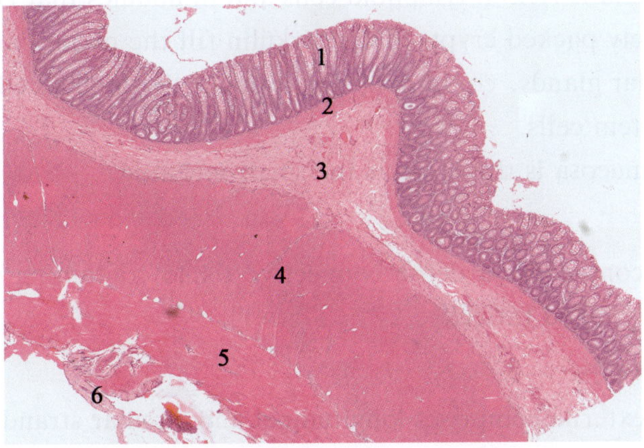

1. Lamina propria; 2. Muscularis mucosae; 3. Submucosa; 4. Circular smooth muscle layer; 5 Longitudinal smooth muscle layer; 6. Adventitia

Figure 14 - 17　Photomicrograph of a section of colon (HE)

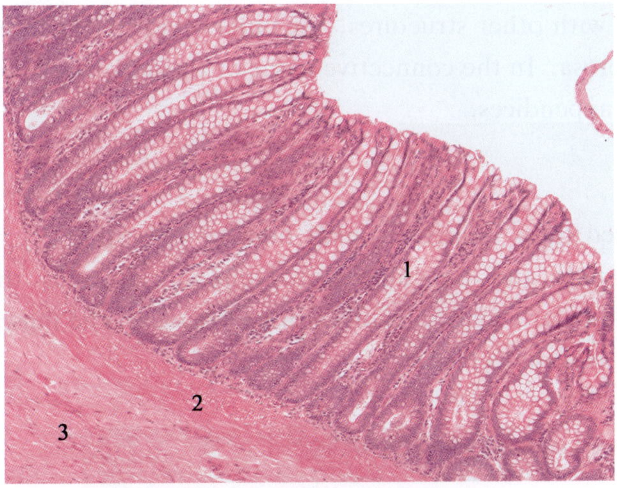

1. Large intestine gland; 2. Muscularis mucosae; 3. Submucosa

Figure 14 - 18　Photomicrograph of a section of colon (HE)

6.1　Cecum, Colons, and Rectum

6.1.1　Mucosa

No villi are present. The mucosa and the submucosa form the semilunar fold. The mucosal epithelium is composed of many goblet cells, surface absorptive cells, stem cells, and occasional enteroendocrine cells. The primary function of the columnar absorptive cells is reabsorption of water and electrolytes. Goblet cells are more numerous in the large intestine than in the small intestine. They produce mucin, and facilitate the passage of the increasingly solid contents.

The lamina propria is rich in lymphoid cells and in nodules that frequently extend into the submucosa. Closely packed crypts of Lieberkühn fill the major part of lamina propria. They are single tubular glands, containing absorption cells, goblet cells, a small number of endocrine cells and stem cells.

The muscularis mucosa is the same as the small intestine.

6.1.2 Submucosa

The submucosa consists of a dense connective tissue containing small arteries, small veins, lymphatic vessels and fat cells.

6.1.3 Muscularis Externa

The Muscularis externa comprises longitudinal and circular strands. The outer layer of the Muscularis externa is, in part, condensed into prominent longitudinal bands of muscle, called teniae coli.

6.1.4 Adventitia

The posterior wall of the ascending colon, descending colon, lower 1/3 of the rectum is directly in contact with other structures, the outer layer of which is fibrous; elsewhere, the outer layer is a serosa. In the connective tissue of the adventitia, adipocytes accumulate to form the epiploic appendices.

6.2 Appendix

It is characterized by a relatively small lumen. The lamina propria has fewer and shorter intestinal glands and has abundant lymphatic nodules that extend into the submucosa, so the muscularis mucosa is often discontinuous. The muscularis externa is very thin, the outer layer is serosa (Figure 14 - 19, 14 - 20).

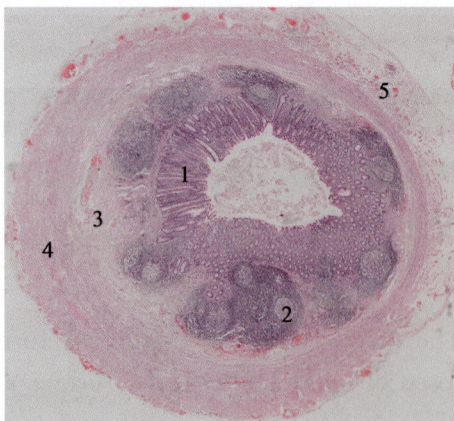

1. Large intestine gland; 2. Lymph nodes; 3. Submucosa; 4. Muscularis; 5. Adventitia

Figure 14 - 19 Photomicrograph of a section of appendix (HE)

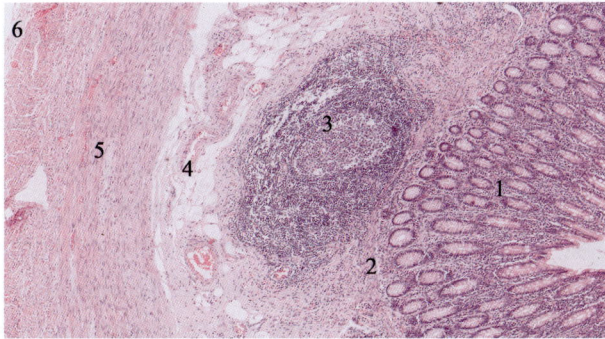

1. Large intestine glands; 2. Muscularis mucosae; 3. Lymph nodes;
4. Submucosa; 5. Muscularis; 6. Adventitia

Figure 14 - 20   Photomicrograph of a section of appendix (HE)

6.3   Anal Canal

The anal mucosa above the dentate line is similar to the rectum. The upper part of the anal canal has longitudinal folds called anal columns. Depressions between the anal columns are called anal sinuses. At the dentate line, the epithelium from the simple columnar epithelium translates to the stratified squamous epithelium, where intestinal glands and muscularis mucosae disappear (Figure 14 - 21). Below the dentate line, the epithelium is stratified squamous epithelium that is continuous with that skin; the lamina propria has anal glands and sebaceous glands. The submucosa contains the rectal venous plexus. Enlargements of these submucosal veins constitute internal hemorrhoids. The circular layer of the muscularis thickens to form the internal anal sphincter. The external anal sphincter is formed by striated muscle of the pelvic floor.

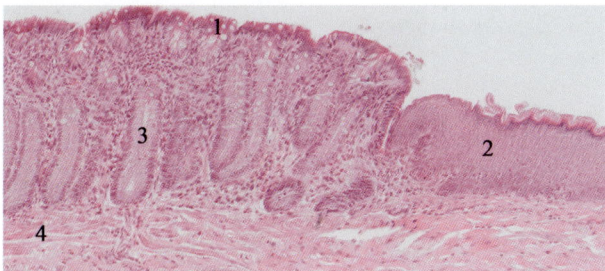

1. Simple columnar epithelium; 2. Non-keratinized stratified squamous epithelium; 3. Large intestine gland; 4. Muscularis mucosae

Figure 14 - 21   Photomicrograph of Junction of rectum and anal canal (HE)

7   Endocrine Cells of Gastrointestinal Tract

More than 40 types of endocrine cells scattered in the surface and glandular epithelium of the gastrointestinal tract (Table 14 - 1, 14 - 2).

Electron microscopy showed that they were irregular pyramidal in shape, with the base attached to the basement membrane and basal lateral processes contacting with adjacent cells; a large number of secretory granules were found in the basal cytoplasm.

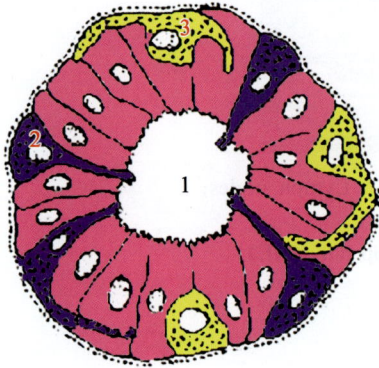

1. Lumen; 2. Open type; 3. Closed type

Figure 14 - 22 Ultrastructural diagram of endocrine cells of gastrointestinal tract

Polypeptide-secreting cells of the digestive tract divide into 2 classes: the open type, in which the apex of the cell presents microvilli and contacts the lumen of the organ (Figure 14 - 22), the chemical contents of the digestive tract (e. g., certain nutrients, pH values) might act on its microvilli and thereby influence secretion of these cells; and the closed type, in which the cellular apex is covered by other epithelial cells (Figure 14 - 22), which mainly regulated by mechanical stimulation of gastrointestinal movement or other hormones to change its endocrine state.

These secretory granules contain peptide and (or) amine hormones, which are mostly released on the basal surface of cells, transported by blood circulation and act on target cells. A few hormones act directly on adjacent cells to regulate function of the target cells in a paracrine manner. At present, the immunohistochemical method is mainly used to show these cells.

(Wang Shanshan)

第十四章　消　化　管

消化管是一条长约 9 米,直径不等的连续性管道,包括口腔、咽、食管、胃、小肠和大肠。这些器官的管壁结构具有某些共同的分层规律,又各具有与其功能相适应的特点。

第一节　消化管壁的一般结构

从食管到大肠,消化管的管壁由内向外依次为:黏膜、黏膜下层、肌层和外膜四层(图 14 - 1)。

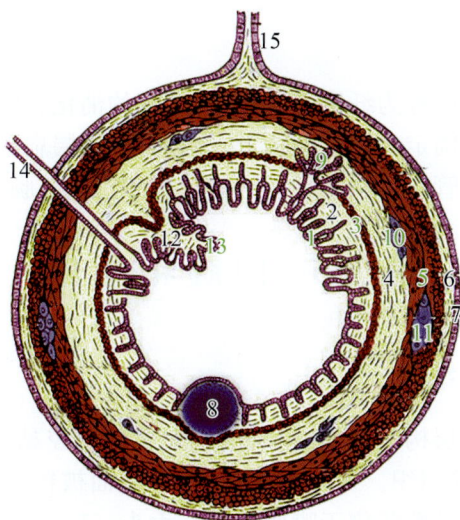

1—上皮；2—固有层；3—黏膜肌层；4—黏膜下层；5—肌层；6—外膜；7—浆膜；8—淋巴小结；9—黏膜下腺；10—黏膜下神经丛；11—肌间神经丛；12—皱襞；13—肠绒毛；14—导管；15—系膜

图 14 - 1　消化管壁的一般结构模式图

一、黏膜

黏膜由上皮、固有层和黏膜肌层组成。黏膜具有三个主要功能：保护、吸收和分泌。

1. 上皮

口腔、咽、食管和肛管上皮是复层扁平上皮，以保护功能为主；胃和肠为单层柱状上皮，以消化吸收功能为主。

2. 固有层

固有层是富含血管、淋巴管和平滑肌纤维的结缔组织。胃肠固有层富含腺体和淋巴组织。

3. 黏膜肌层

一般由薄层平滑肌纤维组成，其收缩可促进黏膜运动。黏膜肌层是黏膜和黏膜下层的分界。

二、黏膜下层

黏膜下层由致密的不规则结缔组织组成，富含血管、淋巴管和淋巴组织。在食管和十二指肠的黏膜下层中分别有食管腺和十二指肠腺。黏膜下层内还有黏膜下神经丛，主要由多极神经元和无髓神经纤维组成，可调节黏膜肌层收缩和腺体分泌。食管、小肠和大肠的黏膜和黏膜下层共同突向管腔，形成皱襞。

三、肌层

一般由内环行和外纵行两层平滑肌纤维组成。相邻两层之间有一层薄薄的结缔组织，其中包括肌间神经丛，结构与黏膜下神经丛相似，调节肌层运动。肌纤维收缩可混合并推动消化管的内容物（图 14 - 2）。

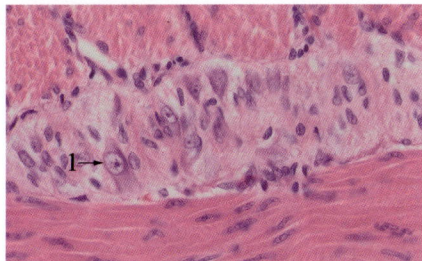

1—神经元

图 14 - 2　肌间神经丛（HE 染色）

四、外膜

仅由结缔组织组成的外膜称为纤维膜,具有纤维膜的消化管(食管、十二指肠、升结肠和降结肠),其管壁可直接附着或固定在邻近结构上。由间皮(单层扁平上皮)和结缔组织组成的外膜称浆膜。具有浆膜的消化管(胃、空肠、回肠、横结肠和乙状结肠)表面光滑,利于器官运动。

第二节 口腔和咽部

一、口腔黏膜的一般结构

口腔黏膜由上皮和固有层构成,无黏膜肌层。大多数口腔黏膜上皮是非角化复层扁平上皮,固有层是富含血管的结缔组织。牙龈、硬腭和舌背表面被覆角化复层扁平上皮,这些区域的固有层直接连接骨组织。骨骼肌位于嘴唇、脸颊、舌头、口底和软腭的黏膜下。

二、舌

舌由表面的黏膜和深部的舌肌组成。舌黏膜由复层扁平上皮和固有层组成。舌肌由纵行、横行及垂直走行的骨骼肌纤维束交织构成。

舌根将舌头固定在舌骨上。舌体背表面被"V"形舌界沟分为前 2/3 和后 1/3。舌背表面后 1/3 由淋巴小结构成的舌扁桃体组成。舌背表面前 2/3 有许多舌乳头,是黏膜上皮和固有层形成的突起。主要有 3 种类型的乳头(图 14-3)。

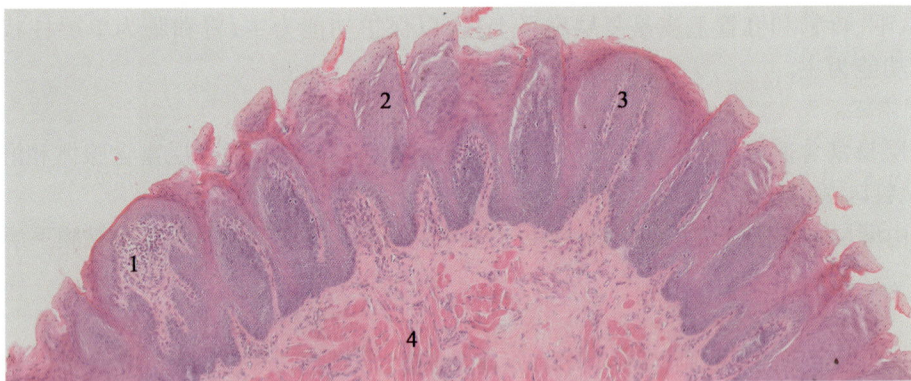

1—轮廓乳头;2—丝状乳头;3—菌状乳头;4—骨骼肌纤维
图 14-3 舌乳头(HE 染色)

1. 丝状乳头

丝状乳头相当多,分布在整个舌背表面。它们呈圆锥形,没有味蕾,尖端稍向咽部倾斜,复层扁平上皮高度角化,外观白色,称舌苔。

2. 菌状乳头

菌状乳头数量较少,多位于舌尖与舌缘,呈蘑菇状,顶部上皮内有少量味蕾。固有层富含毛细血管,外观呈红色。菌状乳头上皮为非角化复层扁平上皮。

3. 轮廓乳头

轮廓乳头是 7～12 个非常大的圆形乳头,位于舌界沟的正前方。固有层中有很多浆液性的味腺。每个乳头周围的黏膜凹陷形成环沟,腺导管开口于沟底,较多味蕾分布在乳头周边上皮内。分泌物可洗去味蕾表面的食物碎渣,使味蕾不断接受新的物质刺激。

味蕾呈卵圆形,主要分布在菌状乳头和轮廓乳头上皮内,少数散在于软腭、会厌及咽部上皮内。味蕾是味觉感受器。每个味蕾主要由 60～80 个纺锤形味细胞聚集而成(图 14-4)。味细胞是一种神经上皮细胞,这些细胞紧密排列在上皮表面形成一个味孔。其游离面有长长的微绒毛,称为味觉毛,穿过味孔,暴露在口腔潮湿的环境中。其基底面含突触小泡样颗粒,基底面与味觉神经末梢形成突触。味蕾深部还有锥体形基细胞,属于未分化细胞,可分化为味细胞。

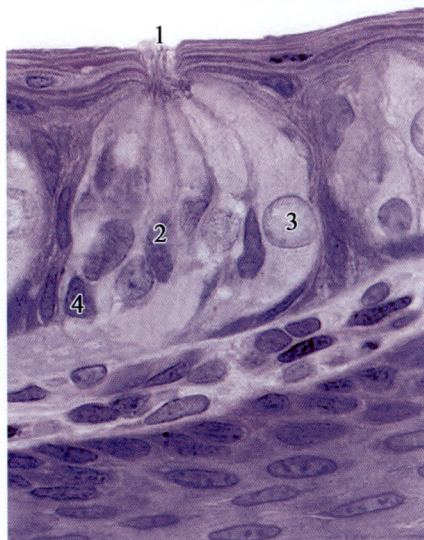

1—味孔;2—支持细胞;3—味细胞;4—基细胞
图 14-4 味蕾(HE 染色)

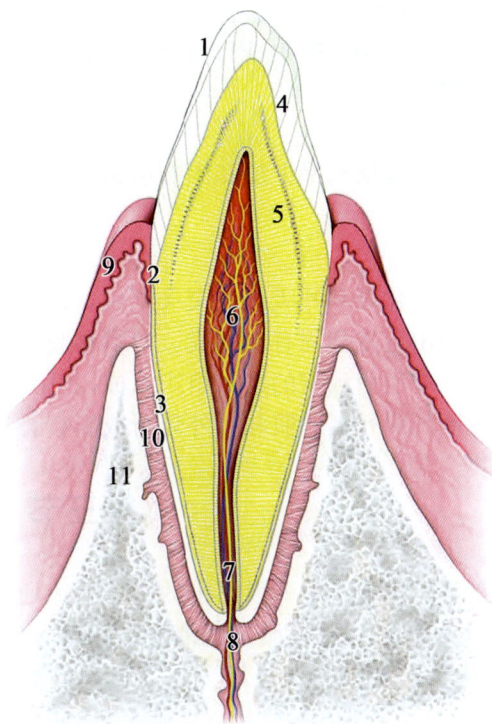

1—牙冠;2—牙颈;3—牙根;4—釉质;5—牙本质;6—牙髓;7—牙根管;8—牙根尖孔;9—牙龈;10—牙周膜;11—牙槽骨
图 14-5 牙的模式图

三、牙齿

牙齿由牙冠、牙根和牙颈组成。露在外面的为牙冠,埋在牙槽骨内的为牙根,两者交界处为牙颈。牙中央有牙髓腔,开口于牙根底部的牙根孔。牙由钙化的硬组织和牙髓软组织构成。牙实质由 3 种钙化物质——牙本质、牙釉质和牙骨质组成。牙周组织是维持上颌骨和齿槽骨中牙齿的结构,包括牙周膜、牙龈和牙槽骨骨膜(图 14-5)。

1. 牙本质

位于牙冠(冠状牙本质)和牙根(根状牙本质)中,并围绕着牙髓腔。牙本质是牙齿的主体,有牙本质小管和间质构成。其间质由 65%～70% 的钙盐和 30%～35% 的 I 型胶原纤维构成。牙髓腔包括位于牙冠中的髓室和牙根中的根管。牙髓填充于牙髓腔,是一种富含血管的结缔组织,对牙本质和釉质具有营养作用。成牙本质细胞排列在牙本质和牙髓之间,可以持续形成牙本质的有机质。

2. 牙釉质

牙釉质覆盖牙冠的牙本质表面。它是体内最硬的组织,由 96% 的钙盐和 4% 的有机质组成,有机质主要为釉蛋白。

3. 牙骨质

牙骨质覆盖牙根的牙本质表面,在牙颈部与牙釉质相连,其组成及结构与骨组织相似。

4. 牙周膜

牙周膜是结缔组织,内含较粗的成束的胶原纤维,连接牙骨质和牙槽骨,将牙齿牢固地固定在牙槽中。

5. 牙龈

牙龈由复层扁平上皮和固有层组成。每颗牙齿的颈部都被牙龈包围。

四、咽

咽是消化管和呼吸道的交叉部位,分为口咽、鼻咽和喉咽三部分。

黏膜由上皮和固有层构成。口咽黏膜为复层扁平上皮,鼻咽和喉咽部为假复层纤毛柱状上皮。固有层由致密的结缔组织组成,其中含有许多小的黏液性唾液腺。此外还有咽扁桃体。肌层由咽内纵行括约肌和咽外环行或斜行骨骼肌组成。外膜为纤维膜。

第三节　食　　管

食管是消化管中一段固定的肌性管道,它是食物从咽运送到胃的通道。管腔内有纵行皱襞。当食物通过时,黏膜皱襞消失,管腔扩张避免黏膜受损伤(图 14-6)。

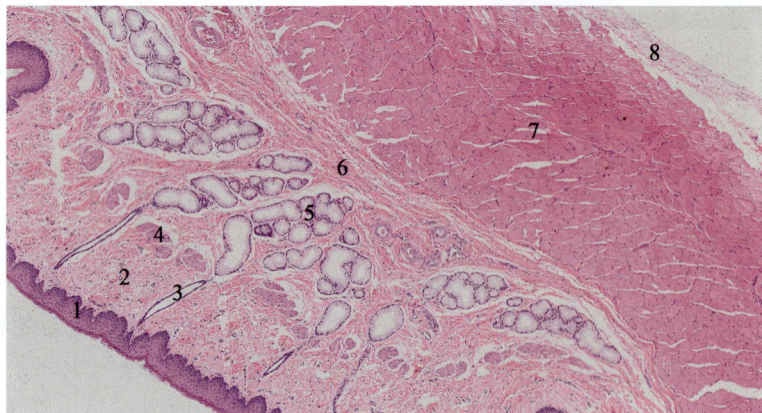

1—上皮;2—固有层;3—食管腺导管;4—黏膜肌层;5—食管腺分泌部;6—黏膜下层;7—肌层;8—纤维膜
图 14-6　食管横断面(HE 染色)

一、黏膜

食管黏膜由非角化复层扁平上皮、固有层和一层纵行平滑肌纤维组成的黏膜肌层构成。

二、黏膜下层

黏膜下层由不规则致密结缔组织组成,其中含有较大的血液和淋巴管、弥漫性淋巴组织和淋巴小结、神经纤维和神经节细胞。黏膜下层含有黏液性腺体,即食管腺。其导管穿过黏膜开口于食管管腔。

三、肌层

肌层由内环行、外纵行两层肌纤维构成。食管上 1/3 由骨骼肌纤维组成,中 1/3 由骨骼肌纤维和平滑肌纤维组成,下 1/3 由平滑肌纤维组成。

四、外膜

食管外表面为纤维膜,它通过结缔组织与邻近结构相连,起固定作用。

第四节 胃

胃是消化管扩张的部分。进入胃的食物,与胃液混合形成食糜。胃可贮存食物,初步消化蛋白质,并吸收部分水、无机盐和醇类。

胃具有消化管的一般结构特征,由黏膜、黏膜下层、肌层和浆膜构成。排空的胃,可见纵行皱襞。当胃充盈时,这些皱襞消失。

一、黏膜

胃的表面被一些浅沟分成许多不规则凸起的区域,称为胃小区。黏膜上皮内陷到固有层形成胃小凹,胃腺开口于胃小凹的底部(图 14-7~图 14-9)。

1. 上皮

胃黏膜表面和胃小凹的上皮为单层单柱状上皮,主要为表面黏液细胞。该细胞核卵圆形,位于基部;顶部胞质充满黏原颗粒。在 HE 染色切片上,因为黏原颗粒在固定和脱水过程中丢失,细胞顶部通常着色浅淡以至透明;细胞间有紧密连接。这些细胞分泌含有高浓度碳酸氢盐的不可溶碱性黏液,覆盖在上皮表面,保护上皮免受胃液中酸性物质的侵害。表面黏液细胞不断脱落,由胃小凹底部的干细胞增殖分化而来,其更新周期为 3~5 天。正常胃上皮无杯状细胞;胃黏膜出现杯状细胞,病理学定义为胃的肠上皮化生,可能是胃癌的前期。

2. 固有层

胃固有层内有胃腺;根据所在部位的不同,分为贲门腺、胃底腺和幽门腺。腺体之间和胃小凹之间有少量结缔组织。除成纤维细胞外,还有许多淋巴细胞、浆细胞、肥大细胞、嗜酸性粒细胞和散在的平滑肌纤维。

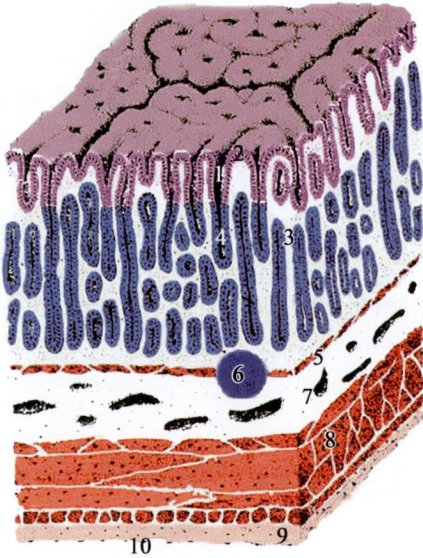

1—胃小凹;2—单层柱状上皮;3—固有层;4—胃底腺;5—黏膜肌层;6—淋巴小结;7—黏膜下层;8—肌膜;9—浆膜;10—间皮

图 14-7 胃底部立体模式图

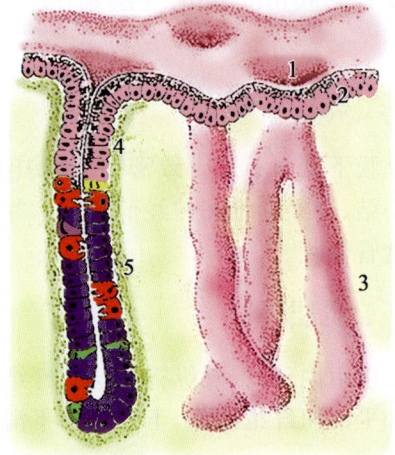

1—胃小凹;2—单层柱状上皮;3—固有层;4—胃小凹;5—胃底腺;黄:干细胞;玫红:颈黏液细胞;红:壁细胞;蓝:主细胞;绿:内分泌细胞

图 14-8 胃底腺模式图

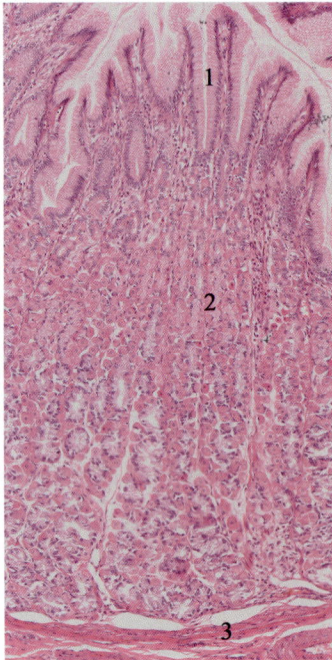

1—胃小凹;2—胃底腺;3—黏膜肌层
图 14-9 胃黏膜光镜图(HE 染色,低倍)

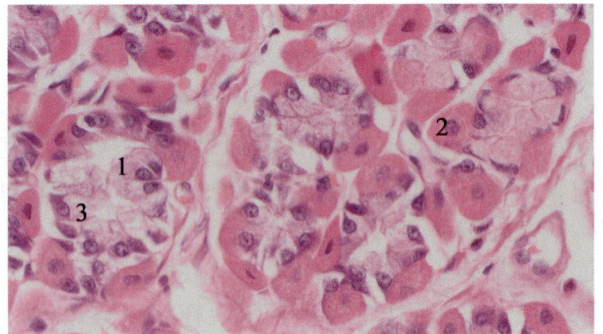

1—胃底腺;2—壁细胞;3—主细胞
图 14-10 胃底腺光镜图(HE 染色,高倍)

(1)胃底腺:胃底腺分布于胃底和胃体的固有层,约有 1500 万条。胃底腺是分支管状腺,可分为峡部、颈部和基部。每个胃小凹的底部与 3～7 条腺体相通。胃底腺由壁细胞、主细胞、颈部黏液细胞、内分泌细胞和干细胞组成(图 14-9~图 14-10)。

壁细胞,又称泌酸细胞,主要分布于胃底腺的上半部分(峡部和颈部)。细胞呈圆形或锥体,核圆形,位于中央,胞质嗜酸性强(图 14-11)。电镜观察,壁细胞游离面胞膜向胞质内深陷,形成细胞内分泌小管。小管表面有许多微绒毛伸向管腔,靠近小管的细胞质中存在光滑的小管或小泡,称为微管泡系统。

壁细胞的这些特异性结构于分泌盐酸(HCl)的过程中而呈显著差异(图 14-11)。在静息细胞中,微绒毛很少,可见许多微管泡结构。在分泌活跃的细胞中,小管与腺腔相通,小管内微绒毛增多,微管泡系统明显减少或消失。所以人们认为,微管泡系统是细胞内小管的储备形式。胞质含有大量线粒体。壁细胞的寿命约为 200 天,由干细胞增殖分化而来。

壁细胞分泌盐酸。细胞内分泌小管的膜含有质子泵(H^+/K^+-ATP 酶)和 Cl^- 通道。它们能将壁细胞形成的 H^+ 和血液吸收的 Cl^- 分别导入小管形成盐酸并分泌到腺腔。线粒体为这一过程提供能量。

壁细胞也分泌内因子,内因子是一种糖蛋白,在胃腔中与维生素 B_{12} 结合并形成复合物。当这种复合物到达回肠时,它与表面吸收细胞上的特定受体结合,维生素被吸收。人体缺乏内因子导致 B_{12} 缺乏,导致红细胞形成障碍,可出现恶性贫血。

主细胞,又称胃酶细胞,位于胃底腺的基部。主细胞具有典型的蛋白质合成细胞的特点(图 14-12)。细胞呈柱状,靠近细胞基部有圆形细胞核。细胞核周围的细胞质强嗜碱性,顶部充满酶原颗粒,HE 切片染色过程中,颗粒多溶解消失,顶部浅染(图 14-10)。这些颗粒含有非活性的胃蛋白酶原,在胃的酸性环境中可转化为具有活性的胃蛋白酶。

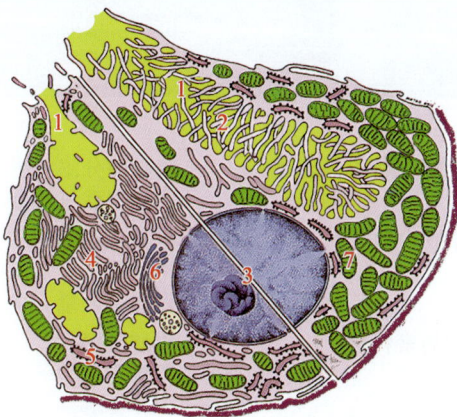

1—细胞内分泌小管;2—微绒毛;3—细胞核;4—微管泡系统;5—粗面内质网;6—高尔基复合体;7—线粒体
图 14-11 壁细胞模式图
静止期(左);活跃期(右)

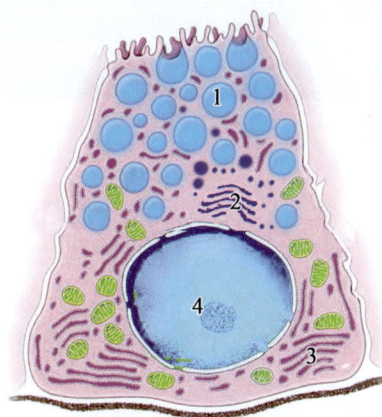

1—黏原颗粒;2—高尔基复合体;3—粗面内质网;4—细胞核
图 14-12 胃主细胞模式图

颈黏液细胞,位于胃底腺的颈部,在壁细胞之间单独或成群出现。该细胞分泌可溶性酸性黏液,成为食糜的一部分并润滑食糜。这些细胞寿命约为 6 天。

干细胞分布于胃小凹底部和胃底腺上部,数量较少。细胞呈柱状,核卵圆形,位于细胞基部。细胞通过有丝分裂增殖分化为胃的上皮细胞和腺细胞。

内分泌细胞将其产物分泌到固有层或黏膜下层的血管中。它们存在于胃底腺的颈部和底部。寿命为60～90天。这些细胞产生激素，如组胺、胃泌素、生长抑素、分泌素和胆囊收缩素（表14-1、表14-2）。

表14-1　常见胃肠激素的生理作用

激素	合成细胞及分布	主要功能	
		促进功能	抑制功能
胃泌素	G 细胞（胃）	胃酸分泌	
生长素	Gr 细胞（胃）	生长激素分泌 食欲和饥饿感	脂质代谢 脂肪组织中的脂肪利用
胆囊收缩素-促胰酶素（CCK）	I 细胞（十二指肠和空肠）	胆囊收缩 胰酶分泌 胰腺碳酸氢根离子分泌 胰腺生长	胃排空
胰泌素	S 细胞（十二指肠）	胰腺酶分泌 胰腺碳酸氢根离子分泌 胰腺生长	胃酸分泌
胃抑制肽（GIP）	K 细胞（十二指肠和空肠）	胰岛素释放	胃酸分泌
胃动素	Mo 细胞（十二指肠和空肠）	胃动力 肠动力	

表14-2　其他胃肠激素的生理作用

激素	合成细胞及分布	主要功能	
		促进功能	抑制功能
候选激素			
胰多肽	PP 细胞（胰腺）	胃排空和肠道运动	胰腺酶分泌 胰腺碳酸氢盐分泌
YY 肽	L 细胞（回肠和结肠）	结肠中的电解质和水吸收	胃酸分泌 胃排空 食物摄入量
胰高血糖素样肽-1（GLP-1）	L 细胞（回肠和结肠）	胰岛素释放	胃酸分泌 胃排空
旁分泌激素			
生长抑素	D 细胞（胃肠黏膜）		胃泌素释放 胃酸分泌 其他胃肠激素释放
组胺	胃肠黏膜	胃酸分泌	
神经内分泌激素			
蛙皮素	胃	胃泌素释放	
脑啡肽类	胃肠黏膜和平滑肌	平滑肌收缩	肠分泌物
血管活性抑制肽（VIP）	胃肠黏膜和平滑肌	胰腺酶分泌 肠分泌	平滑肌收缩 括约肌收缩

（2）贲门腺：分布于近贲门处宽 1～3 cm 区域的固有层，贲门腺为黏液腺。

（3）幽门腺：分布于幽门部 4～5 cm 宽区域的固有层。此处胃小凹较长，幽门腺分泌部短小，为分支且卷曲的管状腺。壁细胞在这里很少。G 细胞散在分布于幽门的黏膜上皮细胞之间，释放胃泌素。胃泌素刺激壁细胞释放胃酸，促进胃肠黏膜细胞增殖。

3 种腺体分泌物的混合，称为胃液。

胃液含有高浓度盐酸，腐蚀力极强，胃蛋白酶能分解蛋白质，而胃黏膜却像陶瓷般耐腐蚀，不受破坏，因为黏液-碳酸氢盐屏障起保护作用。该屏障存在于黏膜的表面。主要是黏膜细胞间的紧密连接和表面黏液层发挥作用。黏液层厚 0.25～0.5 mm，主要由不可溶性黏液凝胶构成，并含有大量的碳酸根离子。黏液层将上皮与胃蛋白酶隔离，高浓度的 HCO_3^- 使局部 pH 值为 7，既抑制了酶的活性，又可中和渗入的 H^+，形成 H_2CO_3，后者被胃上皮细胞的碳酸酐酶迅速分解为 H_2O 和 CO_2。此外，胃上皮细胞的快速更新也能及时修复胃黏膜损伤。胃黏膜屏障保护胃黏膜不被自我消化。如果屏障受到破坏，引发胃组织的自我消化，则形成胃炎或胃溃疡。

3. 黏膜肌层

由内环行和外纵行两层平滑肌纤维组成。

二、黏膜下层

黏膜下层由致密的结缔组织组成，含有脂肪组织和血管，以及神经纤维和黏膜下神经丛。

三、肌层和浆膜

肌层为由外纵行、中环行和内斜行三层平滑肌纤维组成。在幽门和贲门，中层平滑肌增厚，形成幽门括约肌和贲门括约肌。外膜为浆膜。

第五节 小 肠

小肠分为三部分：十二指肠、空肠和回肠。它是消化和吸收的主要场所。

一、黏膜

小肠黏膜表面有绒毛，是由单层柱状上皮和固有层向肠腔突起形成的，长 0.5～1.5 mm。在十二指肠，绒毛呈叶状，到达回肠后逐渐呈指状，在回肠，呈短圆锥形。由黏膜层和黏膜下层突向肠腔形成环形皱襞，此皱襞不会因为食物通过而消失（图 14-13、图 14-14）。

固有层内有小肠腺，是绒毛根部上皮向固有层凹陷形成的。小肠腺为单管状腺，又称利伯屈恩隐窝或肠隐窝。肠腺在绒毛根部开口于肠腔。肠腺与绒毛的上皮相连。

1. 上皮

绒毛上皮由杯状细胞、吸收细胞和内分泌细胞组成。肠腺除上述细胞外，还包含干细胞和帕内特细胞。

吸收细胞是覆盖绒毛表面的主要细胞，肠腺上皮中吸收细胞少。吸收细胞呈柱状，核椭圆形，位于基底部。每个细胞的游离面有 2 000～3 000 根微绒毛，形成光镜下的纹状缘状（刷状缘）。微绒毛表面有一层厚的细胞衣，主要由蛋白多糖构成，富含双糖酶和肽酶等消化酶。小

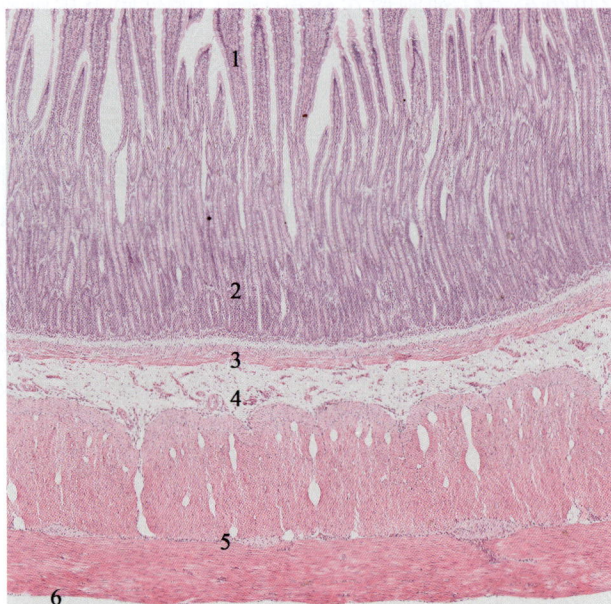

1—小肠绒毛;2—小肠腺;3—黏膜肌层;4—黏膜下层;5—肌层;6—外膜

图 14-13　空肠横断面光镜图(HE 染色,低倍)

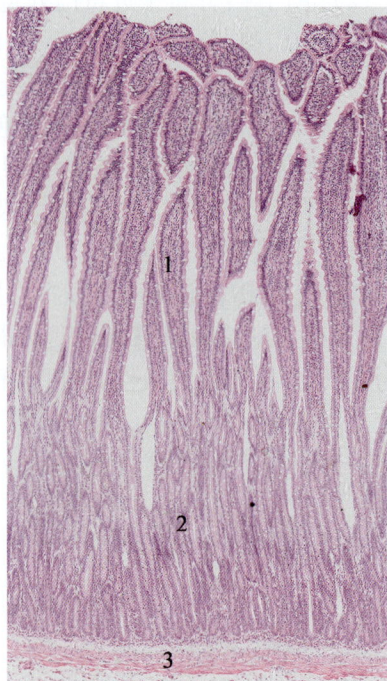

1—小肠绒毛;2—小肠腺;3—黏膜肌层

图 14-14　空肠的黏膜层光镜图

(HE 染色,低倍)

肠摄取的营养物质(糖、蛋白质、脂肪等)几乎全部被吸收细胞消化、吸收。皱襞使肠表面积增加 3 倍,绒毛使肠表面积增加 10 倍,微绒毛使细胞游离面面积扩大约 20 倍,微绒毛、小肠绒毛和皱襞使小肠表面积一共增大了 400～600 倍。

吸收细胞胞质内富含滑面内质网和高尔基复合体,将细胞吸收的脂类物质制造成乳糜微粒。乳糜颗粒在细胞基部释放入细胞侧面间隙中,再经过基膜进入中央乳糜管被吸收。相邻吸收细胞近游离面有紧密连接,可阻止肠腔中的物质从细胞间隙进入组织。

另外,吸收细胞参与分泌型免疫球蛋白 A 的分泌;位于十二指肠和空肠上部的吸收细胞可释放肠激酶,将非活性胰蛋白酶原转化为活性胰蛋白酶。

杯状细胞散布在吸收细胞之间。从十二指肠到回肠末端其数量增加。杯状细胞产生黏液,其功能是保护和润滑肠壁。

帕内特细胞,又称潘氏细胞,位于小肠腺的基部,呈锥体状,核位于基底部,胞质顶部含有大量的嗜酸性分泌颗粒。颗粒中含有溶菌酶和防御素(隐窝素),对肠道微生物有杀灭作用。

肠内分泌细胞(表 14-1、表 14-2)产生激素,如胆囊收缩素、分泌素等,这些激素能增加胰腺和胆囊的活动,抑制胃的分泌功能和运动。

干细胞位于肠隐窝的下半部分,胞体小,呈柱状。细胞通过有丝分裂增殖,分化,迁移来更新上述所有类型的细胞;它们向隐窝基部或绒毛顶端移动,最后从绒毛中脱落进入管腔。肠上皮细胞的更新周期为 4～7 天。

2. 固有层

小肠固有层由疏松的结缔组织构成,除含有大量小肠腺外,还有丰富的血管、淋巴管、神经纤维和平滑肌纤维。

此外,绒毛中轴的固有层含有 1～2 条中央乳糜管,它们是起始段为盲端的毛细淋巴管(图 14-15)。中央乳糜乳管从绒毛顶端开始延伸到黏膜肌层上方,在那里它们形成一个毛细淋巴管丛。中央乳糜管比毛细血管腔大,但它们的管壁柔软,管腔常塌陷。它们对脂质的吸收很重要。通过表面吸收细胞吸收的氨基酸、糖等水溶性物质转运到绒毛中轴的固有层,经此处毛细血管入血。来源于黏膜肌层的平滑肌细胞延伸到绒毛中轴,分布在中央乳糜管和毛细血管周围。平滑肌纤维收缩可使绒毛缩短,有助于将血管和毛细淋巴管中的营养物质输送到全身。

固有层含有分散的淋巴细胞和淋巴小结。十二指肠和空肠有单独的淋巴小结,回肠有发达的淋巴小结,称为集合淋巴小结,可以到达黏膜下层。

3. 黏膜肌层

由薄薄的内环行和外纵行平滑肌纤维组成。

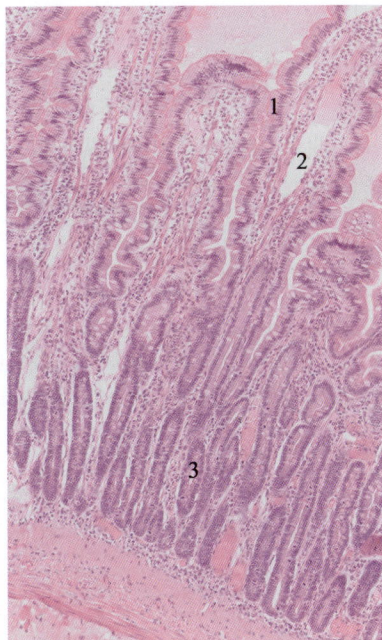

1—小肠绒毛上皮;2—中央乳糜管;
3—小肠腺

图 14-15 中央乳糜管光镜图
(HE 染色,高倍)

二、黏膜下层

由富含血管和淋巴管的致密结缔组织组成。十二指肠黏膜下层含有腺体,即十二指肠腺(Brunner's gland)。它们是弯曲的管状腺体,开口于肠腺。这些腺体由黏液细胞组成,分泌碱性黏液(pH 8.1～9.3),保护十二指肠黏膜免受胃酸侵蚀(图 14-16)。

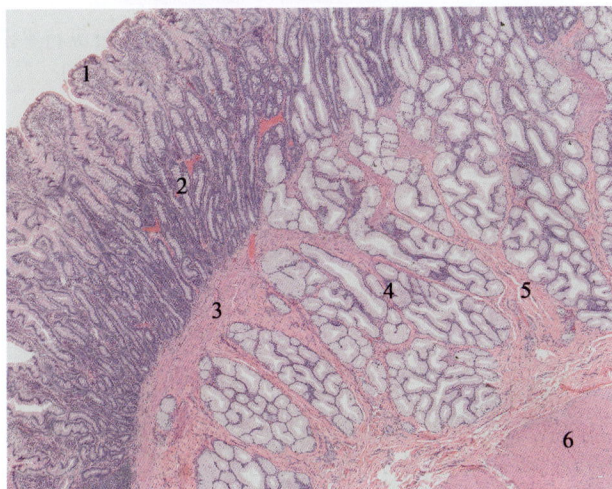

1—小肠绒毛;2—小肠腺;3—黏膜肌层;4—十二指肠腺;5—黏膜下层;6—肌层
图 14-16 十二指肠光镜图(HE 染色,低倍)

小肠上皮和腺体的分泌物称为小肠液。成人每天分泌量为 1～3 L,含有大量的水、NaCl、

KCl 等。

三、肌层和外膜

肌层由内环行和外纵行的平滑肌纤维组成。除了十二指肠部分为纤维膜,小肠大部分被浆膜覆盖。

第六节　大　　肠

大肠分为盲肠、阑尾、结肠、直肠、肛管。大肠的主要功能是水和电解质的重吸收、粪便的形成和储存,以及细菌对某些不可消化食物的发酵。

一、盲肠、结肠和直肠

它们的结构基本相同(图 14-17、图 14-18)。

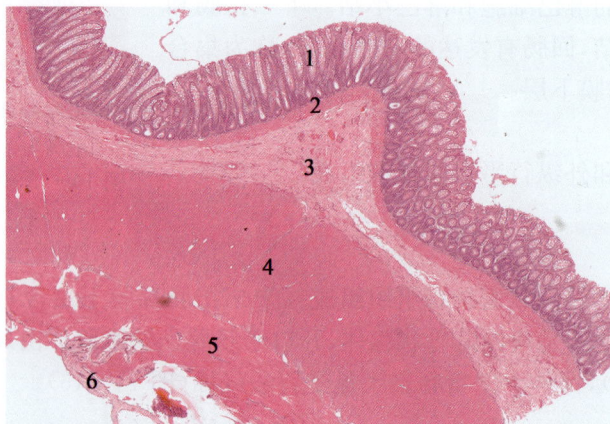

1—固有层;2—黏膜肌层;3—黏膜下层;4—内环形平滑肌;5—外纵行平滑肌;6—外膜
图 14-17　结肠的横断面光镜图(HE 染色,低倍)

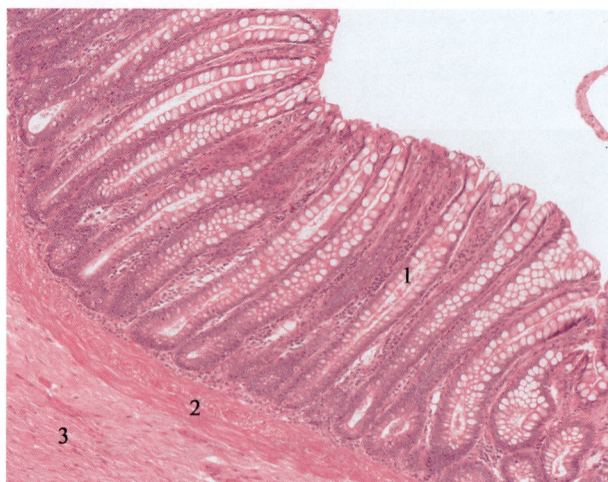

1—大肠腺;2—黏膜肌层;3—黏膜下层
图 14-18　结肠的横断面光镜图(HE 染色,高倍)

1. 黏膜

无绒毛。黏膜层和黏膜下层形成半月形皱襞。黏膜上皮由较多的杯状细胞、吸收细胞、少量干细胞和肠内分泌细胞组成。柱状吸收细胞的主要功能是重吸收水和电解质。大肠中的杯状细胞比小肠中的多,它们分泌黏液,润滑肠道。

固有层富含淋巴细胞和淋巴小结。淋巴小结可延伸到黏膜下层。固有层有密集的大肠腺,呈单管状,开口于肠腔。含有吸收细胞、杯状细胞、少量内分泌细胞和干细胞,无帕内特细胞。黏膜肌层与小肠相同。

2. 黏膜下层

由致密的结缔组织组成,包含小动脉、小静脉、淋巴管和脂肪细胞。

3. 肌层

包括纵行和环行两层平滑肌纤维。外纵行肌局部增厚形成结肠带。由于结肠带短于肠管的长度,使肠管皱缩形成结肠袋。

4. 外膜

升结肠和降结肠后壁,直肠下 1/3 的管壁外层与周围组织直接相连,为纤维膜;其余大部分为浆膜。在外膜的结缔组织中,常有脂肪细胞聚集形成肠脂垂。

二、阑尾

阑尾管腔相对较小。固有层的肠腺较少且短,淋巴小结发达,可延伸至黏膜下层,故黏膜肌层常不连续。肌层很薄,外层是浆膜(图 14-19、图 14-20)。

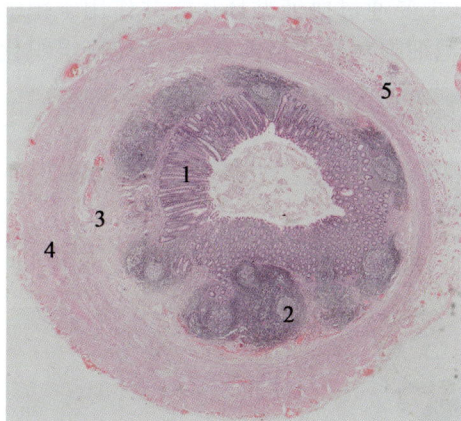

1—大肠腺;2—淋巴小结;3—黏膜下层;4—肌层;5—外膜
图 14-19 阑尾横断面光镜图(HE 染色,低倍)

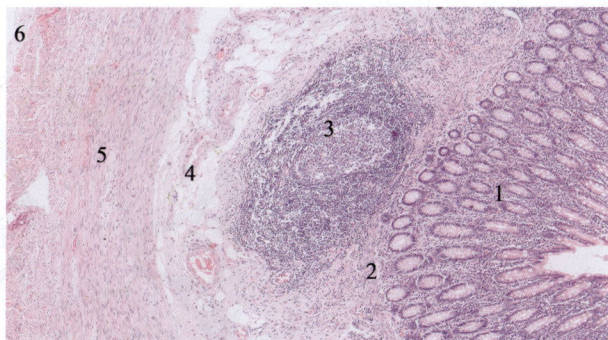

1—大肠腺;2—黏膜肌层;3—淋巴小结;4—黏膜下层;5—肌层;6—外膜
图 14-20 阑尾横断面光镜图(HE 染色,高倍)

三、肛管

齿状线以上的肛管黏膜与直肠相似。肛管的上部有纵向褶皱,称为肛柱。肛柱之间的凹陷称为肛窦。在齿状线处,单层柱状上皮转化为复层扁平上皮,肠腺和黏膜肌层消失(图 14-21)。齿状线以下,上皮为复层扁平上皮,与皮肤连续;固有层有肛门腺和皮脂腺。黏膜下层含有直肠静脉丛。如黏膜下静脉扩张则形成痔。环行肌增厚形成肛门内括约肌。肛门外括约肌由盆底的骨骼肌纤维形成。

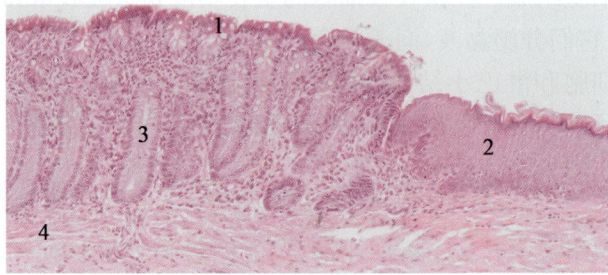

1—单层柱状上皮；2—非角化复层扁平上皮；3—大肠腺；4—黏膜肌层
图 14-21　直肠肛管交界处光镜图(HE 染色，高倍)

第七节　胃肠的内分泌细胞

40 多种内分泌细胞散在分布于胃肠道的黏膜上皮和腺上皮中(表 14-1、表 14-2)。

电镜下这些细胞呈不规则锥体形，基底附着于基膜，基底侧突与邻近细胞接触；基底细胞胞质中有大量分泌颗粒。内分泌细胞分两类：①开放型，细胞顶端有微绒毛，感受管腔内的化学信息(比如营养素、pH 值等)，影响这些细胞的分泌；②封闭型，细胞顶端被其他上皮细胞覆盖，主要通过胃肠运动的机械刺激或其他激素来调节内分泌状态(图 14-22)。细胞内的分泌颗粒含有肽类和(或)胺类激素，通过细胞的基底面释放，主要通过血液循环运输并作用于靶细胞。少数激素以旁分泌方式直接作用于邻近细胞，调节靶细胞功能。目前，主要用免疫组织化学方法鉴定识别这些细胞。

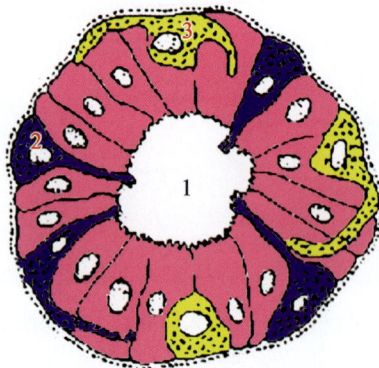

1—管腔；2—开放型内分泌细胞；3—封闭型内分泌细胞
图 14-22　消化管内分泌细胞超微结构模式图

（王姗姗）

Chapter 15

Digestive Glands

The digestive glands include the small digestive glands that are distributed in the wall of digestive tracts and the large glands. The small digestive glands include the minor salivary glands, esophageal glands, gastric glands and intestinal glands, etc. The large glands constitute organs including the 3 pairs of the major salivary glands, the pancreas, the liver and the gallbladder. The large glands are located outside the digestive tracts and deliver their secretory products to the lumen of the digestive tracts by a system of ducts.

1 Major Salivary Glands

The major salivary glands include 3 paired glands: the parotid, submandibular and sublingual glands. They are surrounded by a capsule of connective tissue that is rich in collagen fibers. The parenchyma of the glands consists of secretory portions and a branching duct system (Figure 15 – 1).

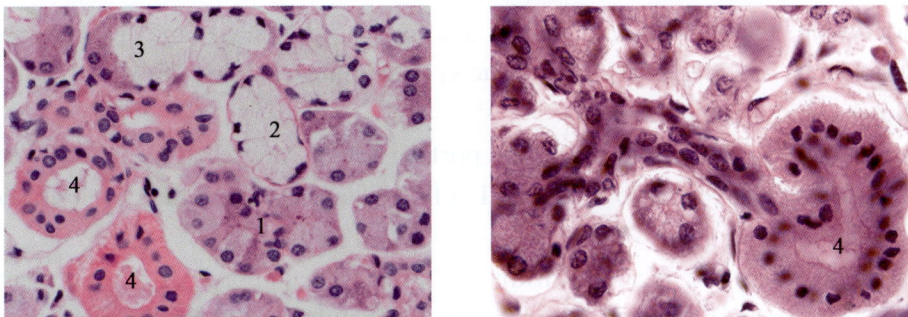

1. Serous acini; 2. Mucous acini; 3. Mixed acini; 4. Striated duct

Figure 15 – 1   Light photomicrograph of submandibular gland

1.1 General Structure of the Major Salivary Glands

The major salivary glands are compound, tubule acinar glands, consisting of many secretory units at the end of a highly branched duct system. The acini and the ducts connected with them constitute lobules. There are connective tissue septa between lobules.

1.1.1 Secretory Portions

The secretory portions of salivary glands are also called acini. They are smaller collection of the secretory cells, composed of serous and mucous secretory cells. According to the components of these 2 cell types, the acini are classified in 3 categories, such as serous acini, mucous acini and mixed acini (Figure 15 - 1).

Serous acini are composed of serous cells. Serous cells are usually pyramidal in shape, with a broad base resting on the basal lamina and a narrow apical surface. They have single, round, basally located nuclei. In the basal region, the cytoplasm tends to be basophilic, and it appears more eosinophilic in the apical area. Serous cells are protein-secreting cells. They have well-developed rough endoplasmic reticulum (RER), Golgi complex, and abundant apically situated secretory granules rich in salivary amylase, which is an enzyme that initiates the digestion of complex carbohydrates.

Mucous acini are composed of mucous cells. Mucous cells are similar in shape to the serous cells. Their nuclei are also basally located but are flattened. The cytoplasm is palely stained with a foamy appearance. Comparing with the serous cells, the mucous cells have a less extensive RER and a considerably greater Golgi apparatus. The apical region of the cytoplasm is occupied by abundant secretory granules. The mucous cells produce a thick glycoprotein-rich secretion (mucus) that lubricates oral cavity and enables food to slide over the mucosa.

Mixed acini are composed of both serous and mucous cells. They often appear to have a small group of the serous cells displaced at the blind end of the mucous acini and form crescent-shaped figure, termed the serous demilune.

1.1.2 Duct Portions

The ducts of major salivary glands are highly branched and range from small intercalated ducts to large principal ducts: the intercalated ducts, striated ducts, interlobular ducts and the main ducts.

The intercalated ducts are the terminal portions of the branched duct system. They are composed of a single layer of low cuboidal cells. Their narrow lumen is continuous with that of the acini.

The striated ducts are located within the lobules, equipped with a simple cuboidal epithelium that gradually becomes columnar epithelium. The nuclei are centrally or apically located. The plasma inholdings are seen as striations (Figure 15 - 1).

The interlobular ducts initially have a simple columnar epithelium, which transform from a stage of pseudostratified epithelium into stratified epithelium in the main excretory duct that opens in the oral cavity.

1.2 Structural Features of the Major Salivary Glands

1.2.1 Parotid Glands

The parotid gland is almost purely serous and has relatively long intercalated ducts and short striated ducts. The secretion contains the enzyme ptyalin.

1. 2. 2　Submandibular Glands

The submandibular glands are mixed glands. In humans, 90% of the endpieces of the submandibular gland are serous acinar, whereas 10% consist of mucous tubules with serous demilunes. The intercalated ducts are less extensive than that in the parotid glands. In contrast, the striated ducts are well developed and long.

1. 2. 3　Sublingual Glands

The sublingual glands are mixed glands with predominantly mucous acini, but occasionally mucous acini with serous demilunes can be seen. Intercalated ducts and striated ducts are rarely seen.

2　Pancreas

The pancreas is covered by a thin capsule of connective tissue that send septa into the pancreas and separate it into lobules. The pancreas gland is mixed, comprising exocrine portion and endocrine portion. The exocrine part constitutes the major part of the gland, which produces digestive enzymes. The endocrine part is also called islet of Langerhans and scatter throughout the exocrine part and constitute approximately 1% of the pancreas (Figure 15 - 2,15 - 3). The endocrine cells in the islets of Langerhans secrete hormones.

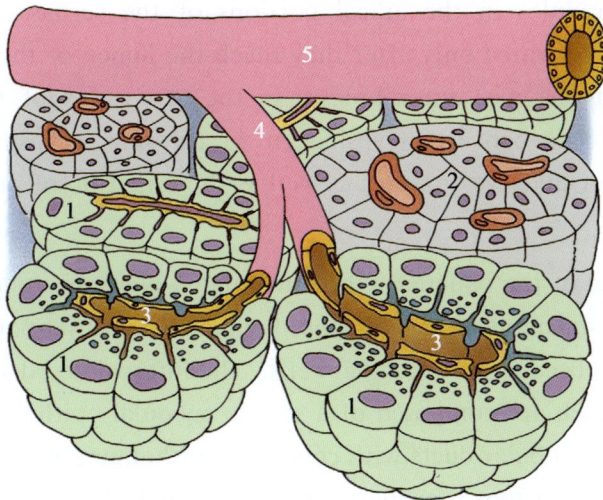

1. Serous cell; 2. Islet of Langerhans; 3. Intercalated duct; 4. Introlobular duct; 5. Interlobular duct
Figure 15 - 2　The structure of pancreas

2.1　Exocrine portion

The exocrine portion of the pancreas is tubuloacinar gland (Figure 15 - 4).

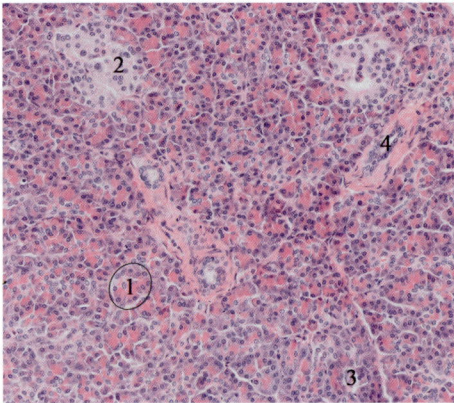

1. Acini; 2. Islet of Langerhans; 3. Intralobular duct; 4. Interlobular duct

Figure 15 - 3　Light photomicrograph of pancreas

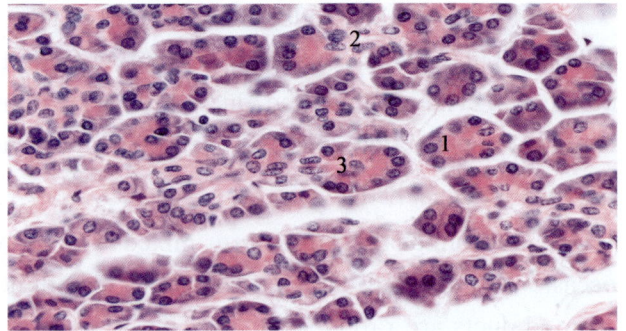

1. Acini; 2. Intercalated duct; 3. Centroacinar cell

Figure 15 - 4　Light photomicrograph of exocrine portion of pancreas

2.1.1　Acini

Each acinus is composed of $40-50$ serous cells. The cells are highly polarized, with a spherical nucleus, and are typical protein-secreting cells. They all have the typical morphological characteristics of serous cells. The acinar cells produce, store and release a large number of digestive enzymes including proteolytic endopeptidases, proteolytic exopeptidases, amylolytic enzymes, lipases, nucleolytic enzymes, etc. The enzymes are stored in zymogen granules in the apical portions of the serous cells. The pancreatic digestive enzymes are activated only after they reach the lumen of the small intestine. The proteolytic activity of enzymes enterokinases in the glycocalyx of the microvilli of the intestinal absorptive cells converts trypsinogen to trypsin. Trypsin then catalyzes the conversion of the other inactive enzymes as well as the digestion of proteins in the chyme.

2.1.2　Duct System

In the duct system of the pancreas, the intercalated ducts are relatively longer and are composed of a simple squamous or cuboidal epithelium. The initial portion extends into the lumen of the acinus to become centroacinar cells. The intercalated ducts drain directly into intralobular ducts, which are composed of a simple cuboidal epithelium. The intralobular ducts unite to form interlobular ducts with columnar epithelium. And the interlobular ducts join a main pancreatic duct that runs longitudinally through the entire length of the organ. Goblet cells are present among the columnar epithelial cells of the pancreatic duct. The pancreatic duct opens into a recess of the duodenal lumen. There are no striated ducts in the pancreatic duct system.

2.2　Endocrine Portion

The endocrine portion of the pancreas is composed of spherical aggregates of cells, which are known as islet of Langerhans. There are about 1 million islets in an adult pancreas. They are scattered throughout the exocrine portion and most numerous in the tail of the pancreas. The sizes of the islets vary 75 – 500 μm in diameter. The islets are extensively vascularized by fenestrate capillaries. In H&E stained sections, the islets appear as clusters of palely stained cells (Figure 15 – 3). It is hard to identify the cell types by routinely prepared specimens. After Zenker-formol fixation and staining by the Mallory-Azan method, however, it is possible to identify 3 principal cell types (Figure 15 – 5): A (alpha), B (beta) and D (delta) cells. About 5% of the cells appear to be unstained in this method.

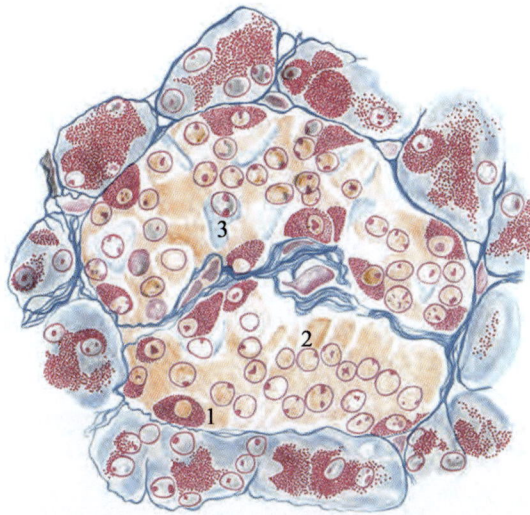

1. A cell; 2. B cell; 3. D cell
Figure 15 – 5　Cell types of islet of Langerhans

2.2.1　A Cells

A cells constitute about 20% of the islet population and are generally located peripherally in the islets. They secrete glucagon, which increases the rate of conversion of liver glycogen to glucose, and stimulates the release of glucose into blood.

2.2.2　B Cells

B cells constitute about 70% of the islet population and are generally located centrally in the islets. They secrete insulin, which is the most abundant endocrine secretion. Insulin facilitates the anabolic processes in muscles, liver and fat, in which it stimulates the synthesis of glycogen, protein and fatty acids. The most important direct effect of insulin is acting antagonistically to glucagon and facilitating the utilization of glucose by increasing glucose oxidation and glycogenesis, thus lowering blood glucose levels.

Absence or inadequate amounts of insulin lead to elevated blood glucose levels and the presence of glucose in the urine, a condition known as diabetes mellitus.

2.2.3 D Cells

D cells constitute about 5% of the islet population and are located peripherally in the islets. They secrete somatostatin, which inhibits the release of glucagon and insulin.

2.2.4 PP Cells

PP cells are small in number and are mostly located peripherally in the islets, and also found in the epithelium of small or middle size of the exocrine duct, and occasionally among acinar cells. The PP cells secrete pancreatic polypeptide. The hormone is inhibitory for the activity and motility in gut, as well as the secretion of the pancreatic enzymes and bicarbonate ions.

3 Liver

The liver is the largest gland of the body. It is covered by a capsule of dense connective tissue rich in elastic fibers. With the exception of a bare area, the liver is almost completely invested with peritoneum. Thin connective tissue septa enter the parenchyma of the liver at the hilum, together with the portal vein, hepatic artery, hepatic ducts, nerves and lymphatics, to divide the liver into lobules. In peripheral regions of the lobules, there are portal areas (Figure 15 - 6).

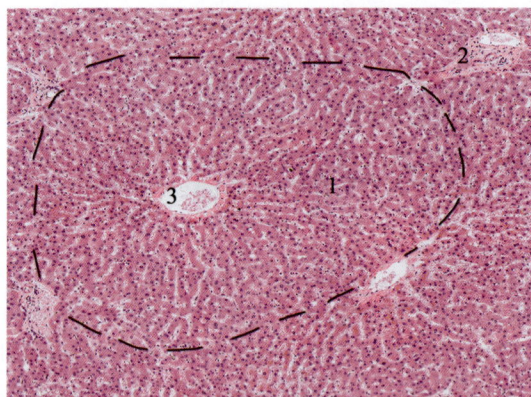

1. Hepatic lobule; 2. Portal area; 3. Central vein
Figure 15 - 6 Hepatic lobule and portal area

3.1 Hepatic Lobules

The hepatic lobule or liver lobule is the basic structural unit of the liver (Figure 15 - 7). There are about 0.5 - 1 million lobules in an adult liver. Each lobule is about 2.0 mm × 1.0 mm in size. Most parts of the lobules contact in close, making it difficult to establish the exact limits between different lobules. But in certain animals (e.g. pigs), the lobules are separated from each other by a layer of connective tissue. At the center of the lobule there is a relatively large venule called the central vein. The hepatocytes arranged in plates radiate from the central vein to the periphery of the lobule, as do the sinusoids.

Hepatocyte plates consist of a row of closely-packed hepatocytes. In cross section, it has been observed that hepatocytes consist of cords, so called hepatic cords. The sinusoids connect the terminal ramification of the hepatic artery and portal vein with the central vein. Tiny channels termed bile canaliculi are present between adjacent hepatocytes. The hepatic plates, sinusoids and bile canaliculi consist of an independent and closely related complex network in the hepatic lobule (Figure 15 – 7).

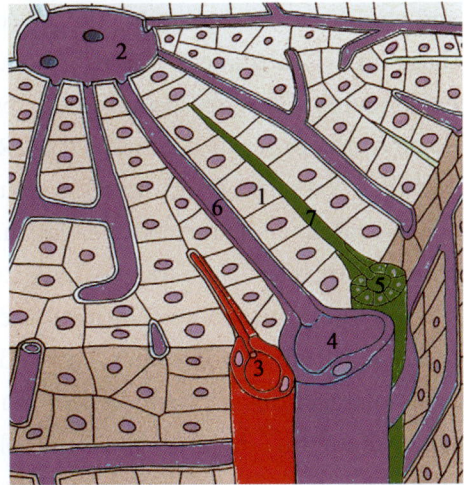

1. Hepatocyte plate; 2. Central vein; 3. Hepatic arteriole; 4. Portal venule; 5. Bile ductile; 6. Hepatic sinusoid; 7. Bile canaliculi

Figure 15 – 7   Structure of hepatic lobule

3. 1. 1 Hepatocyte

Hepatocytes constitute about 80% of the cell population of the liver. They are polygonal cells measuring between 20 and 30 μm in each dimension. The hepatocytic membrane has 3 functional surfaces: the surface facing the sinusoids, the surface facing the bile canaliculi and the surface in contact with adjacent cells. There are many microvilli that cover the surfaces facing sinusoids and bile canaliculi.

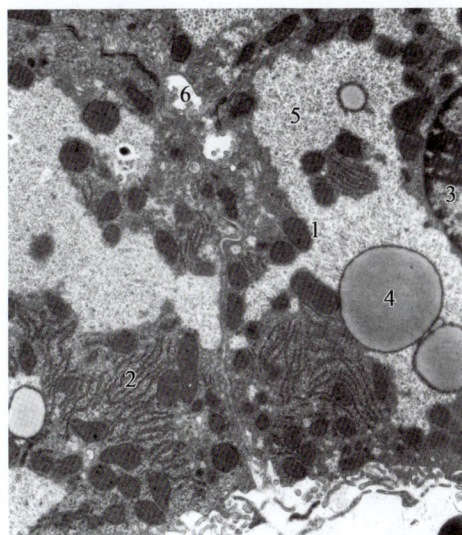

1. Mitochondria; 2. Rough plasma membrane; 3. Nucleus; 4. Lipid droplet; 5. Glycogen particle; 6. Bile canaliculi

Figure 15 – 8   Electron photomicrograph of hepatocyte

Hepatocyte nuclei are large and spherical, and occupy the center of the cells. Many cells in the adult liver are binucleate. Most cells in the adult liver are tetraploid. The hepatocyte cytoplasm is generally acidophilic. Under electron microscope, various organelles are presented. Each organelle plays important roles in the liver's function (Figure 15 – 8).

There are 800 to 1 000 mitochondria in each hepatocyte, which may supply the energy for the cell's metabolic activity. The hepatocyte has an abundant RER and smooth endoplasmic reticulum (SER). The RER usually congregates around the nucleus and mitochondria, synthesizing many important plasma proteins including blood albumin, fibrinogen, prothrombin, lipoprotein and complement proteins. The SER contains enzymes involved in the formation of bile, the synthesis of the lipids and cholesterol compounds，the glycogenolysis and the modification and detoxification of those toxic substances from blood. There are about 50 Golgi apparatuses in each hepatocyte. They are usually distributed around the nucleus or near the bile canaliculi. Some of the proteins synthesized by RER are transferred to Golgi apparatus for processing，and then excreted from hepatic sinusoidal surface in secretory vesicles. Golgi apparatus concentrated near the bile canaliculi are believed to be associated with the exocrine secretion of bile. Hepatocytes have 200 to 300 peroxisomes per cell. Peroxisomes contain a large amount of oxidase that generates toxic hydrogen peroxide. The enzyme catalase，also residing within peroxisomes，degrades hydrogen peroxide to oxygen and water. These types of reactions are involved in many detoxification processes occurring in the liver. In fact，about one half of the ethanol ingested is converted to acetaldehyde by enzymes contained in liver peroxisomes. The lysosomes are quite abundant and active. They are important in the normal replacement of cellular components and organelles，as well as in cellular defense mechanisms. The inclusions such as glycogen particles，lipid droplets and pigments may be present. Their quantity depends on the physiological state of the cells (Figure 15 – 8).

3. 1. 2　Hepatic Sinusoid

The space between the hepatic plates contains the sinusoidal capillaries. The sinusoids receive mixed arterial and venous blood from the interlobular branches of both the portal vein and the hepatic artery at the periphery of a lobule，and then drain into the central veins.

Hepatic sinusoids are lined with a thin discontinuous endothelium. It has a discontinuous basal lamina that is absent over large areas. The discontinuity of the endothelium is evident in two ways：large fenestrae presented within the endothelial cells and large gaps presented between neighboring endothelial cells. The leaky properties of the endothelium of the sinusoids facilitate metabolic exchange between the liver and the blood (Figure 15 – 9,15 – 10).

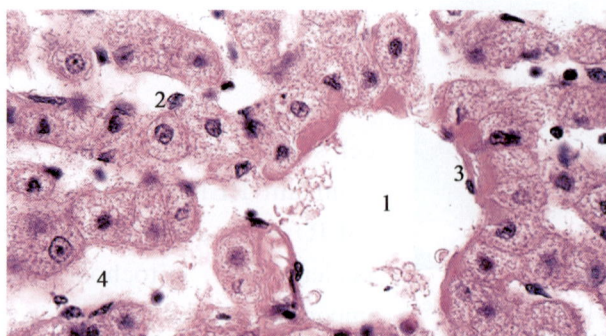

1. Central vein；2. Kupffer cell；3. Endothelial cell；4. Hepatic sinusoid
Figure 15 – 9　Light photomicrograph of hepatic sinusoid

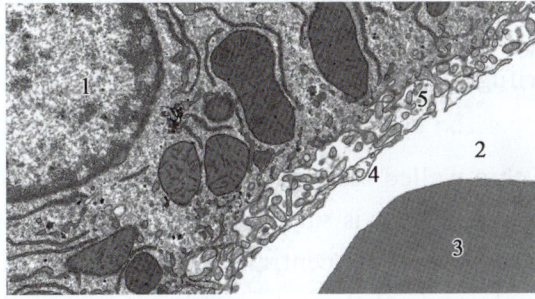

1. Hepatic nucleus; 2. Hepatic sinusoid; 3. Red blood cell; 4. Endothelial cell; 5. Perisinusoidal space

Figure 15 - 10　Electron photomicrograph of hepatic sinusoid

Hepatic sinusoids differ from other sinusoids in that a second cell type, Kupffer cell, which is a regular part of the vessel lining. Kupffer cells are a member of the mononuclear phagocyte system. The transmission electron microscope (TEM) clearly show that the Kupffer cells are from part of the lining of the sinusoid. Processes of Kupffer cells often seem to span the sinusoidal lumen and may even partially occlude it. Their main functions are to metabolize aged erythrocytes, digest hemoglobin, secrete proteins related to immunologic processes and destroy bacteria that eventually enter the portal.

3.1.3　Perisinusoidal Space

The perisinusoidal space, also called Space of Disse, lies between the basal surface of hepatocytes and the basal surfaces of endothelial cells (Figure 15 - 10). Small, irregular microvilli project into this space from the basal surface of the hepatocytes. The microvilli increase the surface area available for exchange of materials between hepatocytes and plasma by 6 times. Blood fluids readily percolate through the endothelial wall and make intimate contact with the surface of the hepatocytes, permitting an easy exchange of macromolecules from the sinusoidal lumen to the hepatocytes and vice versa. Thus, the perisinusoidal space is the site of exchange of materials between blood and hepatocytes.

The other cell type found in the perisinusoidal space is the hepatic stellate cell, also called fat-storing cell or Ito cell. These cells are the primary storage site for hepatic vitamin A in the form of retinyl esters within cytoplasmic lipid droplets. In certain pathologic conditions, such as chronic inflammation or liver cirrhosis, hepatic stellate cells lose their lipid and vitamin A storage capability and differentiate into cells with characteristics of myofibroblasts. These cells appear to play a significant role in hepatic fibrogenesis; they synthesize and deposit type Ⅰ and type Ⅲ collagen within the perisinusoidal space, resulting in liver fibrosis.

3.1.4　Bile Canaliculi

The bile canaliculi are the smallest branches of the biliary tree. They are small intercellular channels formed by invaginating of opposing membrane of adjoining hepatocytes. They are approximately $0.5\,\mu$m in luminal diameter and isolated from the rest of the intercellular compartment by junctional complexes including tight junctions and desmosomes (Figure 15 – 8). Microvilli of the 2 adjacent hepatocytes extend into the canalicular lumen. Bile flow is centrifugal, that is from the central vein toward the portal canal.

3.1.5 Central Vein

The central vein is a thin-walled vessel receiving blood from the hepatic sinusoids. The endothelial lining of the central vein is surrounded by small amounts of spirally arranged connective tissue fibers. Because of its central position in the classic lobule, the central vein is actually the terminal venule of the system of hepatic veins. It leaves the lobule at its base by merging into the larger sublobular vein.

3.2 Portal Area

The portal area occupies a potential space at each of the 6 corners of the lobule. Each area contains 3 main elements surrounded by connective tissue: a hepatic arteriole, a portal venule and a bile ductile (Figure 15 – 7, 15 – 11). Hepatic arteriole is a branch of the hepatic artery, contains blood from the celiac trunk of the abdominal aorta. The portal venule is a branch of the portal vein, contains blood from the superior and inferior mesenteric and splenic veins. The bile ductile is tributary of a bile duct, lined by cuboidal epithelium, carries bile synthesized by hepatocytes and eventually empties into the hepatic duct.

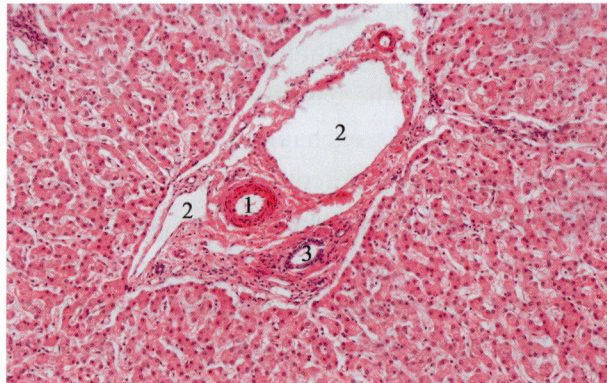

1. Hepatic arteriole; 2. Portal venule; 3. Bile ductile
Figure 15 – 11　Hepatic portal area

3.3 Blood Supply

The liver has a dual blood supply consisting of a venous supply via the hepatic portal vein and an arterial supply via the hepatic artery. Both vessels enter the liver at the hilum, the same site at which the common bile duct, carrying the bile secreted by the liver, and the lymphatic vessels leave the liver. The liver receives its major blood supply (about 75%) from the hepatic portal vein, which carries venous blood that is largely depleted of oxygen. The blood delivered to the liver by the hepatic portal vein comes from the digestive tract and the major abdominal organs, such as the pancreas and spleen. The portal blood carried to the liver contains nutrients and toxic materials absorbed in the intestine, blood cells and breakdown products of blood cells from the spleen, and endocrine secretions of the pancreas and enteroendocrine cells of the gastrointestinal tract. The hepatic artery carries oxygenated blood to the liver, providing the remaining 25% of its blood supply.

3.4 Formation and Transport of the Bile

The bilirubin is a by-product of the hemoglobin catabolism. It is reabsorbed and conjugated with glucuronic acid to form the water-soluble bilirubin glucuronide in sinusoids by hepatocytes. Bilirubin glucuronide, cholic acid, phospholipids, cholesterol, water and electrolytes are secreted as bile. The produced bile flows through the bile canaliculi, bile ductules and bile ducts. These structures gradually merge, forming a network that converges to form the hepatic duct. After receiving the cystic duct from the gall bladder, the hepatic duct continues to the duodenum as the common bile duct.

3.5 Liver Regeneration

One of the most important features of the liver is its remarkable ability to regenerate. The loss of hepatic tissue by surgical removal or from the action of toxic substances triggers a mechanism by which hepatocytes begin to divide, continuing until the original mass of tissue is restored. In humans, this capacity is considerably restricted but is still important, because parts of a liver can be used in surgical liver transplantation.

4 Gallbladder

The gallbladder is a pear-shaped, distensible sac with a volume of about 50 mL in humans. It is attached to the visceral surface of the liver. It stores and concentrates bile and releases it to the duodenum. The wall of the gallbladder is layered similar to the digestive tract with the absence of a submucosa.

The mucosa has abundant folds that are particularly evident when the gallbladder is empty. The mucosal surface consists of simple columnar epithelium. The epithelial cells have short and not well-developed apical microvilli. They can secrete mucus. The lamina propria of the mucosa is particularly rich in fenestrated capillaries and small venules. External to the lamina propria is a muscularis externa that has numerous collagen and elastic fibers among the bundles of smooth muscle cells. The gallbladder does not have a muscularis mucosa or submucosa. External to the muscularis externa is a thick layer of dense connective tissue, the layer of tissue where the gallbladder attaches to the liver surface is referred to as the adventitia. The unattached surface is covered by a serosa.

(Zhang Ling, Wang Lei)

第十五章 消 化 腺

消化腺包括大消化腺及位于消化管各段管壁内的小消化腺,后者包括小唾液腺、食管腺、胃腺和肠腺等。大消化腺包括三对大唾液腺、胰腺、肝脏和胆囊。大消化腺独立于消化管外,其分泌物通过导管输送到消化管腔内。

第一节 大 唾 液 腺

人口腔内有三对大唾液腺:腮腺、颌下腺和舌下腺。它们被富含胶原纤维的结缔组织囊所包裹。唾液腺的实质部分由分泌部和分支的导管系统组成。

一、大唾液腺的一般结构

大唾液腺为复管泡状腺,由高度分支的导管系统末端连接分泌部组成。腺泡和与其相连的导管构成小叶。小叶之间有结缔组织间隔(图 15-1)。

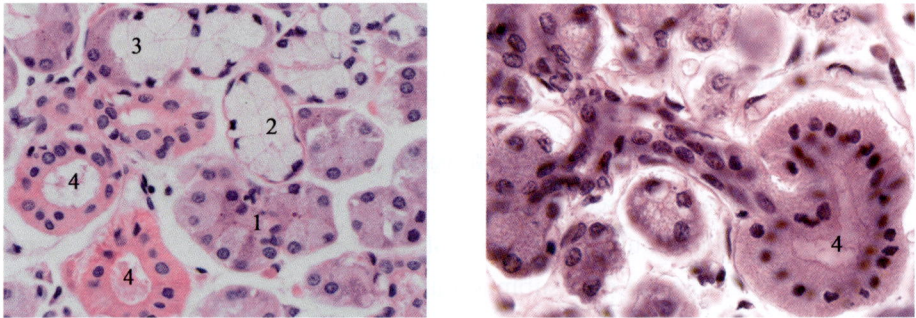

1—浆液性腺泡;2—黏液性腺泡;3—混合性腺泡;4—纹状管

图 15-1 颌下腺光镜结构

(一) 分泌部

唾液腺的分泌部也叫腺泡,它们由分泌细胞聚集而成,包括浆液性腺细胞和黏液性腺细胞。根据组成腺泡的细胞类型,可将腺泡分为浆液性腺泡、黏液性腺泡和混合性腺泡三种类型(图 15-1)。

浆液性腺泡由浆液性腺细胞组成。浆液性腺细胞通常呈锥体形,基部较宽,位于基膜上,顶面较窄。核圆形,位于细胞的基底部。细胞基底部的胞质呈嗜碱性,细胞顶端的胞质则呈嗜酸性。浆液性腺细胞是蛋白质分泌细胞,它们具有丰富的粗面内质网和发达的高尔基复合体,顶部胞质中含大量分泌颗粒,颗粒内富含唾液淀粉酶,该酶的作用是启动碳水化合物复杂的消化反应过程。

黏液性腺泡由黏液性腺细胞组成。黏液性腺细胞与浆液性腺细胞形态类似。其胞核也位于细胞基底部,但呈扁平状。胞质染色浅,呈泡沫状。与浆液性腺细胞相比,黏液性腺细胞的粗面内质网较少,但其高尔基复合体更发达。细胞顶端的胞质内有大量分泌颗粒。黏液性腺细胞产生黏稠的富含糖蛋白的分泌物(黏液),可润滑口腔,使食物更易滑过黏膜。

混合性腺泡由浆液性腺细胞和黏液性腺细胞组成。通常在黏液性腺泡的一侧有一小群浆液性腺细胞覆盖,形成半月形,称为浆半月。

(二)导管

大唾液腺具有高度分支的导管系统,唾液由闰管汇集进入纹状管,再汇合进入小叶间导管,最后汇集进入主导管并开口于口腔。

闰管是导管的起始部,由单层矮立方上皮围成。管腔狭窄,与腺泡腔直接相连。

纹状管位于小叶内,起始部为单层立方上皮,逐渐演变为单层柱状上皮,细胞核位于细胞中央或顶部。细胞基部可见由质膜内褶形成的纵纹。

小叶间导管起始部为单层柱状上皮,逐渐演变为假复层上皮,最终在主导管形成复层上皮与口腔黏膜移行。

二、大唾液腺的结构特点

(一)腮腺

腮腺是纯浆液性腺,闰管较长,纹状管较短,分泌物含唾液淀粉酶。

(二)颌下腺

颌下腺为混合性腺,其中90%的腺泡为浆液性腺泡,10%为混合性腺泡,可见浆半月。与腮腺相比,颌下腺的闰管较短,而纹状管则较发达(图15-1)。

(三)舌下腺

舌下腺为混合性腺,以黏液性腺泡为主,偶见混合性腺泡伴随浆半月。闰管和纹状管均罕见。

第二节 胰 腺

胰腺表面被薄层的结缔组织所覆盖,结缔组织伸入胰腺实质并将其分隔成胰腺小叶。胰腺实质包括外分泌部和内分泌部。外分泌部是腺体的主要部分,可产生消化酶。内分泌部也称为胰岛,散在分布于外分泌部,约占胰腺实质的1%(图15-2、图15-3)。胰岛的内分泌细胞可分泌激素。

一、外分泌部

胰腺的外分泌部为复管泡状腺(图15-4)。

(一)腺泡

每个腺泡由40～50个浆液性腺细胞组成。细胞高度极化,核呈球形,为典型的蛋白质分

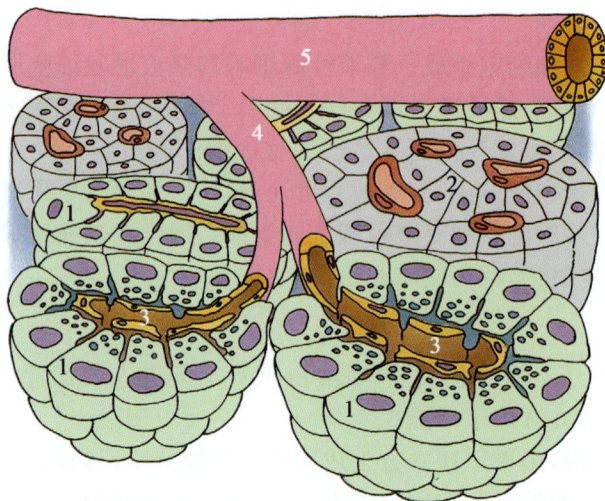

1—浆液性腺细胞；2—胰岛；3—闰管；4—小叶内导管；5—小叶间导管
图 15-2　胰腺结构

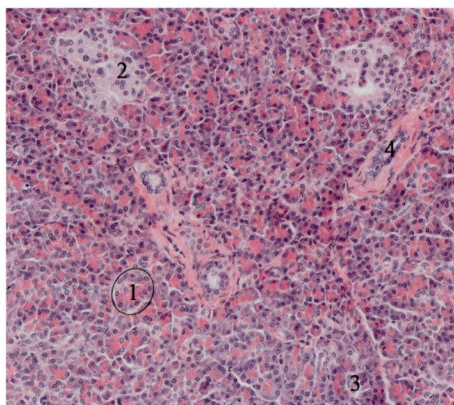

1—腺泡；2—胰岛；3—小叶内导管；4—小叶
间导管

图 15-3　胰腺光镜结构

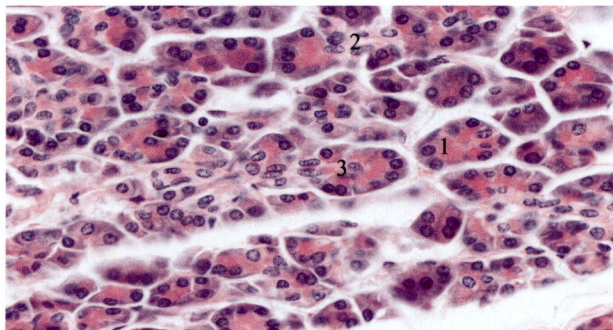

1—浆液性腺细胞；2—闰管；3—泡心细胞
图 15-4　胰腺外分泌部光镜结构

泌细胞,具有典型的浆液性腺细胞形态特征。腺泡细胞可产生、储存和释放大量消化酶,包括蛋白水解内肽酶、蛋白水解外肽酶、淀粉水解酶、脂肪酶和核酸水解酶等。这些酶储存于腺细胞顶部的酶原颗粒内。胰腺内的消化酶只有到达小肠腔后才会被激活,小肠吸收细胞微绒毛内的肠激酶具有蛋白水解活性,可将胰蛋白酶原转化为胰蛋白酶,后者可催化其他非活性酶的转化及食糜中蛋白质的消化。

　　在腺泡腔中央可见一些染色较浅的细胞。它们是延伸入腺泡腔内的闰管起始部分的上皮细胞,这些细胞较小,称为泡心细胞。

(二) 导管

　　胰腺的闰管较长,由单层扁平上皮或立方上皮围成,其起始部延伸入腺泡腔形成泡心细胞。胰腺内无纹状管,闰管直接汇集入小叶内导管。小叶内导管由单层立方上皮组成。小叶内导管汇集为小叶间导管,小叶间导管由单层柱状上皮围成,它最终汇集入主导管贯穿整个胰腺并将分泌物输入小肠腔。

二、内分泌部

胰腺的内分泌部由球形细胞团组成,又称为胰岛。成人胰腺中大约有 100 万个胰岛。它们散布在外分泌部,多位于胰腺尾部。胰岛的直径通常为 $75\sim500\,\mu m$。胰岛内含有丰富的有孔毛细血管。HE 染色下胰岛呈染色浅的团状(图 15-3),无法区分细胞种类,只有用特殊染色才能进行区分,如运用 Mallory-Azan 染色法,可以鉴定 3 种主要的细胞类型(图 15-5):A(α)细胞、B(β)细胞和 D(δ)细胞。但仍有约 5% 的细胞无法用此方法显色。

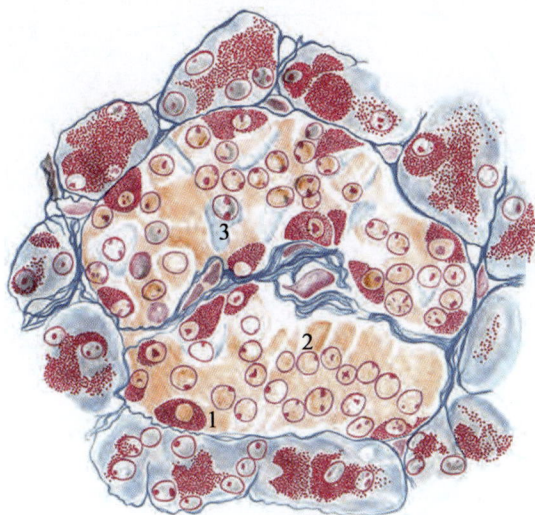

1—A 细胞;2—B 细胞;3—D 细胞
图 15-5 胰岛细胞类型

(一) A 细胞

A 细胞约占胰岛细胞总数的 20%,常分布于胰岛的外周部分。它们可分泌胰高血糖素,能提高肝糖原转化为葡萄糖的速率,从而提高血糖水平。

(二) B 细胞

B 细胞约占胰岛细胞总数的 70%,常分布于胰岛的中央,可分泌胰岛素。胰岛素能够促进肌肉、肝脏和脂肪内的合成代谢过程,从而促进糖原、蛋白质和脂肪酸的合成。胰岛素最重要和直接的作用是拮抗胰高血糖素的作用,通过增加葡萄糖氧化和糖生成作用促进组织对葡萄糖的利用,从而降低血糖水平。

胰岛素缺乏或水平不足会导致血糖水平升高,并从尿液中排出,这种情况称为糖尿病。

(三) D 细胞

D 细胞约占胰岛细胞总数的 5%,位于胰岛的周边部。它们可分泌生长抑素,抑制胰高血糖素和胰岛素的释放。

(四) PP 细胞

PP 细胞数量较少,主要分布于胰岛的外周部,也可见于较小的导管上皮中,偶见于腺泡中。PP 细胞可分泌胰多肽,抑制肠道运动及胰酶和碳酸氢根离子的分泌。

第三节 肝   脏

肝脏是人体内最大的腺体。它表面覆盖有富含弹性纤维的致密结缔组织。肝脏表面大部分区域被腹膜覆盖。结缔组织被膜随着门静脉、肝动脉、肝管、神经和淋巴管一起在肝门处伸入肝脏实质内,将肝脏实质分割成很多肝小叶。在肝小叶周围区域分布有门管区(图 15 - 6)。

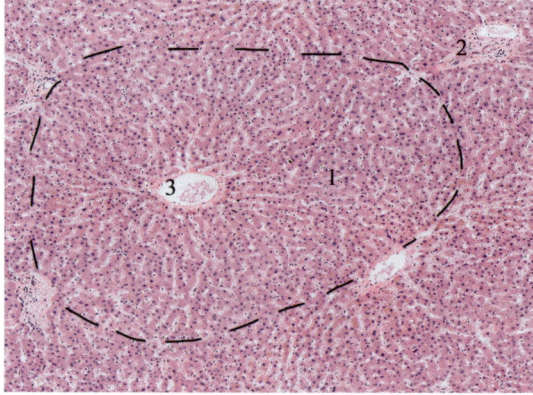

1—肝小叶;2—门管区;3—中央静脉
图 15 - 6 肝小叶和门管区

一、肝小叶

肝小叶是肝脏的基本结构单位(图 15 - 7)。成人肝脏中有 50~100 万个肝小叶,每个肝小叶的大小约为 2.0 mm×1.0 mm。人的肝小叶之间连接紧密,因此肝小叶常连成一片,分界不清。但在一些动物(如猪)中,肝小叶之间结缔组织较丰富,因此肝小叶的界限清晰。肝小叶中央有一个相对较大的小静脉,称为中央静脉。肝细胞呈板状排列,从中央静脉向小叶周围呈放射状排列,肝血窦位于肝板之间也呈放射状排列。

肝细胞板由一排紧密排列的肝细胞组成。在肝小叶横切面上,肝细胞排列呈索状,称为肝索。肝血窦将肝动脉和门静脉的终末分支与中央静脉连接起来。相邻肝细胞之间存在微小管道称为胆小管。肝小叶内的肝板、肝血窦和胆小管是一个相互独立又密切相关的复杂网络。

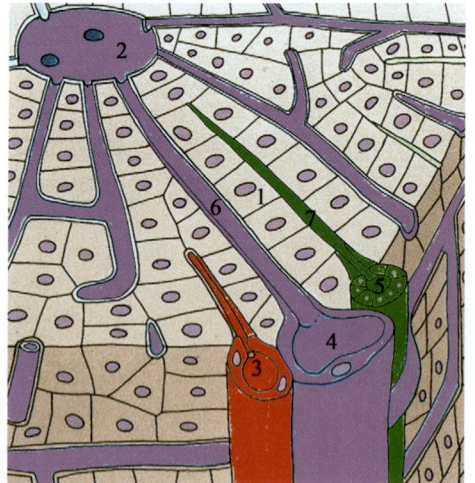

1—肝板;2—中央静脉;3—小叶间动脉;4—小叶间静脉;5—小叶间胆管;6—肝血窦;7—胆小管
图 15 - 7 肝小叶结构

（一）肝细胞

肝细胞约占肝脏细胞总数的 80%。细胞呈多边形,直径 20～30 μm。肝细胞膜有 3 个功能表面:血窦面、胆小管面和与相邻细胞接触面。在血窦面和胆小管面分布有许多微绒毛。

肝细胞的核较大,呈球形,位于细胞中央。成人肝脏内有许多双核肝细胞,且大部分肝细胞为四倍体细胞。胞质常呈嗜酸性。电镜下各种细胞器均丰富,每种细胞器都具有重要作用(图 15-8)。

肝细胞内线粒体丰富,每个肝细胞中存在 800～1 000 个线粒体,它们为细胞的代谢活动提供能量。肝细胞内有丰富的粗面内质网和滑面内质网。粗面内质网通常聚集在核周和线粒体附近,可合成许多重要的血浆蛋白,包括血浆白蛋白、纤维蛋白原、凝血酶原、脂蛋白和补体蛋白等。滑面内质网分布有多种酶系,可参与胆汁的形成、脂类和胆固醇复合物的合成、糖原的分解及血液中有毒物质的修饰和解毒。每个肝细胞中大约有 50 个高尔基复合体,常分布于核周围或胆小管附近。粗面内质网合成的部分蛋白质转运至高尔基复合体进行加工,再以囊泡分泌的方式从肝血窦面排出。分布在胆小管周围的高尔基复合体主要参与胆汁的分泌。每个肝细胞有

1—线粒体;2—粗面内质网;3—肝细胞核;
4—脂滴;5—糖原颗粒;6—胆小管

图 15-8　肝细胞电镜结构

200～300 个过氧化物酶体。过氧化物酶体含有大量的氧化酶,能产生有毒的过氧化氢,而过氧化物酶体中还存在过氧化氢酶,可将过氧化氢降解为氧气和水,从而解除过氧化氢的毒性。肝脏内的许多解毒过程都与这一反应有关,人体摄入的乙醇约一半可被肝脏过氧化物酶体中的酶转化为乙醛。肝细胞内的溶酶体丰富,功能活跃,它们在细胞成分和细胞器的更新过程以及细胞防御机制中发挥重要作用。肝细胞内还存在糖原颗粒、脂滴和色素等内含物。它们的数量取决于肝细胞的生理状态(图 15-8)。

（二）肝血窦

肝血窦填充于肝板之间的空隙内。它接收来自肝小叶周围小叶间静脉和小叶间动脉的动静脉混合血液,然后流入中央静脉。

肝血窦壁由薄层不连续内皮组成。内皮基膜不连续,有大面积缺失。内皮细胞上有较大的窗孔,相邻内皮细胞之间间隙较大。血窦内皮的通透性促进了肝脏和血液之间的物质交换(图 15-9、图 15-10)。

肝血窦与其他血窦的不同之处在于,肝血窦壁除了内皮细胞外,还存在第二种类型的细胞即库普弗细胞(Kupffer 细胞)。库普弗细胞是单核吞噬细胞系统的成员。电镜下可见库普弗细胞镶嵌于窦壁,它的突起常可横跨整个窦腔,甚至可能部分阻塞窦腔。库普弗细胞的主要功能是清除老化的红细胞,分解血红蛋白,分泌免疫相关蛋白,并清除进入门静脉的细菌。

（三）窦周隙

窦周隙,又称 Disse 隙,位于肝细胞膜和肝血窦内皮细胞之间(图 15-10)。肝细胞膜伸出

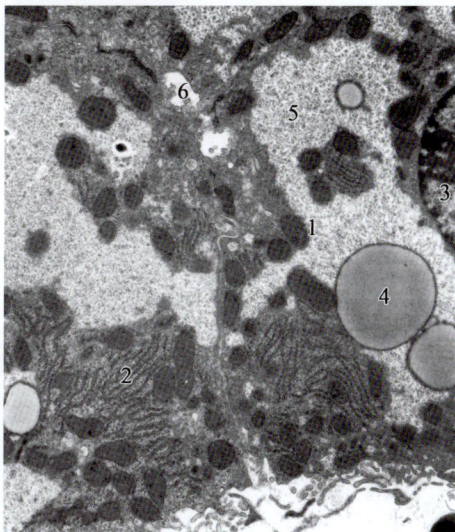

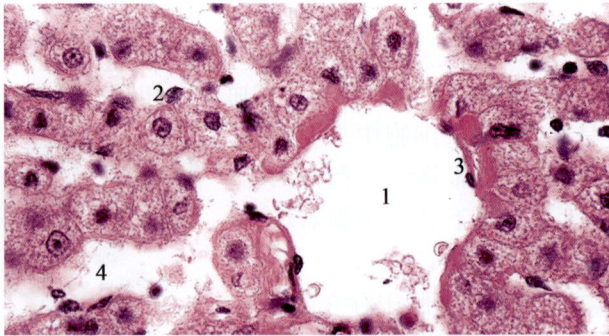

1—中央静脉;2—库普弗细胞;3—内皮细胞;4—肝血窦
图 15-9　肝血窦光镜结构

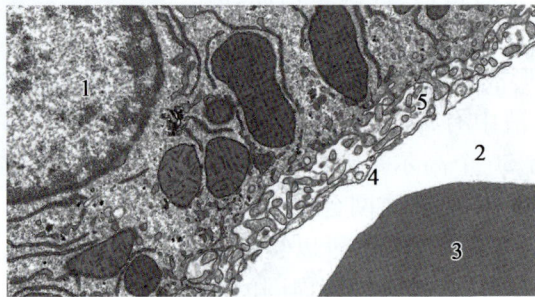

1—肝细胞核;2—肝血窦;3—红细胞;4—内皮细胞;5—窦周隙
图 15-10　肝血窦电镜结构

小而不规则的微绒毛进入窦周隙。微绒毛使肝细胞和血浆之间物质交换的表面积增加了 6 倍。血浆可较易穿出血窦内皮细胞进入窦周隙,窦周隙内充满血浆,大分子物质也能较易在肝血窦和肝细胞之间进行交换。因此,窦周隙是血液和肝细胞之间交换物质的场所。

窦周隙内存在一种星形细胞,也称为贮脂细胞或 Ito 细胞。它是肝内维生素 A 的主要储存场所,维生素 A 以视黄醇酯的形式存在于胞质内的脂滴中。在一些病理条件下,如慢性炎症或肝硬化时,贮脂细胞会丧失脂质和维生素 A 的储存能力,并分化出成纤维细胞的特征。此时贮脂细胞在肝纤维化中起着重要作用:它们可合成Ⅰ型和Ⅲ型胶原,沉积在窦周隙内导致肝纤维化。

(四) 胆小管

胆小管是肝内胆道系统的最小的分支。它们是由相邻肝细胞的细胞膜内陷形成的细胞间微小管道,其管径约为 0.5 μm(图 15-8)。胆小管与肝细胞之间的其他间隙被连接复合体(包括紧密连接和桥粒)隔离开。相邻两个肝细胞的微绒毛伸入小管腔内。肝内胆汁的流向是从肝小叶中央向周边流动。

(五) 中央静脉

中央静脉位于肝小叶中央,是肝静脉系统的末梢静脉,管壁较薄,血液来自肝血窦。中央静脉的内皮被少量螺旋状排列的结缔组织纤维所包围。它离开肝小叶后汇集入小叶下静脉。

二、门管区

肝小叶有 6 个角,每个角都有一个门管区。门管区结缔组织丰富,其内有小叶间动脉、小叶间静脉和小叶间胆管(图 15 - 7、图 15 - 11)。小叶间动脉是肝动脉的分支,其血液来自腹主动脉。小叶间静脉是门静脉的分支,包含来自肠系膜上、下静脉和脾静脉的血液。小叶间胆管则是胆管的分支,由单层立方上皮围成,其内主要为肝细胞合成的胆汁,小叶间胆管最终汇集入肝管。

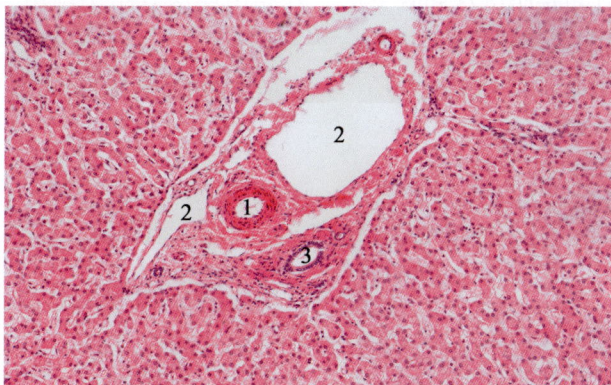

1—小叶间动脉;2—小叶间静脉;3—小叶间胆管

图 15 - 11 肝门管区

三、肝脏的血液供应

肝脏具有双重血供,血供来源包括肝门静脉和肝动脉,它们都从肝门处进入肝脏。肝脏的主要血液供应(约 75%)来自肝门静脉,静脉血氧含量低。肝门静脉输送到肝脏的血液主要来自消化管和一些重要的腹腔内器官,如胰腺和脾脏。因此门静脉血液中含有肠道吸收的营养物质和有毒物质、脾血细胞和血细胞分解产物、胰腺和胃肠道内分泌细胞分泌的激素。肝动脉则将含氧量高的血液输送到肝脏,提供其余 25% 的血液供应。

四、胆汁的形成和运输

胆红素是血红蛋白分解代谢的产物,它被肝细胞重新吸收并与葡萄糖醛酸结合,在肝血窦中形成水溶性胆红素葡萄糖醛酸。胆汁的成分主要有胆红素葡萄糖醛酸苷、胆酸、磷脂、胆固醇、水和电解质。肝细胞产生的胆汁流经胆小管、闰管和小叶间胆管,最后汇聚进入肝管。肝管与胆囊的胆囊管汇合后形成胆总管进入十二指肠。

五、肝再生

肝脏最重要的特征之一是其显著的再生能力。不管是外科手术切除或有毒物质的作用而导致的肝组织丢失,都能触发肝细胞的分裂机制,且这种分裂会一直持续到肝组织恢复至原来的重量。因此,在临床上,只需要一部分肝脏即可以用作外科手术肝脏移植的来源。

第四节 胆 囊

胆囊呈梨形,可扩张,人胆囊容积约 50 ml。它附着于肝脏的内脏面。胆囊的功能是储存和浓缩胆汁并将其释放到十二指肠。胆囊壁的结构与消化管相似,但无黏膜下层。黏膜层形成了丰富的皱褶,当胆囊排空时尤为明显。上皮为单层柱状,上皮细胞游离面微绒毛短而不发达,可分泌黏液。固有层富含有孔毛细血管和小静脉。肌层的平滑肌细胞束间有大量的胶原和弹性纤维。胆囊没有黏膜肌层及黏膜下层。外膜由厚层致密结缔组织构成,附着于肝的表面,未附着于肝的表面则被浆膜覆盖。

（张 玲 王 蕾）

Chapter 16

Respiratory System

The respiratory system consists of the paired lungs and a series of air passages including nasal cavity, pharynx, larynx, trachea and bronchi. Respiratory system has 3 principal functions: air conduction, air filtration and gas exchange (respiration). The air passage of the respiratory system consists of a conducting portion and a respiratory portion. The conducting portion consists of those air passages that lead to the sites of respiration in the lung for gas exchange, including: nasal cavity, nasopharynx, larynx, trachea, paired primary bronchi, and the bronchi and bronchioles in the lung. The bronchioles represent the terminal part of the conducting passages. Collectively, the

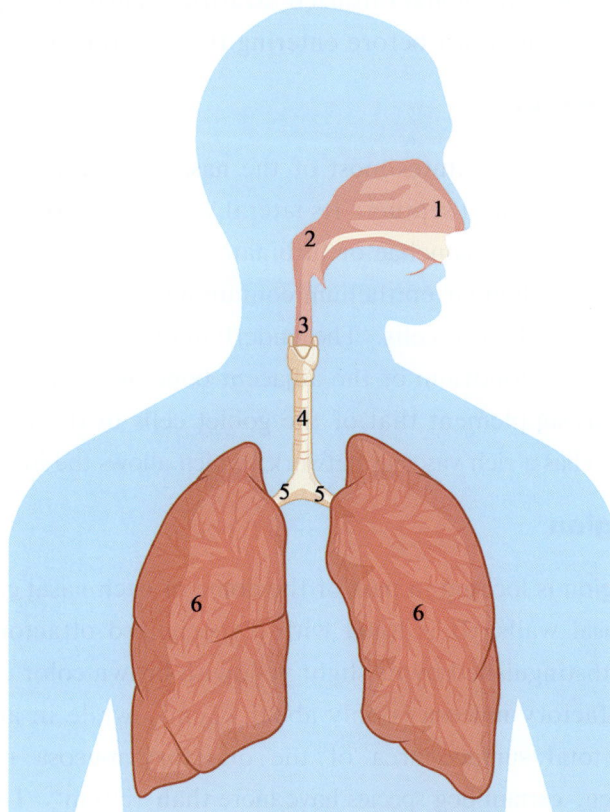

1. Nasal cavity; 2. Pharynx; 3. Larynx; 4 Trachea; 5. Primary bronchi; 6. Lung

Figure 16 - 1   Organs of respiratory system

internal bronchi and the bronchioles constitute the bronchial tree. The respiratory portion is part of the respiratory tract where gas exchange occurs. Sequentially, it includes respiratory bronchioles, alveolar ducts, alveolar sacs and alveoli.

1 Nasal Cavity

The nasal cavities are paired chambers separated by a bony and cartilaginous septum. Each cavity or chamber communicates anteriorly with the external environment through the anterior nares, posteriorly with the nasopharynx through the choanae, and laterally with the paranasal sinuses and nasolacrimal duct, which drains tears from the eye into the nasal cavity. The chambers are divided into 3 regions: nasal vestibule, respiratory region and olfactory region.

1.1 Nasal Vestibule

The nasal vestibule forms a part of the external nose and communicates anteriorly with the external environment. It is lined with stratified squamous epithelium, which is continuous to the skin of the face. Sebaceous glands are also present, and their secretions assist in the entrapment of particulate matter. Deeper in the vestibule, the keratinized epithelium transforms into the nonkeratinized stratified squamous epithelium, and then becomes respiratory epithelium just before entering the respiratory region.

1.2 Respiratory Region

The respiratory region constitutes most of the nasal cavities. The medial wall of the respiratory region is termed nasal septum. Its lateral walls are thrown into folds by 3 shelf-like and bony projections called conchae or turbinates. The respiratory region is lined by a ciliated, pseudostratified columnar epithelium containing ciliated cells, goblet cells, brush cells, small granule cells and basal cells. The underlying lamina propria is firmly attached to the periosteum and perichondrium of the adjacent bone or cartilage. It contains mucous glands. Their secretions supplement that of the goblet cells in the respiratory epithelium. The lamina propria also has a rich vascular network, which allows the inhaled air to be warmed.

1.3 Olfactory Region

The olfactory region is located in part of the dome of each nasal cavity, the contiguous lateral and medial nasal walls. It is lined with a specialized olfactory mucosa. In living tissue, this mucosa is distinguished by its slight yellowish brown color. In humans, the total surface area of the olfactory mucosa is only about $10\,cm^2$, while in animals with an acute sense of smell, the total surface area of the olfactory mucosa is considerably more extensive. For instance, certain dog species have more than $150\,cm^2$. The olfactory region is lined by pseudostratified columnar epithelium, which is composed of olfactory receptor cells, supporting or sustentacular cells and basal cells (Figure 16 - 2).

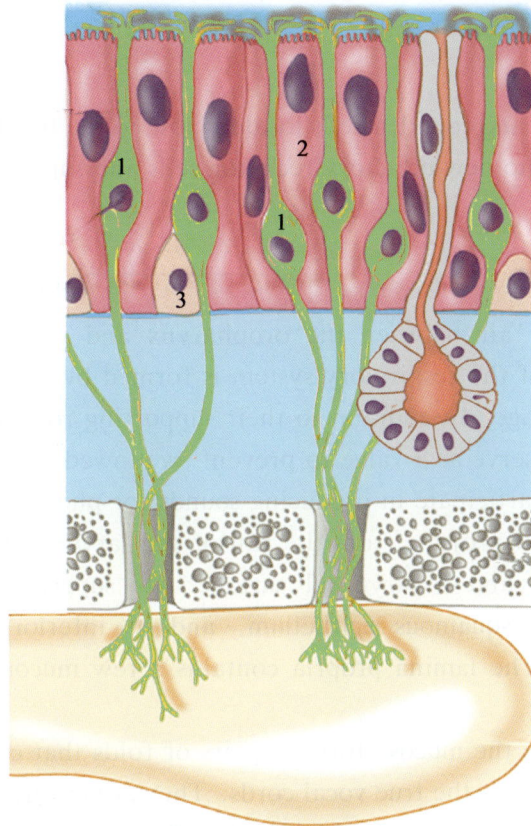

1. Olfactory receptor cell; 2. Supporting cell; 3. Basal cell

Figure 16 – 2   Olfactory mucosa of nasal cavity

1.3.1   Olfactory Receptor Cells

Olfactory receptor cells are bipolar neurons that span the thickness of the epithelium and enter the central nerve system. The apical domain of each olfactory receptor cell has a single dendritic process that projects above the epithelial surface as a knoblike structure called the olfactory vesicle. A number of long and thin cilia with typical basal bodies arise from the olfactory vesicle and extend radially in a plane parallel to the epithelial surface. These cilia are nonmotile and respond to odoriferous substances by generating a receptor potential. The basal domain of the cell gives rise to an unmyelinated axonal process that leaves the epithelial compartment. Bundles of axons from olfactory receptor cells pass through a thin cribriform plate of the ethmoid bone, and then the dura and arachnoid matters, and finally the olfactory bulb of the brain.

1.3.2   Supporting Cells

Supporting cells are the most numerous cells in the olfactory epithelium. They are columnar cells with numerous microvilli on their apical surface and abundant mitochondria. Well-developed junctional complexes bind the supporting cells to the adjacent olfactory cells. The supporting cells provide both metabolic support and physical support to the olfactory receptor cells.

1.3.3 Basal Cells

Basal cells are small and rounded cells located close to the basal lamina. They are stem cells that differentiate into new olfactory receptor cells and supporting cells.

2 Larynx

The passageway for air between the oropharynx and trachea is the larynx. This complex tubular region of the respiratory system is formed by irregularly shaped plates of hyaline and elastic cartilage. In addition to their supporting role for maintaining an open airway, these cartilages serve as a valve to prevent swallowed food or fluid from entering the trachea. They also participate in producing sounds for phonation.

The epiglottis, which projects from the rim of the larynx, extends into the pharynx and has both a lingual and a laryngeal surface. Its superior surface is covered by nonkeratinized stratified squamous epithelium, and its inferior surface is covered by respiratory epithelium. The lamina propria contains a few mucous glands and an elastic cartilage plate.

Below the epiglottis, the mucosa forms 2 pairs of folds that extend into the lumen of the larynx. The lower pair is the true vocal cords. They are covered by stratified squamous epithelium. Each contains a large elastic fiber bundle running front to back, called the vocal ligament, and a parallel skeletal muscle bundle, called the vocalis muscle. Ligaments and intrinsic laryngeal muscles join the adjacent cartilaginous plates, which are responsible for generating tension in the vocal folds, opening and closing the glottis. The upper pair of folds constitute the false vocal cords (vestibular folds). They are covered by respiratory epithelium, and numerous serous glands are observed within the lamina propria.

3 Trachea and Primary Bronchi

3.1 Trachea

The trachea is a short, flexible air tube about 2.5 cm in diameter and 10 cm in length. The trachea extends from the larynx to about the middle of the thorax, where it divides into 2 primary bronchi. The wall of the trachea consists of 3 layers: mucosa, submucosa and adventitia (Figure 16 - 3).

3.1.1 Mucosa

The mucous membrane of the trachea is composed of a ciliated pseudostratified columnar epithelium and an elastic fiber-rich lamina propria. The epithelium is composed of ciliated columnar cells, goblet cells, brush cells, basal cells and small granule cells (Figure 16 - 4).

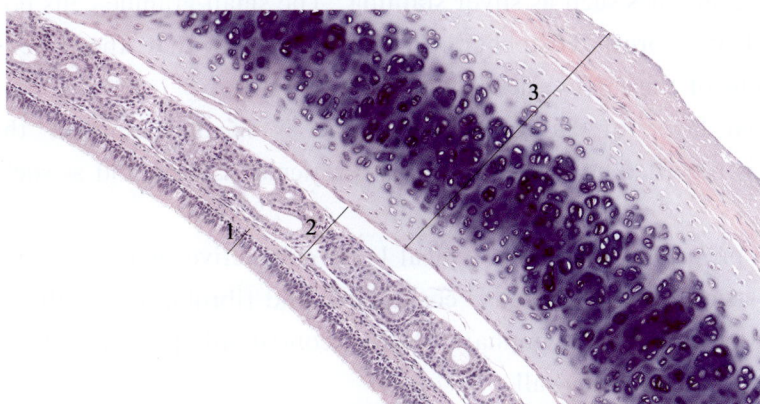

1. Mucosa; 2. Submucosa; 3. Adventitia

Figure 16 - 3   Light photomicrograph of trachea

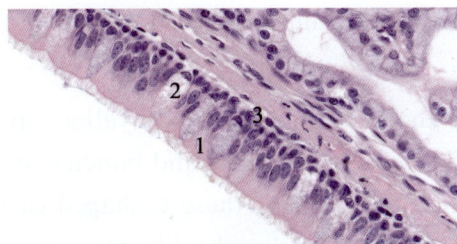

1. Ciliated columnar cell; 2. Goblet cell; 3. Basal cell

Figure 16 - 4   Light photomicrograph of trachea epithelium

Ciliated columnar cells are the most of the tracheal cell types. Cilia appear in histologic sections as short and hair-like profiles projecting from the apical surface. The cilia provide a coordinated sweeping motion of the mucous coat from the farthest reaches of the air passages toward the pharynx. So ciliated cells serve as important protective mechanism for removing small inhaled particles from the lungs.

The goblet cells are the second abundant cells in the trachea, which are similar in appearance to intestinal goblet cell. They are readily seen in the light microscope after they have accumulated mucinogen granules in their cytoplasm. They secrete the mucus that cover the epithelium, and trap and remove bacteria and other particles from inspired air.

Brush cells are columnar cells bearing blunt microvilli. The basal surface of the cells is in synaptic contact with an afferent nerve ending. Thus, the brush cells are regarded as receptor cells.

Basal cells are small round cells that lie on the basal lamina but do not reach the lumen. They serve as a reserve cell population that maintains individual cell replacement in the epithelium.

Small granule cells usually occur singly in the trachea and are sparsely dispersed among other cell types. They are difficult to distinguish from basal cells in the light microscope without special techniques such as silver staining. The small granule cells possess numerous granules with dense cores. Histochemical studies reveal that these cells constitute a population of cells of the diffuse neuroendocrine system.

A distinctive layer of basement membrane is located beneath the epithelium. Structurally, it is regarded as a thick and dense reticular lamina and as such is part of the lamina propria.

The lamina propria appears as a typical loose connective tissue. It contains numerous lymphocytes. Plasma cells, mast cells, eosinophils and fibroblasts are the other cell types readily observed in this layer. Lymphatic tissue is consistently present in the lamina propria and submucosa of the tracheal wall.

3.1.2 Submucosa

The submucosa is loose connective tissue similar in appearance to the lamina propria, which makes it difficult to determine where it begins. Submucosal glands composed of mucus-secreting acini with serous demilunes are also present in the submucosa.

3.1.3 Adventitia

The adventitia contains the C-shaped rings of hyaline cartilage, smooth muscle and fibroelastic ligament. The fibroelastic ligament and bundles of smooth muscle bind to the perichondrium and bridge the open ends of these C-shaped cartilages. Contraction of the muscle and the resultant narrowing of the tracheal lumen are used in the cough reflex. The smaller bore of the trachea after contraction provides for increased velocity of expired air, which aids in clearing the air passage.

3.2 Primary Bronchi

At the level of the sternal angle, trachea is divided into 2 primary branches: the right and left primary bronchi. Initially, the bronchi have the same general histologic structure as the trachea. At the point where the bronchi enter the lungs to become intrapulmonary bronchi, the structure of the bronchial wall changes and the bronchi decrease in size because of branching. The cartilage rings are replaced by cartilage plates of irregular shape. And the smooth muscle becomes an increasingly conspicuous layer as the amount of cartilage diminishes.

4 Lungs

The lung is covered by a serous membrane that is the visceral layer of the pleura. The structure of lungs can be divided into 2 portions: substantiality and interstitial substance. The interstitial substance consists of connective tissue, blood vessels, lymphatic vessels and nerve tissue. The substantiality of the lungs is customarily divided into 2 principal portions: a conducting portion and a respiratory portion.

On entering the hilum of the lung, the primary bronchi course downward and outward, giving rise to 3 bronchi in the right lung and 2 in the left lung, each of which supplies a pulmonary lobe. These lobar bronchi divide repeatedly, giving rise to smaller bronchi, whose terminal branches are called bronchioles. Each bronchiole enters a pulmonary lobule, where it branches to form 5 – 7 terminal bronchioles. The pulmonary lobules are pyramid-shaped with the apex directed toward the pulmonary hilum. Each lobule is delineated by a thin connective tissue septum. Terminal bronchioles are the smallest components of the conducting portion of the lungs. Respiratory bronchioles are the first region of the respiratory portion of the lung. Subsequent to several branches, each respiratory bronchiole terminates in an alveolar duct. And each of the resultant alveolar ducts usually ends as blind outpouching that is composed of 2 or more small clusters of alveoli. Each cluster is known as an alveolar sac. Alveoli are the terminal air spaces of the respiratory portion and the actual sites of gas exchange between the air and the blood (Figure 16 – 5).

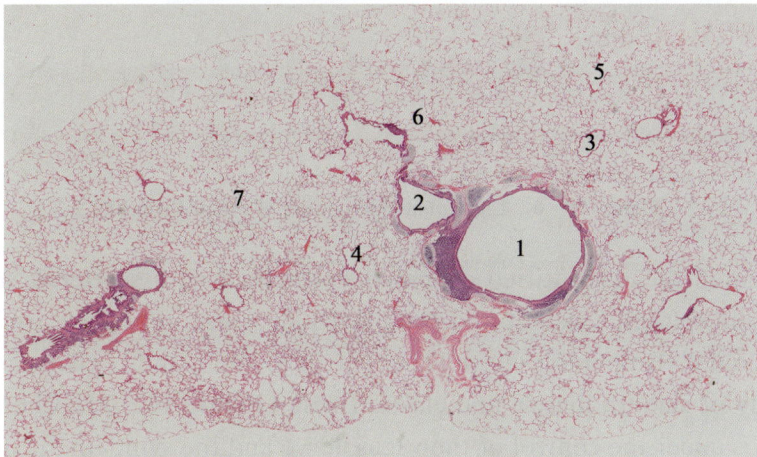

1. Small bronchi; 2. Bronchiole; 3. Terminal bronchiole; 4. Respiratory bronchiole; 5. Alveolar duct; 6. Alveolar sac; 7. Alveoli

Figure 16 – 5　Light photomicrograph of lung

4.1　Conducting Portion

4.1.1　Lobar Bronchi, Segmental Bronchi and Small Bronchi

The mucosa of the bronchi is structurally similar to the mucosa of the trachea. With the branching of the bronchi, several trends are observed, including the decrease of the height of epithelium, the number of goblet cells and glands, and the amount of cartilage plates, and the increase of smooth muscle (Figure 16 – 6).

4.1.2　Bronchioles

Bronchioles are intralobular airways with diameters of 1 mm or less. Large bronchioles

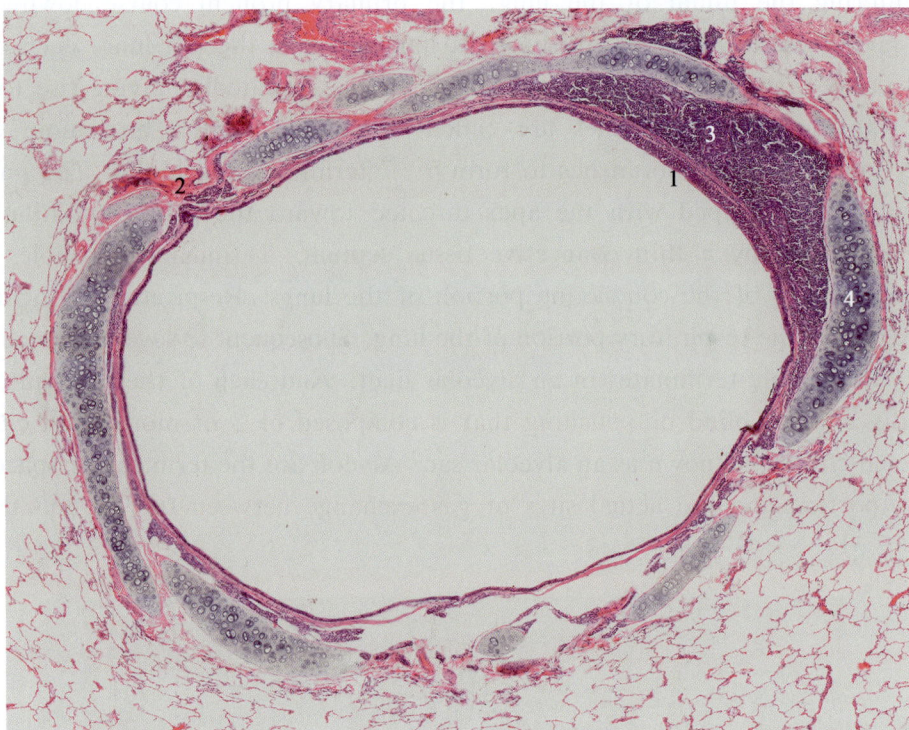

1. Pseudostratified ciliated columnar epithelium; 2. Smooth muscle; 3. Gland; 4. Cartilage plate

Figure 16 - 6　Light photomicrograph of Small Bronchi

are lined by ciliated pseudostratified columnar epithelium with scattered goblet cells. As they branch, their epithelial height and complexity decrease until they are simple ciliated columnar or cuboidal. Bronchioles have lesser cartilage and glands. Their lamina propria is composed largely of smooth muscle and elastic fibers (Figure 16 - 7). The musculature of the bronchioles is under the control of the vagus nerve and the sympathetic nervous system. Stimulation of the vagus nerve decreases the diameter of these structure while sympathetic stimulation produces the opposite effect.

4.1.3　Terminal Bronchioles

Terminal bronchioles are the smallest conducting bronchioles. They are lined with a simple cuboidal epithelium in which Clara cells are interspersed among the ciliated cells (Figure 16 - 8). Clara cells increase in number as the ciliated cells decrease along the length of the bronchiole. Clara cells are non-ciliated cells that have a characteristic rounded or dome-shaped apical surface projection. The cytoplasm contains glycogen granules, lateral and apical Golgi apparatus, elongated mitochondria and a few secretory granules. Clara cells are known to secret proteins that protect the bronchiolar lining against oxidative pollutants and inflammation. Terminal bronchioles have a moderate content of smooth muscle cells, but neither cartilage nor glands in their walls.

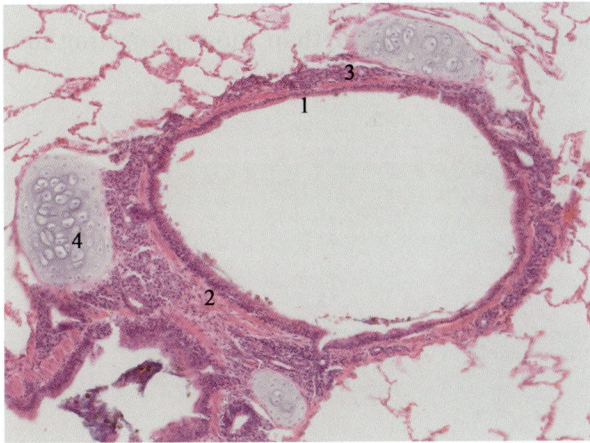

1. Simple columnar epithelium; 2. Smooth muscle;
3. Gland; 4. Cartilage plate
Figure 16 - 7   Light photomicrograph of bronchiole

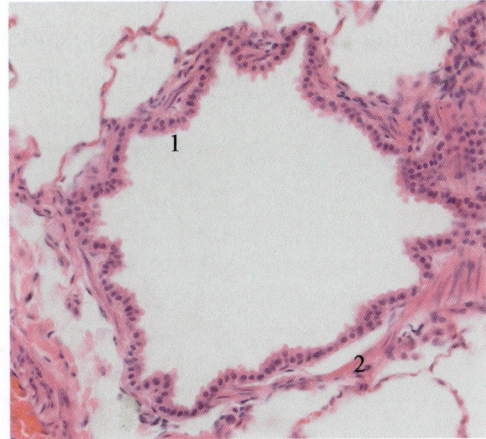

1. Simple cuboidal epithelium; 2. Smooth muscle
Figure 16 - 8   Light photomicrograph of terminal bronchiole

4.2 Respiratory Portion

4.2.1 Respiratory Bronchioles

Respiratory bronchioles serve as a transitional zone between the conducting and respiratory portions of the respiratory system. The wall of the respiratory bronchioles is interrupted by numerous saclike alveoli where gas exchange occurs. They have narrow diameter and are lined by cuboidal epithelium (Figure 16 - 9). The epithelium of the initial segments of the respiratory bronchioles contains both ciliated cells and Clara cells. Distally, Clara cells predominate. At the rim of the alveolar openings the bronchiolar epithelium becomes continuous with the squamous alveolar lining cells.

4.2.2 Alveolar Ducts

Alveolar ducts do not have walls of their own. They are merely continuous sequence of alveoli. An alveolar duct that arises from a respiratory bronchiole forms branches and each of the resultant alveolar ducts usually ends as blind outpouching composed of 2 or more small clusters of alveoli. Both the alveolar ducts and the alveoli are lined with squamous alveolar cells. A network of smooth muscle cells is in the lamina propria surrounding the rim of the alveoli. These sphincter-like smooth muscle bundles appear as knobs between adjacent alveoli (Figure 16 - 9).

4.2.3 Alveolar Sacs

Alveolar sacs are spaces surrounded by clusters of alveoli. The surrounding alveoli open into these spaces. Usually, the alveolar ducts and sacs are cut in oblique or cross-section and only the openings to the alveoli are seen, making it hard to distinguish them.

In such cases, the best clue is the size of the knobs projecting in the passageways. The projecting into alveolar sacs lack smooth muscle and are smaller than those projecting into either the alveolar ducts (Figure 16 – 9).

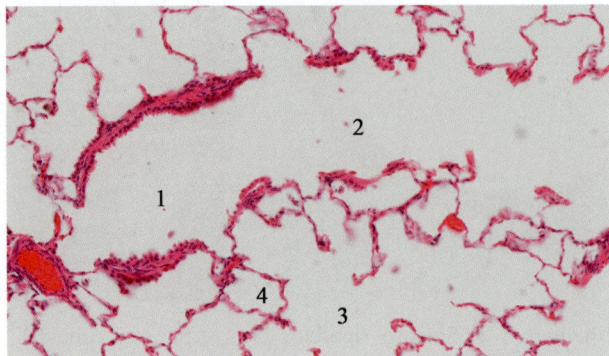

1. Respiratory bronchiole; 2. Alveolar duct; 3. Alveolar sac; 4. Alveoli

Figure 16 – 9   Light photomicrograph of respiratory portion

4.2.4　Alveoli

Alveoli are the terminal air spaces of the respiratory system and are the actual sites of gas exchange between the air and the blood. Alveoli are sac-like evaginations of the respiratory bronchioles. The diameter of an alveolus is about 200 μm. About 150 – 250 million alveoli are found in each adult lung. Their combined internal surface area is approximately 75 m^2. Alveoli are surrounded and separated from one another by an exceedingly thin connective tissue layer that contains blood capillaries. Alveoli have a continuous lining of alveoli epithelium, which is composed of 2 specialized cells: simple squamous cells (type I) and cuboidal cells (type II) (Figure 16 – 10). The tissue between adjacent alveolar air space is called the alveolar septum or septal wall.

4.2.4.1　Alveolar epithelium

Type I alveolar cells, also known as type I pneumocytes, comprise only 40% of the entire alveolar lining cells. They are extremely thin squamous cells. They line 95% of the surface of the alveoli. These cells are joined to one another and to the other cells of the alveolar epithelium by tight junctions. The junctions form an effective barrier between the air space and the components of the septal wall.

Type II alveolar cells, also called type II pneumocytes, are cuboidal and interspersed among the type I cells. Type II cells account for 60% of the alveolar lining cells. However, because of the different shape, type II cells cover only about 5% of the alveolar air surface. They are identifiable in paraffin sections of lung because the nucleus is large, ovoid to round, and light-staining, and the cytoplasm appears vacuolated or foamy. On electron microscopy, they have the appearance of secretory cells with granular reticulum, mitochondria, Golgi apparatus, apical surface microvilli and in apical cytoplasm, multi-

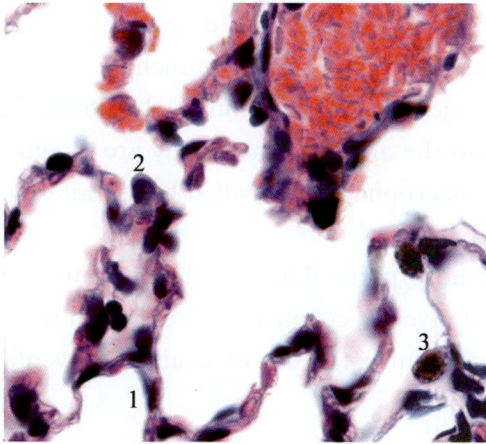

1. Type Ⅰ alveolar cell; 2. Type Ⅱ alveolar cell;
3. Dust cell

**Figure 16 – 10   Light photomicrograph of
alveoli**

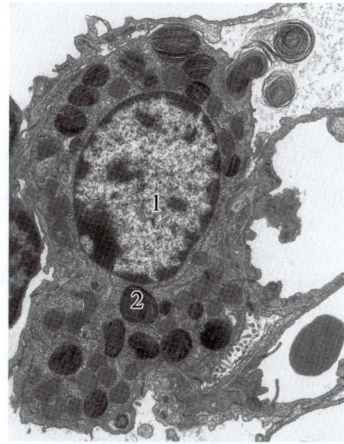

1. Nucleus; 2. Lamellar body

**Figure 16 – 11   Electron photomicrograph
of type Ⅱ alveolar cell**

lamellar bodies (Figure 16 – 11). Lamellar bodies, which average 1 – 2 μm in diameter, contain concentric or parallel lamellae limited by a unit membrane.

Histochemical studies show that these bodies, which contain phospholipids, glycosaminoglycans, and proteins, are continuously synthesized and released at the apical surface of the cells. The lamellar bodies give rise to a material that spreads over the alveolar surfaces, providing an extracellular alveolar coating, pulmonary surfactant that lowers alveolar surface tension. The reduction of surface tension means that less inspiratory force is needed to inflate the alveoli, and thus the work of breathing is reduced. In addition, without surfactant, alveoli would tend to collapse during expiration. In fetal development, surfactant appears in the last weeks of gestation and coincides with the appearance of lamellar bodies in the type Ⅱ cells. A deficiency of surfactant of the newborn can cause the respiratory distress syndrome, which is a life-threatening disorder.

4.2.4.2   Interalveolar Septa

The interalveolar septa is the sparse connective tissue around alveoli and consists of capillaries, elastic and reticular fibers. The capillaries and connective tissue constitute the interstitium, in which is found the richest capillary network in the body. The anastomosing pulmonary capillaries are supported by a meshwork of reticular and elastic fibers. These fibers are arranged to permit expansion and contraction of the interalveolar septum. Gas exchange occurs between the air in the alveolar lumen and the blood in the interstitial capillaries. The basement membrane, leukocytes, macrophages and fibroblasts can also be found within the interstitium of the septum.

Pulmonary macrophages are also called dust cells. They are found in the interior of the interalveolar septum and are often seen on the surface of the alveolus (Figure 16 – 10).

Pulmonary macrophages are derived from blood monocytes and belong to the mononuclear phagocytotic system. These cells serve as phagocytes and remove debris, such as carbon particles, from the lumen of the alveolus. They migrate up the bronchial tree and are ultimately swallowed with the mucus. In congestive heart failure, the lungs become congested with blood, and erythrocytes pass into the alveoli, where they are phagocytized by alveolar macrophages. In such cases, these macrophages are called heart failure cells.

4.2.4.3 Alveolar Pores

Each septum may be interrupted by 1 or more pores that vary from 10 to 15 μm in diameter. These alveolar pores connect adjacent alveoli, equalize air pressure in the alveoli and promote the collateral circulation. They maximize the use of available alveoli when some small airways are blocked.

4.2.4.4 Blood-Air Barrier

The blood-air barrier is the structure for the exchange of oxygen and CO_2. It is 0.2 - 0.5 μm in thickness and comprises 5 layers: ①surfactant-containing fluid produced by the type Ⅱ alveolar cells, ②the type Ⅰ alveolar cells and their basement membrane, ③a minute tissue space, ④the blood capillary basement membrane, and ⑤ the capillary endothelium. Gas exchange between the air in alveolar lumen and the blood in the capillary takes place in the blood-air barrier (Figure 16 - 12).

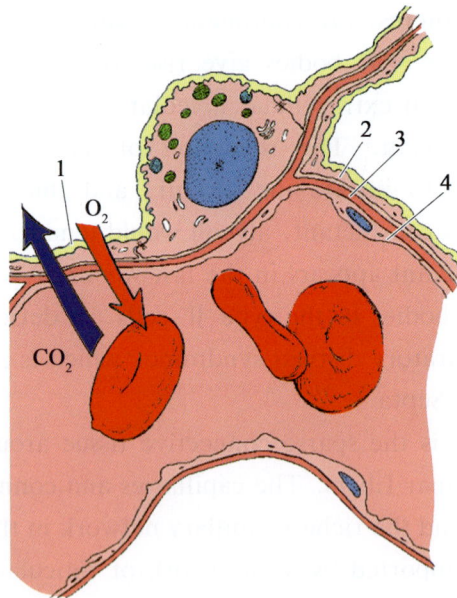

1. Surface fluid; 2. Type Ⅰ alveolar cell with basement membrane; 3. Connective tissue; 4. Capillary epithelium and basement membrane

Figure 16 - 12 Blood-air barrier

4.3 Pulmonary Blood Vessels

The lungs have a dual blood supply: the pulmonary (functional) circulation and systemic (nutrient) circulation.

The functional circulation is provided by the pulmonary arteries and veins. Pulmonary arteries arise from the heart's right ventricle as large-diameter elastic arteries. The pulmonary arteries branch and enter the lung at the pulmonary root. They follow the bronchial tree's branching pattern to carry oxygen-poor blood to the lungs' capillary beds for oxygenation. Pulmonary veins collect oxygenated blood from the lungs capillaries and return it to the heart's left atrium for distribution through the aorta and its branches.

The systemic circulation is provided by the bronchial arteries and veins. Bronchial arteries enter at the pulmonary root and follow the bronchial tree's branching pattern to the respiratory bronchial level. Branches of the bronchial arteries carry oxygen-rich blood to capillaries in the bronchi, bronchioles, interstitium and pleura. Bronchial veins are typical small veins that carry blood from the submucosal bronchial venous plexuses and accompany the bronchial tree.

(Zhang Ling, Wang Lei)

第十六章　呼 吸 系 统

　　呼吸系统由鼻、咽、喉、气管、主支气管和肺组成。呼吸系统主要有三个功能：空气传导、过滤和气体交换（呼吸）。鼻腔、鼻咽、喉、气管、主支气管、肺内支气管和细支气管组成导气部，其中终末细支气管是导气部的末端。肺内支气管和细支气管共同构成支气管树。从呼吸性细支气管、肺泡管、肺泡囊到肺泡组成呼吸部，是发生气体交换的场所。

第一节　鼻　　腔

　　鼻腔是由骨性和软骨性的鼻中隔隔开的成对腔室，前端与外界相通，后端与鼻咽后方相连，侧面与副鼻窦和鼻泪管相通，可将眼泪引流至鼻腔。鼻腔可分为鼻前庭、呼吸部和嗅部。

一、鼻前庭

　　鼻前庭是外鼻的一部分，直接与鼻腔外部相通。它内衬复层扁平上皮，与面部皮肤相连，

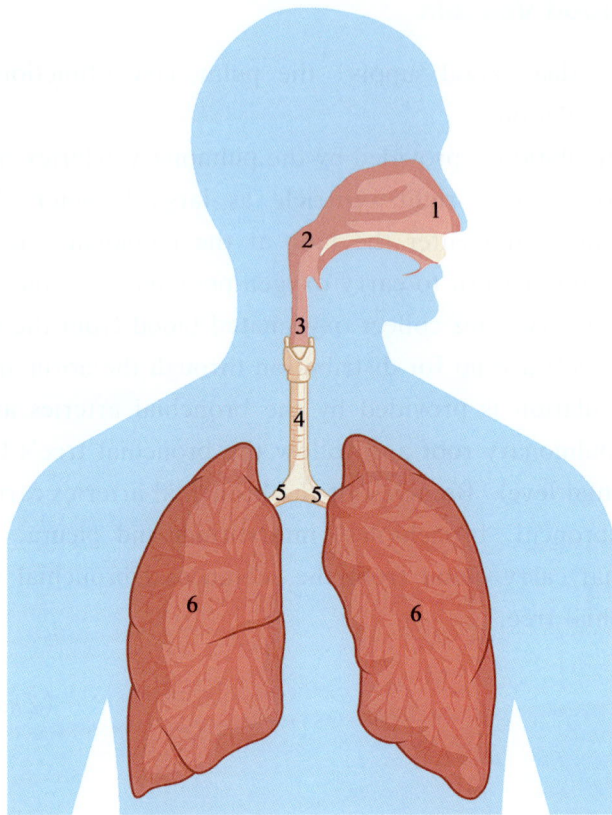

1—鼻腔;2—咽;3—喉;4—气管;5—主支气管;6—肺
图 16‐1 呼吸系统组成

可见皮脂腺,其分泌物有助于阻挡微尘颗粒。在前庭深部,与呼吸部相邻的上皮组织由角化演变为非角化的复层扁平上皮。

二、呼吸部

呼吸部占鼻腔容积的大部分。呼吸部的内侧壁为鼻中隔。它的外侧壁称为鼻甲,鼻甲由三个骨性折叠突起组成。呼吸部表面覆盖假复层纤毛柱状上皮,上皮由纤毛细胞、杯状细胞、刷细胞、小颗粒细胞和基细胞组成。上皮下方的固有层牢固地附着在邻近骨或软骨的骨膜和软骨膜上,固有层内有黏液腺,其分泌物与杯状细胞的分泌物共同形成一层黏液覆盖于上皮表面。固有层内血管丰富,可升高吸入空气的温度。

三、嗅部

嗅部位于鼻腔顶部及相邻的鼻腔外侧和内侧壁。它内衬一层特殊的嗅觉黏膜,在活体组织中呈浅黄棕色。人类嗅黏膜的表面积只有 $10\,cm^2$ 左右,而在嗅觉敏锐的动物中,嗅黏膜的表面积大得多,如狗的嗅黏膜面积可超过 $150\,cm^2$。嗅部表面覆盖假复层柱状上皮,由嗅细胞、支持细胞和基细胞组成(图 16‐2)。

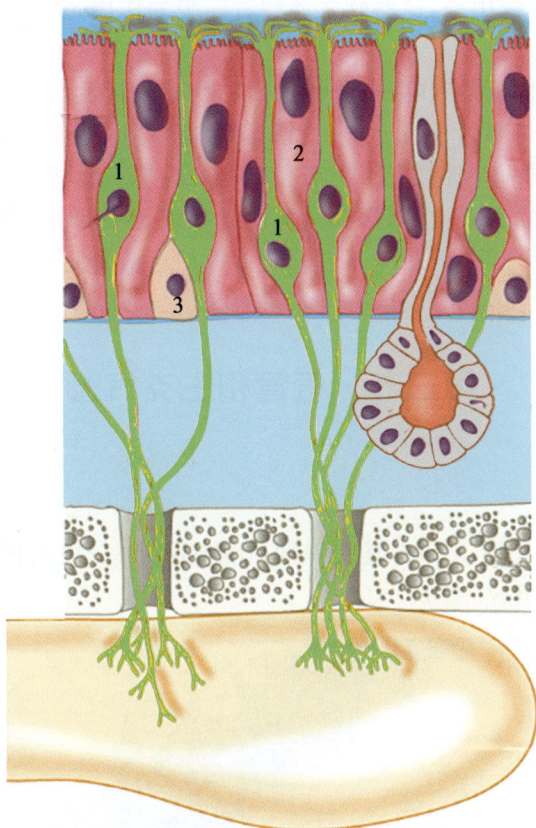

1—嗅细胞；2—支持细胞；3—基细胞
图 16-2　鼻腔嗅黏膜

（一）嗅细胞

嗅细胞是双极神经元，穿越嗅上皮进入中枢神经系统。嗅细胞的树突伸出嗅上皮表面，末端膨大形成球状结构，称嗅泡。从嗅泡伸出许多细长纤毛，称为嗅毛，这些纤毛不能摆动，它们能够接收气味的化学刺激。从嗅细胞的基部发出一根无髓鞘的轴突，离开嗅上皮。多个嗅细胞的轴突集合成束，穿过筛骨的筛板，硬脑膜和蛛网膜，最后被软脑膜包围，进入大脑的嗅球。

（二）支持细胞

支持细胞是嗅上皮中数量最多的细胞。细胞呈柱状，游离面有大量微绒毛，线粒体丰富。发达的连接复合体将支持细胞与邻近的嗅细胞紧密连接。支持细胞可为嗅细胞提供支持、分隔和代谢作用。

（三）基细胞

基细胞位于基膜上，细胞小而圆，是干细胞，可分化为嗅细胞和支持细胞。

第二节　喉

喉位于口咽和气管之间，是一个复杂的管腔性器官，由不规则的透明和弹性软骨板构成。

除了维持气道开放的支持作用外,这些软骨还起着瓣膜的作用,防止吞咽的食物或液体进入气管,并且也参与发声。

会厌从喉部边缘突出,延伸到咽部,分为舌面和喉面。其舌面及喉面上部的黏膜上皮为未角化复层扁平上皮,喉面基部为呼吸上皮。固有层含有少量黏液腺和弹性软骨板。

会厌下方的黏膜形成两对皱襞突出于喉腔。上一对是室襞(假声带),下一对是声襞(真声带)。声襞表面覆盖复层扁平上皮,内含大量弹性纤维束和平行排列的骨骼肌束,前者为声带韧带,后者为声带肌。韧带和声带肌与邻近的软骨板相连从而使声带产生张力,并负责开关声门。室襞表面覆盖呼吸上皮,固有层内有许多浆液腺。

第三节　气管和主支气管

一、气管

气管直径约 2.5 cm,长约 10 cm,具有弹性,在胸腔中部分成两根主支气管。气管壁由黏膜、黏膜下层和外膜三层组成(图 16-3)。

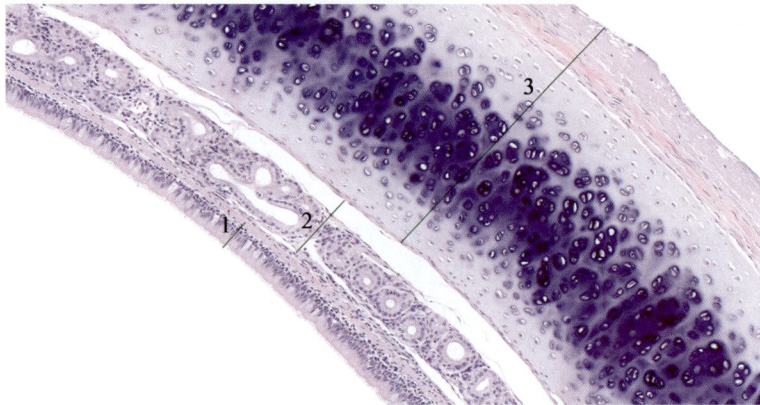

1—黏膜;2—黏膜下层;3—外膜
图 16-3　气管光镜结构

(一) 黏膜

气管黏膜由假复层纤毛柱状上皮和富含弹性纤维的固有层组成。上皮由纤毛柱状细胞、杯状细胞、刷细胞、基细胞和小颗粒细胞组成(图 16-4)。

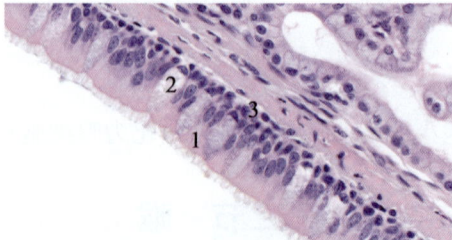

1—纤毛柱状细胞;2—杯状细胞;3—基细胞
图 16-4　气管上皮光镜结构

1. 纤毛柱状细胞

数量最多,纤毛呈短毛发状,位于细胞游离面。纤毛可将黏膜表面的黏液及其黏附的灰尘细菌等扫向喉部。因此,纤毛细胞是清除肺部吸入性微粒的重要保护因素。

2. 杯状细胞

气管内数量第二的细胞,其形态与肠杯状细胞相似。它们的胞质中含有大量黏原颗粒,因此光镜下易见。杯状细胞分泌的黏液覆盖在上皮表面,捕获并清除吸入空气中的细菌和其他颗粒。

3. 刷细胞

呈柱状,表面分布有微绒毛。细胞的基底面与传入神经纤维末端形成突触。因此刷状细胞被认为是受体细胞。

4. 基细胞

位于基膜上,细胞小,呈圆形。它们是干细胞,可增殖分化为上皮中的其他细胞类型。

5. 小颗粒细胞

数量少,散在分布在其他细胞之间。光镜下难以与其他细胞区分,只有用银染等特殊技术才能显色。小颗粒细胞有很多颗粒。组织化学染色提示,小颗粒细胞是弥散神经内分泌系统的成员。

上皮基底部为基膜。从结构特征来看,这层基膜具有非常厚而致密的网状层,因此通常认为它是固有层的一部分。

固有层为典型的疏松结缔组织,含有大量淋巴细胞。在该层也经常能看到浆细胞、肥大细胞、嗜酸性粒细胞和成纤维细胞。淋巴组织则始终存在于固有层和黏膜下层。

(二)黏膜下层

黏膜下层为疏松结缔组织,结构与固有层类似,因此两者无明显界限,不易区分。黏膜下层的腺体为混合性腺,即黏液性腺泡一侧覆盖有浆半月。

(三)外膜

外膜主要由C形的透明软骨环构成,还含有平滑肌和弹性纤维。C形缺口部位由纤维韧带、平滑肌束与软骨膜连接所封闭。咳嗽反射时,肌组织收缩引起气管腔变小,使呼出空气流速加快,有助于清理气道。

二、主支气管

气管在胸骨角水平分为两支,即左右主支气管。主支气管起始段组织结构与气管相同。当支气管进入肺成为肺内支气管时,支气管壁结构开始发生改变,支气管管径因分支开始减小。软骨环被不规则形状的软骨片代替。随着软骨片数量的减少,平滑肌变得越来越多。

第四节 肺

肺表面覆盖浆膜,为胸膜脏层,可分为实质和间质两部分。间质由结缔组织、血管、淋巴管和神经组织组成。肺实质通常包含两个主要成分:导气部和呼吸部。

主支气管进入肺门后在右肺分为3支,左肺分为2支,每根支气管供应一个肺叶。这些肺叶支气管反复分支,形成肺段支气管和小支气管。小支气管末端分支为细支气管,每个细支气管进入一个肺小叶,并继续分支形成5～7个终末细支气管。肺小叶呈金字塔形,尖端朝向肺门,外周被薄层结缔组织包裹。终末细支气管是肺内导气部最小的组成部分。从呼吸性细支气管开始进入肺呼吸部,在数次分支之后,呼吸性细支气管分支为肺泡管,后者通常开口于肺泡囊。肺泡囊由肺泡围成,肺泡是肺呼吸部的最末端成分,是空气和血液之间气体交换的实际场所(图16-5)。

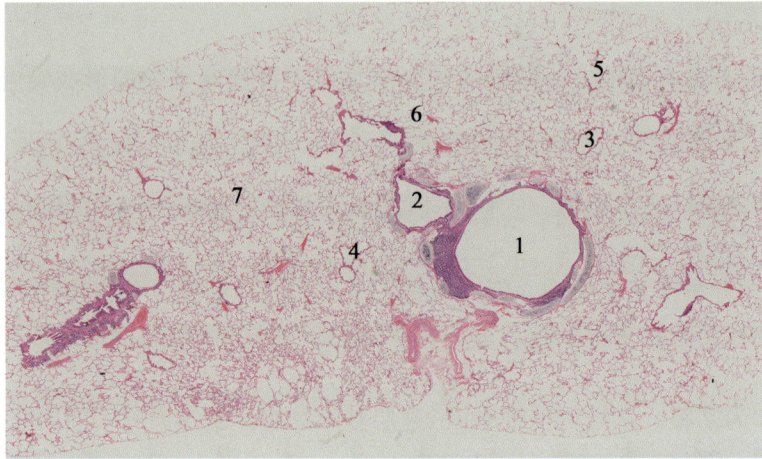

1—小支气管;2—细支气管;3—终末细支气管;4—呼吸性细支气管;5—肺泡管;6—肺泡囊;7—肺泡

图16-5 肺光镜结构

一、导气部

(一) 叶支气管、段支气管和小支气管

这几段支气管的黏膜层结构上与气管黏膜相似。但随着支气管分支,上皮高度降低,杯状细胞和腺体数量减少,软骨片数量减少,平滑肌增多(图16-6)。

(二) 细支气管

细支气管直径等于或小于1 mm。较大的细支气管上皮为假复层纤毛柱状上皮,杯状细胞散在分布。随着它们不断分支,其上皮高度降低,细胞种类减少,最终形成单层纤毛柱状或立方上皮。细支气管的软骨片和腺体较少,其固有层主要由平滑肌和弹性纤维组成(图16-7)。细支气管壁内的肌组织受迷走神经和交感神经系统的调控。刺激迷走神经可使管径减小,而刺激交感神经则扩张管腔。

(三) 终末细支气管

终末细支气管是导气部的终末部,也是最细的分支,管壁被单层立方上皮所覆盖,上皮以纤毛细胞为主,可见克拉拉细胞散布其间(图16-8)。随着终末细支气管的延伸,克拉拉细胞的数量逐渐增加。克拉拉细胞无纤毛,游离面具有特征性的圆形或穹顶状隆起,胞质内含有糖原颗粒、高尔基复合体、线粒体和少量的分泌颗粒。克拉拉细胞能分泌蛋白质,保护支气管壁免受氧化污染物和炎症的影响。终末细支气管有完整的平滑肌,没有软骨片和腺体。

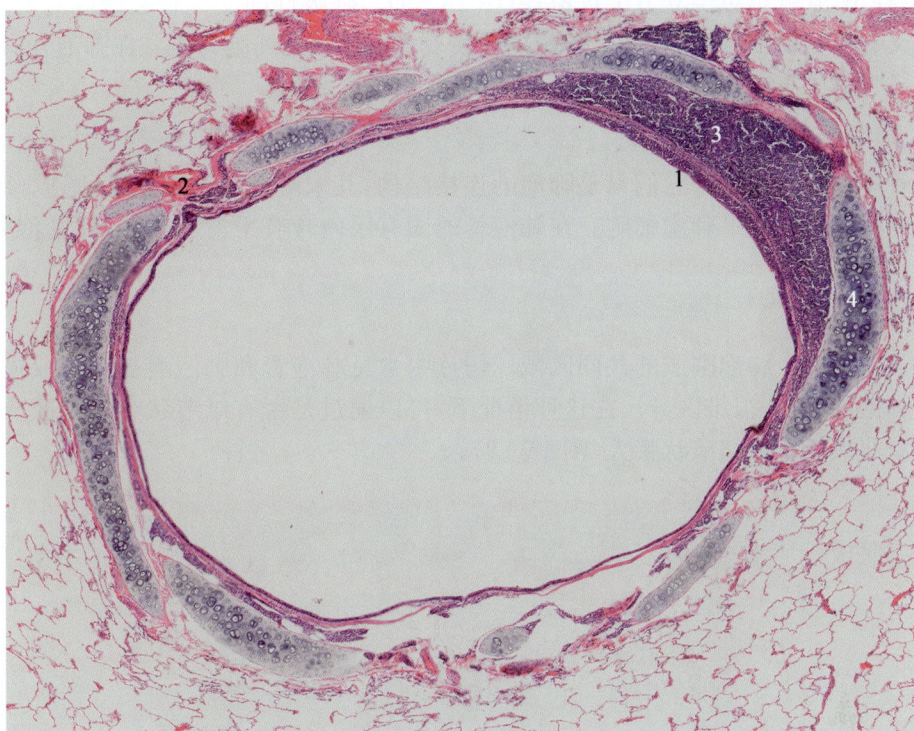

1—假复层纤毛柱状上皮；2—平滑肌；3—黏膜下腺；4—透明软骨片

图 16-6　肺小支气管光镜结构

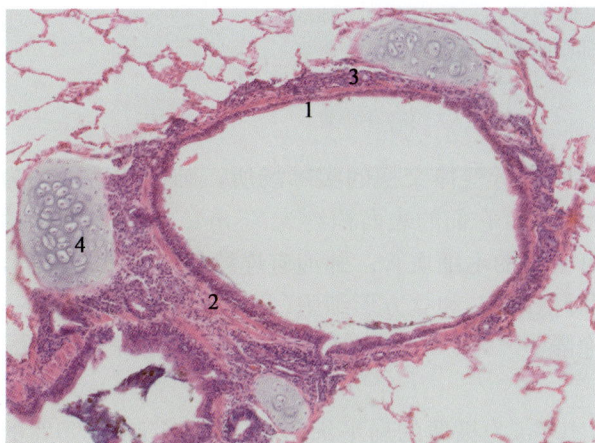

1—纤毛柱状细胞；2—平滑肌；3—黏膜下腺；4—透明软骨片

图 16-7　肺细支气管光镜结构

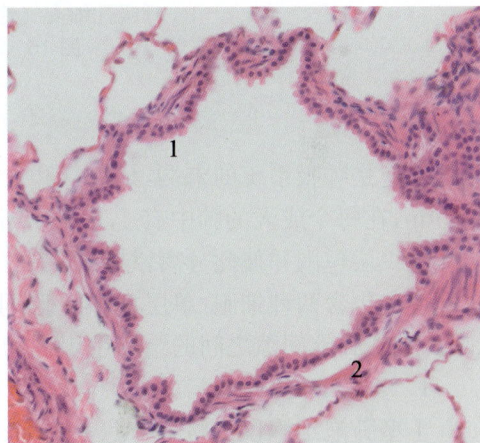

1—单层立方上皮；2—平滑肌

图 16-8　肺终末细支气管光镜结构

二、呼吸部

(一) 呼吸性细支气管

呼吸性细支气管是呼吸系统导气部和呼吸部之间的过渡结构，管壁有肺泡开口，可进行气体交换,管径小,管壁由单层立方上皮覆盖(图 16 - 9)。呼吸性细支气管起始段的上皮中既有纤毛细胞又有克拉拉细胞,随着支气管的延伸演变为以克拉拉细胞为主。在肺泡开口的边缘,呼吸性细支气管的上皮与肺泡的肺泡上皮相延续。

(二)肺泡管

肺泡管本身没有管壁。它们只是肺泡的连接结构,其末端通常与肺泡囊相连。肺泡管和肺泡壁都衬有极薄的扁平肺泡细胞。在肺泡管的固有层内含有平滑肌成分,使肺泡管呈现结节状突起(图 16 - 9)。

(三)肺泡囊

肺泡囊是由多个肺泡围成的共同区域。切片中常见肺泡管和肺泡囊被斜切或横切,因此只能看到肺泡的开口,很难区分。在这种情况下,可以通过是否有结节状突起来区分两者,肺泡囊无平滑肌故不形成结节状膨大(图 16 - 9)。

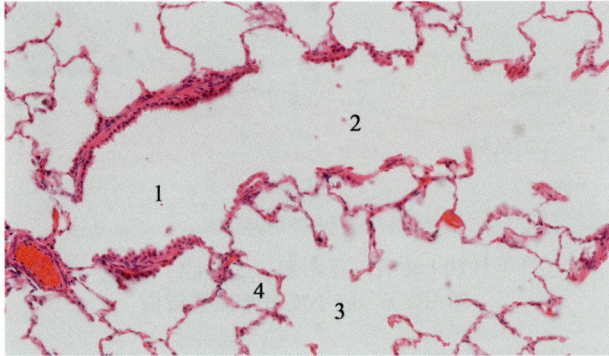

1—呼吸性细支气管;2—肺泡管;3—肺泡囊;4—肺泡
图 16 - 9　肺呼吸部光镜结构

(四)肺泡

肺泡是呼吸系统的末端,是空气和血液之间进行气体交换的实际场所。肺泡的直径约为 $200\,\mu m$,在每个成人的肺中有 1.5～2.5 亿个肺泡。它们的表面积约为 $75\ m^2$。肺泡被超薄的结缔组织层包围并彼此分离,结缔组织内含有丰富的毛细血管。肺泡有连续的肺泡上皮覆盖,肺泡上皮包含两种细胞:单层扁平细胞(Ⅰ型肺泡细胞)和立方形细胞(Ⅱ型肺泡细胞)(图 16 - 10)。相邻肺泡间隙之间的结缔组织称为肺泡隔。

1. 肺泡上皮

Ⅰ型肺泡细胞仅占整个肺泡上皮细胞的 40%,为极薄的扁平细胞,占据整个肺泡 95% 的表面积。这些细胞彼此相连,并通过紧密连接与肺泡上皮的其他细胞相连,紧密连接在肺泡和肺泡隔之间形成屏障结构。

Ⅱ型肺泡细胞呈立方形,散布在Ⅰ型肺泡细胞之间。Ⅱ型肺泡细胞占肺泡上皮细胞的 60%,但是仅占肺泡表面积的 5%。细胞核较大,卵圆形或圆形,染色浅,细胞质呈空泡状或泡沫状,因此石蜡切片中可见。电镜下呈现分泌细胞的特点,细胞游离面可见微绒毛,胞质内有分泌颗粒、线粒体、高尔基复合体,顶部胞质内见板层小体(图 16 - 11)。板层小体直径为 1～ $2\,\mu m$,包含同心圆或平行排列的板层状结构。组织化学染色显示其含有磷脂、糖胺聚糖和蛋

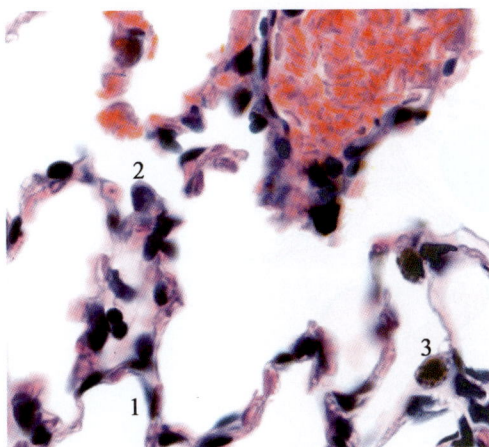

1—Ⅰ型肺泡细胞；2—Ⅱ型肺泡细胞；3—尘细胞
图 16‐10 肺泡光镜结构

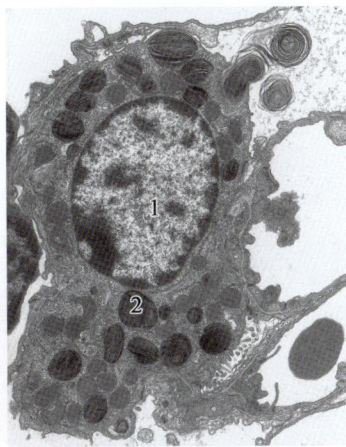

1—细胞核；2—板层小体
图 16‐11 Ⅱ型肺泡细胞电镜结构

白质，合成后释放于细胞表面。板层小体产生的这种物质能够降低肺泡表面张力，被称为肺泡表面活性物质，它能防止肺泡过度扩张或塌陷。在胎儿发育过程中，Ⅱ型肺泡细胞在妊娠的最后几周才会发育成熟形成板层小体分泌肺泡表面活性物质。因此早产儿常因缺乏肺泡表面活性物质导致呼吸窘迫综合征，可能导致夭折。

2. 肺泡隔

肺泡周围的薄层结缔组织，由毛细血管、弹性纤维和网状纤维组成。间质内毛细血管网最为丰富。肺毛细血管由网状纤维和弹性纤维网包裹，这些纤维有助于肺泡隔的扩张和收缩。气体交换在肺泡腔中的空气和间质毛细血管中的血液之间进行。间质内还可见基膜、白细胞、巨噬细胞和成纤维细胞。

肺巨噬细胞也被称为尘细胞，可见于肺泡隔，常见于肺泡表面（图 16‐10）。肺巨噬细胞来源于血液的单核细胞，属于单核吞噬细胞系统。它们具有吞噬功能，能清除肺泡腔内的尘粒，还可沿着支气管树向上迁移，最终与黏液一起被吞噬。充血性心力衰竭时，肺部充血，红细胞进入肺泡，被肺巨噬细胞吞噬形成心衰细胞。

3. 肺泡孔

隔膜上有肺泡孔，直径为 $10\sim15\ \mu m$。这些肺泡孔连接肺泡，平衡相邻肺泡内的气压。当一些小气道阻塞，他们可最大限度地利用所有可用的肺泡。

4. 气‐血屏障

指 O_2 和 CO_2 进行交换必须通过的结构。厚度从 $0.2\sim0.5\ \mu m$ 不等，包括 5 层：①肺泡表面含表面活性物质的液体层；②Ⅰ型肺泡细胞及其基膜；③薄层结缔组织；④毛细血管基膜；⑤毛细血管内皮。在气‐血屏障处，肺泡腔中的空气与毛细血管内的血液发生气体交换（图 16‐12）。

三、肺的血液循环

肺有双重血液供应：肺（功能性）循环和体（营养性）循环。

1. 肺循环

血液来源于肺动脉。肺动脉起源于心脏的右心室，是直径较大的弹性动脉。肺动脉分支

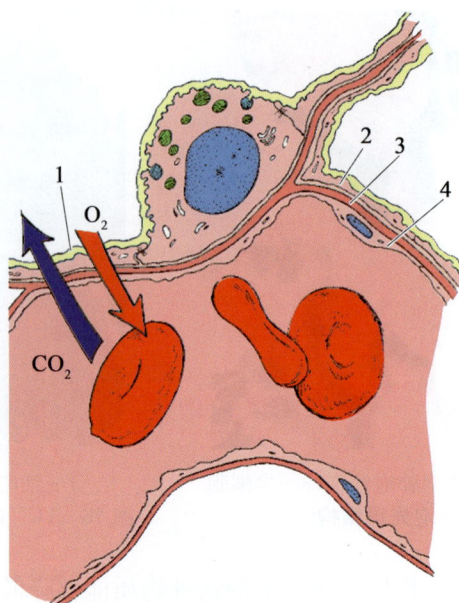

1—液体层;2—Ⅰ型肺泡细胞及基膜;3—薄层结缔组织;4—毛细血管内皮细胞及基膜

图 16 - 12　肺气血屏障

从肺门部进入肺,沿着支气管树的分支,将含氧量低的血液输送到肺部的毛细血管。而肺静脉则收集肺毛细血管内含氧量高的血液并返回心脏左心房,通过主动脉及其分支将血液输送全身。

2. 体循环

血液来源于支气管动脉。支气管动脉从肺门部进入,沿着支气管树的分支走行。支气管动脉的分支将富含氧气的血液输送到支气管、细支气管管壁及间质和胸膜内的毛细血管。支气管静脉是典型的小静脉,通过伴随支气管树分布的黏膜下支气管静脉丛回流血液。

（张　玲　王　蕾）

Chapter 17

Urinary System

The urinary system consists of the paired kidneys, the ureters, the unpaired bladder, and the urethra. Its major function is to maintain the homeostasis of water, electrolytes and acid-base balance by regulating the production of urine. Additionally, multiple bioactive substances including renin, erythropoietin, prostaglandin that are produced in the kidneys play important roles in regulating the physiological function of the body.

1　Kidneys

The renal parenchyma consists of the cortex and the medulla. The outer cortex is dark red, composed of the medullary ray and the cortical labyrinth. Each medullary ray plus the surrounding cortical labyrinth constitutes a renal lobe. The inner medullar is a lighter region that consists of 10 − 18 renal pyramids. The bottom of the pyramids connects with the cortex, and the tip stretches into the minor calyx that collects urine, called the renal papilla. Each renal pyramid plus surrounding cortex constitutes the renal lobe. The cortex between the renal pyramid is called the renal column (Figure 17 − 1).

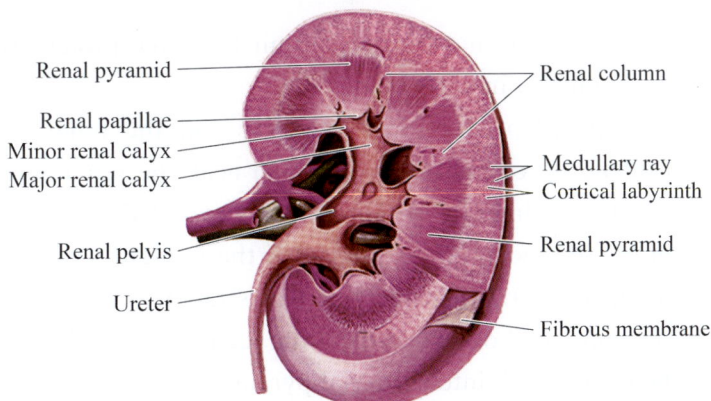

Figure 17 − 1　Diagram of coronal kidney

The renal medulla consists of the nephron and the collecting duct with a few connective tissue, blood vessels and nerves. Each nephron consists of a renal corpuscle and a renal tubule connecting the corpuscle, constituting the structural and functional unit for urine production. Renal tubules will converge in the collecting duct, which are all single-layered epithelial ducts, called the urinary tracts. The distribution of the nephron and the collecting duct in the renal parenchyma is regular. The convoluted parts of the renal corpuscle and the renal tubule are located in the cortical labyrinth and the renal column. The straight part of the renal tubules and the collect ducts are located in the medullary ray and the renal pyramid (Figure 17 - 2).

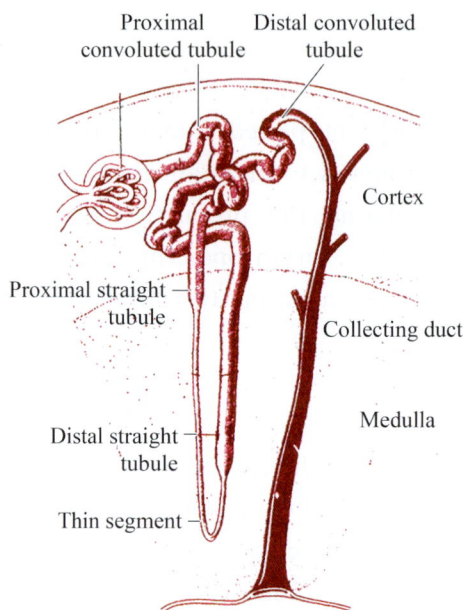

Figure 17 - 2　Diagram of nephron and collecting duct

1.1　Nephron

The nephron is the structural and functional unit for urine production and excretion. There are 1 - 2 million nephrons in each kidney.

The nephron is composed of the renal corpuscle and the renal tubule. The initial segment of the renal tubule is convoluted and located near the renal corpuscle, called the convoluted segment of the proximal tubule (proximal convoluted tubule). The straight part of the renal tubule enters the medulla, and is called the straight segment of the proximal tubule (proximal straight tubule). Then the proximal straight tubule suddenly narrows and continues as the thin segment. Following the thin segment, the diameter of the tubule suddenly increases and comes back into the renal pyramid and the medullary ray, called the straight segment of the distal tubule (distal straight tubule). The proximal straight tubule, the thin segment and the distal straight tubule constitute a U-shaped structure, called the loop of Henle. The segment of the loop of Henle that descends from the cortex to the medulla is called the descending limb, and the segment that ascends from the medulla to the cortex is called the ascending limb. The loops are different in the length, the longer ones can reach the renal papilla, and the shorter ones are only present in the medullary ray. The distal straight tubule will convolute near the renal corpuscle in the cortex when leaves the medullary ray, called the convoluted segment of the distal tubule (distal convoluted tubule), and finally enters the collecting ducts (Table 17 - 1).

Table 17 - 1　Component of Kidney

Nephron
- Renal corpuscle
  - Glomerulus (Cortical labyrinth, Renal column)
  - Renal capsule
- Renal tubule
  - Proximal tubule
    - Proximal convoluted tubule (Cortical labyrinth, Renal column)
    - Proximal straight tubule
  - Thin segment — Loop of Henle (Medullary ray, Renal pyramid)
  - Distal tubule
    - Distal straight tubule
    - Distal convoluted tubule (Cortical labyrinth, Renal column)

Urinary tubule
- Collecting duct
  - Arcuate renal tubule (Cortical labyrinth)
  - Straight collecting tubule (Medullary ray, Renal pyramid)
  - Paillary duct (Renal papilla)

Depending on the location of the renal corpuscle in the cortex, the nephron can be classified as the cortical nephron and the juxtamedullary nephron. The majority of the nephron (85% of the total) is the cortical nephron. Their renal corpuscles are located in the middle and superficial layer of the cortex. The renal corpuscles are small, the loop of Henle and the thin segment are both short. The cortical nephron plays an important role in the production of urine. The juxtamedullary nephron is less (15% of the total). Their renal corpuscles are larger and located near the medulla. The loop of Henle and the thin segment are longer. The juxtamedullary nephron is critical to the urine concentration.

1.1.1　Renal Corpuscle

The renal corpuscle is spherical, about 200 μm in diameter, and consists of the glomerulus and the glomerular (Bowman) capsule. The renal corpuscle has 2 poles. The side where the arteriole enters and leaves is called the vascular pole. The other side, where the renal corpuscle connects with the proximal convoluted, is called the tubular pole (Figure 17 - 3).

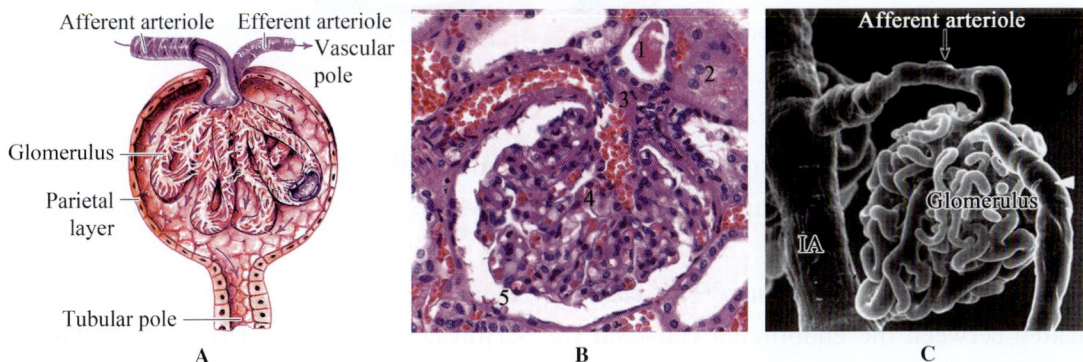

Figure 17 - 3　Renal corpuscle
A. Diagram of renal corpuscle; B. LM of renal corpuscle; C. SEM of renal corpuscle

1.1.1.1　Glomerulus

The glomerulus is a spherical tuft of capillaries between the afferent arteriole and the efferent arteriole (Figure 17 - 4). A thicker afferent arteriole enters from the vascular pole into the renal capsule, forms 4 - 5 branches, then each branch forms many capillaries that match with each other. The gap among capillaries is filled with the mesangium. These capillaries eventually converge into a thinner efferent arteriole that leaves the glomerular (Bowman) capsule from the vascular pole. Because the afferent arteriole is thicker than the efferent arteriole, the blood pressure in the glomerulus is higher than the normal capillaries. When the blood flows through the glomerulus, a large amount of water and small molecules will be filtered out from the capillary and move into the renal capsule. Moreover, the negatively charged glycoprotein (cell coat) with enriched sialic acid on the lumen surface of the endothelial cell can selectively filter out the substances in the blood.

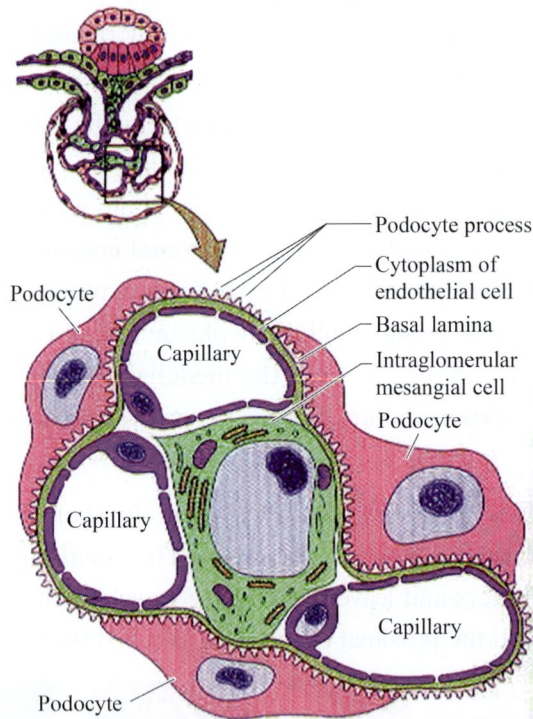

Figure 17 - 4　Glomerulus

Under the electron microscope, the glomerular capillaries are finely fenestrated (50 - 100 nm in diameter, no diaphragm) for filtering out substances in the blood. There is basement membrane on the basal surface of the endothelium except for the place that contacts with the mesangium. The basement membrane is thick (about 330 nm), and located between the endothelial cells and the Sertoli cells or between the mesangium and the Sertoli cells. There is no basement membrane between the endothelial cells and the mesangial cells. Under the light microscope, the basement membrane is homogeneous, and

PAS positive. Under the electron microscope, the basement membrane consists of 3 layers with thick and dense middle layer, while the other 2 layers are thin and loose.

The basement membrane mainly contains type IV collagen, proteoglycan and laminin, forming a molecular sieve with type IV collagen as the skeleton. The negatively charged heparan sulfate is attached to the skeleton, which can prevent the passage of negatively charged substances, so the basement membrane has selective permeability to macromolecules in the filtrate.

The mesangium is composed of the mesangial cells and the mesangial matrix, which is distributed between the capillaries. The mesangial cells are star-like in shape, and have protrusions that can stretch into the place between the endothelium and the basement membrane, or into the capillaries from the endothelial cells. Their nuclei are small and often darkly stained. Developed rough endoplasmic reticulum, Golgi complex, lysosomes, phagocytic vesicles can be observed in the mesangial cells. Sometimes a few secretory granules are also visible. There are microtubules, microfilaments and intermediate filaments in the cell body and the protrusion.

The mesangial cells can synthesize substances forming the basement membrane and the mesangial matrix, phagocytize and degrade the immune complex deposited on the basement membrane so as to maintain its permeability, and also participate in the renewal and repair of the basement membrane. The contractile property of the mesangial cells can affect the blood flow in the glomerulus by regulating the diameter of the capillaries. The mesangial cells can also secret bioactive substances including renin and enzymes, which may be related to the regulation of blood flow in the glomerulus. The mesangial matrix fills among the mesangial cells, with the effects of supporting and transparency in the glomerulus. There are also a few macrophages in the mesangium.

1.1.1.2 Glomerular (Bowman) Capsule

The glomerular capsule is a double-walled epithelial capsule formed by the swelling and depression of the beginning part of the renal tubule. It is a cup-like sac and composed of the parietal layer and the visceral layer. The space between these 2 layers is named the capsular space, which connects with the lumen of the proximal convoluted tubule (Figure 17 - 5).

The outer layer (parietal layer) is a simple squamous epithelium with few organelles in the cytoplasm. These organelles are small mitochondria, Golgi complexes and some vesicles. The outer parietal layer is connected with the epithelium of the proximal tubule at the tubular pole, and reflexed to be the internal layer (visceral layer) of the glomerular capsule at the vascular pole.

The visceral layer of the renal corpuscle consists of the highly specialized podocytes. The podocyte has a large cell body and a lightly stained nucleus. Developed rough endoplasmic reticulum, abundant free ribosomes, and larger Golgi complex in their cytoplasm suggest the active function of protein synthesis. There are also endocytic vesicles,

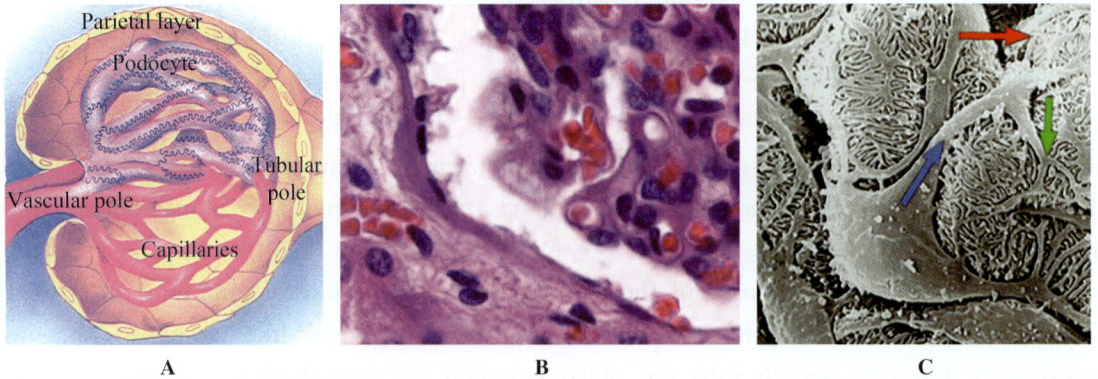

Figure 17 - 5   Glomerular capsule
A. Diagram of glomerular capsule; B. LM of glomerular capsule; C. SEM of podocyte

multivesicular bodies and lysosomes in their cytoplasm, which suggest the active endocytosis. Under the scanning electron microscope, several primary processes extend from the cell body of the podocyte. Each primary process gives rise to many interdigitating secondary processes or pedicels. Adjacent pedicels are embedded in each other to be palisade-shaped, and contact closely with the basal lamina. Between the pedicels are spaces with the width of 25 nm, which are named slit pores. The slit pores are covered with the 4 - 6 nm thick slit diaphragms. The contraction of the microfilaments in the processes of podocytes can regulate the width of the slit pores.

1.1.1.3   Filtration Barrier

The renal corpuscle is like a filter. When blood flows through the glomerular capillaries, high pressure will push the substances in plasma to go through the filtration barrier or filtration membrane, which is composed of the fenestrated capillary endothelium, the glomerular basement membrane, and slit diaphragms (Figure 17 - 6). The liquid filtered into the capsular space is primary urine. The composition of the primary urine is similar to that of the blood plasma except for the large proteins. The filtration membrane can selectively filter the substances in blood plasma. Water, solutes, and small molecules can pass the filtration membrane easily, whereas it is difficult for plasma proteins

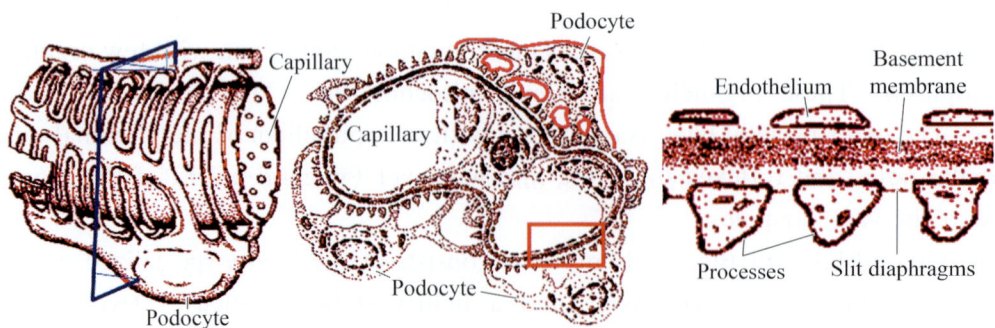

Figure 17 - 6   Ultrastructure of the filtration barrier

and other large molecules. The reason is the difference of filtrates in molecular size, electric charge, shape and so on. Normally, the substances smaller than 70 kDa and less than 4 nm in diameter can pass the filtration membrane. Meanwhile, the substances with positive charge will pass the filtration membrane more easily, such as glucose, polypeptides, urea, electrolytes, water and so on.

In the adult, 2 kidneys produce 180 L primary urine (125 ml/min) every day. If the filtration membrane is damaged, large plasma proteins or even red blood cells will also pass through the membrane, forming proteinuria or hematuria. When the mesangial cells remove the sediments in the basement membrane, endothelial cells and podocytes will reconstitute basement membrane, and the function of filtration membrane will recover.

1.1.2   Renal Tubule

The renal tubule is composed of the simple cuboidal epithelium. There are basement membrane and little amount of connective tissue outside the epithelial cells. The renal tubules consist of the proximal tubule, the thin segment, and the distal tubule. These tubules are different in diameter, length and cell morphology.

1.1.2.1   Proximal Tubule

The proximal tubule is the beginning of the renal tubule, and characterized as the longest and the thickest tubule. It is 14 mm in length and $50 - 60 \ \mu m$ in diameter, accounting for half of the renal tubule (Figure $17 - 7$). According to the morphology, the proximal tubule can be divided into the proximal convoluted tubule and the proximal straight tubule.

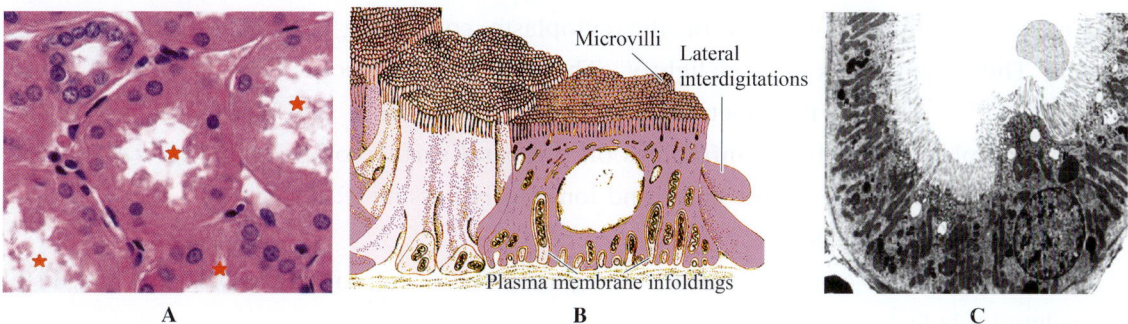

Figure $17 - 7$ Proximal tubule

A. LM of proximal tubule; B. Microstructure of proximal tubule; C. TEM of proximal tubule

Proximal convoluted tubule is located in the cortical labyrinth, and highly convoluted near the renal corpuscle. Under the light microscope, proximal convoluted tubule has thick wall and small, irregular lumen. The wall of the tubule is composed of simple cuboidal cells or conical cells, which are large with unclear border. The cells have very acidophilic cytoplasm, and a brush border in the lumen. The nucleus located near the base is large and round, and stained light with an obvious nucleolus. The wall of the proximal convoluted tubule is generally surrounded by $6 - 12$ epithelial cells, but only $3 - 4$ nuclei can be observed on one cross section because these cells are too large. Under the electron microscope, the cell apex has many long microvilli that can form a brush border. The membrane invaginations on the basal surface of the cell forms many plasma membrane infoldings. There are many large, longitudinally-arranged rod-shaped or curved mitochondria in the cytoplasm among the infoldings. The unclear border of tubule cells observed under the light microscope is caused by the lateral interdigitations between neighboring cells. The lateral interdigitations and plasma membrane infoldings increase the cell surface area. There are tight junctions, intermediate junctions, desmosomes and slit junctions on the side of epithelial cells near the lumen. The cell apex has many tubules, vesicles, lysosomes, phagosomes and multivesicular bodies that related to the reabsorption and decomposition of proteins.

The proximal straight tubule is located in the medullary ray and renal pyramid. Its structure is similar to that of the proximal convoluted tubule. However, the epithelial cells of the proximal straight tubule are shorter, with fewer microvilli, lateral interdigitations and plasma membrane infoldings compared to the proximal convoluted tubule.

At least 85% Na^+ and water, all of small molecular proteins, peptides, glucose, amino acids, 50% bicarbonate, phosphate, urea, and vitamins of primary urine are reabsorbed in the proximal tubule. Furthermore, the epithelium of the proximal tubule can secrete H^+, NH_3, creatinine, hippuric acid, and transport and discharge phenol red, penicillin and organic iodide in blood.

1.1.2.2 Thin Segment

The tubule is thin and only $10 - 15\,\mu$m in diameter, which is surrounded by the simple squamous epithelium. The part of the cytoplasm containing nuclei protrudes into the lumen. The cytoplasm is stained lightly. There is no brush border on the epithelial cell (Figure 17 - 8). Under the electron microscope, there are a few microvilli on the free surface and plasma membrane infoldings on the basal surface of epithelial cells. The thin wall of the thin segment allows water and ions easily passing it.

1.1.2.3 Distal Tubule

The distal tubule can be divided into 2 parts: the distal straight tubule and the distal convoluted tubule.

Under the light microscope, the distal tubule has some characteristics when compared to the proximal tubule: ①The distal tubule is shorter, so fewer sections will be observed. ②Because the cuboidal epithelia cells are smaller and flatter, the lumen of the distal tubule is larger with more nuclei seen. ③The simple cuboidal cells have basal longitudinal stripes but no brush border. ④ The cytoplasm of the cell is less acidophilic and lightly colored. ⑤The nucleus stays close to the lumen. The distal straight tubule is about $30\,\mu$m in diameter and about $9\,$mm in length. Under the electron microscope, there are a few short and small microvilli on the surface of cells, and the plasma membrane infoldings of epithelial cells are well-developed. The mitochondria of the plasma membrane infoldings are long and

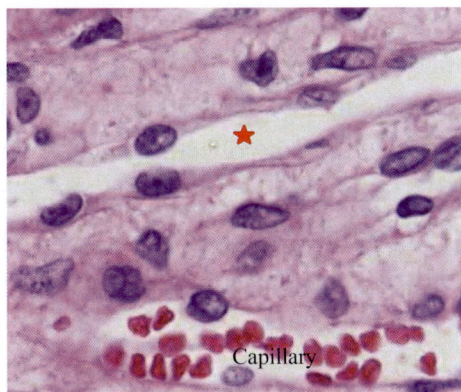

Figure 17 - 8　Thin segment (Red star. The lumen of thin segment)

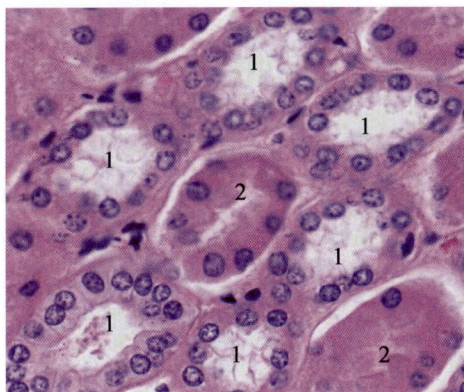

1. Distal tubule; 2. Proximal tubule
Figure 17 - 9　Distal tubule (HE)

thin, and arranged in the same direction as the longitudinal axis of cells (Figure 17 - 9). The distal straight tubule can reabsorb Na^+ and repel water, making the tubular fluid in a hypotonic state. Reabsorbed Na^+ will move to the interstitial substance, making the interstitial substance in a hypertonic state, which is critical for the concentration of the urine. The functions of the distal straight tubule are regulated by several hormones including antidiuretic hormone, parathyroid hormone, calcitonin and hyperglycemia, in a way that affect the reabsorption of ions through activation of adenylate cyclase.

The distal convoluted tubules are $35 - 45\,\mu m$ in diameter and $4.6 - 5.2\,mm$ in length. Its structure is similar to that of the distal straight tubule, however, the plasma membrane infoldings are less developed. The distal convoluted tubule is an important location for ions exchange. The reabsorption of Na^+, Ca^{2+} and discharge of K^+, H^+, NH_3 present in the distal convoluted tubule, which is important for maintaining the acid-base balance of body fluid. Aldosterone, as a kind of adrenal cortex hormones, can regulate this process by facilitating the reabsorption of Na^+ and the discharge of K^+.

1.2　Collecting Duct

Collecting ducts are $20 - 38\,mm$ in length, and consist of arched collecting ducts, straight collecting ducts and papillary ducts (Figure 17 - 10). Arched collecting ducts are very short, which locate in the cortical labyrinth. They connect with the distal convoluted tubule and then move into the medullary ray to form an arcade, and finally connect with the straight collecting ducts. The latter runs parallelly with the medullary ray to the renal papillae to become papillary ducts. In the apex of the renal pyramid, many arched collecting ducts

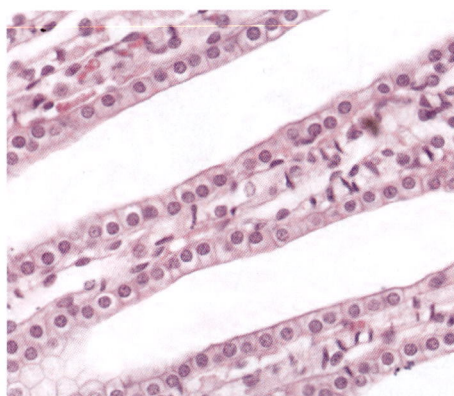

Figure 17 - 10　LM of collecting ducts (HE)

merge further as a papillary duct.

The diameter of the straight collecting duct increases gradually. Its wall turns from the simple cuboidal epithelium to simple columnar epithelium, and finally become simple tall columnar epithelium in the renal papillae. The epithelial cells of collecting ducts have clear border, pale-staining cytoplasm, round and dark staining nuclei. Under the electron microscope, there are a few short microvilli on the free surface of the epithelial cells, and some lateral protrusions and short plasma membrane infoldings. Collecting ducts are composed of cells with few organelles.

Collecting ducts can concentrate filtrate through water reabsorption and ions exchange. Their functions are regulated by aldosterone and antidiuretic hormone, just as distal convoluted tubules. However, atrial natriuretic peptide can block collecting ducts from reabsorbing water to increase the urine.

Taken together, when filtrate formed in the renal corpuscle goes through the renal tubules and collecting ducts, most water, nutrients and inorganic salts will be reabsorbed into the blood, and some ions exchange also take place here. Epithelial cells of the renal tubules also discharge some metabolites to form concentrated urine, which runs from the papillary ducts into the calyces in a daily amount of $1-2$ L accounting for about 1% of the filtrate. Therefore, the kidney not only discharges metabolic wastes, but also plays important roles in maintaining water-salt balance and homeostasis of internal environment.

1.3 Juxtaglomerular Complex

The juxtaglomerular complex, also known as the juxtaglomerular apparatus, is composed of juxtaglomerular cells, macula densa and extraglomerular mesangial cells (Figure 17 - 11). It is located at the vascular pole of the renal corpuscle, and is triangular in shape. The macula densa is the base of the "triangle", and afferent and efferent arterioles

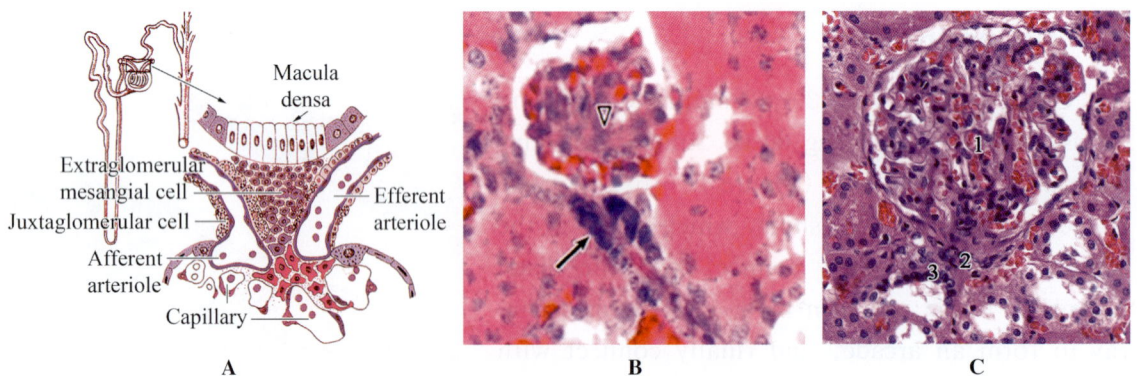

Figure 17 - 11 Juxtaglomerular complex
A. Diagram of juxtaglomerular complex; B. LM of juxtaglomerular cells (HE; △. Glomerulus; ↑. Juxtaglomerular cells); C. LM of juxtaglomerular complex (HE; 1. Glomerulus; 2. Extraglomerular mesangial cells; 3. Macula densa)

form the 2 lateral sides of the "triangle", and the extraglomerular mesangial cells are located in the center of the "triangle".

1.3.1   Juxtaglomerular Cell

The smooth muscle cells of afferent arterioles near the vascular pole of the renal corpuscle are transformed into epithelioid cells called juxtaglomerular cells (Figure 17 – 11B). They are large, cuboidal or polygonal, with large and round nuclei and light staining. The rich cytoplasm containing abundant PAS-positive secretory granules is weakly basophilic. Under the electron microscope, the cytoplasm has few myofilaments, abundant rough endoplasmic reticulum and free ribosomes, well-developed Golgi complex, and many membrane-encapsulated secretory granules containing renin. Renin is a type of enzyme that can transform angiotensinogen into angiotensin I , which can be transformed into angiotensin II with the effect of transferase secreted by pulmonary vascular endothelial cells. Angiotensin II will activate zona glomerulosa to produce more aldosterone, which will promote distal tubules to reabsorb Na^+. Angiotensin is a vasoconstrictor with the effect of increasing blood pressure. Juxtaglomerular cells also produce erythropoietin that can induce erythropoiesis.

The major function of the juxtaglomerular cells is to synthesize and secrete renin. Released renin will induce the increase of blood pressure when it enters into the blood circulation through the renal interstitium near the small arteries.

1.3.2   Macula Densa

The epithelial cells in the end of the distal tubule near vascular pole are elevated, narrowed, and arranged closely to form an oval structure called macula densa (Figure 17 – 11C). The nucleus is oval and located in the cell apex. There are digitations on the basal surface of cells that stick to juxtaglomerular cells to make the basement membrane incomplete. Macula densa is a type of ion sensor that can monitor the concentration of Na^+ in the filtrate of distal tubule and deliver "message" to other cells in the juxtaglomerular complex. For example: when the concentration of Na^+ in the filtrate decreases, the message will be transferred to the juxtaglomerular cells and extracellular mesangial cells, promote them to secret more renin to enhance the reabsorption of Na^+ and discharge of K^+ in the distal tubule.

1.3.3   Extraglomerular Mesangial Cell

Extraglomerular mesangial cells, also known as polar cushion cells, are located in the triangular area surrounded by the afferent artery, the efferent artery and the macula densa (Figure 17 – 11C). Their morphology is similar to that of intraglomerular mesangium. Extraglomerular mesangial cells are located in the center of the juxtaglomerular complex. They stay close to the macula densa, and also connect juxtaglomerular cells and intraglomerular mesangial cells through gap junctions. Therefore, they may play a role as information transfer in the juxtaglomerular complex.

1.4　Renal Interstitium

The renal interstitium includes connective tissue, blood vessels, nerves and so on. There is less connective tissue in the renal cortex and more near the renal papillae. Except for the connective tissue, the renal interstitium contains a special type of cell called the interstitial cell, which is star-link in shape with long protrusions. The long axis of the interstitial cell is vertical to the adjacent renal tubules and vasa recta. Under the electron microscope, there are characteristic osmiophilic lipid droplets in the cytoplasm, as well as abundant rough endoplasmic reticulum, Golgi complexes, lysosomes, phagosomes and mitochondria. These cells can form fibers and ground substances, and produce prostaglandins. Prostaglandins can induce vasodilation, improve blood flow, accelerate the transfer of reabsorbed water, and finally promote the concentration of urine.

1.5　Blood Circulation

The kidney has a rich blood supply and low vascular resistance. About 1 200 ml/min of blood is pumped into the kidney in a quiet normal person, which is 1/4 - 1/3 of the cardiac output, and about 90% of blood will be distributed in the cortex.

The kidney's renal artery divides into several interlobular arteries when enters the kidney through the hilum. Around the renal pelvis, interlobular arteries divide into the arcuate artery. Arcuate arteries divide into several smaller interlobular arteries, which radiate and extend into the cortex. The end of the smaller interlobular artery reaches the capsule to form the capillary network. The branch of interlobular arteries forms the microvascular afferent arterioles, which enter the renal corpuscle to form the glomerulus. Then blood leaves the renal corpuscle via the efferent artery, which branches to form the peritubular capillary network that is distributed near the renal tubule. The capillary network converges into interlobular veins, arcuate veins, and interlobular veins in order. These veins run parallel with the corresponding arteries, and finally form the renal vein and leave the kidney. The efferent arteries of nephrons near the medulla not only form the peritubular capillary network, but also branch to form the capillary network in the medulla. These branches return and ascend to become straight venules, which form "U" shaped straight vascular loops running parallel with the medullary loop. Both loops are closely related in the function. The straight venules converge into the interlobular veins or arcuate veins (Figure 17 - 12).

The kidney blood circulation is closely related to its function, and the characteristics are as follows: the renal artery starts from the abdominal aorta. They are short and thick, with high blood flow. Moreover, the blood vessels in the kidney run straight, and blood can reach the glomerulus quickly. Blood flow is different in the different regions of the kidney. 90% of the blood supplies the cortex and is filtered after entering the glomerulus. The 2 ends of the capillaries of the glomerulus are both arterioles. The diameter of the

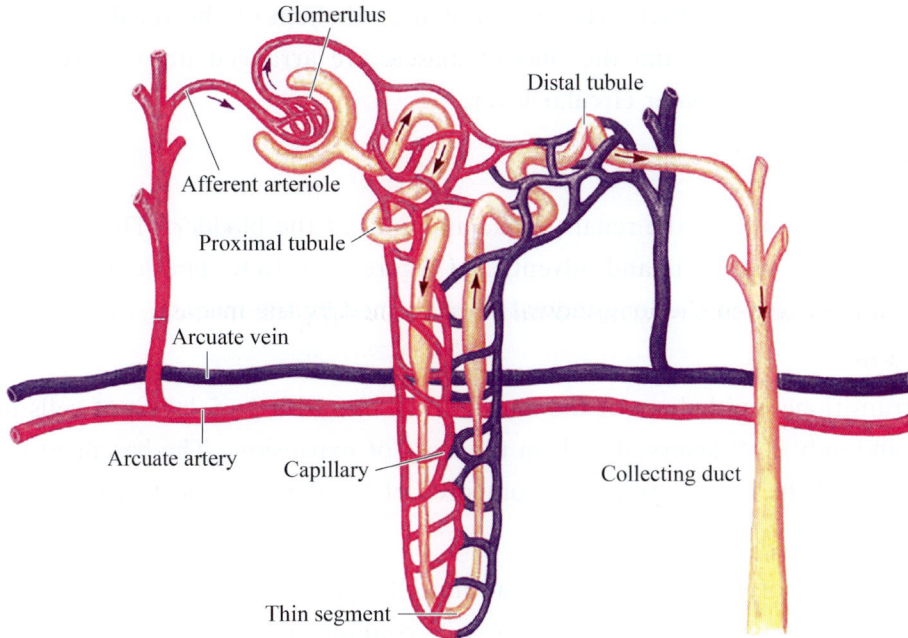

Figure 17 – 12   Blood supply to the kidney

afferent artery is thicker than that of the efferent artery, resulting in high blood flow and high blood pressure, which is good for filtration. There are 2 types of capillaries in the kidney blood circulation: capillaries in the glomerulus and the peritubular capillary network. Because much water is filtered out when blood flows through the glomerulus, the colloid osmotic pressure of blood in the peritubular capillary near the renal tubule is very high, which is beneficial to the movement of the reabsorbed substances into the blood. Straight vascular loops run parallel with the medullary loop in the medulla, which is beneficial to the reabsorption of renal tubules and collecting ducts, and the concentration of urine.

2   Urination Ducts

Urination ducts include calyces, renal pelvis, ureters, bladder and urethra. Its function is to eliminate urine from the body. The calyces, renal pelvis, ureter, and bladder have similar histological structure except for the urethra. They all consist of the mucosa, muscularis and adventitia. The walls become gradually thicker from the calyces to the bladder.

2.1   Calyces and Renal Pelvis

The calyces and pelvis are the ducts of urination in the kidney. The epithelium of the calyces migrates with that of the papillary ducts, which is transitional epithelium consisting of 2 – 3 layers of cells. There is a little amount of connective tissue and smooth muscle outside the epithelium. The connective tissue and smooth muscle will push the urine to flow downwards when they contract. The transitional epithelium of the renal pelvis is thicker with 3 - 4 layers of cells, and the smooth muscle are arranged into 2 layers: an inner longitudinal layer and an outer circular layer.

2.2 Ureter

The ureter starts from the renal pelvis, and ends at the bladder. The walls consist of 3 layers: mucosa, muscularis and adventitia (Figure 17 - 13). The lumen of the ureter looks like star because of the longitudinal plica formed by the mucosa.

2.2.1 Mucosa

The transitional epithelium of the mucosa is thick, with 4 - 5 layers of cells in normal condition and only 2 - 3 layers of cells in the state of expansion. The basement membrane is indistinct, and the lamina propria is composed of the dense connective tissue.

2.2.2 Muscularis

The upper 2/3 of the ureter contains an inner longitudinal smooth muscle and an outer circular smooth muscle, while the lower 1/3 contains the inner longitudinal, middle circular and outer longitudinal smooth muscle. The contraction and relaxation of the muscularis facilitate the movement of the urine into the bladder.

2.2.3 Adventitia

The adventitia is the fibrosa that migrates with the surrounding connective tissue.

The ureter runs obliquely through the bladder wall and forms a valve in the opening. When the bladder is full, the walls and valve are blocked by pressure, preventing urinary reflux.

2.3 Bladder

The bladder is a hollow organ that stores urine. Its structure is similar to that of the ureter, although the muscularis is thicker (Figure 17 - 14).

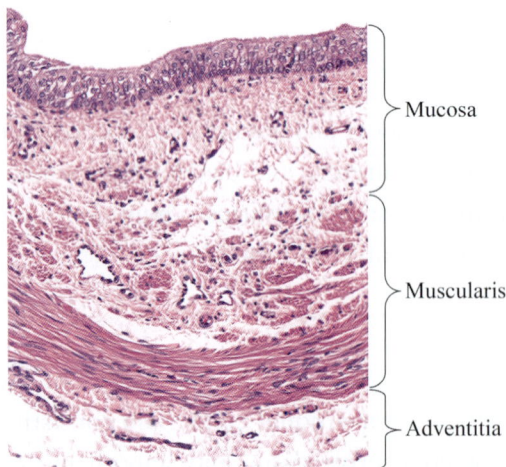

Figure 17 - 13   LM of ureter (HE)

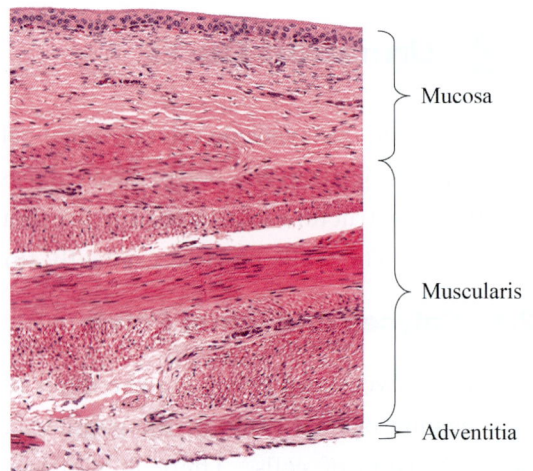

Figure 17 - 14   LM of bladder (HE)

2.3.1 Mucosa

The mucosa produces many plicae that will decrease or disappear when the bladder is full. The epithelium of the mucosa is transitional epithelium whose cell morphology and layers vary depending on the distension and contraction of the bladder. When the bladder is empty, the epithelium becomes thick with 8 – 10 layers of cells. Umbrella cells are large and rectangular. When the bladder is full, the epithelium has only 2 – 3 layers of cells and umbrella cells become oblate. There is a very thin basement membrane under the epithelium, which is not easy to be observed using light microscope. Under the electron microscope, there are infoldings and vesicles on the membrane of umbrella cells. The infoldings can be unfolded and flattened when the bladder is full. The cytoplasm near the free surface is denser to prevent the erosion of urine in the bladder. There are well-developed tight junctions between the cells, preventing the transfer of ions and water between the tissue and urine.

The lamina propria is dense connective tissue containing collagenous fibers, elastic fibers, and abundant blood vessels.

2.3.2 Muscularis

The muscularis is thick and composed of spiral-shaped smooth muscle bundles, much loose connective tissue, and blood vessels. Although the layers of the muscularis are not clear, it can be roughly divided into 3 layers: the inner longitudinal layer, the middle circular layer, and the outer longitudinal layer. The arrangement of the muscularis can eliminate all urine from the bladder when the bladder contracts. The middle circular smooth muscle is getting thicker to become the sphincter at the urethral orifice.

2.3.3 Adventitia

The adventitia is composed of the loose connective tissue containing blood vessels, lymphatic vessels and nerves. Only the top of the bladder is covered by the serosa.

(*Xu Linwei, Yang Lin, Yang Fan*)

第十七章　泌尿系统

泌尿系统包括肾、输尿管、膀胱和尿道等器官,主要功能是生成和排出尿液,通过对尿液生成过程的调节,维持机体的水、电解质及酸碱平衡。另外,肾分泌的多种生物活性物质,如肾素、促红细胞生成素、前列腺素等,对机体的生理功能起着重要的调节作用。

第一节　肾

　　肾形似蚕豆,外缘隆起,内缘中部凹陷为肾门,是肾动脉、肾静脉、淋巴管、神经和输尿管出入之处。肾表面外包致密性结缔组织被膜,称肾纤维膜。

　　肾实质由皮质和髓质两部分构成。肾冠状剖面上,皮质位于外周,呈暗红色,由髓放线和皮质迷路组成。每条髓放线及其周围的皮质迷路构成一个肾小叶。髓质色淡,位于肾的深部,由10~18个肾锥体构成。肾锥体的底与皮质相连,顶部钝圆,伸入肾小盏内,为肾乳头,其上有10~25个小孔,为乳头孔,是乳头管的开口,尿液由此排至肾小盏内。每个肾锥体及其周围的皮质构成一个肾叶,肾锥体之间的肾皮质称为肾柱(图17-1)。

　　肾实质由肾单位和集合管构成,其间有少量结缔组织、血管和神经等构成的间质。每个肾单位包括一个肾小体和一条与它相连的肾小管,是尿液形成的结构和功能单位。肾小管汇入集合管,它们都是单层上皮性管道,合称泌尿小管。肾单位和集合管在肾实质内的分布是有规律的。肾小体和肾小管的曲部位于皮质迷路和肾柱内,肾小管的直部与集合管位于髓放线和肾锥体内(图17-2)。

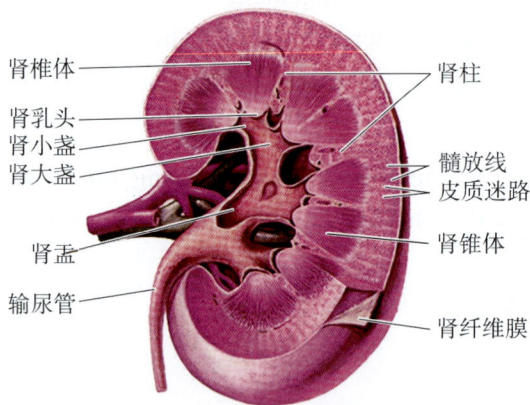

图17-1　肾冠状剖面模式图

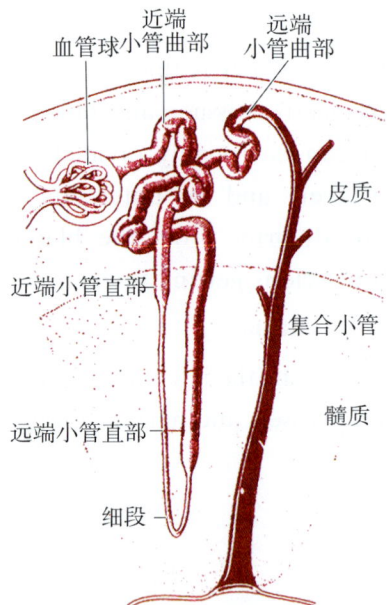

图17-2　肾单位及集合管结构模式图

一、肾单位

　　肾单位是尿液生成与排泄的基本结构和功能单位。每个肾有100万~200万个肾单位。肾单位由肾小体及肾小管两部分构成。肾小管的起始段在肾小体附近盘曲走行,称近端小管曲部(又称近曲小管)。继而进入髓放线或髓质直行,称近端小管直部(近直小管)。随后管径骤然变细,称细段。细段之后,管径又骤然增粗,并返折向上走行于肾锥体和髓放线内,称远端小管直部或远直小管。近端小管直部、细段和远端小管直部三者构成"U"形的襻,称髓襻。髓襻由皮质向髓质方向下行的一段称降支,而由髓质向皮质方向上行的一段称升支。髓襻长短不一,长者可达乳头部,短者只存在于髓放线中。远端小管直部离开髓放线后,在皮质迷路内盘曲走行于肾小体附近称远端小管曲部(或称远曲小管),最后汇入集合管(表 17-1)。

表 17-1 肾实质的组成

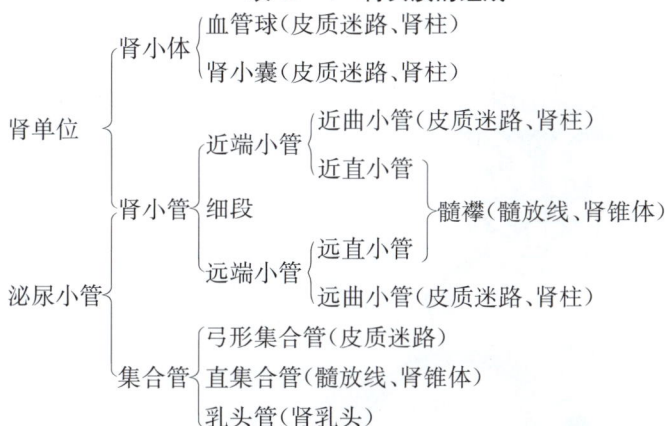

```
                ┌ 肾小体 ┌ 血管球(皮质迷路、肾柱)
                │        └ 肾小囊(皮质迷路、肾柱)
       ┌ 肾单位 │        ┌ 近端小管 ┌ 近曲小管(皮质迷路、肾柱)
       │        │        │          └ 近直小管 ┐
       │        └ 肾小管 ┤ 细段      ├ 髓襻(髓放线、肾锥体)
泌尿小管┤                 │          ┌ 远直小管 ┘
       │                 └ 远端小管 └ 远曲小管(皮质迷路、肾柱)
       │        ┌ 弓形集合管(皮质迷路)
       └ 集合管 ┤ 直集合管(髓放线、肾锥体)
                └ 乳头管(肾乳头)
```

根据肾小体在皮质中的位置,肾单位可分为浅表肾单位和髓旁肾单位两种。浅表肾单位数量多,约占肾单位总数的 85%,其肾小体位于皮质中部和浅层,体积较小,髓襻较短,髓襻中的细段也短。浅表肾单位在尿液形成中起重要作用。髓旁肾单位数量较少,约占肾单位总数的 15%。其肾小体靠近髓质,体积较大,髓襻和细段均较长。髓旁肾单位对尿液浓缩具有重要的生理意义。

(一) 肾小体

肾小体呈圆球状,直径约 200 μm,由血管球和肾小囊两部分组成。肾小体有两个极,有微动脉出入的一端称血管极,在血管极的对侧,肾小体与近端小管曲部相连处为尿极(图 17-3)。

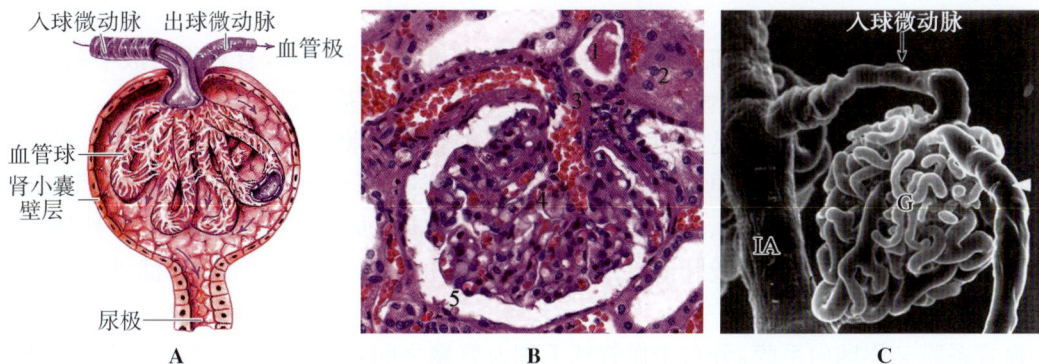

图 17-3 肾小体

A. 肾小体结构模式图;B. 肾小体光镜结构(HE 染色;1—远端小管;2—近端小管;3—血管极;4—血管球;5—肾小囊腔);C. 血管球电镜结构

1. 血管球

位于入球微动脉与出球微动脉之间的盘曲成球的毛细血管襻(图 17-4)。一条较粗的入球微动脉从肾小体血管极处进入肾小囊,先分成 4~5 支,每支再分支形成许多相互吻合的毛细血管襻,其间充填有血管系膜。这些毛细血管最终汇合成一条较细的出球微动脉,由血管极处离开肾小囊。由于入球微动脉管径较出球微动脉粗,故血管球内的血压较一般毛细血管的高。当血液流经血管球时,大量水和小分子物质易于滤出毛细血管壁而进入肾小囊腔内。另外,在内皮细胞的腔面覆有一层带负电荷的、富含唾液酸的糖蛋白(细胞衣),对血液中的物质有选择性通透作用。

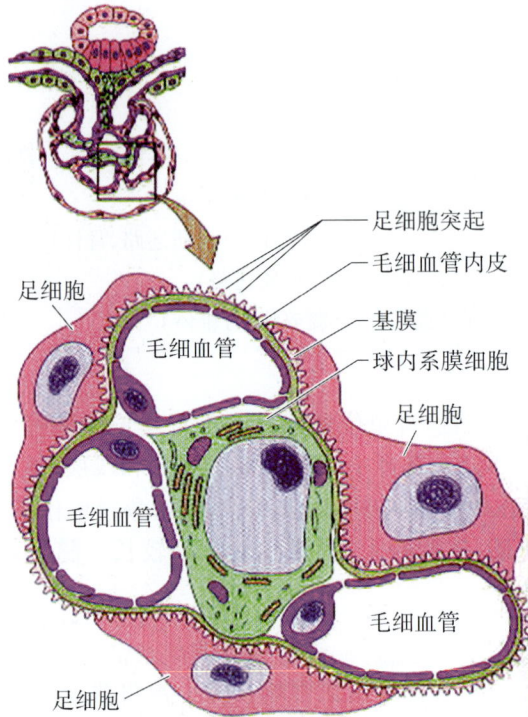

图 17-4　血管球结构模式图

　　电镜下,血管球为有孔毛细血管,其孔径为 50~100 nm,无隔膜,有利于血液中物质滤过。内皮基底面除与血管系膜相接触的部位外,都有基膜。血管基膜较厚,约 330 nm。位于内皮细胞与足细胞之间,或系膜与足细胞之间。在内皮细胞和系膜细胞之间没有基膜。光镜下基膜为均质状,PAS 反应阳性。电镜下基膜分为三层,中层较厚而致密,内、外层较薄而稀疏。

　　基膜主要含Ⅳ型胶原蛋白、蛋白聚糖和层粘连蛋白,形成以Ⅳ型胶原蛋白为骨架的分子筛,骨架上附有带负电荷的硫酸肝素,可阻止带负电荷的物质通过,故基膜对滤液中的大分子物质有选择性通透作用。

　　血管系膜又称球内系膜,分布于血管球毛细血管襻之间,由系膜细胞和系膜基质组成。系膜细胞呈星形,有突起,细胞突起可伸至内皮与基膜之间,或经内皮细胞之间伸入毛细血管腔内。其细胞核较小,染色较深,细胞内有较发达的粗面内质网及高尔基复合体、溶酶体、吞噬体等,有时还可见少量分泌颗粒;胞体和突起内有微管、微丝和中间丝。

　　系膜细胞能合成基膜和系膜基质的成分;还可吞噬和降解沉积在基膜上的免疫复合物,以维持基膜的通透性,并参与基膜的更新和修复;系膜细胞的收缩活动可调节毛细血管的管径以影响血管球内血流量;系膜细胞还可分泌肾素和酶等生物活性物质,可能与血管球内血流量的局部调节有关。系膜基质填充在系膜细胞之间,在血管球内起支持和通透作用。血管系膜内还可有少量巨噬细胞。

2. 肾小囊

又称鲍曼囊,由肾小管起始部膨大并凹陷而成的双层扁囊,似杯状,分为壁层和脏层两层,两层间的狭窄腔隙为肾小囊腔,与近曲小管腔相通(图17-5)。

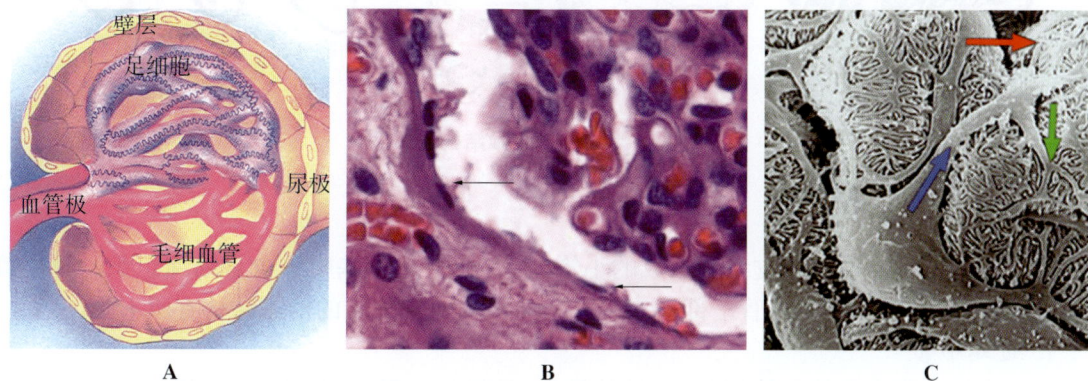

图17-5 肾小囊

A.肾小囊结构模式图;B.肾小囊壁层光镜结构;C.肾小囊脏层足细胞电镜结构

肾小囊外层(肾小囊壁层)为单层扁平上皮,胞质内细胞器稀少,有体积较小的线粒体、高尔基复合体及一些小泡。在肾小体尿极处与近端小管上皮相延续,在血管极处返折为肾小囊内层(肾小囊脏层)。

肾小囊脏层由高度特化的足细胞构成。足细胞胞体较大,细胞核染色较浅,细胞质内有发达的粗面内质网、丰富的游离核糖体和体积较大的高尔基复合体,提示足细胞具有活跃的合成蛋白质的功能。胞质内常见吞饮小泡及溶酶体,提示足细胞有较强的胞吞活动。扫描电镜下,可见从足细胞胞体伸出几个较大的初级突起,从初级突起上再分出许多指状的次级突起,相邻次级突起相互镶嵌,形成栅栏状,紧贴在毛细血管基膜外,突起之间有宽约25 nm的裂隙,称裂孔,孔上覆盖一层厚4~6nm的裂孔膜。足细胞的突起内含有微丝,微丝的收缩可调节裂孔的宽度。

3. 滤过屏障

肾小体类似一个滤过器。当血液流经血管球毛细血管时,其内压力较高,血液中的部分物质将穿过下列结构进入肾小囊腔,这些结构包括:有孔毛细血管内皮、基膜和足细胞裂孔膜,称为滤过屏障或滤过膜(图17-6)。滤入肾小囊腔的液体称为原尿。原尿除不含大分子蛋白质外,其成分与血浆相似。滤过膜对血浆成分具有选择性的通透作用,血浆中的水、离子和小分子物质很容易通过滤过膜,而血浆蛋白和其他大分子物质则不易通过滤过膜,这与滤过物的分子大小、电荷及性状等因素有关。一般情况下,分子量7万以下、直径4 nm以下的物质可通过滤过膜,其中又以带正电荷的物质易于通过,如葡萄糖、多肽、尿素、电解质和水等。

在成人,一昼夜两肾可形成原尿约180 L(每分钟125 ml)。若滤过膜受损害,则血浆中的大分子蛋白质、红细胞等亦可通过滤过膜漏出,出现蛋白尿或血尿。当血管系膜细胞清除了基膜内沉积物,内皮细胞和足细胞重建新的基膜后,滤过膜功能又可恢复。

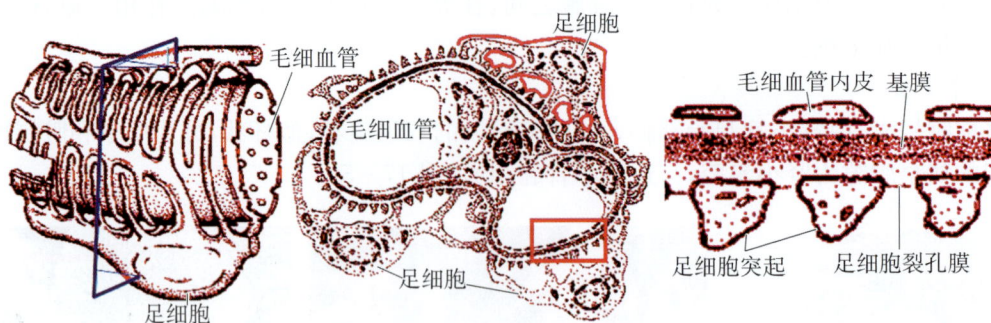

图 17-6　滤过屏障超微结构模式图

(二) 肾小管

肾小管是由单层立方上皮细胞围成的小管,上皮细胞外为基膜及少量结缔组织。肾小管包括近端小管、细段和远端小管三部分,各段的管径、长度及细胞的形态结构有所不同。

1. 近端小管

近端小管是肾小管的起始部分,也是其最长、最粗的一段,长约 14 mm,管径 50~60 μm,约占肾小管总长的一半(图 17-7)。根据近端小管的形态结构,将其分为曲部(近曲小管)和直部(近直小管)两段。

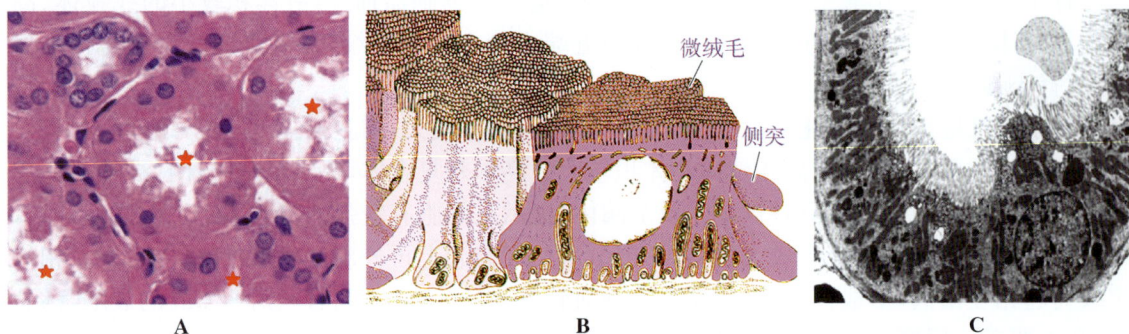

图 17-7　近端小管
A.近端小管光镜结构(HE 染色);B.近端小管电镜结构模式图;C.近端小管透射电镜结构

近曲小管位于皮质迷路内,在肾小体附近高度盘曲。光镜下,管壁厚,管腔小而不规则,管壁由单层立方或锥体形细胞构成,细胞体积较大、分界不清。胞质强嗜酸性,细胞基底部有纵纹,游离面有刷状缘。核大而圆,位于近基底部,着色浅,核仁明显。近曲小管一般由 6~12 个细胞围成管壁,但由于细胞体积较大,通常在一个横断面上只能见到 3~4 个细胞核。电镜下可见近曲小管上皮细胞的游离面有密集细长的微绒毛,构成光镜下所见的刷状缘。细胞基底面的胞膜向内凹陷,形成许多质膜内褶。褶间胞质内有许多体积较大、纵行排列的杆状或弯曲状的线粒体。相邻细胞的侧面可发出侧突,呈指状交叉,细胞基部的侧突可伸入邻近细胞质膜内褶的空隙内,故光镜下细胞分界不清。线粒体和质膜内褶共同形成光镜下所见的基底纵纹。侧突和质膜内褶的存在也大大扩大了细胞的表面积。相邻上皮细胞近腔的侧面有紧密连接、中间连接、桥粒和缝隙连接。细胞的顶部胞质内有许多小管和小泡,以及大量溶酶体和吞噬体,这些结构与蛋白质的重吸收和分解有关。

近直小管位于髓放线和肾锥体内,结构与近曲小管相似,但上皮细胞略矮,微绒毛、侧突和质膜内褶均不如近曲小管发达。

近端小管是原尿重吸收的主要场所,原尿中85%以上的钠离子和水,全部的小分子蛋白、多肽、葡萄糖和氨基酸,50%的碳酸氢盐、磷酸盐和尿素,以及维生素等都在此处被重吸收。另外,近端小管上皮还向管腔内分泌 H^+、NH_3、肌酐和马尿酸等物质,并能转运和排出血液中的酚红、青霉素及有机碘化物等。

2. 细段

管径细,直径 $10\sim15\,\mu m$。管壁薄,由单层扁平上皮围成,含细胞核的部分突向管腔,胞质着色浅,无刷状缘(图 17-8)。电镜下,上皮细胞游离面有少量短微绒毛,基底面质膜内褶少。由于细段管壁极薄,有利水和离子的透过。

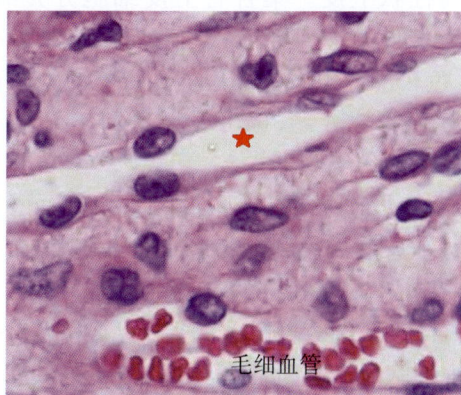

图 17-8 细段光镜结构(红色五角星:细段管腔)

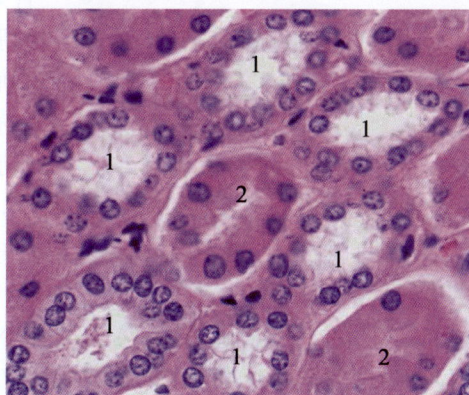

1—远端小管;2—近端小管
图 17-9 远端小管(HE 染色)

3. 远端小管

远端小管可分为直部(远直小管)和曲部(远曲小管)两个部分。

光镜下,与近端小管相比,远端小管有以下几个特点:①远端小管较短,故切片中它的断面较少;②上皮细胞较矮,立方形,且细胞体积较小,因此管腔相对较大,且在远端小管的横断面上,核的数量相对较多;③细胞的游离缘无刷状缘,但细胞的基部有基底纵纹;④细胞的胞质嗜酸性较弱,着色较浅;⑤细胞核的位置靠近腔面。远直小管管径约 $30\,\mu m$,长约 $9\,mm$。电镜下,细胞表面有少量短小的微绒毛,基底部的质膜内褶发达,褶深可达细胞高度的 2/3 或更多。质膜内褶的线粒体细长,其排列方向与细胞纵轴相一致(图 17-9)。远直小管能主动重吸收 Na^+,而对水不通透,使小管液呈低渗状态。重吸收的 Na^+ 排至间质,使间质呈高渗状态,在尿液浓缩过程中起重要作用。远直小管的功能活动受多种激素的调节,包括抗利尿激素、甲状旁腺激素、降钙素和高血糖素,这些激素通过刺激细胞内腺苷酸环化酶的活性来影响小管对离子的重吸收。

远曲小管直径 $35\sim45\,\mu m$,长 $4.6\sim5.2\,mm$。其结构与直部相似,但质膜内褶和线粒体不如直部发达。远曲小管是离子交换的重要部位,有重吸收 Na^+、Ca^{2+} 和排出 K^+、H^+ 和 NH_3 等功能,对维持体液的酸碱平衡发挥重要作用。此过程受肾上腺盐皮质激素的调节,醛固酮能促进此段重吸收 Na^+ 和排出 K^+。

二、集合管

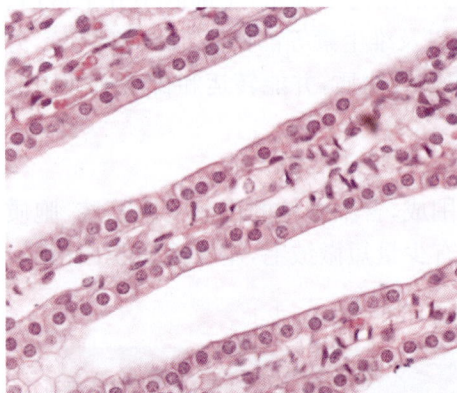

图 17-10　集合管光镜结构(HE 染色)

集合管全长 20～38 mm,由弓形集合管、直集合管和乳头管组成(图 17-10)。弓形集合管很短,位于皮质迷路内,一端连接远曲小管,呈弧形弯入髓放线,与直集合管相连。直集合管沿髓放线下行至肾锥体乳头,改称乳头管,开口于肾小盏。直集合管在髓放线下行时沿途有许多弓形集合管汇入。

直集合管的管径由细逐渐变粗,管壁上皮也由单层立方上皮逐渐变为单层柱状上皮组成,至乳头管处成为高柱状上皮。集合管上皮细胞分界清楚,细胞质着色淡而明亮,细胞核圆形,位于中央或靠近基底部,着色较深。电镜下,集合管上皮细胞游离面仅有少量短小的微绒毛,也可见少量侧突和短小的质膜内褶。细胞内细胞器少。

一方面,集合管能重吸收水和交换离子,使原尿进一步浓缩,并与远曲小管一样,受醛固酮和抗利尿激素的调节。另一方面,集合管还可受心房钠尿肽的作用,减少对水的重吸收,导致尿量增多。

综上所述,肾小体形成的原尿,经过肾小管和集合管后,绝大部分水、营养物质和无机盐被重吸收入血,部分离子也在此进行交换。肾小管上皮细胞还排出机体部分代谢产物,最后形成浓缩的终尿,经乳头管排入肾小盏,其量为每天 1～2 L,仅占原尿总量的 1% 左右。因此,肾在泌尿过程中不仅排出了机体的代谢废物,还对维持机体水盐平衡和内环境的稳定起重要作用。

三、球旁复合体

球旁复合体也称肾小球旁器,由球旁细胞、致密斑和球外系膜细胞组成(图 17-11)。位于肾小体的血管极处,大致呈三角形。致密斑为三角形的底,入球微动脉和出球微动脉分别形成三角形的两个侧边,球外系膜细胞则位于三角区的中心。

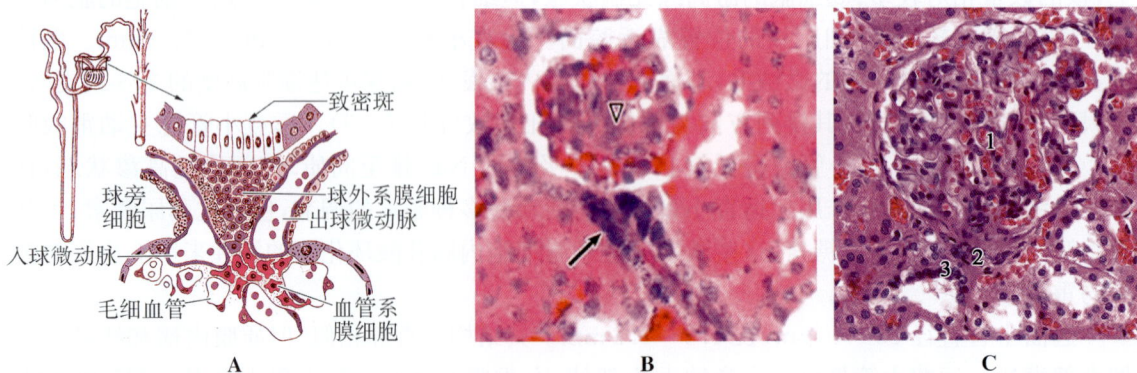

图 17-11　肾球旁复合体
A. 肾球旁复合体结构模式图;B. 球旁细胞光镜结构(HE 染色;△—血管球;↑—球旁细胞);C. 肾球旁复合体光镜结构(HE 染色;1—血管球;2—球外系膜细胞;3—致密斑)

（一）球旁细胞

入球微动脉靠近肾小体血管极处，管壁平滑肌细胞转变为上皮样细胞，称球旁细胞（图 17 - 11B）。球旁细胞的体积较大，呈立方或多边形，细胞核大而圆，着色浅。胞质丰富，呈弱嗜碱性，内含有丰富的 PAS 反应阳性的分泌颗粒。电镜下，胞质内肌丝少，含有丰富的粗面内质网和游离核糖体，发达的高尔基复合体，含大量的膜包被分泌颗粒，内含肾素。肾素是一种酶，能使血浆中的血管紧张素原转变为血管紧张素 I，在肺血管内皮细胞分泌的转换酶作用下转变为血管紧张素 II，刺激肾上腺皮质球状带产生更多的醛固酮，促进肾远端小管对钠离子的重吸收。血管紧张素是血管收缩剂，有升高血压的作用。球旁细胞还能产生红细胞生成素，是红细胞生成的诱导因子。

球旁细胞的主要功能是合成和分泌肾素，释放的肾素经小动脉周围的肾间质进入血液循环，致血压升高。

（二）致密斑

远端小管末端靠近血管极侧的上皮细胞增高、变窄，密集排列而形成的椭圆形结构，称致密斑（图 17 - 11C）。细胞核椭圆形，位于细胞顶部，细胞基底面有指状突起伸至球旁细胞，两者之间的基膜常不完整。致密斑是一种离子感受器，能感受远端小管滤液内 Na^+ 的浓度变化，并将"信息"传递给球旁复合体的其他细胞，如当滤液内 Na^+ 浓度降低时，可将信息传递给球旁细胞和球外系膜细胞，促使球旁细胞分泌肾素，增强远端小管对 Na^+ 的重吸收和排出 K^+ 的作用。

（三）球外系膜细胞

球外系膜细胞又称极垫细胞，位于入球微动脉、出球微动脉和致密斑围成的三角形区域内（图 17 - 11C）。细胞形态结构与球内系膜相似。球外系膜细胞位于球旁复合体的中央，一方面与致密斑相贴，另一方面与球旁细胞、球内系膜细胞之间有缝隙连接，因此，其在球旁复合体的功能活动中可能起到信息传递的作用。

四、肾间质

肾间质包括肾内的结缔组织、血管和神经等。肾皮质内的结缔组织较少，越接近肾乳头结缔组织越多。肾间质中除一般结缔组织成分外，有一种特殊的细胞，称为间质细胞，呈星形，有较长的突起。细胞长轴与邻近肾小管、直小血管相垂直。电镜下，胞质内有特征性的嗜锇性脂滴，还有丰富的粗面内质网、高尔基复合体、溶酶体、吞噬体及线粒体。该细胞可以合成间质内的纤维和基质，还可以产生前列腺素。前列腺素可舒张血管，促进周围血管内的血液流动，加快重吸收水分的转运，从而促进尿液浓缩。

五、肾的血液循环

肾的血液供应丰富，血管阻力小，正常人安静时每分钟约有 1 200 mL 血液供应两侧肾脏，相当于心输出量的 1/4～1/3，其中约 90% 的血液分布在皮质。

肾动脉直接由腹主动脉分出，经肾门入肾后分为数支叶间动脉，在肾柱内上行至皮质与髓质交界处，横行分支为弓形动脉。弓形动脉分出若干小叶间动脉，呈放射状走行于皮质迷路内，其末端抵达被膜下形成毛细血管网。小叶间动脉沿途向两侧分出许多入球微动脉进入肾小体,形成血管球。再汇合成出球微动脉离开肾小体后,又分支形成球后毛细血管网,分布在肾小管周围。毛细血管网依次汇合成小叶间静脉、弓形静脉和叶间静脉,它们与相应动脉伴行,最后形成肾静脉出肾。髓旁肾单位的出球微动脉不仅形成球后毛细血管网,还发出若干直小动脉直行降入髓质,在髓质的不同深度形成毛细血管网,又返折直行上升为直小静脉,构成"U"形直血管襻,并与髓襻伴行,二者功能关系密切。直小静脉汇入小叶间静脉或弓形静脉(图 17 - 12)。

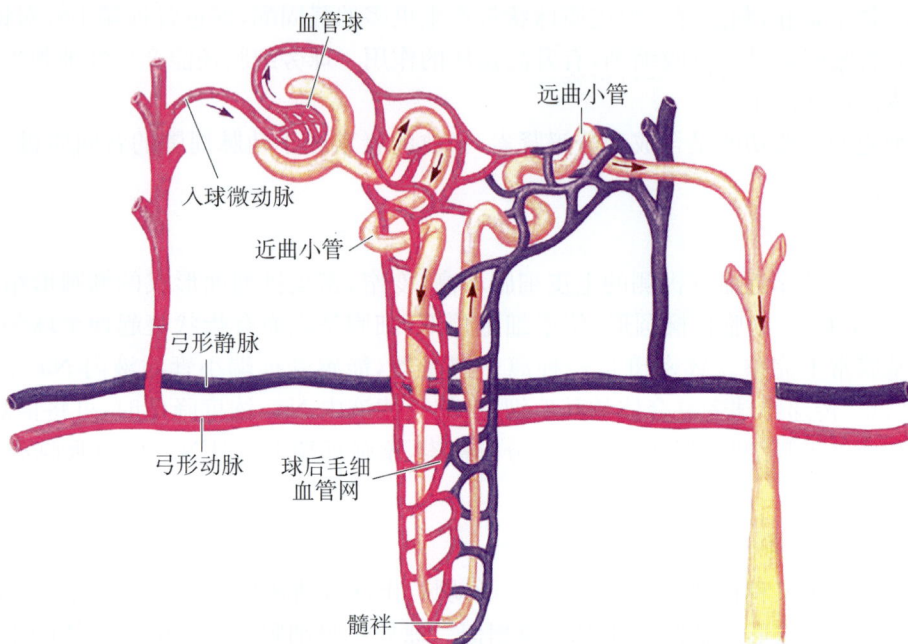

图 17 - 12 肾血液循环模式图

肾的血液循环与肾功能密切相关,其特点是:①肾动脉直接起始于腹主动脉,短而粗,血流量大,流速快。此外,肾内血管走行较直,血液能很快抵达血管球。②肾内不同区域的血流不同,肾血流量的 90%供应皮质,进入血管球后被滤过。③肾小体血管球的毛细血管两端皆为微动脉,入球微动脉管径比出球微动脉粗,使血管球内血流量大,血压高,有利于滤过。④肾内血管通路中出现两次毛细血管,即血管球毛细血管和球后毛细血管网,由于血流经血管球时大量水分被滤出,分布在肾小管周围的球后毛细血管内血液的胶体渗透压甚高,有利于肾小管上皮细胞重吸收的物质进入血流。⑤髓质内直小血管襻与髓襻伴行,有利于肾小管和集合管的重吸收和尿液浓缩。

第二节 排 尿 管 道

排尿管道包括肾盏、肾盂、输尿管、膀胱及尿道。其功能是将肾产生的尿液排出体外。除尿道外,排尿管道各部分的组织结构基本相似,均由黏膜、肌层和外膜构成。从肾小盏至膀胱,此三层结构逐渐增厚。

一、肾盏和肾盂

肾盏和肾盂为肾内排尿管道。肾盏的上皮与乳头管上皮相移行,上皮较薄,由2～3层细胞组成,为变移上皮。上皮外有少量的结缔组织和平滑肌,收缩时使尿液向下流动。肾盂的变移上皮略厚,有3～4层细胞,平滑肌可分为内纵、外环两层。

二、输尿管

输尿管起自肾盂,终于膀胱,管壁结构可分为黏膜、肌层和外膜三层(图17-13)。由于黏膜形成多条纵行的皱襞,使管腔呈星形。

(一)黏膜

黏膜表面的变移上皮较厚,有4～5层细胞,扩张时只有2～3层细胞,基膜不清楚,固有层为细密的结缔组织。

(二)肌层

输尿管上2/3段的肌层为内纵、外环两层平滑肌,下1/3段为内纵、中环和外纵三层平滑肌。肌层的收缩和舒张,可促使尿液进入膀胱。

(三)外膜

输尿管外膜是纤维膜,与周围的结缔组织相移行。输尿管斜穿膀胱壁,开口处黏膜折叠成瓣。当膀胱充盈时,输尿管壁和瓣膜受压封闭,可防止尿液反流。

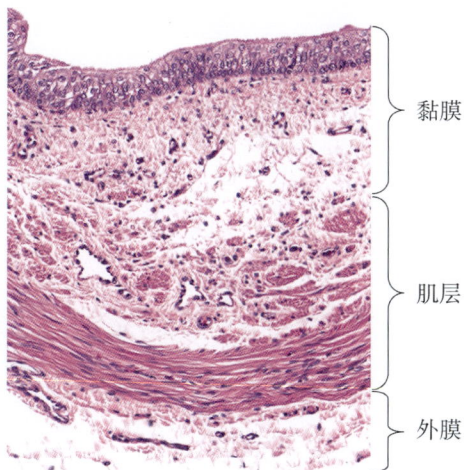

图17-13 输尿管光镜结构(HE染色)

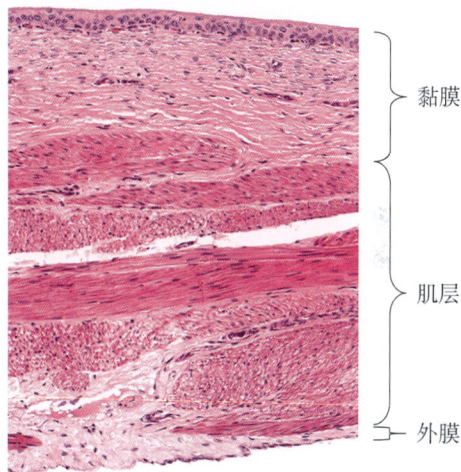

图17-14 膀胱光镜结构(充盈膀胱,HE染色)

三、膀胱

膀胱是贮尿器官,其结构与输尿管大体相同,但肌层特别厚(图17-14)。

(一)黏膜

黏膜形成许多皱襞,膀胱充盈时,皱襞减少或消失。

黏膜上皮为变移上皮,其细胞形态及层次的多少随膀胱的胀缩而变化。膀胱空虚时,上皮增厚,细胞可达 8～10 层,表层的盖细胞大,呈矩形;膀胱充盈时上皮细胞仅 2～3 层,盖细胞变扁。上皮下有一层很薄的基膜,光镜下不易分辨。电镜下,盖细胞游离面细胞膜有内褶和囊泡,膀胱充盈时内褶可展开拉平。细胞近游离面的细胞质较为浓密,可防止膀胱内尿液的侵蚀。细胞间有极为发达的紧密连接,防止了高度浓缩的尿液中各种离子进入组织及组织内的水进入尿液。

固有层为较细密的结缔组织,含有胶原纤维和弹性纤维,有丰富的血管。

(二) 肌层

肌层厚,由许多螺旋形平滑肌束组成,其间有较多的疏松结缔组织及血管。各肌层分界不明显,但大致能分为内纵、中环和外纵三层,肌层的排列使膀胱收缩时能将其所容纳的尿液完全排出。中层环形肌在尿道口处增厚为括约肌。

(三) 外膜

外膜由疏松结缔组织组成,含有血管、淋巴管和神经。仅膀胱顶部为浆膜。

(郑 英 牛长敏)

Chapter 18

Male Reproductive System

The male reproductive system consists of the testis, genital ducts, accessory glands, and penis. Testis produce sperm and male hormones principally testosterone. The genital ducts and accessory glands produce secretions required for sperm maturation and activity and assist in propelling sperm toward the exterior; these secretions provide nutrients for spermatozoa. Spermatozoa and the secretions of the genital ducts and accessory glands make up the semen, which is introduced into the female reproductive tract by the penis.

1 Testes

The testis, an ovoid gland weighing about 15 g, is encased in a thick capsule of dense connective tissue known as the tunica albuginea. A visceral layer of the tunica vaginalis invests the capsule externally. The tunica albuginea thickens on the posterior side to form the mediastinum testis. From this fibrous region, septa penetrate the organ and divide it into about 250 pyramidal compartments or testicular lobules. Each lobule contains loose connective tissue with endocrine interstitial cells (or Leydig cells) secreting testosterone, and one to four highly convoluted seminiferous tubules in which sperm production occurs. Near mediastinum the seminiferous tubules continue in short and straight segments, known as tubuli recti, which connect to rete testis in the mediastinum (Figure 18 − 1, 18 − 2).

1.1 Seminiferous Tubules

In the adult, the seminiferous tubule measures 150 to 250 μm in diameter and 30 to 70 cm in length. Each seminiferous tubule is lined with a complex, specialized stratified epithelium called spermatogenic epithelium. The basement membrane of this epithelium is covered by fibrous connective tissue, with an innermost layer containing fusiform myoid cells, which allow weak contractions of the tubule. The spermatogenic epithelium consists of two types of cells: large nondividing Sertoli cells; dividing cells of the spermatogenic lineage, which comprise five to eight concentric cell layers (Figure 18 − 3, 18 − 4).

1.1.1 Spermatogenic Cells

From the basement toward the lumen of the seminiferous tubules, the germ cells are at various developmental stages, including spermatogonia, primary spermatocytes, secondary

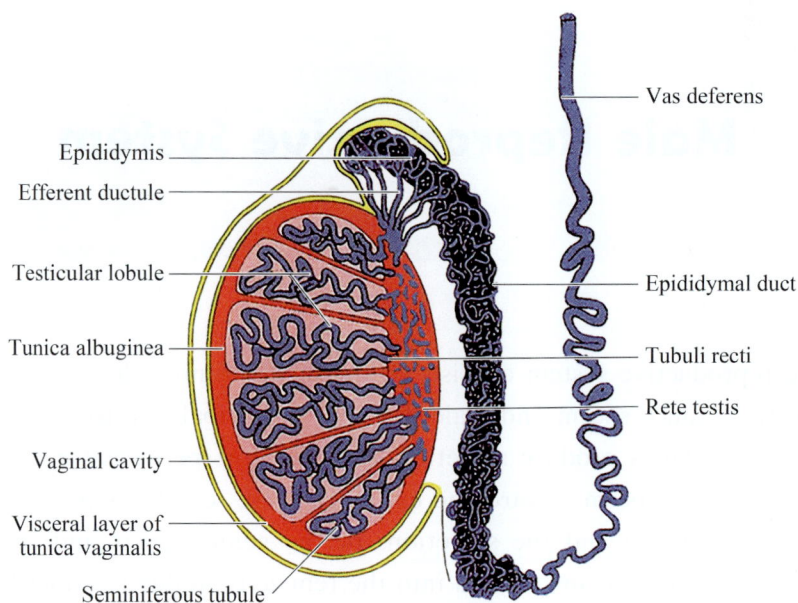

Figure 18 - 1　Schematic of testis and epididymis

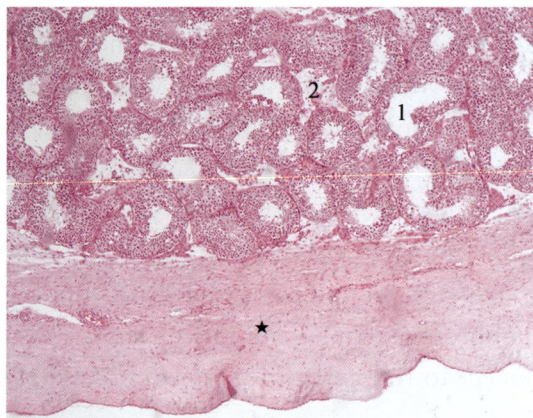

★. Tunica albuginea; 1. Seminiferous tubule; 2. Testicular interstitium
Figure 18 - 2　Light micrograph of part of the testis (HE, 40×)

spermatocytes, spermatids and spermatozoa. These cells undergo the process of spermatogenesis, in which diploid spermatogonia give rise to haploid spermatozoa. This process takes 64 ± 4.5 days, involving spermatogonia mitosis, spermatocyte meiosis, and the final differentiation of spermatids called spermiogenesis (Figure 18 - 5).

1.1.1.1　Spermatogonia

Spermatogonia are round or ovoid cells about 12μm in diameter, occupy a basal niche in the epithelial wall of the tubules, next to the basement membrane. At puberty, spermatogonia enlarge and become mitotically active. A subpopulation called type A spermatogonia act as stem cells, dividing to produce new stem cells and other type A

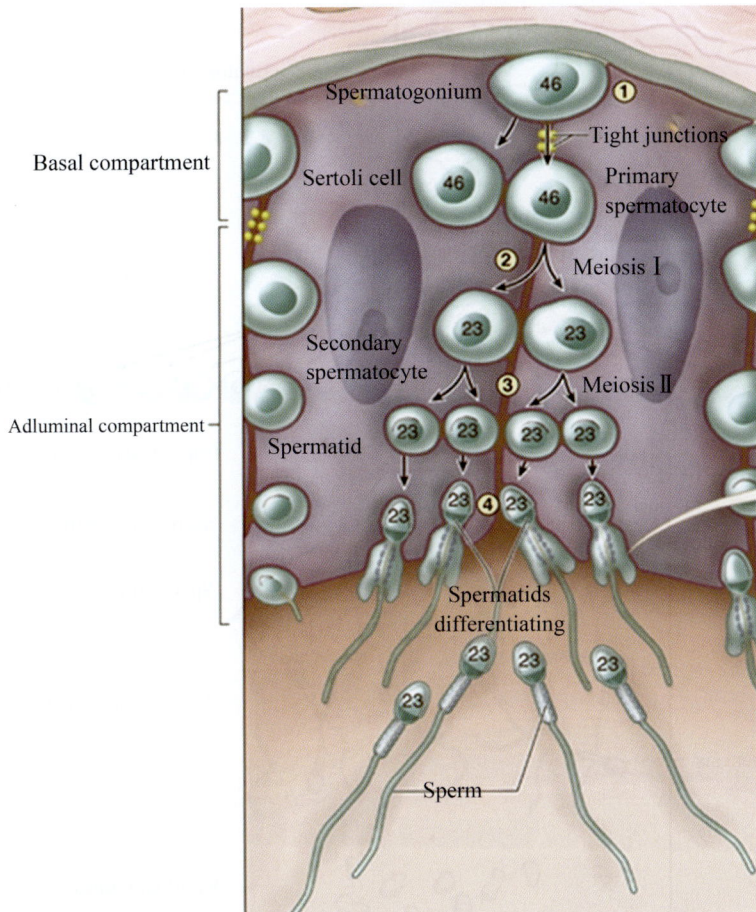

Figure 18 - 3　The diagram of spermatogenic cells and Sertoli cells

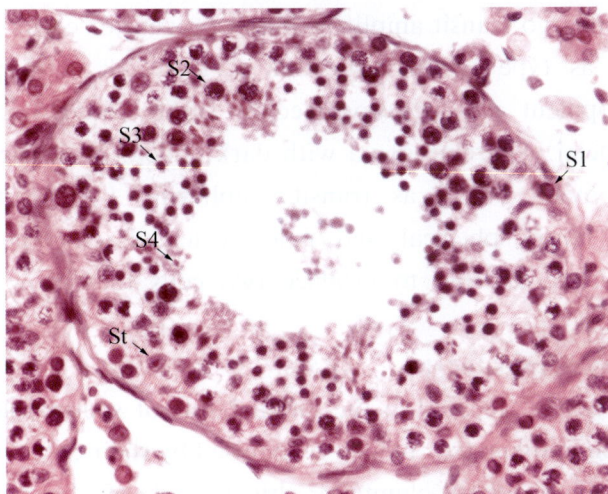

S1. Spermatogonium; S2. Primary spermatocyte; S3. Spermatid; S4. Spermatozoon; St. Sertoli cell

Figure 18 - 4　Light micrograph of seminiferous tubule in transverse section (HE, 400×)

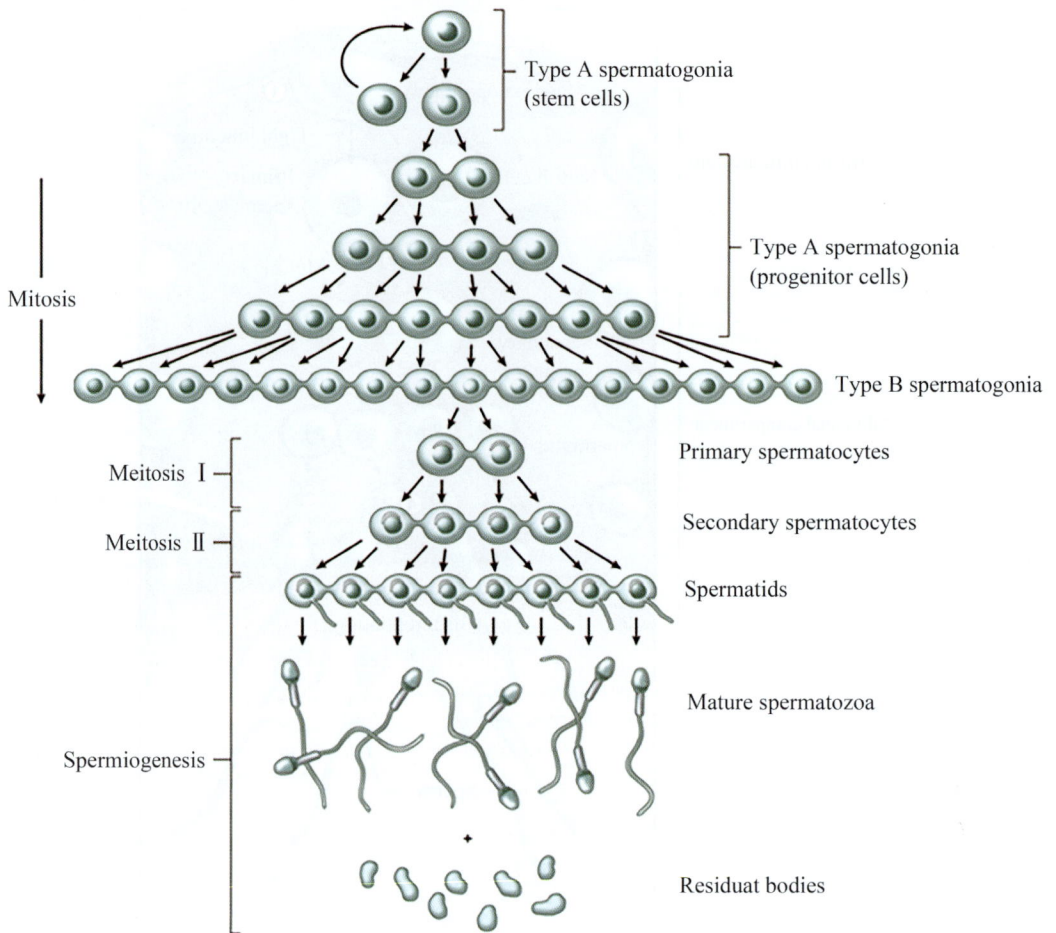

Figure 18 – 5   The diagram of spermatogenesis

spermatogonia that undergo transit amplification as progenitor cells; these progenitor cells further differentiate as type B spermatogonia (Figure 18 – 5). Different stages of spermatogonia development can be recognized by subtle changes in shape and staining properties of their nuclei. Spermatogonia with dark, ovoid nuclei act as stem cells; with more pale-staining, ovoid nuclei as transit amplifying (progenitor) cells. Type B spermatogonia have more spherical and pale nuclei. Each type B spermatogonium undergoes a final mitotic division to produce two cells that grow in size and become primary spermatocytes.

1.1.1.2   Primary Spermatocytes

Primary spermatocytes, located in the luminal side of spermatogonia, are round and large cells about 18 μm in diameter, readily recognised by their copious cytoplasm and large spherical nuclei containing coarse clumps or thin threads of chromatin (Figure 18 – 4). Primary spermatocytes replicate their DNA, so each cell has 46 (44＋XY) chromosomes, and a DNA content of 4N. Soon after their formation, the primary spermatocytes enter the first meiotic prophase that lasts about 3 weeks. Most spermatocytes seen in sections of testis are in this phase of meiosis. The first meiotic division of the primary spermatocytes produces smaller cells called secondary spermatocytes.

1.1.1.3   Secondary Spermatocytes

The secondary spermatocyte is about 12 μm in diameter, with a spherical and dark nucleus; it has only 23 chromosomes ($22+X$ or $22+Y$), but each still consists of two chromatids so the amount of DNA is 2N. Secondary spermatocytes are rare in testis sections because they are very short-lived cells that remain in interphase only briefly and quickly undergo the second meiotic division. Division of each secondary spermatocyte separates the chromatids of each chromosome and produces two haploid cells called spermatids (Figures 18-3 and 18-5).

1.1.1.4   Spermatids

Spermatids can be distinguished by their small size (7-8 μm in diameter) and by nuclei with areas of condensed chromatin. Their position within the seminiferous tubules is close to the lumen. Each spermatid contains 23 chromosomes, and a DNA content of 1N. The spermatid will transform into a sperm. This process is called spermiogenesis. No cell division occurs during this process, but the spermatid undergoes obviously morphological development. The principal changes of spermiogenesis are described as below (Figure 18-6): ① The nucleus becomes more condensed and elongated, with the histones of nucleosomes replaced by protamines. ② Golgi complex transforms the acrosomal vesicle, the latter will further become into the acrosome which like a cap and spreads over the anterior of nucleus. ③ The centrioles migrate to a position near the cell surface and opposite the forming acrosome. One of the centrioles forms the flagellum which is structurally

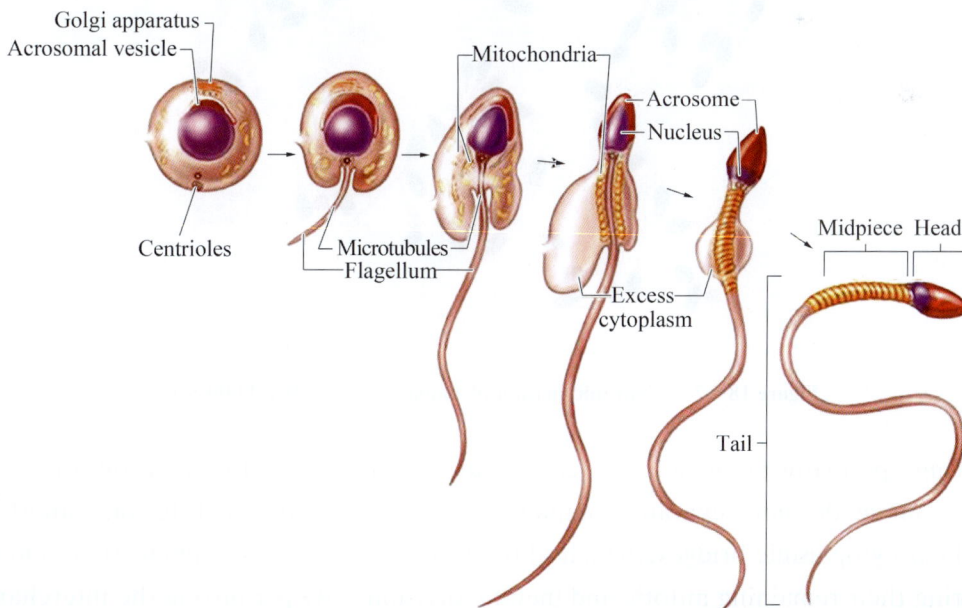

Figure 18-6   The diagram of spermiogenesis

and functionally similar to that of a cilium. ④Mitochondria aggregate around the proximal part of the flagellum, forming mitochondrial sheath where the ATP for flagellar movements is generated. ⑤Unneeded cytoplasm is shed as a residual body from each spermatozoon and phagocytized by Sertoli cells.

1.1.1.5 Spermatozoa

The human spermatozoon is like tadpole in shape, and approximately $60\,\mu$m long and may be subdivided into two parts, the head and the tail (Figure 18 - 7). The shape of the head is oval in anterior view and flattened pyriform in lateral view. The principal components of the head are the nucleus and the acrosome. The condensed nucleus is a compact mass of chromatin. The acrosome overlies the anterior two-thirds of the nucleus; it is a specialized type of lysosome containing hydrolytic enzymes such as hyaluronidase, acrosin, etc. These enzymes play an important role in fertilization (See Chapter 20). Segments of the tail, in order of their proximity to the head, are designated the neck, the middle piece, the principal piece, and the end piece. The axial core of whole tail is called axoneme which is consists of $9+2$ microtubules and surrounded by the nine outer dense fibers arranged in longitudinal. The axoneme is a main movement device of spermatozoa. The neck region of the tail has a pair of centrioles. The middle piece has a mitochondrial sheath which is the energy supply center for spermatozoa. The principal piece is the longest segment in the tail; the outer dense fibers are enclosed in the fibrous sheath, both of these structures assist sperm motility. The end piece is short and only has the axoneme (Figure 18 - 8).

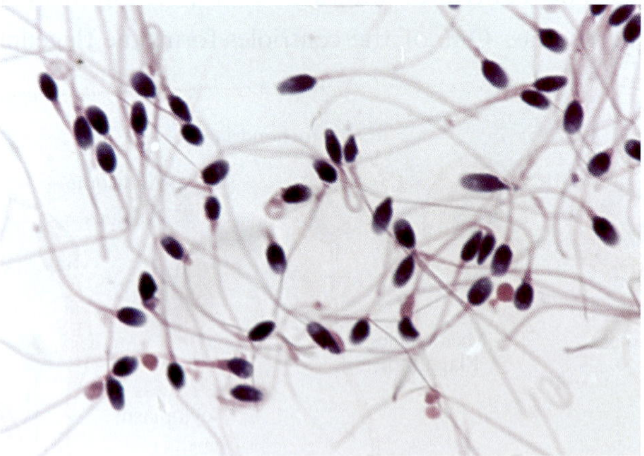

Figure 18 - 7   Light micrograph of human sperm (HE, $1\,000\times$)

During spermatogenesis all the cells that derived from the division of a single spermatogonium do not separate completely but remain attached to one another by intercellular cytoplasmic bridges, which allow free cytoplasmic communication among the cells during their remaining mitotic and meiotic divisions. By permitting the interchange of information from cell to cell, these bridges play an important role in coordinating the

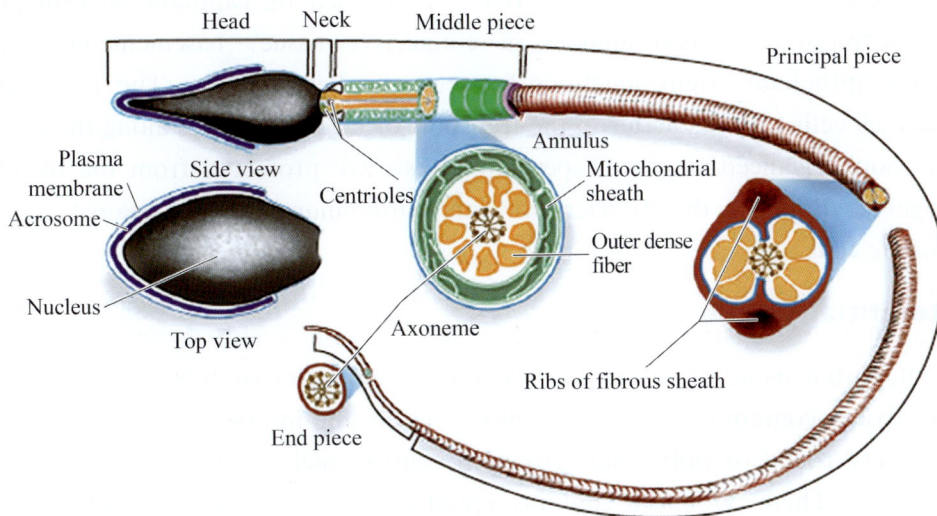

Figure 18 - 8   Ultrastructural schematic of a sperm

sequence of events in spermatogenesis.

1.1.2   Sertoli Cells

Sertoli cells, also called sustentacular cells, are tall pyramidal epithelial cells that form the basal lamina of the seminiferous tubules and partially envelop cells of the spermatogenic lineage. The bases of the Sertoli cells adhere to the basal lamina, and their apical ends extend to the lumen of the seminiferous tubule (Figure 18 - 3). In the light microscope, the outlines of Sertoli cells are poorly defined because of the numerous lateral processes that surround spermatogenic cells. Their nuclei are typically ovoid or triangular, euchromatic, and have a prominent nucleolus (Figure 18 - 4). Ultrastructurally Sertoli cells contain abundant smooth endoplasmic reticulum, some rough endoplasmic reticulum, well-developed Golgi complexes, numerous mitochondria, and lysosomes, as well as microtubules and intermediate filaments forming cytoskeleton. Adjacent Sertoli cells are bound together by tight junctions between their basolateral membranes, such that the seminiferous epithelium is divided into basal compartment and adluminal compartment. Spermatogonia lie in a basal compartment, below the tight junctions. The spermatocytes, spermatids and spermatozoa lie in the adluminal compartment, above the tight junctions (Figure 18 - 3).

Sertoli cells have several functions: ① Supply many plasma factors needed for spermatogenic cell growth and differentiation. ②Assist spermatogenic cells movement and spermatozoa release. ③ Secrete testicular fluid contributing to sperm transport; secrete androgen-binding protein (ABP) (promoted by FSH), which concentrates testosterone to a level required for spermatogenesis; secrete inhibin and activin, the former suppresses synthesis and release of FSH, the latter has antagonistic effects to the former. ④Phagocytize and digest the residual bodies that shed during spermiogenesis. ⑤Form a blood-testis barrier: the blood-testis barrier is composed of capillary endothelium and basement membrane, a small amount of connective tissue, basement membrane of seminiferous epithelium, tight junctions between the Sertoli cells. The tight junctions between Sertoli cells form a barrier to the transport of large molecules along the cell space. Thus, the more advanced stages of spermatogenesis are protected from the blood-borne noxious agents. Besides, this barrier prevents autoimmune attacks against the unique spermatogenic cells.

1.2　Interstitial Tissue

The interstitial tissue of the testis between the seminiferous tubules consists of loose connective tissue, containing lymphatics, blood vessels and interstitial cells (Leydig cells). Leydig cells are round or polygonal cells with central nuclei and eosinophilic cytoplasm (Figure 18 - 9). Their cytoplasm contains abundant, tightly packed smooth endoplasmic reticulum (SER), numerous scattered mitochondria with tubulovesicular cristae, and many spherical lipid droplets of various sizes, a typical feature of steroid-secreting cells. Leydig cells produce the androgen (mainly testosterone), which is responsible for spermatogenesis, the development and differentiation of the male reproductive organs, maintenance of the secondary sex characteristics and the sexuality.

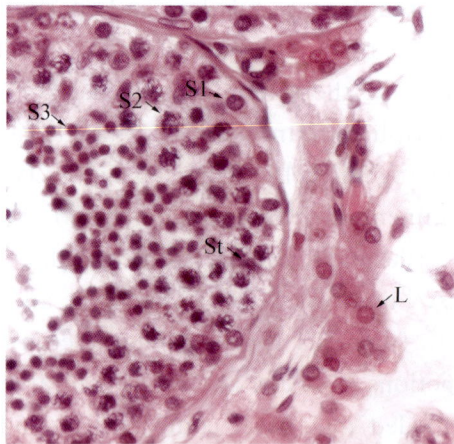

S1. Spermatogonium; S2. Primary spermatocyte; S3. Spermatid; St. Sertoli cell; L. Leydig cell
Figure 18 - 9　Light micrograph of a clump of Leydig cells (HE, 400×)

1.3　Straight Tubule and Rete Testis

Near mediastinum the seminiferous tubules continue in short and straight segments, known as straight tubule. This portion of the tubule is loss of spermatogenic cells and lied by the simple cuboidal or short columnar epithelium. Straight tubule confluent with the rete testis, contained within the mediastinum. The rete testis is a highly anastomotic network of channels lined with simple cuboidal epithelium. These ducts drain testicular fluid and spermatozoa to the epididymis (Figure 18 - 1).

1.4　Endocrine Regulation of Testis Function

Spermatogenesis depends on the action of two kinds of hormone secreted by the hypophysis, FSH and luteinizing hormone (LH), on the testicular cells. LH acts on the interstitial cells, stimulating the production of testosterone necessary for the normal development of spermatogenic cells. FSH is known to act on the Sertoli cells, promoting the synthesis and secretion of androgen-binding protein; this protein combines with testosterone and transports it into the lumen of the seminiferous tubules, ensuring the hormone level required for spermatogenesis. Meanwhile, the inhibin secreted by Sertoli cells and the androgen secreted by interstitial cells feedback suppresses secretion of GnRH, FSH and LH.

2　Genital Ducts

Genital ducts include the epididymis, vas deferens, and urethra, which provide a beneficial environment for spermatozoon maturation, storage and transportation.

2.1　Epididymis

The epididymis caps the superior and posterior sides of each testis, which divided into three parts: an initial (head) segment, a body, and a caudal (tail) region (Figure 18 - 1). The head consists of 8 - 12 efferent ducts that extend from the rete testis. The efferent duct has an unusual epithelium in which groups of nonciliated cuboidal cells alternate with groups of taller ciliated cells and give the epithelium a characteristic scalloped appearance (Figure 18 - 10). The nonciliated cells absorb some of the fluid secreted by the Sertoli cells. This absorption and the ciliary activity create a fluid

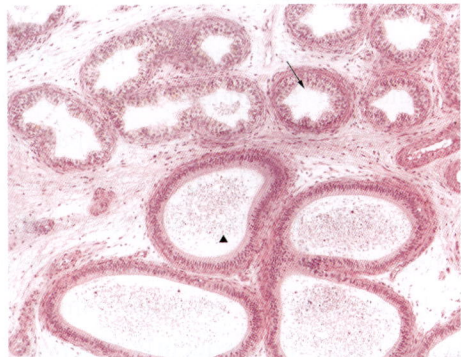

↑. Efferent duct; ▲. Epididymal duct

Figure 18 - 10　Light micrograph of the epididymis (HE, 100×)

flow that carries sperm out of the testis and sweeps toward the body and tail of epididymis.

The efferent ducts gradually fuse to form the epididymal duct, a single highly coiled tube about 4 - 6 m in length. Together with surrounding connective tissue and blood vessels, this long canal forms the body and tail of the epididymis. It is lined with pseudostratified columnar epithelium consisting of tall columnar (principal) cells with characteristic long stereocilia, and small basal (stem) cells (Figure 18 - 10). The principal cells secrete glycolipids and glycoproteins, but also absorb water and remove residual bodies or other debris not removed earlier by Sertoli cells. The duct epithelium is surrounded by a few layers of smooth muscle cells, whose peristaltic contractions move the sperm along the duct and empties the body and tail regions at ejaculation. While passing through this duct, sperm become motile and their surfaces and acrosomes undergo final maturation steps, which is closely related to the secretion of epididymal epithelium.

2.2 Vas Deferens

The vas deferens, a continuation of the epididymis, is a long straight tube with a thick wall and a relatively small lumen, composed of mucosa, muscularis, and adventitia. The mucosa epithelial is pseudostratified; the lamina propria contains many elastic fibers. The very thick muscularis consists of longitudinal inner and outer layers and a middle circular layer; they produce strong peristaltic contractions during ejaculation, which rapidly move sperm along this duct from the epididymis. The outermost adventitia is loose connective tissue containing blood vessels and nerves.

3　Accessory Glands

Accessory glands include prostate, seminal vesicle and bulbourethral gland. The secretions of accessory gland and genital ducts form the semen together with sperm.

3.1 Prostate

The prostate encircles the initial segment of urethra, is surrounded by a fibroelastic capsule rich in smooth muscle, from which septa extends and divides the gland into indistinct lobes. The prostate parenchyma is a collection of 30 – 50 branched compound tubuloacinar glands. Ducts from individual gland may converge but all empty directly into the prostatic urethra, which runs through the center of the prostate. The acinus is lined alternately by simple cuboidal, simple columnar or pseudostratified columnar epithelial cells, forming the irregular lumen. Small spherical acidophilic bodies, named prostatic concretions, are frequently observed in acinar lumina (Figure 18 – 11); their significance is not understood, but their number increases with age and often calcified as prostatic calculus.

The glands are arranged in three major zones around the urethra (Figure 18 – 12): The periurethral zone (also named mucosal gland) is minimum and locates in the urethral mucosa; this zone is the site where most benign prostatic hyperplasia originates. The inner zone (also named submucosal gland) locates in the submucosa. The outer zone contains the prostate's main glands, which is the major site of prostatic cancer.

The prostate can produce fluid that contains various glycoproteins, enzymes, and small molecules such as prostaglandins, which participates in semen composition and affects sperm motility and fertilization ability.

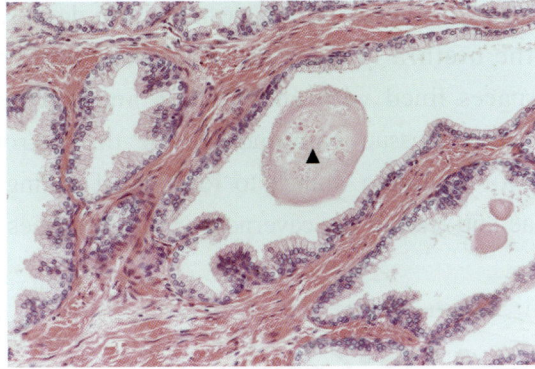

▲. prostatic concretion

Figure 18－11   Light micrograph of the prostate（HE，200×）

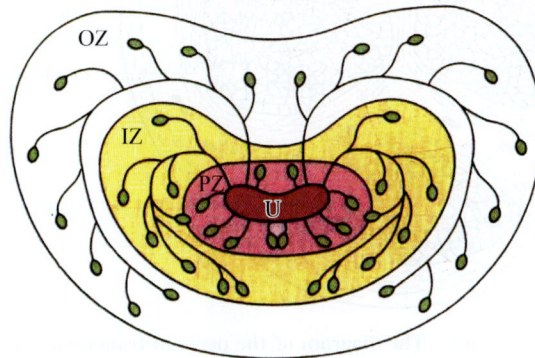

OZ. Outer zone；IZ. Inner zone；PZ. Periurethral zone；U. Urethra

Figure 18－12   The diagram of the prostate structure

3.2 Seminal Vesicles

The seminal vesicles are pair of convoluted saccular organs. The mucosa displays a great number of folds and is lining with pseudostratified columnar epithelial cells rich in secretory granules. A small amount of smooth muscle and connective tissue adventitia overlay the outside of mucosa. The seminal vesicles produce a viscid, yellowish secretion containing fructose, prostaglandins, etc, among which fructose is a major energy source for sperm motility.

3.3 Bulbourethral Glands

The bulbourethral glands are pair of pea-like compound tubuloacinar glands. During erection they release a clear mucus-like secretion that coats and lubricates the urethra in preparation for the imminent passage of sperm.

4 Penis

The penis consists of three erectile tissues, plus the penile urethra, surrounded by skin. Two of the erectile masses, the corpora cavernosa, are dorsal; the corpus spongiosum is ventral and surrounds the urethra (Figure 18 - 13). All three erectile tissues consist of many venous cavernous spaces lined with endothelium and separated by trabeculae with smooth muscle and connective tissue continuous with the surrounding tunic. Arteriae profunda penis in the corpora cavernosa branch to form small coiling helicine arteries, which travel through the trabeculae and lead to the cavernous vascular spaces of erectile tissue.

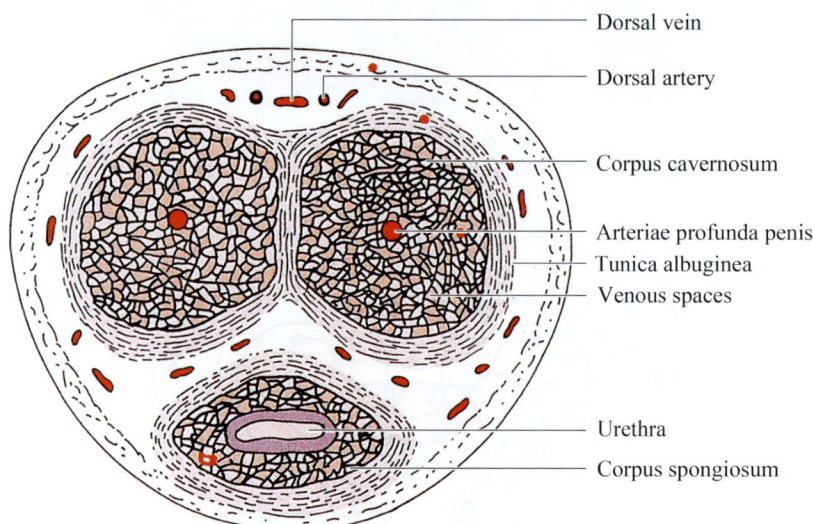

Figure 18 - 13 The diagram of the penis in transverse section

Penile erection involves blood filling the cavernous spaces in the three masses of erectile tissue, which is controlled by autonomic nerves in these vascular walls. Parasympathetic stimulation relaxes the trabecular smooth muscle and dilates the helicine arteries, allowing increased blood flow and filling the cavernous spaces. This enlarges the corpora cavernosa and causes them to compress the dorsal veins against the dense tunica albuginea, which blocks the venous outflow and produces tumescence and rigidity in the erectile tissue.

(Zhu Hui)

第十八章　男性生殖系统

　　男性生殖系统由睾丸、生殖管道、附属腺和阴茎组成。睾丸产生精子并分泌雄激素(主要是睾酮)。生殖管道是储存和运送精子的器官,其与附属腺的分泌物能促进精子成熟、营养精子并保障其功能。生殖管道和附属腺的分泌物与精子一起构成精液,通过阴茎进入女性生殖道。

第一节　睾　丸

睾丸呈扁椭圆形,重约15g,包裹在一层较厚的致密结缔组织囊即白膜中,表面覆以鞘膜脏层。白膜在睾丸后缘增厚形成睾丸纵隔,纵隔的结缔组织呈放射状伸入睾丸实质将其分成约250个锥形睾丸小叶。每个小叶内有1～4条细长弯曲的生精小管,它们在接近纵隔处变为短而直的直精小管,进入纵隔内相互吻合形成睾丸网。生精小管之间的疏松结缔组织称睾丸间质,其中有分泌激素的Leydig细胞(图18-1、图18-2)。

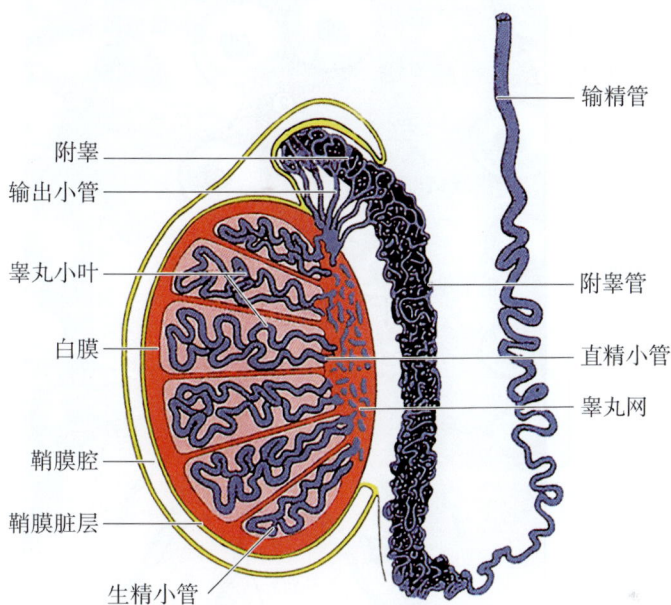

图18-1　睾丸与附睾模式图

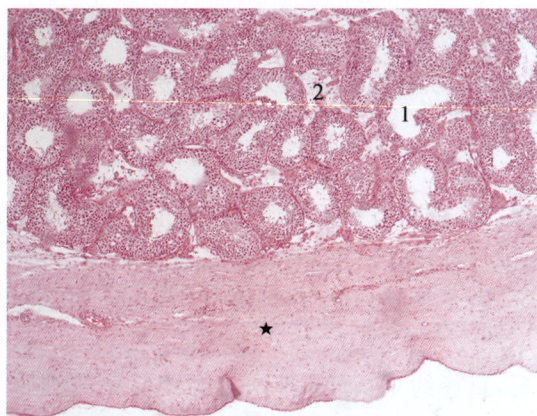

★—白膜;1—生精小管;2—睾丸间质
图18-2　睾丸光镜图(HE染色,40×)

一、生精小管

成人的生精小管长 30~70 cm,直径 150~250 μm,管壁由特殊的复层上皮构成,即生精上皮。生精上皮由支持细胞和 5~8 层生精细胞组成。上皮基膜外侧有纤维结缔组织和梭形的肌样细胞,肌样细胞收缩有助于精子排出(图 18-3、图 18-4)。

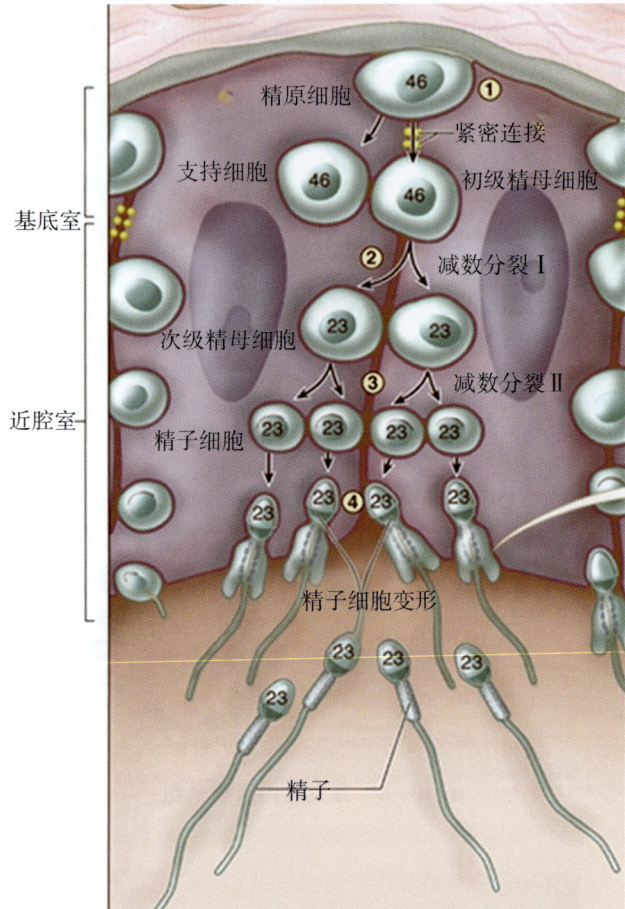

图 18-3 生精小管中生精细胞和支持细胞模式图

(一) 生精细胞

自生精小管基底部至腔面,依次有精原细胞、初级精母细胞、次级精母细胞、精子细胞和精子。精原细胞形成精子的过程称精子发生,人需要 64±4.5 天完成,该过程经历了精原细胞有丝分裂、精母细胞减数分裂、精子细胞分化(精子形成)三个阶段(图 18-5)。

1. 精原细胞

靠近基膜,圆或卵圆形,直径约 12 μm。进入青春期后精原细胞呈现有丝分裂活跃状态,其中 A 型精原细胞为干细胞,不断地分裂增殖,一部分子细胞仍为干细胞,另一部分则为祖细胞、可增殖分化为 B 型精原细胞(图 18-5)。不同发育阶段的精原细胞在细胞核形状和染色特性上有细微差别:A 型精原细胞核为卵圆形,染色较深者为干细胞,染色较浅的为祖细胞;B

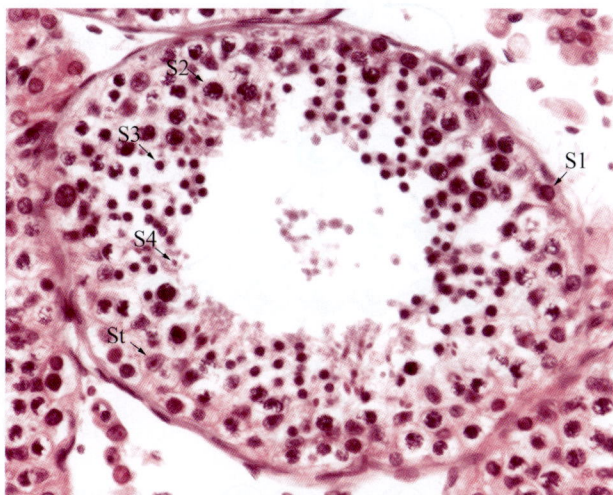

S1—精原细胞；S2—初级精母细胞；S3—精子细胞；S4—精子；St—支持细胞

图 18 - 4　生精小管光镜图(横断面,HE 染色,400×)

型精原细胞核多为球形,染色较淡。B 型精原细胞经过数次分裂后,分化为初级精母细胞。

2. 初级精母细胞

位于精原细胞近腔侧,圆形,直径约 18 μm。细胞核大而圆,丝球状,内含或粗或细的染色质丝,核型为 46,XY(图 18 - 4)。初级精母细胞经过 DNA 复制后(4nDNA),进行第一次减数分裂,形成两个次级精母细胞。第一次减数分裂前期历时较长(持续约 3 周),睾丸切片中大多数精母细胞都处于这个阶段。

3. 次级精母细胞

直径约 12 μm,细胞核呈球形,染色较深。细胞核型为 23,X 或 23,Y;每条染色体仍由两个染色单体组成,因此 DNA 数量是 2n。因次级精母细胞只在间期短暂存在即进入第二次减数分裂,故在睾丸切片中不易见到。次级精母细胞分裂时将每条染色体的染色单体分开,产生两个单倍体的精子细胞(图 18 - 3、18 - 5)。

4. 精子细胞

靠近管腔,直径约 8 μm,细胞核圆,染色质浓缩。细胞核型为 23,X 或 23,Y (1nDNA)。精子细胞不再分裂,而是经过复杂的形态发育转化为精子,这一过程称精子形成,主要包括(图 18 - 6):①细胞核浓缩、伸长,成为精子头部主要结构,核小体中组蛋白被鱼精蛋白取代。②高尔基复合体形成顶体小泡,后者融合形成顶体覆盖于细胞核前端。③中心粒迁移到细胞核另一端,与顶体相对,其中一个中心粒形成轴丝,是精子尾部(或称鞭毛)的主要结构。④线粒体聚集在鞭毛的近端,形成线粒体鞘,产生精子运动所需的 ATP。⑤多余的细胞质脱落形成残余体,被支持细胞吞噬。

5. 精子

人的精子形似蝌蚪,长约 60 μm,可分为头、尾两部分(图 18 - 7)。头部正面观为卵圆形,侧面观呈梨形。头部有一个高度浓缩的细胞核,其前 2/3 有顶体覆盖。顶体是特殊的溶酶体,内含各种水解酶,如透明质酸酶、顶体酶等,在受精过程中发挥重要作用(见第二十章)。尾部分为颈段、中段、主段和末段四部分。构成尾部全长的轴心是轴丝,由 9＋2 排列的微管组成,

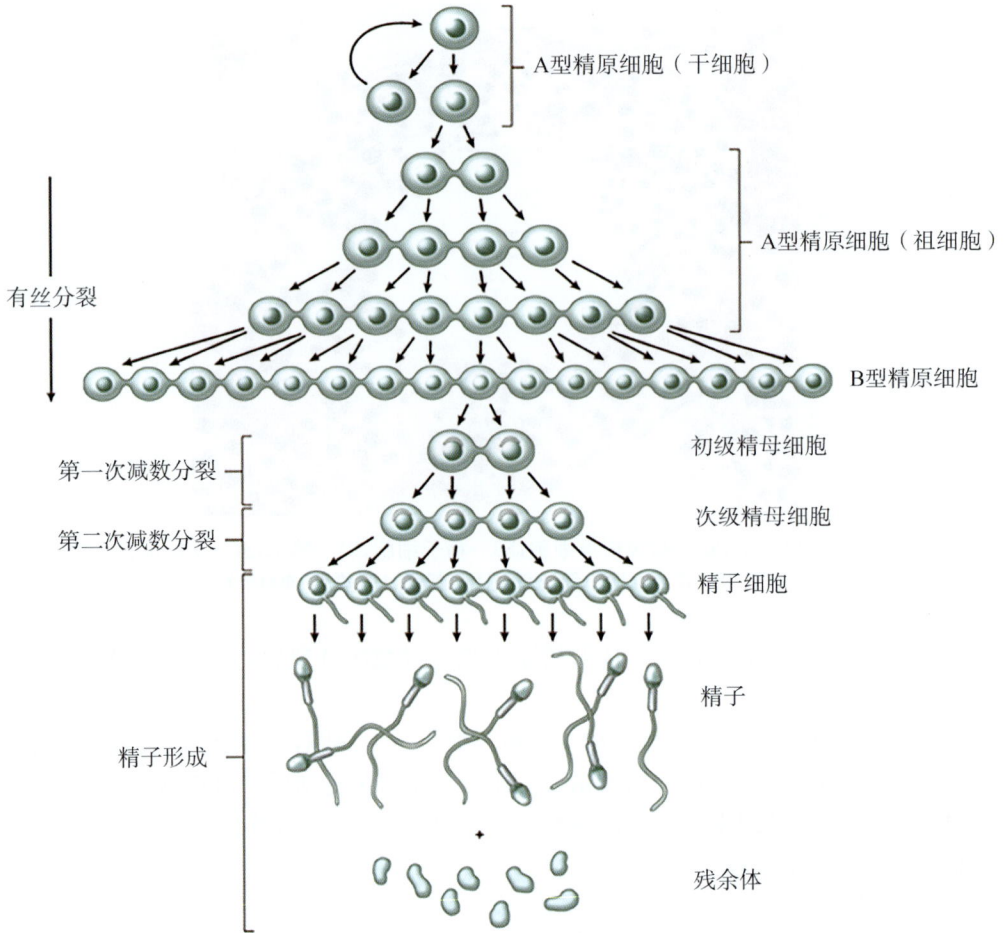

图 18-5　精子发生示意图

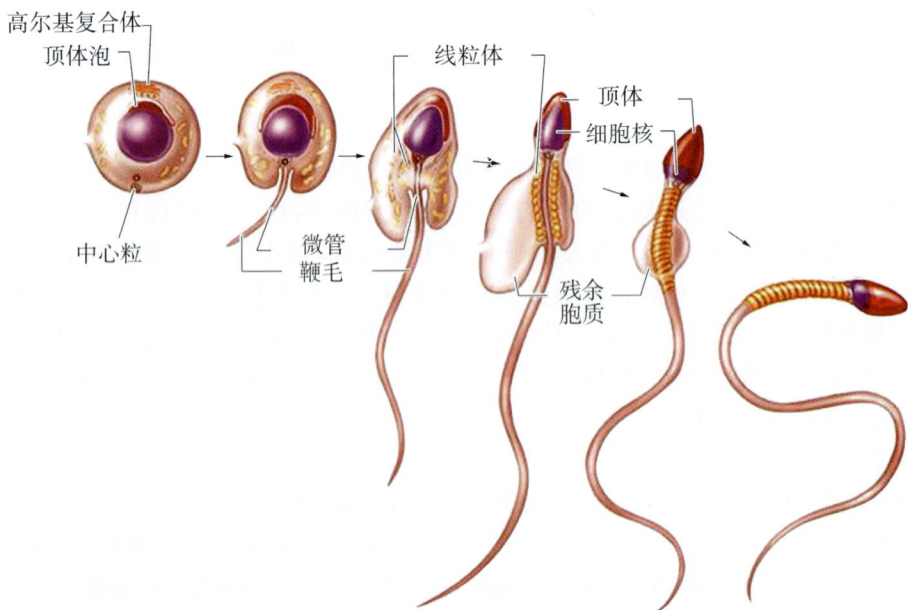

图 18-6　精子形成模式图

是精子运动的主要装置;轴丝外有 9 根纵行的外周致密纤维。颈段有中心粒。中段的外侧包有线粒体鞘,是精子的能量供应中心。主段最长,外周致密纤维外方有纤维鞘,这两种结构均辅助精子运动。末段短,其内仅有轴丝(图 18-8)。

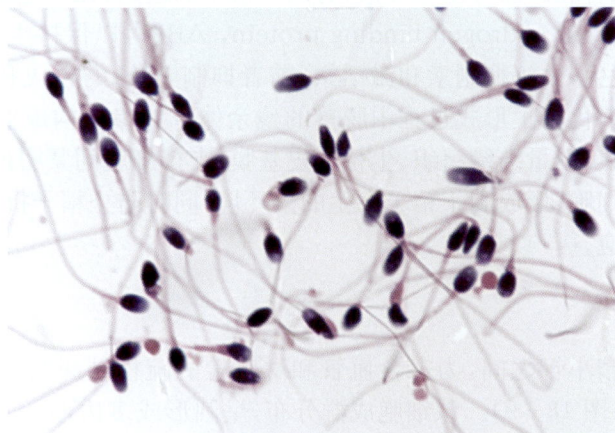

图 18-7　人精子光镜图(HE 染色,1 000×)

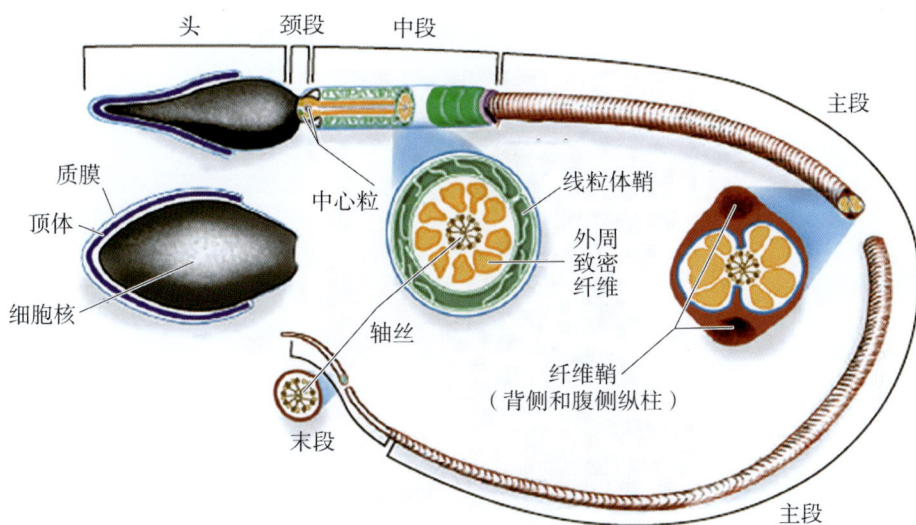

图 18-8　精子超微结构模式图

在精子发生过程中,一个精原细胞增殖分化所产生的各级生精细胞,其细胞质并未完全分开,有胞质桥相连,形成同步发育的同源细胞群。胞质桥的存在有利于细胞间信息传递,协调精子发生的有序进行。

(二) 支持细胞

支持细胞,又称 Sertoli 细胞。细胞为长锥体形,其基部附着于生精小管基膜,顶端伸达小管腔面(图 18-3)。光镜下支持细胞轮廓不清,因其侧面伸出突起,其间镶嵌各级生精细胞;细胞核为卵圆形或三角形,染色浅,核仁明显(图 18-4)。电镜下,细胞质内有丰富的滑面内质网、粗面内质网,高尔基复合体发达,线粒体和溶酶体较多,并有许多微丝和微管。相邻支持细胞侧面在近基底部形成紧密连接,将生精上皮分成基底室和近腔室两部分。精原细胞位于紧密连接下方的基底室,精母细胞、精子细胞和精子位于紧密连接上方的近腔室内(图 18 - 3)。

支持细胞发挥重要功能,包括:①对生精细胞起支持和营养作用。②协助生精细胞向腔面移动,并使精子释放入管腔。③分泌睾丸液,有助于精子的运送;在卵泡刺激素(FSH)作用下,合成分泌雄激素结合蛋白(androgen binding protein,ABP),以保持生精小管内有较高的雄激素水平,促进精子发生;分泌抑制素和激活素,前者抑制 FSH 的合成和分泌,后者对前者有拮抗作用。④吞噬和消化精子形成过程中脱落的残余体。⑤参与构成血-睾屏障:血-睾屏障由毛细血管内皮和基膜、少量结缔组织、生精上皮基膜、支持细胞间紧密连接组成;可阻止血液中有害物质接触生精细胞、形成利于精子发生的微环境,同时防止精子抗原物质逸出生精小管外而引发自身免疫反应。

二、睾丸间质

睾丸间质位于生精小管之间,为富含血管和淋巴管的疏松结缔组织,其中有睾丸间质细胞,又称 Leydig 细胞(图 18 - 9)。该细胞成群分布,呈圆形或多边形,细胞核圆,胞质嗜酸性,具有类固醇激素分泌细胞的超微结构特点(富含滑面内质网、管状嵴线粒体和脂滴)。睾丸间质细胞分泌雄激素(主要是睾酮),可启动和维持精子发生和男性生殖器官发育,以及维持第二性征和性功能。

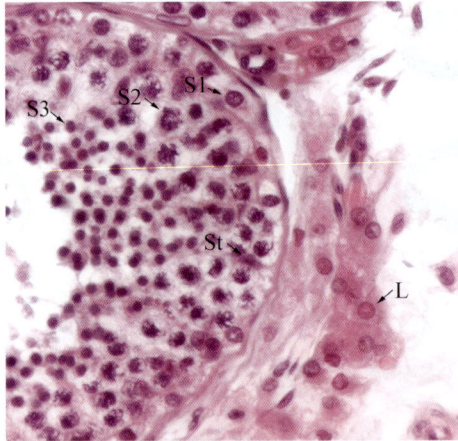

S1—精原细胞;S2—初级精母细胞;S3—精子细胞;St—睾丸支持细胞;L—睾丸间质细胞
图 18 - 9　睾丸间质及生精小管局部光镜图(HE 染色,400×)

三、直精小管和睾丸网

生精小管近睾丸纵隔处延伸为短而细的直行管道,称直精小管,管壁上皮为单层立方或矮柱状,无生精细胞。直精小管进入睾丸纵隔内分支吻合成网状管道,为睾丸网,由单层立方上皮组成。这些小管把睾丸液和精子运送入附睾(图 18 - 1)。

四、睾丸功能的内分泌调节

精子发生依赖于垂体分泌的两种激素 FSH 和黄体生成素(LH)对睾丸细胞的作用。LH

作用于 Leydig 细胞,促进睾酮的合成和分泌。FSH 作用于支持细胞,促进 ABP 的合成和分泌;ABP 与睾酮结合,保持生精小管内高浓度的雄激素环境,促进精子发生。同时,支持细胞分泌的抑制素和 Leydig 细胞分泌的雄激素反馈抑制下丘脑 GnRH 和腺垂体 FSH、LH 的分泌。

第二节 生殖管道

包括附睾、输精管和尿道,为精子的成熟、贮存和输送提供有利的环境。

一、附睾

附睾位于睾丸的后外侧,分头、体、尾三部(图 18-1)。头部由 8～12 条从睾丸网延伸来的输出小管组成;管壁上皮由无纤毛立方细胞和高柱状纤毛细胞交替排列构成,故腔面不规则(图 18-10)。无纤毛细胞能吸收管腔内一些物质,这种吸收作用和纤毛运动共同产生液体流,将精子带出睾丸并扫向附睾体、尾部。

输出小管融合成一根附睾管,长约 4～6 米,高度盘曲并与周围结缔组织和血管一起形成附睾体、尾部。管壁上皮为假复层纤毛柱状上皮,由主细胞和基细胞组成(图 18-10);主细胞较高,表面有静纤毛,具分泌和吸收功能;基细胞矮小,是干细胞。上皮外侧有薄层平滑肌,其收缩有助于精子在管道中的运送。精子通过附睾后,获得运动能力及功能上的成熟,这与附睾上皮的分泌物密切相关。

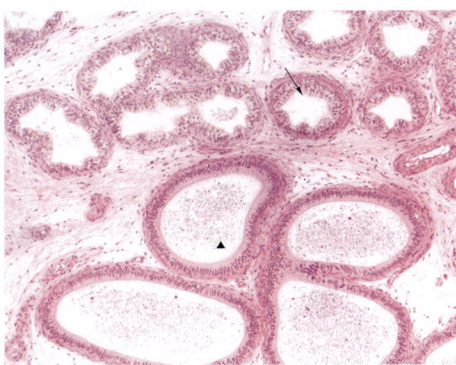

↑—输出小管;▲—附睾管

图 18-10 附睾光镜图(HE 染色,100×)

二、输精管

输精管是附睾的延续,是一个腔小壁厚的长直管,管壁由黏膜、肌层和外膜组成。黏膜上皮为假复层,固有层含有大量弹性纤维。肌层厚,由内纵行、中环行和外纵行排列的平滑肌组成,它们在射精时强烈收缩,将精子快速排出。外膜是含有血管和神经的疏松结缔组织。

第三节 附属腺

附属腺包括前列腺、精囊和尿道球腺,它们和生殖管道的分泌物一起与精子共同组成精液。

一、前列腺

环绕于尿道起始段,表面覆盖富含弹性纤维和平滑肌的结缔组织被膜,并伸入腺内分隔组织。腺实质主要由 30～50 个复管泡状腺组成,它们的导管汇集后开口于前列腺尿道部(穿过前列腺中心)。腺泡由单层立方、单层柱状或假复层柱状上皮细胞交替排列构成,故腺腔不规则；腔内可见球形嗜酸性小体，称为前列腺凝固体(图 18 - 11)。这些小体的意义尚不清楚，但它们随年龄的增长而增加，并常钙化为前列腺结石。

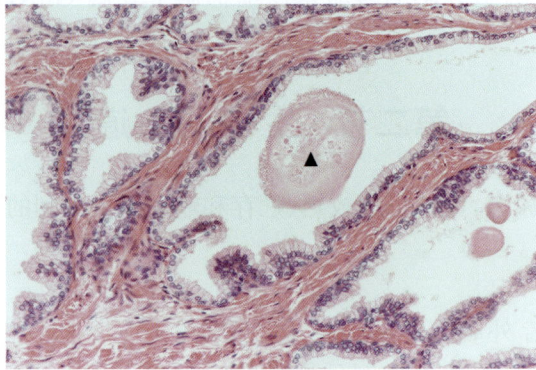

▲—前列腺凝固体
图 18 - 11　前列腺光镜图(HE 染色，200 ×)

腺体可分三个带(图 18 - 12)：①尿道周带(又称黏膜腺)，最小，位于尿道黏膜内，该区域是大多数良性前列腺增生的起源地；②内带(又称黏膜下腺)，位于黏膜下层；③外带(又称主腺)，构成前列腺的大部，前列腺癌主要发生在该部位。

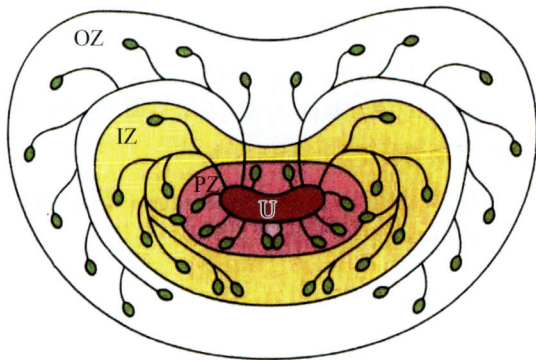

OZ—外带；IZ—内带；PZ—尿道周带；U—尿道
图 18 - 12　前列腺整体结构示意图

前列腺的分泌液含各种糖蛋白、酶及前列腺素等小分子，它们参与精液的组成，影响精子的运动和受精能力。

二、精囊

精囊是一对盘曲的囊状器官。黏膜向腔内突起形成皱襞，表面覆盖假复层柱状上皮，其细胞内含有很多分泌颗粒。黏膜外有少量平滑肌和结缔组织外膜。精囊分泌黏稠的黄色液体，内含果糖、前列腺素等，其中果糖为精子运动提供能量。

三、尿道球腺

尿道球腺是一对豌豆状的复管泡状腺。在勃起过程中，它们释放出一种透明的黏液样分泌物,覆盖并润滑尿道,为精子即将通过做准备。

第四节　阴　茎

　　阴茎由三个勃起组织、阴茎尿道及周围的皮肤构成。背侧的勃起组织为两个阴茎海绵体;腹侧勃起组织环绕尿道,为 1 个尿道海绵体(图 18-13)。这三个勃起组织均由许多静脉海绵窦组成,窦之间由含平滑肌和结缔组织(与周围白膜延续)的小梁分隔,窦腔内衬内皮。阴茎深动脉分支形成螺旋动脉,穿行于小梁并与静脉海绵窦通连。

　　阴茎勃起时,在副交感神经刺激下,小梁平滑肌放松,螺旋动脉扩张,血流量增加而填充海绵窦腔,使得海绵体增大,压迫背静脉抵住致密的白膜,从而阻断静脉流出,使勃起组织肿胀和僵硬。

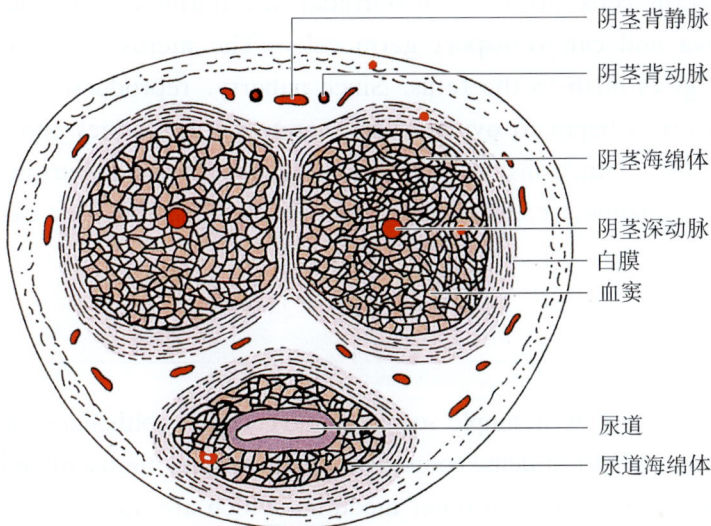

图 18-13　阴茎横断面模式图

标注:阴茎背静脉、阴茎背动脉、阴茎海绵体、阴茎深动脉、白膜、血窦、尿道、尿道海绵体

（祝　辉）

Chapter 19

Female Reproductive System

The female reproductive system consists of the paired ovaries and oviducts (fallopian tubes, or uterine tubes), the uterus, the vagina, and the external genitalia. Ovaries produce female germ cells (ova) and steroidal sex hormones. Oviducts are sites for fertilization of ova and can transport germ cells. The uterus is the organ that forms menstruation and gives birth to the fetus. Since puberty, reproductive organs and breasts mature rapidly, ovaries begin to ovulate and secrete sex hormones and the endometrium changes periodically. Functions of ovaries gradually decline during menopause. In addition, mammary glands are included in this chapter because they can secrete milk to feed babies.

1 Ovary

Each ovary is covered by a simple squamous or cuboidal epithelium, surface epithelium, which is overlying a thin layer of dense connective tissue capsule, tunica albuginea. An ovary is divided into an outer cortex and an inner medulla, which are not clearly demarcated. The cortex is thick and consists of follicles and the corpus luteum at different developmental stages, as well as connective tissue rich in fusiform stromal cells and reticular fibers, while the medulla is thin and is composed of loose connective tissue, containing lots of elastic fibers, blood vessels, lymphatic vessels and nerves. One side of the ovary is the ovarian hilum, where there are some smooth muscles and hilus cells; the hilus cell is similar to the Leydig cell and is generally believed to secrete androgen (Figure 19 – 1).

The development of follicles in the ovarian cortex changes periodically. Seven hundred thousand to 2 million primordial follicles begin to develop in newborns. At the beginning of puberty, there are about 40,000 follicles, and only a few hundred follicles remain at the age of 40 to 50 years old. From puberty to menopause, ovaries ovulate periodically according to the menstrual cycle under the influence of gonadotropins secreted by the pituitary gland. There are 15 to 20 follicles growing and developing every 28 days, and generally only one dominant follicle can mature and ovulate. Normal women ovulate more than 400 times in their lifetime and most of the remaining follicles degenerate into atretic follicles at different stages of development. Ovaries no longer ovulate after menopause.

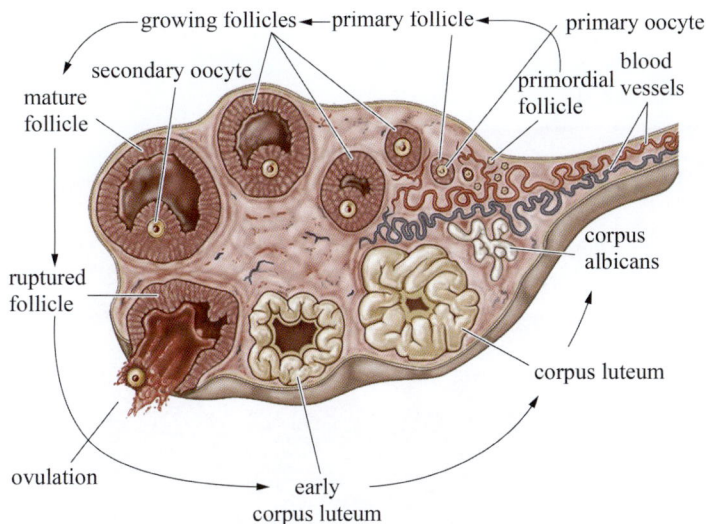

Figure 19 - 1　Schematic of an ovary

1.1　Development and Maturation of Follicles

A follicle is composed of an oocyte and multiple surrounding follicle cells, and is spherical in shape. The follicular development is a continuous change process, roughly going through four stages: primordial follicle, primary follicle, secondary follicle and mature follicle. Primary follicles and secondary follicles are also called growing follicles.

1.1.1　Primordial Follicle

Primordial follicles are resting follicles located in the superficial cortex, with small sizes and a large number. Each primordial follicle consists of a primary oocyte enveloped by a single layer of fattened follicular cells. The primary oocyte is round and large, with a big, spherical and eccentric nucleus, in which the chromatin is sparse and lightly stained, and the nucleolus is prominent. The cytoplasm is rich and eosinophilic (Figure 19 - 2). The primary oocyte is derived from the division and differentiation of the oogonia during the embryonic period, and then enters the first meiosis and stays in the prophase for a long time. The division would not be completed until ovulation. The monolayer follicular cells are surrounding the primary oocyte, which are flat, with small cell bodies and oblate and dark nuclei. There is a thin basement membrane between the follicular cells and the surrounding connective tissue, while many gap junctions connect the follicular cells and the oocyte, enabling the follicular cells to support and nourish the oocyte.

1.1.2　Primary Follicle

Primary follicles develop from primordial follicles, located in the deep part of the cortex. The main structural changes are as follows: ①Former flattened follicular cells are transformed into cuboidal or columnar, and then proliferate and differentiate from monolayer to multilayer. Under electron microscope, their rough endoplasmic reticula,

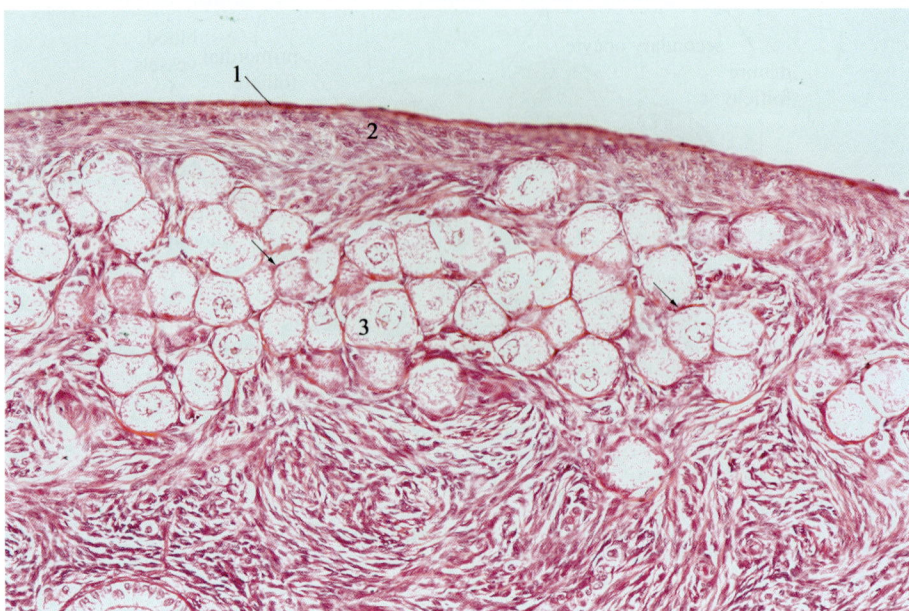

1. Surface epithelium; 2. Tunica albuginea; 3. Primary oocytes; Arrows. Follicular cells

Figure 19 - 2   Light micrograph of primordial follicles

free ribosomes and mitochondria become more extensive, and the Golgi complex is more developed. ②The primary oocyte expands, with increased cytoplasm. Its nucleus becomes larger and bubbly, and the nucleolus is deeply stained. Under electron microscope, there are more Golgi complex, rough endoplasmic reticula and free ribosomes. Cortical granules appear in the superficial cytoplasm, a kind of lysosome that can prevent polysperm fertilization during fertilization. ③There is a perivitelline space between the primary oocyte and the follicular cells, into which the processes of the inner follicular cells and the microvilli of the primary oocytes extend. Extracellular materials accumulate as zona pellucida in the interspace, forming a thick eosinophilic membrane, which is composed of zona pellucida proteins, mainly including ZP1, ZP2, ZP3 and ZP4. The zona pellucida proteins play an important role in recognition and specific binding between sperm and ovum. Gap junctions link the processes of the follicular cells and the primary oocyte membrane, assisting material exchange and information communication. ④Stromal cells immediately outside each growing primary follicle differentiate to form the follicular theca (Figure 19 - 3).

1.1.3 Secondary Follicle

The primary follicle continues to grow and differentiate, and then becomes secondary follicle when a fluid cavity appears between the follicular cells. The main features of the secondary follicle structure are as follows: ① Liquid cavities of different sizes appear between the follicular cells, and then merge into a large cavity called follicular cavity, which is filled with fluid named follicular fluid, containing a variety of hormones and

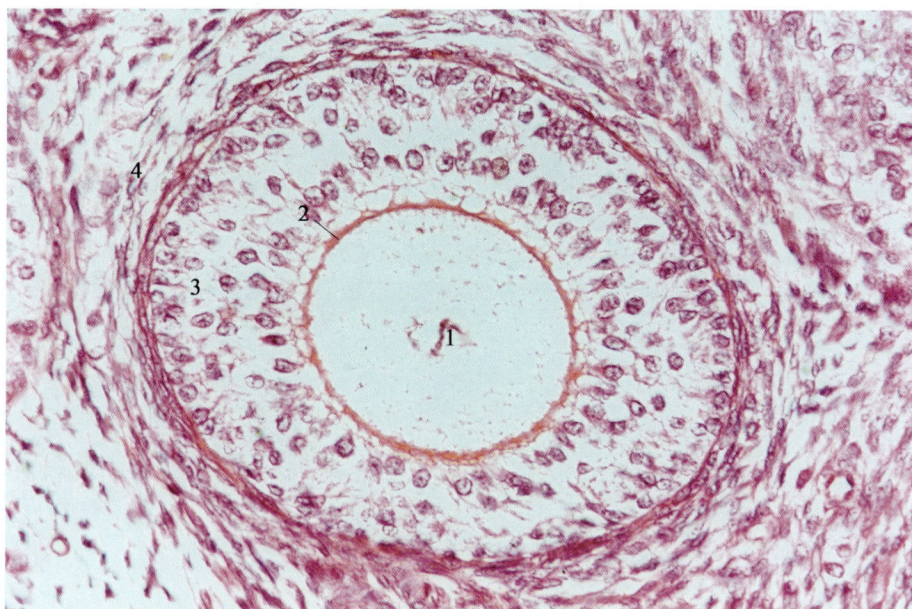

1. Primary oocyte; 2. Zona pellucida; 3. Follicular cells; 4. Follicular theca

Figure 19 - 3　Light micrograph of a primary follicle

biologically active substances. ②The primary oocyte reaches its maximum volume, 125 - 150 μm in diameter, and is surrounded by a layer of zona pellucida about 5 μm thick. Close to the zona pellucida, a layer of tall columnar follicular cells are arranged in a radial pattern, therefore named corona radiata. Due to the continuous expansion of the follicular cavity, the primary oocyte, the zona pellucida, and the surrounding follicular cells gradually occupy one side of the follicular cavity and protrude into the follicular cavity, which is called cumulus oophorus. ③The follicular cells distributed around the follicular cavity, small in size and densely arranged in a granular shape, constitute the follicular wall, which is called granulosa layer. Follicular cells in the granulosa layer are called granulosa cells. ④The follicular theca differentiates into inner and outer layers: the inner layer contains more blood vessels and polygonal theca cells, which have the structural characteristics of cells secreting steroid hormones. There are more fibers, fewer blood vessels and a few smooth muscle fibers in the outer layer (Figure 19 - 4).

1.1.4　Mature Follicle

From puberty, a number of secondary follicles, located on both ovaries, enter into periodic development under the stimulation of FSH secreted by the pituitary gland simultaneously. Usually only one of the best developed follicles can mature, and so called dominant follicle. The mature follicle can release inhibin to negatively feed back to the pituitary gland, reducing the secretion of FSH, leading to the degeneration of other secondary follicles. The mature follicle is large in size, up to 2 cm in diameter, together with enlarged follicular cavity and swelled follicular fluid, occupying the entire cortex and

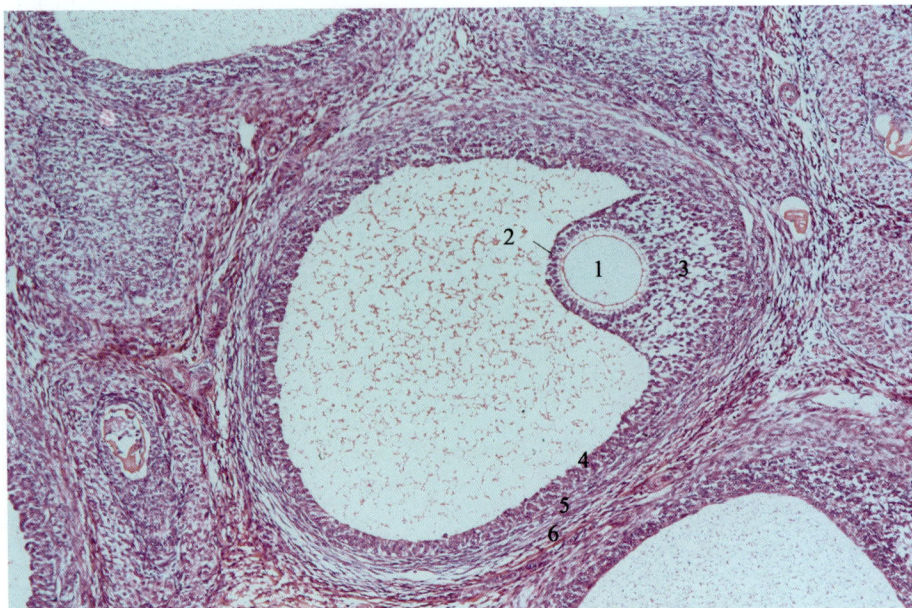

1. Primary oocyte; 2. Corona radiata; 3. Cumulus oophorus; 4. Granulosa layer; 5. Theca interna; 6. Theca externa

Figure 19 - 4　Light micrograph of a secondary follicle

protruding toward the surface of the ovary. Due to the ceased proliferation of the granulosa cells, the granulosa layer becomes thinner, and the cumulus oophorus is gradually separated from the follicular wall and is in the pre-ovulation stage. At 36 - 48 hours before ovulation, the primary oocyte completes the first meiosis, forming a secondary oocyte and a first polar body. Immediately after expulsion of the first polar body, the nucleus of the oocyte begins the second meiotic division, but arrests at metaphase and never completes meiosis unless fertilization occurs, while the first polar body, a very small nonviable cell, is located in the perivitelline space between the secondary oocyte and the zona pellucida.

Secondary follicles and mature follicles function as endocrine glands, in which theca cells and granulosa cells could cooperate to secrete estrogen. Androgen synthesized by the theca cells enters the granulosa cells through the basement membrane, which then is converted into estrogen under the action of the aromatase system. A small portion of the synthesized estrogen enters the follicular cavity, while the rest is released into the blood, regulating the physiological activities of target organs such as the endometrium.

1.2　Ovulation

As follicular fluid in mature follicles increases sharply, the follicular wall, tunica albuginea and the surface epithelium become thinner, and the ovarian surface is ischemic to form transparent follicular stigma. Collagen in the stigma is depolymerized and digested by collagenase and hyaluronidase, coupled with the contraction of the smooth muscle in the outer layer of the theca, resulting in the rupture of mature follicles, following which the secondary oocytes exfoliated from the follicular wall are discharged from the ovary together with the zona pellucida, corona radiata and follicular fluid. The whole process is called ovulation (Figure 19 − 5).

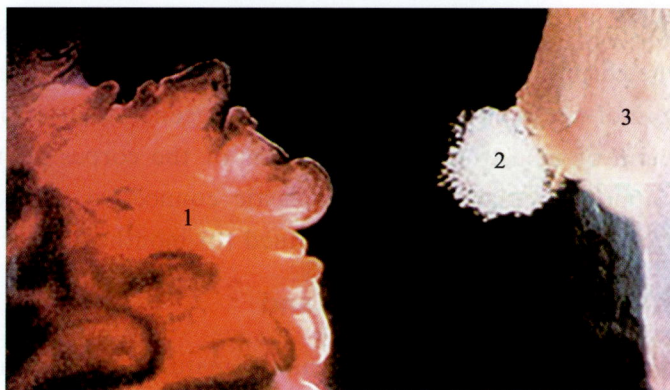

1. Oviduct; 2. The secondary oocyte and corona radiata; 3. Ovary
Figure 19 − 5　Ovulation (Intraperitoneal photograph)

During the child-bearing period, women ovulate once every 28 days, carried out alternately by ovaries on both sides. Usually only one oocyte is liberated during each cycle, but sometimes either no oocyte or two or more simultaneous oocytes may be expelled. Ovulation generally occurs around the 14th day of the menstrual cycle, after which, if the secondary oocyte is fertilized within 24 hours, it will continue to complete the second meiosis, producing a haploid ovum and a second polar body, otherwise it will be degenerated and absorbed. The ovulation process is regulated by neuroendocrine.

1.3　Development and Degeneration of Corpus Luteum

After ovulation, the residual follicular wall, together with the follicular theca and blood vessels, collapses into the follicular cavity, and gradually develops into a large endocrine cell mass rich in blood vessels under the regulation of LH, which is yellow when fresh. It is called corpus luteum, consisting of granulosa lutein cells and theca lutein cells (Figure 19 − 6).

The granulosa lutein cells are enlarged granulosa cells, which contain more lipid droplets in the cytoplasm, and are lightly stained. They account for the majority of the corpus luteum, occupying

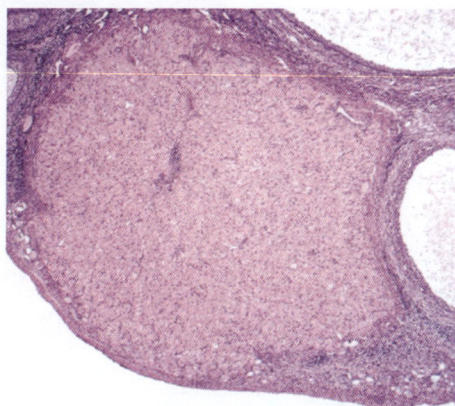

Figure 19 − 6　Light micrograph of a corpus luteum

the central region of the gland, and are responsible for secreting progesterone and relaxin. Relaxin can inhibit the contraction of uterine smooth muscles. The theca lutein cells, which are derived from theca cells, are smaller in volume than granular lutein cells, with darker staining and fewer numbers. They are located on the periphery of the corpus luteum, synthesizing and secreting estrogen. Both cell types have features in common with steroid-secreting cells.

The development of the corpus luteum depends on whether ovum is fertilized or not. If it is fertilized, the corpus luteum can be maintained for 6 months or even longer, which is called corpus lutein of pregnancy, otherwise it will degenerate after only two weeks and is named corpus lutein of menstruation. Both types of the corpus luteum will eventually degenerate and disappear, replaced by hyperplastic connective tissue, corpus albicans, which display as white scars, and can be maintained for months or years.

1.4 Atretic Follicle and Interstitial Gland

The majority of follicles in the ovaries cannot mature, and degenerate at different stages of development. Degenerated follicles are called atretic follicles.

When primordial follicles and primary follicles degenerate, the morphology of oocytes becomes irregular, and follicular cells become smaller and scattered. Finally, all the follicles disappear. When secondary follicles and mature follicles become atretic, oocytes and follicular cells will similarly degenerate and vanish. Nevertheless, theca cells increase in volume and form polygonal cells, whose cytoplasm is filled with lipid droplets, resembling corpus luteum cells and separated by connective tissue and blood vessels into scattered cell clusters, which are called interstitial glands. The interstitial glands will eventually degenerate and be replaced by connective tissue (Figure 19 – 7).

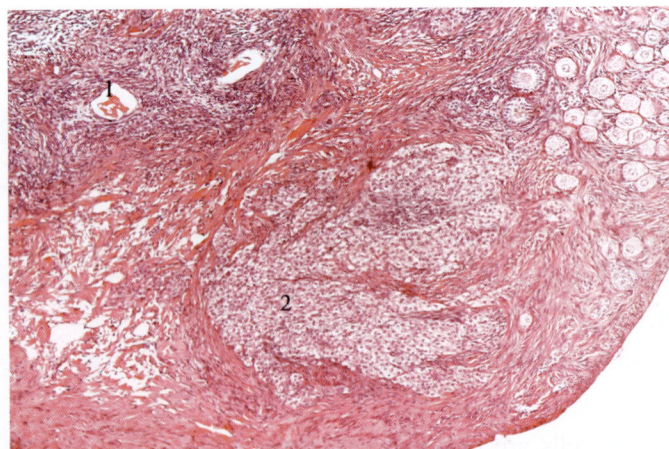

1. Atretic follicle; 2. Interstitial gland

Figure 19 – 7   Light micrograph of the atretic follicle and the interstitial gland

2   Oviduct

The wall of oviducts is composed of mucosa, muscularis and serosa. The mucosa forms many longitudinal and branched plicae toward the lumen, many of which exist in the ampulla. On the transverse section of oviducts, the lumen is quite irregular.

The mucosa is composed of a simple columnar epithelium, which mainly consists of ciliated cells and secretory cells, and lamina propria. The lamina propria is a thin layer of connective tissue, containing many blood vessels and a few smooth muscles. Smooth muscles comprise the muscularis, while the serosa consists of loose connective tissue rich in blood vessels and mesothelia (Figure 19 - 8).

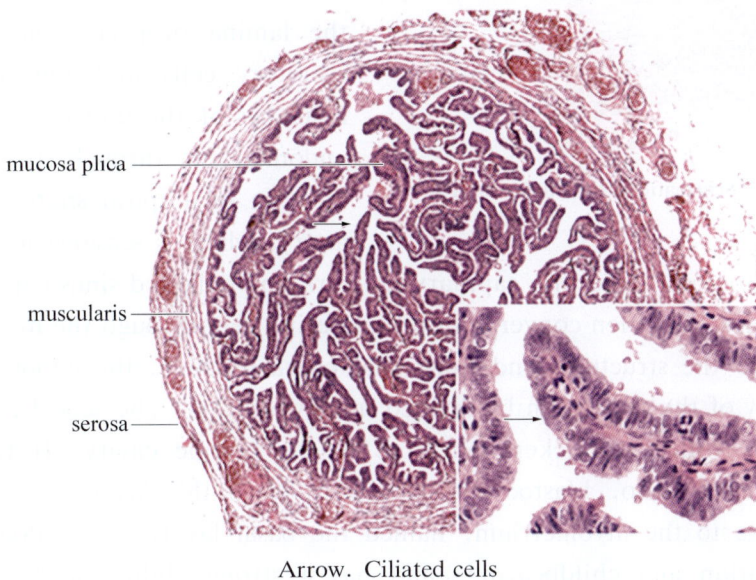

Arrow. Ciliated cells
Figure 19 - 8   Light micrograph of the oviduct

3   Uterus

The uterus is a muscular organ with small cavity and thick wall. The structure of the uterine wall can be divided into three layers from inside to outside: endometrium, myometrium and perimetrium (Figure 19 - 9).

3.1   Structure of Uterine Wall

3.1.1   Endometrium

The endometrium (mucosa) changes in structure and thickness with age and functional status, and is composed of a simple columnar epithelium and lamina propria. The epithelium

endometrium — epithelium

lamina propria

uterine gland

myometrium

perimetrium

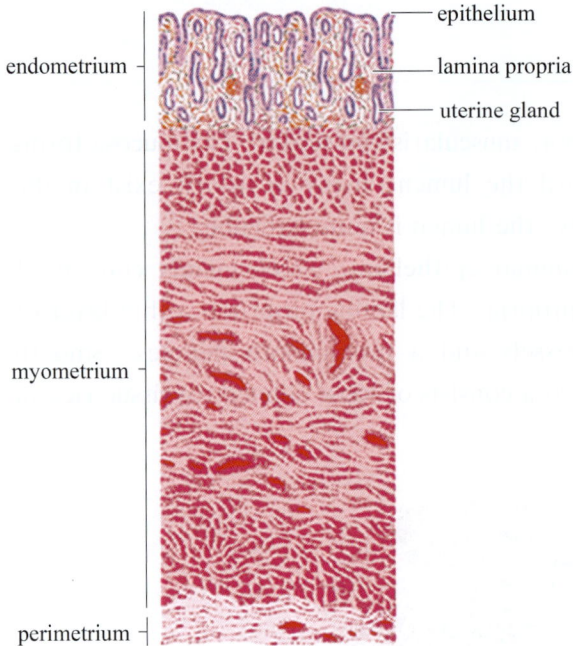

Figure 19-9　Schematic of the uterine wall

consists of ciliated cells and secretory cells, while the lamina propria is composed of connective tissue, uterine glands and blood vessels. In the connective tissue, there are many poorly differentiated fusiform or stellate cells, called stromal cells, which can synthesize and secrete collagen, and proliferate and differentiate with the periodic changes of endometrium. The uterine gland is a single tubular or branched tubular gland formed by the indentation of the surface epithelium into the lamina propria, containing lots of secretory cells and few ciliated cells. Branches of the uterine artery enter the endometrium through the myometrium and run in a spiral shape, named spiral artery, which is sensitive to sex hormones. This artery anastomoses to form a capillary network and enlarged sinus capillaries, which merge into venules, and then converge into the uterine vein through the myometrium.

According to the structural and functional characteristics, the endometrium at the bottom and body of the uterus can be divided into two layers. The superficial layer is the functional layer, which is thicker and close to the uterine cavity. It falls off when menstruation occurs. Also, blastocysts are implanted in this layer. The deep layer is thinner and close to the myometrium, named the basal layer, which does not fall off during menstruation and childbearing, and has a strong ability of proliferation and renovation to produce a new functional layer (Figure 19-10).

3.1.2　Myometrium

The myometrium is the thickest, as long as 1 cm, and is composed of smooth muscle bundles and connective tissue, in which there are blood vessels and various connective tissue cells, especially undifferentiated mesenchymal cells. The contraction of the myometrium contributes to the movement of sperm into the oviduct, the excretion of blood and the delivery of fetuses. The length of the smooth muscle fibers of the adult female uterus is $30-50\,\mu\text{m}$. During pregnancy, these smooth muscles proliferate, growing dozens of times to $500-600\,\mu\text{m}$ long, and the myometrium is thickened. The proliferating smooth muscle fibers come from the division of undifferentiated mesenchymal cells or smooth muscle fibers themselves. Estrogen can increase the number of smooth muscle cells, while progesterone can expand the volume, but inhibit the contraction of smooth muscle cells. After delivery, the uterine smooth muscle fibers can gradually become smaller and return

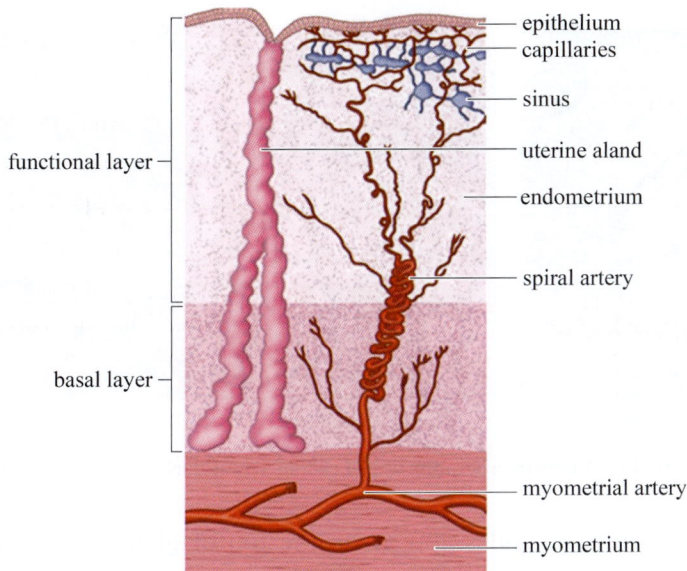

Figure 19 – 10　Schematic of endometrial blood vessels and uterine glands

to their original state, some of which can be autolyzed and absorbed.

3.1.3　Perimetrium

The perimetrium at most of the bottom and body of the uterus is a serosa, while the cervix part is a fibrosa.

3.2　Periodic Changes of Endometrium

Since puberty, the endometrium (except the cervix part) undergoes periodic changes under the regulation of hormones secreted by ovaries. A series of alterations, including exfoliation, bleeding, repair and proliferation of the endometrium, occur every 28 days, and this cycle is called menstrual cycle, which is lasting from the first day of menstruation to the day before the next menstrual onset, and can be divided into three periods: menstrual phase, proliferative phase and secretory phase (Figure 19 – 11).

3.2.1　Proliferative Phase

The proliferative phase refers to the 5th to 14th days of the menstrual cycle. It is also called follicular phase, because some secondary follicles in ovaries begin to grow towards mature follicles, and secrete estrogen during this period. Under the regulation of estrogen, the endometrium is repaired by the proliferation of the remaining basal layer, which is characterized by the division and proliferation of endometrial fusiform stromal cells and the production of a large number of fibers and matrix, and the endometrium thickened from 1 mm to 2 – 4 mm.

In the early stage of the proliferative phase, there are few uterine glands which are short, straight and thin; in the middle stage, the uterine glands increase and bend slightly;

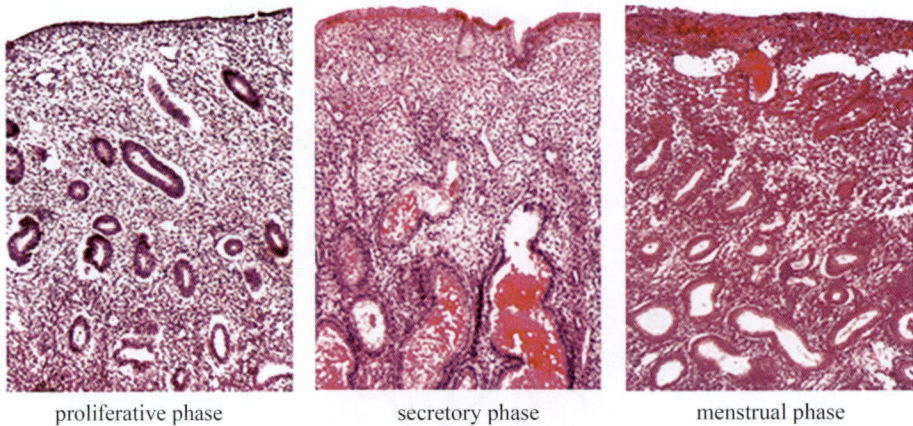

proliferative phase   secretory phase   menstrual phase

Figure 19 – 11　Light micrographs of the endometrium during the menstrual cycle

in the late stage, secretory granules appear on the top of glandular cells, while glycogen gathers in the subnuclear area. In the end of this phase, the uterine glands grow and bend further, and begin to secrete, with enlarged glandular cavities. The spiral arteries are more elongated and curved. On the 14th day of the menstrual cycle, usually one follicle in ovaries can mature and the ovulation takes place. Then the endometrium enters the secretory phase.

3.2.2　Secretory Phase

The secretory phase refers to the 15th to 28th days of the menstrual cycle, during which the corpus luteum is formed, so it is also called luteal phase. Under the regulation of progesterone and estrogen secreted by the corpus luteum, the endometrium continues to proliferate and thicken up to 5 – 7 mm. Meanwhile, the uterine glands become longer and more bent, with larger glandular cavities. Glycogen is transferred from the subnuclear area to the supranuclear area of the glandular cells, which then is excreted into the gland cavities by apocrine secretion, leading to that the gland cavities are filled with viscous liquid containing nutrients such as glycogen. The lamina propria contains much more tissue fluid and is in a state of edema, while the spiral arteries continue to grow and become more bend, extending into the superficial endometrium. At the late stage of secretory phase, some of the cells become larger and rounded, whose cytoplasm is filled with glycogen and lipid droplets, which are called predecidual cells. These cells become decidual cells during pregnancy. If not pregnant, the functional endometrial layer will fall off. The endometrium will then enter the menstrual phase.

3.2.3　Menstrual Phase

The menstrual phase refers to the 1st to 4th days of the menstrual cycle. During this period, due to the sudden drop of estrogen and progesterone caused by degeneration of the corpus luteum of menstruation, spiral arteries in the functional layer of endometrium contract continuously, resulting in endometrial ischemia, cessation of uterine gland secretion and reduction of tissue fluid. The functional layer becomes atrophic and necrotic. Subsequently, the spiral arteries dilate suddenly and briefly, leading to rupture of blood vessels in the functional layer. Blood flows out and accumulates in the superficial part of the endometrium, which is finally exfoliated and expelled through the vagina together with the necrotic endometrium. This discharge is menstruation. Before the end of menstrual phase, the remaining glandular epithelium in the basal layer of the endometrium begins to proliferate rapidly and moves to the surface of the uterine cavity, repairing the endometrial epithelium. When the menstrual phase is over, other tissues also begin to proliferate and endometrium enters the proliferative phase.

3.3 Cervix

The cervical wall is composed of mucosa, muscularis and adventitia. The mucosa consists of epithelium and lamina propria, protruding into the lumen to form plicae. The luminal surface of the cervix is a simple columnar epithelium, composed of secretory cells, ciliated cells and reserve cells. The mucosal epithelium of the cervicovaginal region is a stratified squamous epithelium. A few smooth muscle fibers in the muscularis are dispersed, which are distributed in dense connective tissue. The adventitia is a fibrosa composed of connective tissue.

The cervical mucosa does not peel off periodically, but the quality of its secretions changes with the cycle of ovarian activity. During ovulation, the secretion of cervical glands is increased and thin, which is conducive to sperm movement. When the corpus luteum is formed, the secretion of cervical glandular epithelial cells is reduced and sticky, making it difficult for sperm to pass. During pregnancy, the cervical mucosa thickens, with more plicae, and the secretion is more viscous, which acts as a barrier to prevent sperm and microorganisms from entering the uterus.

3.4 Neuroendocrine Regulation of Periodic Changes of Ovary and Endometrium

The periodic changes of the endometrium are regulated by the hypothalamus-pituitary-gonad axis. Gonadotropin-releasing hormone produced by hypothalamic neuroendocrine cells causes basophils in the pars distalis of the pituitary gland to secrete FSH and LH. FSH can promote the growth and maturation of ovarian follicles and make them secrete large amounts of estrogen, which can transfer the endometrium from the menstrual phase to the proliferative period. Estrogen at a certain concentration in the blood will feed back to the hypothalamus and the pituitary gland, inhibiting the secretion of FSH, but promoting the secretion of LH. Under the synergistic effect of LH and FSH, follicles mature, ovulate and form corpus luteum. The corpus luteum produces progesterone and estrogen, which can propel the endometrium to enter the secretory phase. When the progesterone in the blood increases to a certain concentration, it will feed back to the hypothalamus and the pituitary gland, inhibiting the release of LH. Consequently, the corpus luteum degenerates, inducing a sudden decrease of progesterone and estrogen in the blood, and the endometrium enters the menstrual phase. Due to the reduction of estrogen and progesterone in the blood, which feeds back to the hypothalamus and the pituitary gland, FSH is secreted and the follicles begin to grow and develop again.

The above cycle repeats itself. The hypothalamus and the pituitary gland rhythmically regulate the ovarian activity cycle and the menstrual cycle, keeping them in synchronization to satisfy the requirements of ovulation, fertilization, blastocyst implantation, growth and development (Figure 19 - 12).

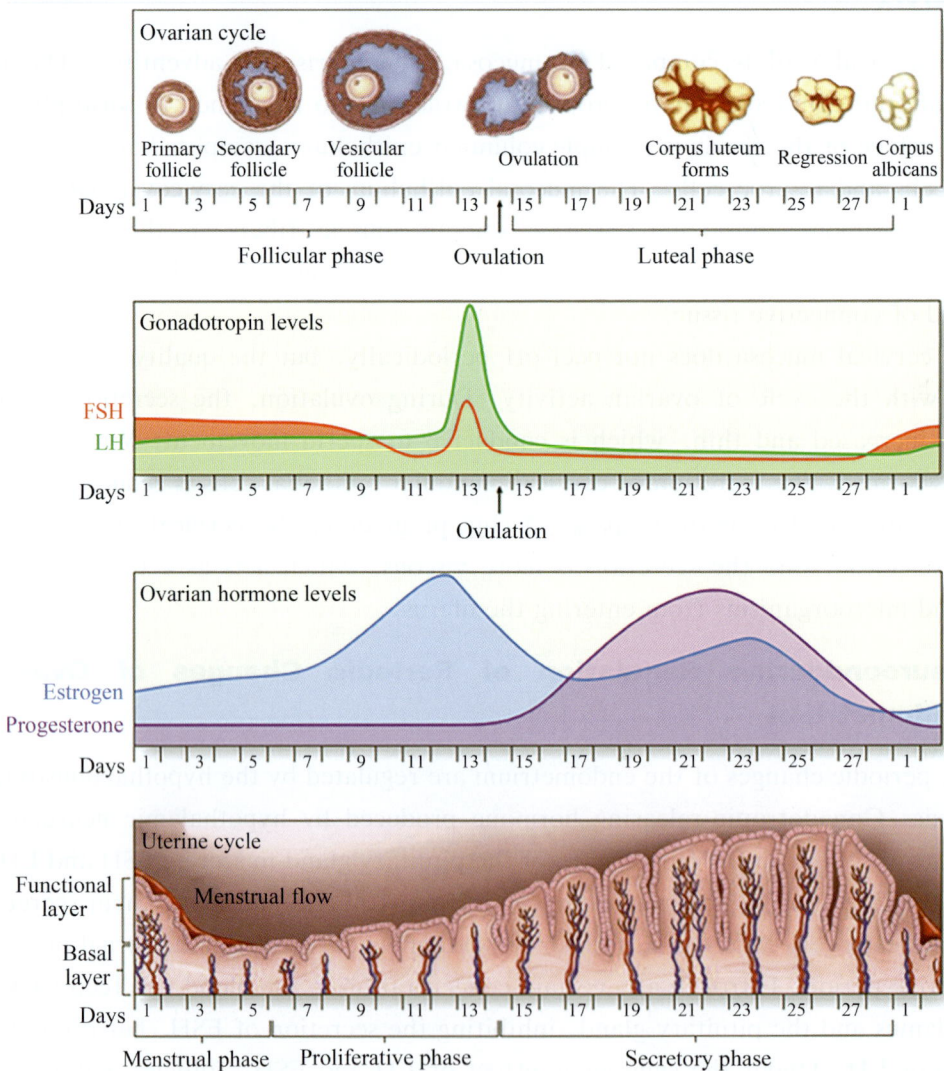

Figure 19 - 12 Relationship between periodic changes of follicular development and endometrium and hormones

4 Vagina

The vaginal wall is composed of mucosa, muscularis and adventitia. The mucosa consists of epithelium and lamina propria, protruding into the vaginal cavity to form many horizontal plicae. The epithelium is an unkeratinized stratified squamous epithelium. The muscularis contains a thin layer of smooth muscles. There is a sphincter made up of circular skeletal muscles in the external orifice of vagina. The adventitia is dense connective tissue rich in elastic fibers.

5 Mammary Gland

Mammary glands are developed to secrete milk and feed babies, whose structures vary with age and physiological conditions, and do not belong to female reproductive organs. They begin to develop in puberty. Mammary glands during pregnancy and lactation have lactation activities, which are named active mammary glands, while those without lactation activities are called resting mammary glands.

One mammary gland is divided into 15 – 25 lobes by connective tissue, and each lobe is divided into several lobules. Each lobule is a compound tubuloacinar gland. The acinar epithelium is a single layer of cubic or columnar cells, and the glandular cavity is very small. There is a basement membrane beneath glandular cells, between which myoepithelial cells exist. Ducts include intralobular ducts, interlobular ducts and lactiferous ducts (Figure 19 – 13, 19 – 14, 19 – 15).

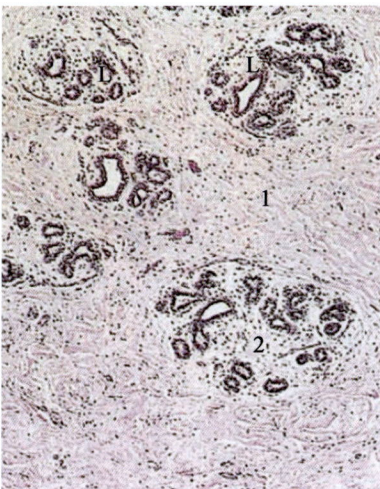

1. Connective tissue; 2. Lobules

Figure 19 – 13 Light micrograph of the resting mammary gland

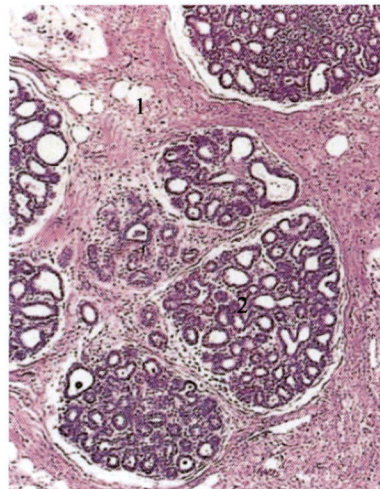

1. Connective tissue; 2. Lobules

Figure 19 – 14 Light micrograph of the active mammary gland during pregnancy

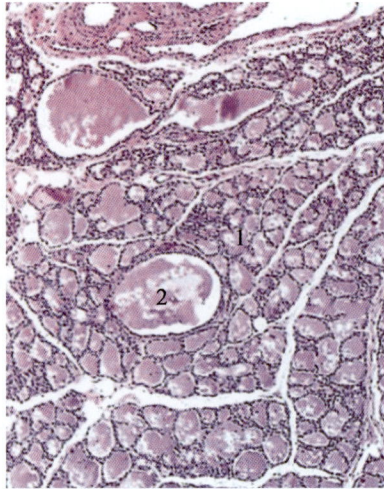

1. Acini; 2. Ducts

Figure 19 - 15　Light micrograph of the active mammary gland during lactation

(*Situ Chenghao*)

第十九章　女性生殖系统

　　女性生殖系统由卵巢、输卵管、子宫、阴道和外生殖器组成。卵巢具有产生卵细胞和分泌性激素的功能;输卵管是受精的场所,并输送生殖细胞;子宫是形成月经和孕育胎儿的器官。自青春期开始,生殖器官和乳房迅速发育成熟,卵巢开始排卵并分泌性激素,子宫内膜出现周期性变化。围绝经期的卵巢功能逐渐减退。此外,因乳腺分泌乳汁,哺育婴儿,故列入本章叙述。

第一节　卵　　巢

　　卵巢表面覆有单层扁平或立方形的表面上皮,上皮深部为薄层致密结缔组织构成的白膜。卵巢实质分为外周的皮质和中央的髓质,二者分界不明显。皮质较厚,由不同发育阶段的卵泡、黄体,以及富含梭形基质细胞和网状纤维的结缔组织等构成;髓质较薄,为疏松结缔组织,其中含有较多的弹性纤维、血管、淋巴管和神经。卵巢一侧为卵巢门部,此处基质内有少量平滑肌和门细胞(与睾丸间质细胞相似,可能分泌雄激素)(图 19-1)。

　　卵巢皮质中卵泡发育呈周期性改变。新生儿有 70 万～200 万个原始卵泡开始发育,青春

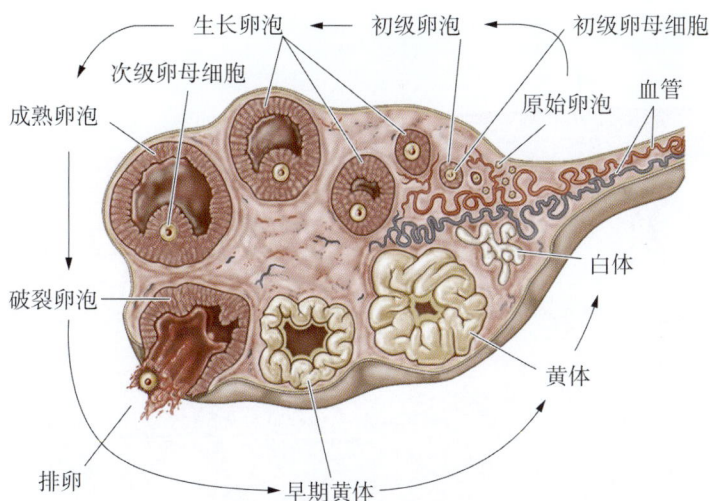

图 19-1 卵巢结构模式图

期开始约 4 万个卵泡,至 40~50 岁时仅剩几百个卵泡。从青春期至围绝经期,卵巢在垂体分泌的促性腺激素影响下,按月经周期呈周期性排卵。每 28 天有 15~20 个卵泡生长发育,一般只有一个优势卵泡能发育成熟并排卵。正常女性一生中排卵 400 余个,其余大部分卵泡均在发育的不同阶段退化为闭锁卵泡。绝经期后卵巢不再排卵。

一、卵泡的发育与成熟

卵泡是由一个卵母细胞和周围的多个卵泡细胞组成,呈球形。卵泡发育是一个连续变化的过程,大致经过原始卵泡、初级卵泡、次级卵泡和成熟卵泡四个阶段,其中初级卵泡和次级卵泡又称为生长卵泡。

(一)原始卵泡

原始卵泡是处于静止状态的卵泡,体积小,数量多,位于浅层皮质,由一个初级卵母细胞和周围一层扁平的卵泡细胞组成。初级卵母细胞呈圆形,体积大;核大而圆,略偏位,染色质稀疏浅染,核仁清楚;胞质丰富,嗜酸性(图 19-2)。初级卵母细胞是在胚胎时期由卵原细胞分裂分化而来,随即进入第一次减数分裂并长期停留在分裂前期,直至排卵前才完成分裂。卵泡细胞围绕初级卵母细胞单层排列,细胞呈扁平形,胞体小,核扁圆,着色深。卵泡细胞和周围结缔组织之间有较薄的基膜,与卵母细胞之间有较多的缝隙连接,具有支持和营养卵母细胞的作用。

(二)初级卵泡

由原始卵泡发育形成,移向皮质深部。其主要结构变化是:①卵泡细胞由扁平形分化为立方形或柱状,进而增殖,由单层分化为多层;电镜下胞质内粗面内质网、游离核糖体及线粒体都增多,高尔基复合体也更发达。②初级卵母细胞增大,胞质增多;核变大,呈泡状,核仁染色深;电镜下胞质内高尔基复合体、粗面内质网、游离核糖体等均增多;浅层胞质出现皮质颗粒,这是一种溶酶体,在受精过程中有防止多精受精的作用。③初级卵母细胞和卵泡细胞之间出现卵周间隙,内层卵泡细胞的突起和初级卵母细胞的微绒毛均伸向间隙,二者共同的分泌物形成较

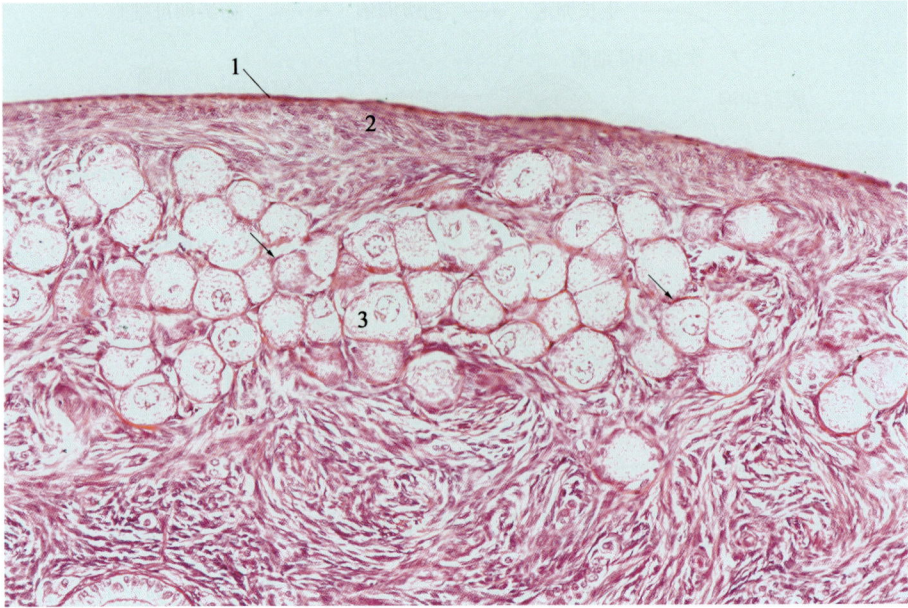

1—表面上皮;2—白膜;3—初级卵母细胞;箭头—卵泡细胞
图 19-2　原始卵泡光镜图

厚嗜酸性膜,即透明带。透明带由透明带蛋白(zona pellucida protein,ZP)组成,主要有ZP1、ZP2、ZP3、ZP4,它们在精子与卵细胞的识别和特异性结合中具有重要作用。卵泡细胞的突起与初级卵母细胞膜可形成缝隙连接,有利于物质交换,信息沟通。④随着初级卵泡体积增大,卵泡周围基质中的梭形细胞增殖分化形成卵泡膜(图 19-3)。

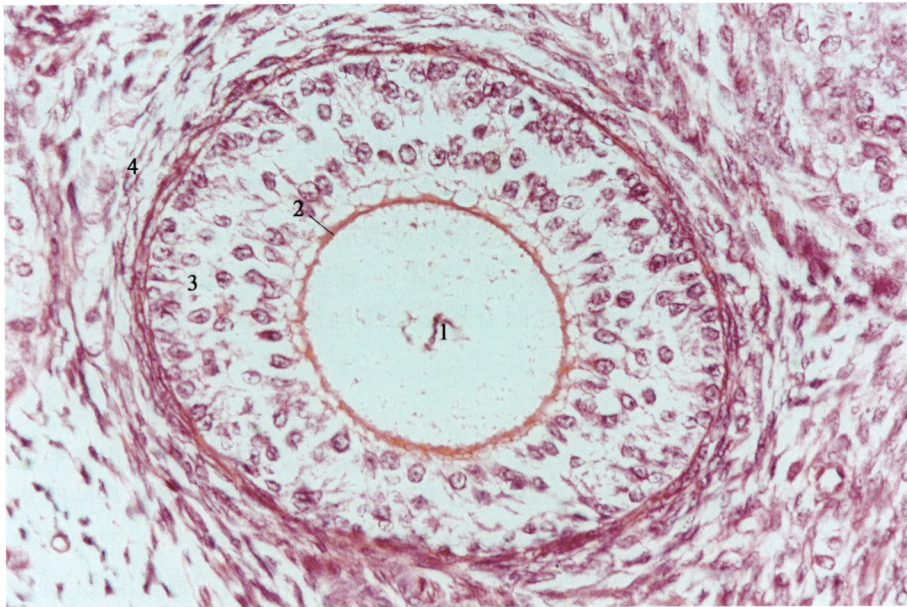

1—初级卵母细胞;2—透明带;3—卵泡细胞;4—卵泡膜
图 19-3　初级卵泡光镜图

（三）次级卵泡

初级卵泡继续生长分化，当卵泡细胞间出现液腔时，称为次级卵泡。次级卵泡结构的主要特点是：①卵泡细胞间出现大小不等的液腔，继而汇合成一个大腔，称为卵泡腔。卵泡腔内液体为卵泡液，内含多种激素与生物活性物质。②初级卵母细胞达到最大体积，直径 $125\sim150\,\mu m$，其周围包裹一层约 $5\,\mu m$ 厚的透明带；紧贴透明带的一层高柱状卵泡细胞呈放射状排列，故名放射冠；由于卵泡腔不断扩大，迫使初级卵母细胞、透明带、放射冠与其周围的卵泡细胞逐渐居于卵泡腔一侧，突入卵泡腔，称为卵丘。③分布于卵泡腔周边的卵泡细胞构成卵泡壁，由于此处卵泡细胞体积较小，排列密集呈颗粒状，故又称颗粒层。颗粒层的卵泡细胞称为颗粒细胞。④卵泡膜分化成内、外两层，内膜层含有较多的血管和多边形的膜细胞，该细胞具有分泌类固醇激素细胞的结构特点；外膜层内的纤维较多、血管少，并有少量平滑肌纤维（图 19-4）。

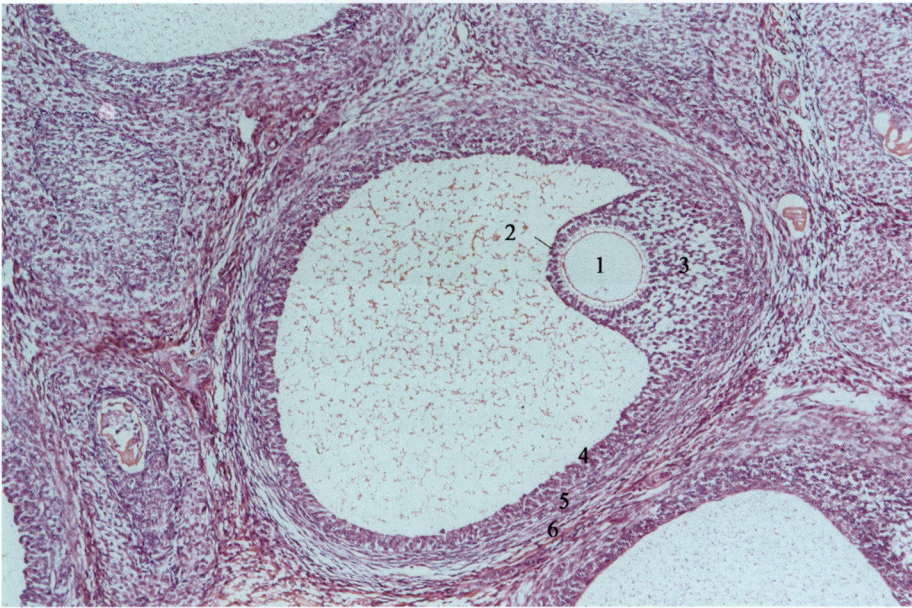

1—初级卵母细胞；2—放射冠；3—卵丘；4—颗粒层；5—卵泡膜内层；6—卵泡膜外层
图 19-4　次级卵泡光镜图

（四）成熟卵泡

在两侧卵巢同时存在一批次级卵泡，青春期开始，在垂体分泌的卵泡刺激素的作用下，这些次级卵泡进入周期性发育，通常仅一个发育最佳的卵泡能够成熟，故称为优势卵泡。成熟卵泡可释放抑制素，负反馈作用于垂体，使卵泡刺激素分泌水平降低，导致其他次级卵泡退化。成熟卵泡体积大，直径可达 2 cm，占据皮质全层并突向卵巢表面。卵泡腔变得很大，卵泡液增多；由于颗粒细胞停止增殖，颗粒层相应变薄，卵丘与周围卵泡细胞出现裂隙，逐渐与卵泡壁分离，处于排卵前期。在排卵前 36～48 h，初级卵母细胞完成第一次减数分裂，形成一个次级卵母细胞和第一极体，次级卵母细胞迅速进入第二次减数分裂，并停滞在分裂中期。第一极体是一个很小的细胞，位于次级卵母细胞与透明带之间的卵周间隙内。

次级卵泡与成熟卵泡具有内分泌功能,主要是膜细胞和颗粒细胞协同合成分泌雌激素。膜细胞合成的雄激素透过基膜进入颗粒细胞,在芳香化酶系的作用下雄激素转变为雌激素。合成的雌激素小部分进入卵泡腔,大部分释放入血,调节子宫内膜等靶器官的生理活动。

二、排卵

随成熟卵泡的卵泡液剧增,卵泡壁、白膜和表面上皮变薄,卵巢表面局部缺血形成透明的卵泡小斑,继而小斑处的胶原被胶原酶、透明质酸酶等解聚和消化,再加上卵泡膜外层的平滑肌收缩等因素,导致成熟卵泡破裂,从卵泡壁脱落的次级卵母细胞连同透明带、放射冠与卵泡液一起从卵巢排出的过程称为排卵(图 19-5)。

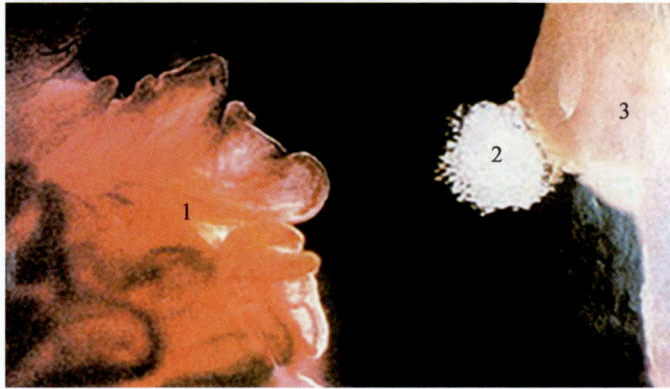

1—输卵管漏斗部;2—次级卵母细胞和放射冠;3—卵巢
图 19-5 卵巢排卵(腹腔内摄影)

生育期妇女,每隔 28 天左右排一次卵;两侧卵巢交替进行,一般一次只排一个卵,偶见排两个或两个以上者。排卵一般发生在月经周期的第 14 天左右。排卵后,次级卵母细胞若受精将继续完成第二次减数分裂,产生一个单倍体的卵细胞和一个第二极体;次级卵母细胞若 24 h 内未受精,则退化被吸收。排卵过程受神经内分泌的调节。

三、黄体的形成与退化

成熟卵泡排卵后,残留的卵泡壁连同卵泡膜及其血管一起向卵泡腔内塌陷,在 LH 的作用下逐渐发育成一个体积较大、富含血管的内分泌细胞团,新鲜时呈黄色,故称为黄体(图 19-6)。其中颗粒层卵泡细胞体积变大,胞质内含较多脂滴,着色浅,占黄体细胞的多数,位于黄体的中央,此即颗粒黄体细胞,主要分泌孕酮和松弛素,松弛素有抑制子宫平滑肌收缩的作用。膜细胞体积较颗粒黄体细胞小,染色较深,数量较少,位于黄体的周边,此即膜黄体细胞,主要分泌雌激素。这两种黄体细胞都具有分泌类固醇激素细胞的结构特征。

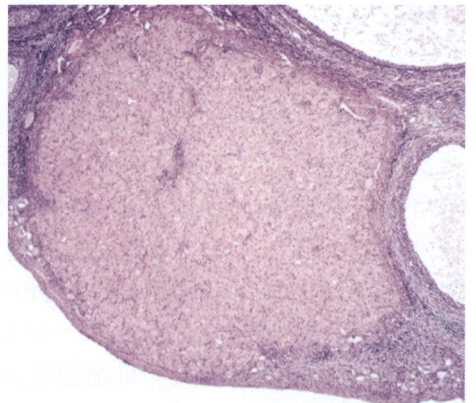

图 19-6 黄体光镜图

黄体发育取决于排出的卵是否受精。如未受精,仅维持两周即退化,称为月经黄体。如受精则可维持 6 个月,甚至更长时间,称为妊娠黄体。两种黄体最终都将退化消失,逐渐被增生的结缔组织取代,变成白色瘢痕,即白体。白体可维持数月或数年。

四、闭锁卵泡与间质腺

卵巢内的绝大多数卵泡不能发育成熟,它们在发育的不同阶段退化。退化的卵泡称为闭锁卵泡。

原始卵泡和初级卵泡退化时,卵母细胞形态变为不规则,卵泡细胞变小而分散,最后变性消失。次级卵泡和成熟卵泡闭锁时,卵母细胞与卵泡细胞同样地变性消失;而膜细胞体积增大,形成多边形细胞,胞质中充满脂滴,形似黄体细胞并被结缔组织和血管分隔成分散的细胞团索,称为间质腺。间质腺最后退化,由结缔组织所代替(图 19 - 7)。

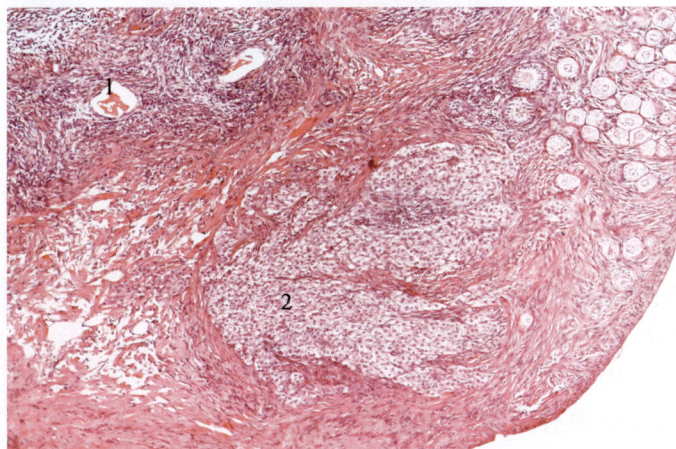

1—闭锁卵泡;2—间质腺
图 19 - 7　闭锁卵泡和间质腺光镜图

第二节　输　卵　管

输卵管管壁由黏膜、肌层和浆膜组成。黏膜向管腔形成许多纵行且分支的皱襞,壶腹部较多,横切面上管腔极不规则。

黏膜由单层柱状上皮和固有层构成,上皮主要由纤毛细胞和分泌细胞组成。固有层为薄层结缔组织,内含较多的血管和少量平滑肌。肌层由平滑肌构成。浆膜由富含血管的疏松结缔组织和间皮构成(图 19 - 8)。

第三节　子　宫

子宫为肌性器官,腔小壁厚。子宫壁的结构由内向外可分内膜、肌层和外膜三层(图 19 - 9)。

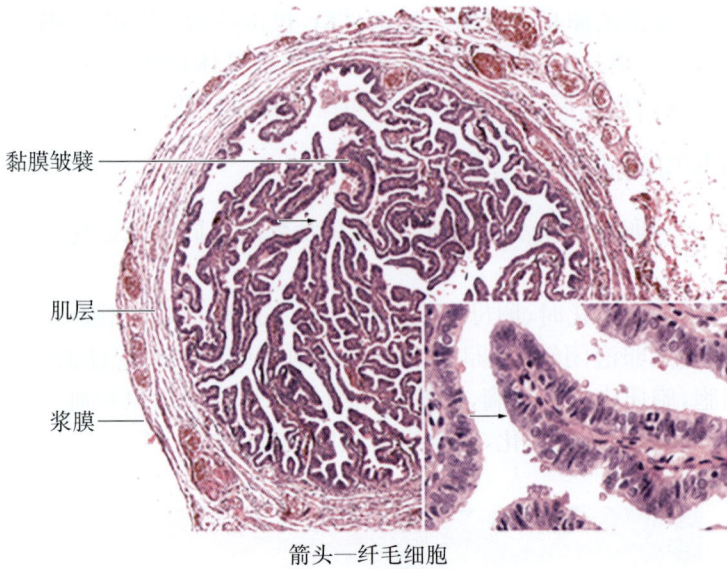

黏膜皱襞

肌层

浆膜

箭头—纤毛细胞

图 19-8　输卵管光镜图

一、子宫壁的结构

(一) 内膜

　　子宫内膜随年龄和功能状态的不同而发生结构和厚薄改变,由单层柱状上皮和固有层组成。上皮由纤毛细胞和分泌细胞构成。固有层由结缔组织及子宫腺和血管等组成。在结缔组织中有大量分化程度较低的梭形或星形细胞,称为基质细胞,可合成及分泌胶原蛋白,并随子宫内膜的周期性变化而增生与分化。子宫腺为内膜表面上皮向固有层内凹陷形成的单管或分支管状腺;腺上皮主要是分泌细胞,纤毛细胞较少。子宫动脉分支通过肌层进入内膜,呈螺旋状走行,称为螺旋动脉,其对性激素反应敏感而迅速。此动脉至内膜浅部分支吻合形成毛细血管网和扩大的窦状毛细血管,然后汇入小静脉,经肌层汇合为子宫静脉。

　　子宫底部和体部的内膜,根据其结构和功能特点,可分浅、深两层:浅层为功能层,较厚,为靠近子宫腔的内膜部分,每次月经来潮时发生脱落,胚泡也在此层内植入;深层为靠近肌层较薄的内膜部分,称为基底层,该层在月经期和分娩时均不脱落并有较强的增生和修复能力,可以产生新的功能层(图 19-10)。

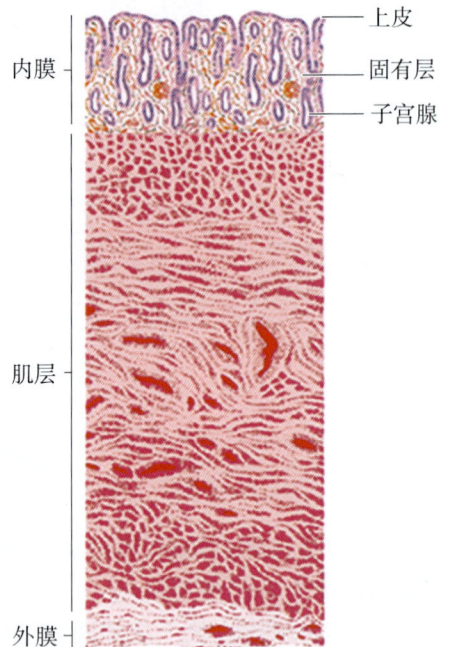

内膜 { 上皮
固有层
子宫腺

肌层

外膜

图 19-9　子宫壁模式图

(二) 肌层

　　最厚,约1cm,由平滑肌束和束间结缔组织组成;结缔组织中有血管和各种结缔组织细胞,其中未分化间充质细胞尤为丰富。肌层大致可分三层,即黏膜下层、中间层和浆膜下层。

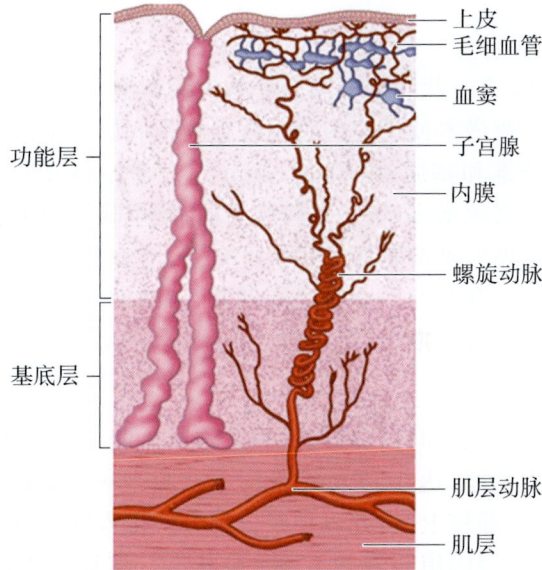

图 19-10 子宫内膜血管和子宫腺模式图

子宫肌层的收缩活动,有助于精子向输卵管运行和经血排出及胎儿娩出。成年女性子宫平滑肌纤维长 30~50 μm,在妊娠时肌纤维增生,可增长数十倍,长达 500~600 μm,肌层增厚。增生的平滑肌纤维来自未分化间充质细胞或平滑肌纤维自身的分裂。雌激素能促使平滑肌细胞数量增加;黄体酮能使平滑肌细胞体积增大,并有抑制平滑肌收缩的作用。分娩后子宫平滑肌纤维可逐渐变小,恢复原状,有部分平滑肌纤维自溶分解而被吸收。

(三) 外膜

大部分子宫底和体部为薄层结缔组织和间皮构成的浆膜,宫颈处为纤维膜。

二、子宫内膜的周期性变化

自青春期开始,子宫内膜(宫颈除外)在卵巢分泌的激素作用下出现周期性变化,即每隔 28 天左右发生一次内膜剥落、出血、修复和增生,称为月经周期。每个月经周期是从月经第 1 天起至下次月经来潮前一天止,可分为增生期、分泌期和月经期三个时期(图 19-11)。

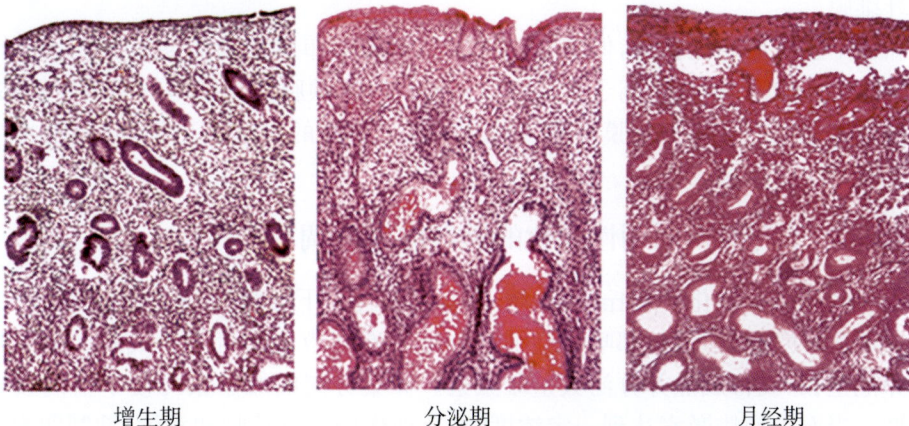

| 增生期 | 分泌期 | 月经期 |

图 19-11 月经周期子宫内膜光镜图

（一）增生期

指月经周期的第5～14天。此间卵巢内有一些次级卵泡开始生长，向成熟卵泡发育，并分泌雌激素，故又称卵泡期。雌激素使子宫内膜由残存的基底层增生修复，表现为内膜梭形基质细胞分裂增殖，产生大量纤维和基质，内膜由1 mm左右增厚达2～4 mm。增生早期子宫腺短、直、细而少；增生中期子宫腺增多、增长并轻度弯曲；增生晚期腺细胞顶部有分泌颗粒，核下区糖原聚集，在染色切片上糖原被溶解而显示核下空泡；增生末期子宫腺增长弯曲，腺腔增大，开始分泌；螺旋动脉更加伸长和弯曲。至月经周期第14天时，卵巢内通常有一个卵泡发育成熟并排卵，子宫内膜随之转入分泌期。

（二）分泌期

指月经周期第15～28天。此时黄体形成，故又称黄体期。在黄体分泌的孕激素和雌激素作用下，子宫内膜继续增生变厚，达5～7 mm，此时子宫腺进一步变长、弯曲、腺腔扩大，糖原由腺细胞核下区转移到细胞顶部核上区，并以顶浆分泌方式排入腺腔，使腺腔内充满含有糖原等营养物质的黏稠液体。固有层内组织液增多呈水肿状态。螺旋动脉继续增长变得更弯曲并伸入内膜浅层。基质细胞继续分裂增殖，到分泌晚期部分细胞增大变圆，胞质内充满糖原和脂滴，称为前蜕膜细胞。妊娠时此细胞变为蜕膜细胞。如未妊娠，内膜功能层将脱落，转入月经期。

（三）月经期

指月经周期的第1～4天。此期由于卵巢月经黄体退化，雌激素和孕激素骤然下降，引起子宫内膜功能层的螺旋动脉持续性收缩，使内膜缺血，子宫腺分泌停止，组织液减少，从而功能层发生萎缩坏死。继而螺旋动脉又突然短暂扩张，致使功能层的血管破裂，血液流出并积聚在内膜浅部，最后与坏死的内膜一起剥落并经阴道排出，此即月经。在月经期结束之前，内膜基底层残留的子宫腺上皮开始迅速增生，并向子宫腔表面推移，使子宫内膜上皮得到修复。待月经期结束，其他组织也开始增生而转入增生期。

三、子宫颈

子宫颈壁由黏膜、肌层和外膜组成。黏膜由上皮和固有层组成，并突向管腔形成皱襞。子宫颈管腔面上皮为单层柱状上皮，由分泌细胞，纤毛细胞和储备细胞构成。宫颈阴道部的黏膜上皮为复层扁平上皮。肌层平滑肌纤维较少且分散，分布于致密结缔组织中。外膜是结缔组织构成的纤维膜。

宫颈黏膜不发生周期性剥落，但其分泌物的质量却随卵巢活动周期发生变化。排卵时宫颈腺分泌物增多而稀薄，有利于精子运动。黄体形成时宫颈腺上皮细胞分泌减少且黏稠，使精子难以通过。妊娠期间子宫颈黏膜增厚，皱襞增多，分泌物的黏稠度更高，起到阻止精子和微生物进入子宫的屏障作用。

四、卵巢和子宫内膜周期性变化的神经内分泌调节

子宫内膜的周期性变化受下丘脑-垂体-性腺轴调控。下丘脑神经内分泌细胞产生的促性腺激素释放激素，使腺垂体远侧部嗜碱性细胞分泌卵泡刺激素和黄体生成素。卵泡刺激素可促进卵巢卵泡生长、发育成熟并分泌大量雌激素。卵巢分泌的雌激素可使子宫内膜从月经期转入增生期。当血中的雌激素达到一定浓度时，反馈作用于下丘脑和垂体，抑制卵泡刺激素的

分泌,但促进黄体生成素的分泌。在黄体生成素和卵泡刺激素的协同作用下,卵泡成熟、排卵并形成黄体。黄体产生孕激素和雌激素,可促使子宫内膜进入分泌期变化。当血中的孕激素增加到一定浓度时,反馈作用于下丘脑和垂体,抑制黄体生成素的释放,于是黄体发生退化,血中孕激素和雌激素骤然减少,子宫内膜进入月经期。由于血中雌、孕激素的减少,又反馈作用于下丘脑和垂体,促使下丘脑和垂体释放卵泡刺激素,卵泡又开始生长发育。上述循环周而复始,下丘脑垂体有节律地调节卵巢活动周期与子宫内膜周期保持同步变化,以适应排卵、受精、胚泡植入和生长发育的需要(图 19 - 12)。

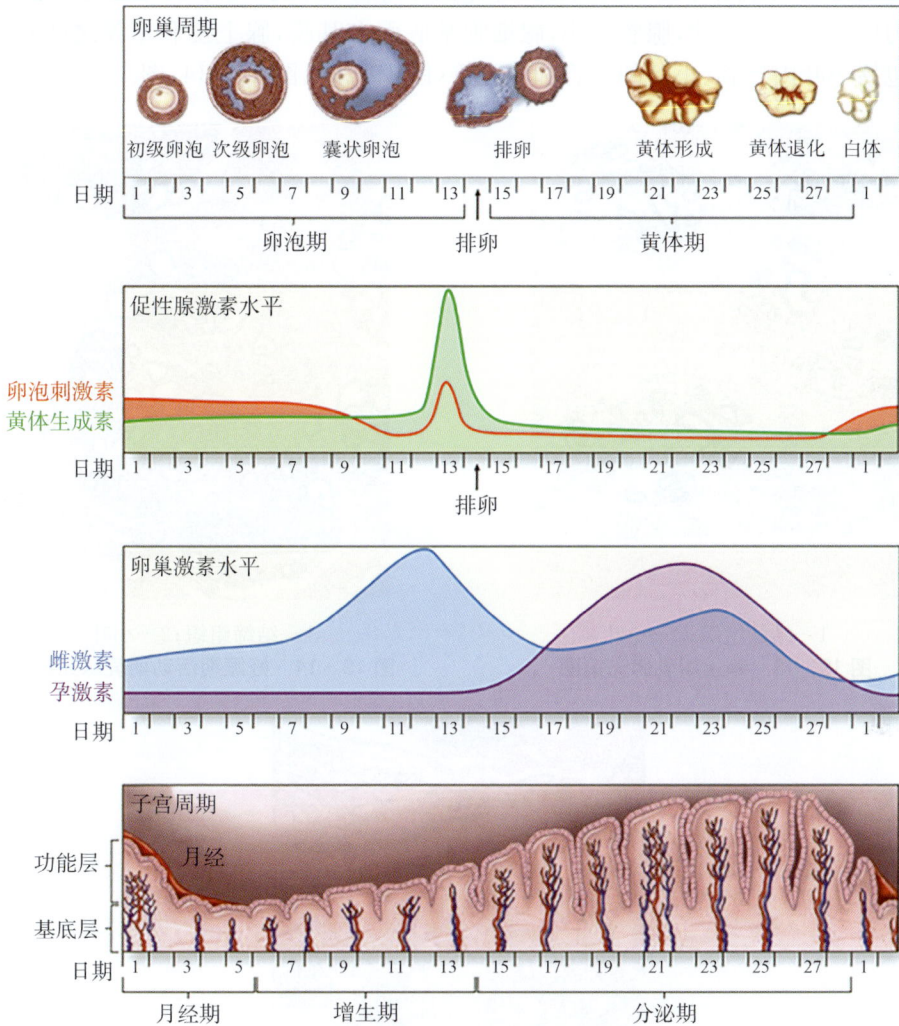

图 19 - 12　卵泡发育和子宫内膜周期性变化与激素的关系

第四节　阴　　道

阴道壁由黏膜、肌层和外膜组成。黏膜向阴道腔内突起形成许多横行皱襞,由上皮和固有层构成。上皮为未角化的复层扁平上皮。肌层由薄层平滑肌构成;阴道外口有环形的骨骼肌构成的括约肌。外膜为富含弹性纤维的致密结缔组织。

第五节 乳　　腺

　　乳腺的主要功能是分泌乳汁、哺育婴儿，不属于女性生殖器官。乳腺的结构因年龄和生理状况的变化而异。乳腺发育始于青春期，妊娠和哺乳期的乳腺有泌乳活动，称为活动期乳腺。无泌乳活动的乳腺，称为静止期乳腺。

　　乳腺由结缔组织分隔为 15～25 个叶，每叶又分为若干小叶，每个小叶属一个复管泡状腺。腺泡上皮为单层立方或柱状，腺腔很小，腺细胞基底面有基膜，腺上皮和基膜之间有肌上皮细胞。导管包括小叶内导管、小叶间导管和输乳管（图 19 - 13、图 19 - 14、图 19 - 15）。

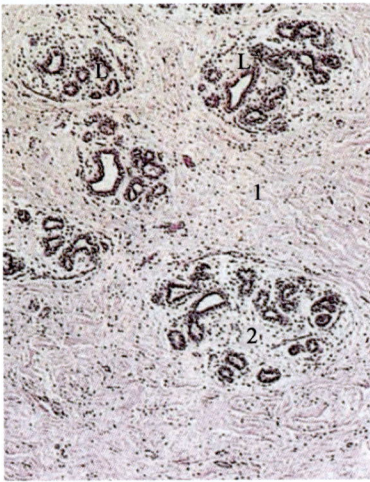

1—结缔组织；2—小叶
图 19 - 13　静止期乳腺光镜图

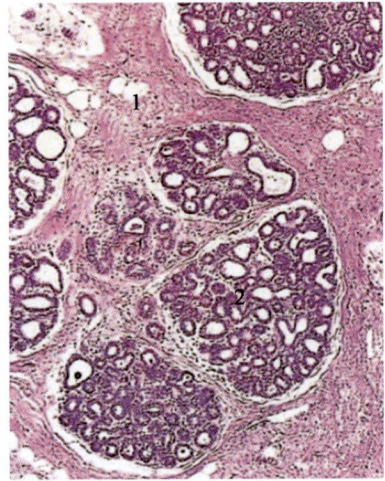

1—结缔组织；2—小叶
图 19 - 14　妊娠期活动期乳腺光镜图

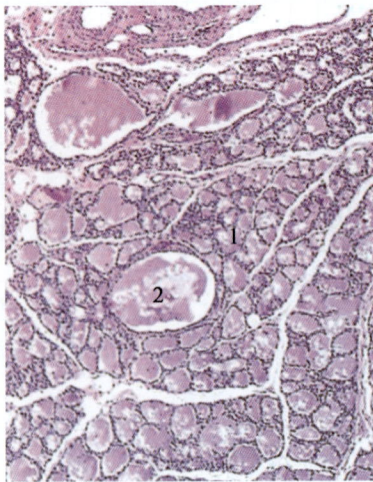

1—腺泡；2—导管
图 19 - 15　哺乳期活动期乳腺光镜图

（司徒成昊）

Chapter 20

Introduction to Embryology

Embryology is the science studying the formation and development of an embryo and fetus, whose content includes the germ cell formation, fertilization, embryonic development, maternal-fetal relationship, congenital malformation, etc.

1 Content of Embryology

Human embryonic development in the maternal uterus lasts for about 38 weeks (266 days), which can be divided into three stages: preembryonic period, embryonic period and fetal period. The preembryonic period is from fertilization to the appearance of bilaminar blastoderm at the end of the second week; the embryonic period is from the 3rd week to the 8th week, during which the embryonic organs, systems and appearance develop; the fetal period is from the 9th week to the birth, during which the fetus grows up gradually, and the organs and systems continue to develop, and some organs perform partial functions.

Embryology includes the following fields: ①Descriptive Embryology uses anatomical or histological methods to observe the development of morphological structures such as the formation of organs and systems, and the proliferation, migration and apoptosis of cells in embryonic development. It is the basic content of Embryology. ②Comparative Embryology compares the embryonic development of different species of animals to explore the biological evolution process. ③Experimental Embryology applies chemical, physical stimulation or microsurgery to the embryo or embryo tissues to observe the influence on embryonic development. ④Chemical Embryology uses chemical, biochemical and histological techniques to study the changes of some chemical substances in embryonic cells and tissues to explore the chemical mechanisms in embryonic development. ⑤Molecular Embryology uses the techniques of molecular biology to study the molecules in fertilization, implantation, cell differentiation, tissue induction, cell migration, etc., to clarify the molecular mechanism of embryonic development. ⑥Reproductive Engineering interferes with the early reproductive process to obtain the desired new-born individuals through in vitro fertilization, early embryo culture, nuclear injection, animal cloning, etc.

2　Brief History of Embryology

Hippocrates (460 B.C.-377 B.C.) and Aristotle (384 B.C.-322 B.C.), two ancient Greek scholars, studied the embryonic development. In 1651, Harvey (1578 - 1658), a British scholar, put forward the hypothesis that all life comes from eggs. Two Dutch scholars, Leeuwenhoek (1632 - 1723) and Graaf (1641 - 1673), discovered sperm and follicle, respectively. In 1855, Mark (1815 - 1865), a German scholar, proposed the theory of three germ layers in embryonic development. Spemann (1869 - 1941), another German scholar, carried out microsurgical experiments on separation, cutting, transplantation, and recombination of amphibian embryos, laying the foundation of Experimental Embryology. In the 1950s, with the development of Molecular Biology, scientists began to study gene expression and its regulation in embryonic development, creating Molecular Embryology. Reproductive Engineering was developed by applying embryologic techniques such as in vitro fertilization and embryo transplantation to treat female infertility. In 1978, the first in vitro fertilization baby in the world was born in Manchester. In 1988, the first in vitro fertilization baby on the Chinese mainland was born in Beijing.

3　Research Methods of Embryology

Scientific progress is usually achieved by the improvement of experimental methods and technological innovation. Embryology benefits form the progress of the following research methods.

3.1　Observation of Chicken Embryos

Chick embryos are incubated to a specific stage of development, then microscopic observation and description or surgery is carried out. The chicken embryo experiment is done in a short period and is easy to operate. With the development of molecular biology technology such as RNA interference, gene transfection and genome sequencing, it lays a good experimental foundation for studying the function of genes related to embryonic development.

3.2　Sectioning Techniques

The serial sections of embryos are made by using slicing technology. The image of each section is processed by a computer with image-analysis technology; thus, the three-dimensional structure image of an embryo can be obtained.

3.3　Transgenic Animals

After cloned genes are inserted into the genome by microinjection, the newly fertilized eggs of experimental animals are implanted into the uterus of the pseudopregnant host and develop into offspring. This method has been widely used in gene function analysis, genetic disease research, disease animal model establishment, etc.

3.4　Tracing Methods

To study the dynamic migration, settlement, and differentiation processes of specific cells during embryonic development, retrovirus-carrying fluorescent protein genes can be transferred into these cells. Non-cytotoxic dyes such as trypan blue and horseradish peroxidase are also commonly used in vivo.

3.5　Microsurgical Techniques

Microsurgery can be used for tissue transplantation or tissue resection. In clinical practice, microsurgical techniques are often used to isolate and cut blastomeres for preimplantation genetic testing.

3.6　Embryonic Stem Cell Technology

Embryonic stem cells are undifferentiated diploid pluripotent stem cells with unlimited proliferation, self-renewal and multi-directional differentiation potential. They can differentiate into nerve cells, myocardial cells, blood cells, etc., which lays the foundation for cell therapy.

3.7　Gene-Editing Techniques

Gene-editing techniques refer to the genetic operations of inserting, removing, or replacing the target genes so as to transfer DNA fragments or repair mutated genes, achieving the purpose of controlling biological characters and behaviors.

3.8　Somatic Cell Cloning Technology

Animal somatic cells are cultured to a dormant state, then their nuclei are transferred into the enucleated oocytes. The somatic nucleus is reprogrammed in the cytoplasm of the oocyte to start cleavage. Then the embryo develops to produce a cloned animal.

4　Congenital Malformations

Congenital malformation (CM) is the morphological and structural abnormality that occurs due to embryonic developmental disorders. The science of studying CMs is called teratology, which is an important branch of embryology.

The incidence of CMs in the world is 1.3%–1.7%, of which limb malformation accounts for 26%; neural tube malformation accounts for 17%; genitourinary malformation accounts for 14%; facial malformation accounts for 9%; digestive system malformation accounts for 8%; cardiovascular malformation accounts for 4%; and multiple malformations account for 22% (Figure 20 - 1).

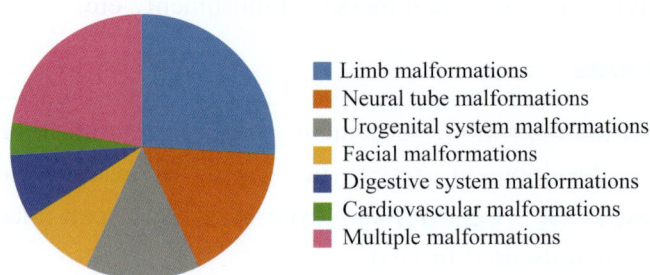

Figure 20 - 1   Incidence of Congenital malformations

CMs can be divided into whole developmental malformations, local developmental malformations, organ or organ locality malformations, poorly differentiated tissue malformations, overdeveloped malformations, incomplete absorption malformations, supernumerary and ectopic developmental malformations, developmental retention malformations, double malformations and parasitic malformations.

The causes of CMs include genetic factors (25%), environmental factors (10%), and the interaction between genetic and environmental factors (65%).

CMs caused by genetic factors include chromosomal abnormalities and genetic mutations. Chromosomal aberrations include abnormalities in the number of chromosomes and structural abnormalities in chromosomes. The abnormalities caused by abnormal number of chromosomes include Turner syndrome, Down syndrome, Edward syndrome, etc. Chromosomal structural abnormalities can also cause deformities such as cat cry syndrome. The occurrence of genetic mutations is rare, mainly including chondrodysplasia, polycystic kidney disease, testicular feminization syndrome, etc.

The environmental factors causing CMs are called teratogens, which mainly affect the external and internal environment of the mother, the microenvironment around the embryo. Environmental teratogenic factors mainly include biological teratogenic factors, physical teratogenic factors, teratogenic drugs, teratogenic chemicals, and other teratogenic factors.

Most deformities are caused by the interaction between environmental and genetic factors. Environmental teratogenic factors can cause congenital deformities by causing chromosomal abnormalities and gene mutations, but the genetic characteristics of embryos can also affect or determine their susceptibility to teratogenic factors.

Embryonic development is a continuous process, but there are also certain stages. Embryos at different stages have different degrees of susceptibility to teratogens. The embryonic period (from the 3rd to the 8th week) is the most susceptible to teratogens, which is called susceptible period.

The World Health Organization has proposed a strategy of three-level prevention for

CMs. The primary prevention refers to preventing the occurrence of defective infants, including premarital examinations, genetic counseling, and prenatal care. The secondary prevention refers to preventing the birth of severely deformed infants. Many deformities can be diagnosed clearly through prenatal amniocentesis, chorionic villus examination, fetal endoscopy, and image examination, some of which can be treated in utero. The tertiary prevention refers to the postnatal treatments of the defects after birth.

5 Significance of Studying Embryology

In the development from one cell (i.e., zygote) to a fetus, there are many complex dynamic changes. Learners should understand the three-dimensional morphology of embryos in a certain period, as well as the temporal and spatial changes of these structures in different periods. This is not only necessary to learn Embryology well, but also helpful to establish scientific thinking methods.

Embryology is an important basic medical course. Only after learning Embryology, can we master how the cells, tissues, organs, and systems are formed and how a newborn is developed and understand some contents of other courses such as Anatomy, Histology, Pathology, and Genetics. Embryology provides the necessary basic knowledge for Obstetrics, Gynecology, Andrology, Reproductive Engineering, Pediatrics, Orthopedics, Oncology, Eugenics, etc.

(Yue Haiyuan)

第二十章　胚胎学绪论

第一节　胚胎学的内容

胚胎学是研究个体发生和发育的过程及其机制的科学,其研究内容包括生殖细胞产生、受精、胚胎发育、母胎关系、先天性畸形等。

人类胚胎在母体子宫中的发育一般经历约 38 周(266 天),可分为 3 个时期。从受精到第 2 周末二胚层胚盘出现,称胚前期;从第 3 周初至第 8 周末,胚的各器官、系统与外形发育,称胚期;从第 9 周初至出生,胎儿逐渐长大,各器官、系统继续发育,部分器官出现一定的功能活动,称胎期。

胚胎学包括以下分支学科。

（1）描述胚胎学：应用解剖学和组织学方法观察胚胎发育中的形态结构演变，如器官和系统的形成、细胞增殖、迁移及凋亡等，是胚胎学的基础内容。

（2）比较胚胎学：比较不同种系动物的胚胎发育，探讨生物进化过程。

（3）实验胚胎学：观察化学或物理因素、显微手术对胚胎发育的影响，研究胚胎发育的规律和机制。

（4）化学胚胎学：应用化学和组织学技术研究胚胎发生过程中胚体内某些化学物质的变化，探讨胚胎发育的化学基础及机制。

（5）分子胚胎学：用分子生物学的理论和技术研究受精、植入、细胞分化、细胞迁移等过程的分子基础，阐明胚胎发育的分子机制。

（6）生殖工程：采用基因技术、克隆技术、胚胎移植、免疫技术等人工干预早期生殖过程，孕育符合期望的新生个体。试管婴儿和克隆动物是该领域中最著名的成就。

第二节　胚胎学发展简史

古希腊学者 Hippocrates(前 460—前 377)和 Aristotle(前 384—前 322)很早就进行过胚胎研究。1651 年，英国学者 Harvey(1578—1658)提出"一切生命皆来自卵"的假设。荷兰学者 Leeuwenhoek(1632—1723)与 Graaf(1641—1673)分别发现了精子与卵泡。1855 年，德国学者 Remark(1815—1865)提出胚胎发育的三胚层学说。另一德国学者 Spemann(1869—1941)应用显微操作技术研究胚胎发育，奠定了实验胚胎学。20 世纪 50 年代，随着分子生物学的诞生，科学家们开始用分子生物学的观点和方法研究胚胎发生过程中基因表达及其调控，建立了分子胚胎学分支。后来在利用体外受精、胚胎移植等实验胚胎学技术治疗女性不孕症的基础上兴起了生殖工程。1978 年世界上第一例试管婴儿在英国曼彻斯特诞生，1988 年中国大陆第一例试管婴儿在北京出生。

第三节　胚胎学的研究方法

科学的发展离不开实验方法、技术的改良和创新。胚胎学的常用研究方法有下面几种。

1. 鸡胚实验

将鸡胚孵化至特定的发育阶段，进行显微镜观察、描述或显微操作。鸡胚实验周期短，容易操作。随着分子生物学技术的发展与应用，鸡胚实验为研究胚胎发育中相关基因的功能奠定了良好的实验基础。

2. 胚胎切片

制作胚胎的连续切片，然后将每张切片的图像用图像分析技术进行计算机处理，就可以得到胚胎立体结构图像。

3. 转基因动物实验

用显微注射等方法将外源基因注入实验动物的受精卵，然后将此受精卵植入受体动物的子宫，使子代动物携带有外源基因。该实验方法被广泛应用在基因功能分析、遗传病研究和疾病动物模型建立等领域。

4. 示踪技术

把带有荧光蛋白基因的逆转录病毒导入胚胎细胞，通过观察胚胎发育过程中荧光蛋白的表达来研究细胞的迁移、定居和分化的动态过程。示踪技术也常用无细胞毒性的活体染料，如台盼蓝、辣根过氧化酶等。

5. 显微操作技术

应用显微手术进行组织移植或组织切除。在临床上，常应用显微操作技术分离、切割卵裂球以进行植入前遗传学检测。

6. 胚胎干细胞技术

胚胎干细胞具有无限增殖、自我更新和多向分化的潜能，可以分化出神经细胞、心肌细胞、血细胞等，可用于细胞治疗。

7. 基因编辑技术

基因编辑指根据实际需要对目的基因进行插入、移除或替换等操作，以导入 DNA 片段或修复突变基因，从而控制生物性状和行为。

8. 体细胞克隆技术

体细胞克隆技术是指将动物的体细胞经过抑制培养，使其达到休眠状态后，再将其细胞核取出并移入细胞核被去除的卵母细胞内，然后再使这些细胞核重新编程，启动卵裂，开始胚胎发育过程，最终产生子代克隆动物的技术。

第四节 先天性畸形

先天性畸形是由胚胎发育紊乱导致出生时出现的形态结构异常。研究先天性畸形的科学称畸形学，是胚胎学的一个重要分支。

一、先天性畸形的概况

全世界先天性畸形的发生率为 1.3%～1.7%，其中四肢畸形占 26%，神经管畸形占 17%，泌尿生殖系统畸形占 14%，颜面畸形占 9%，消化系统畸形占 8%，心血管畸形占 4%，多发畸形占 22%（图 20 - 1）。

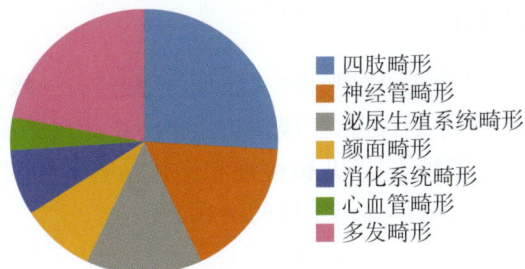

图 20 - 1 先天性畸形的发生率

二、先天性畸形的分类

先天性畸形分为整胚发育畸形、胚胎局部发育畸形、器官和器官局部畸形、组织分化不良性畸形、发育过度性畸形、吸收不全性畸形、超数和异位发生性畸形、发育滞留性畸形、重复畸形和寄生畸形。

三、先天性畸形的发生原因

先天性畸形的发生原因包括遗传因素(25%),环境因素(10%),以及遗传因素与环境因素的相互作用(65%)。

(一)遗传因素

引起的先天性畸形包括染色体畸变、基因突变。

1. 染色体畸变

包括染色体数目的异常和染色体结构异常。染色体数目异常产生的畸形有 Turner 综合征、Down 综合征、Edward 综合征等。染色体的结构异常也可引起猫叫综合征等畸形。

2. 基因突变

导致的畸形较少,主要有软骨发育不全、多囊肾、睾丸女性化综合征等。

(二)环境因素

能引起先天性畸形的环境因素统为致畸因子,主要影响母体周围的外环境、母体的内环境和胚体周围的微环境这三个方面。环境致畸因子主要有生物性致畸因子、物理性致畸因子、致畸性药物、致畸性化学物质和其他致畸因子。

(三)环境因素与遗传因素的相互作用

多数畸形的发生是环境因素与遗传因素相互作用的结果。环境致畸因子可通过引起染色体畸变和基因突变而导致先天性畸形,但胚胎的遗传特性也可以影响或决定胚胎对致畸因子的易感程度。

四、胚胎的致畸敏感期

胚胎发育是一个连续的过程,但也有着一定的阶段性。处于不同发育阶段的胚胎对致畸作用的敏感程度也不同。胚胎发育中最易受到致畸因子作用的时期在胚期,即受精后第 3 周至第 8 周,这一阶段称致畸敏感期。

五、先天性畸形的预防

世界卫生组织提出了干预先天性畸形的"三级预防"策略。一级预防是指防止畸形儿的发生,包括婚前检查、遗传咨询和孕期保健;二级预防是指防止严重畸形儿的出生,很多畸形可以在出生前通过羊水检查、绒毛膜检查、胎儿镜检查和影像检查等做出明确诊断,其中有些可以进行宫内治疗;三级预防是指对畸形儿出生后的治疗。

第五节　学习胚胎学的意义

从一个细胞(受精卵)发育为足月胎儿的过程中存在很多复杂的动态变化。学习者既要了解某一时期胚胎的立体形态,也要掌握这些结构在不同时期的时间与空间的变化。这不仅对学好胚胎学十分必要,而且对建立科学的思维方法也很有益。

　　胚胎学是一门重要的医学基础课程。只有在学习了胚胎学之后，医学生才能掌握人体细胞、组织、器官和系统的产生与演化过程，才能了解整个个体的发生与发育，进而理解解剖学、组织学、病理学、遗传学等学科中的某些内容。胚胎学还为妇产科学、男性学、生殖工程学、儿科学、矫形外科学、肿瘤科学和优生学等临床学科提供了必要的基础知识，同时也是优生学赖以发展的学科之一。

（岳海源）

Chapter 21

General Embryology

The development of a human embryo includes the preembryonic period, embryonic period and fetal period, lasting for about 266 days. The preembryonic period and embryonic period are very crucial for embryonic development, in which a zygote develops into a human-looking fetus. In this chapter, the general process of the development of a human embryo as well as the maternal-fetal relationship is described.

1   Gametes and Fertilization

1.1   Gametes

Human gametes include the sperm and ovum, both of which are haploid cells. Gametes are produced from the precursor germ cells. The ovum is a massive cell and almost immotile, whereas the sperm is highly motile. Half of sperms contain Y chromosome (23, Y) and the other half contain X chromosome (23, X), while the ovum only contains X chromosome (23, X).

1.2   Fertilization

Fertilization is the process to form a zygote by a sperm and an ovum. The fertilization usually occurs in the ampulla of the uterine tube. The secondary oocyte is usually fertilized within 12 – 24 hours after ovulation. If not, they degenerate shortly thereafter. Sperms undergo a process called capacitation before they are capable of fertilizing an oocyte. Capacitation lasts for approximately 7 hours in the uterus or uterine tubes, in which a glycoprotein coat and seminal proteins are removed from the surface of sperm. Most sperms maintain the fertilization ability for about 24 hours in the female genital tract.

Fertilization is a sequence of coordinated events (Figure 21 – 1). First, dispersal of the follicular cells and the corona radiata results mainly from the action of the enzymes released from the acrosome of the many capacitated sperms. The sperm first reaching the zona pellucida combines with the sperm receptor and keeps releasing acrosome enzymes to disperse the zona pellucida, so that a pathway is formed. The process that sperms release enzymes from the acrosome to disperse the corona radiata and zona pellucida is called

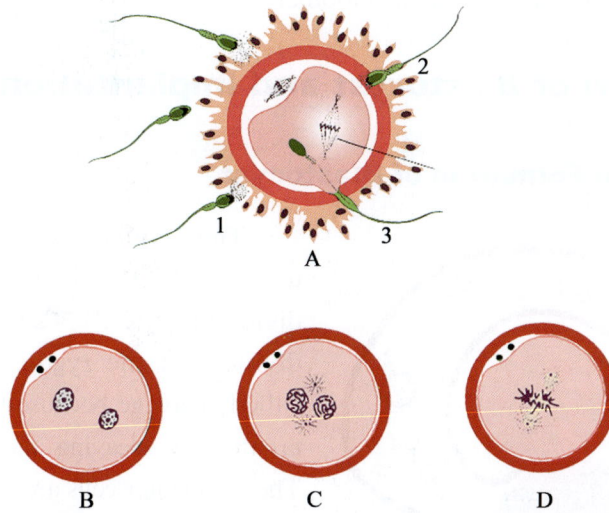

Figure 21 - 1　Drawings showing the process of fertilization

A1. Dispersal of follicular cells; A2. Penetration of zona pellucida; A3. Fusion of plasma membranes of gametes; B. Completion of the second meiotic division of oocyte; C. Formation of the pronuclei; D. Fusion of the pronuclei

acrosome reaction. Second, the plasma membranes of the oocyte and sperm fuse with each other and break down at the area of fusion. The head and tail of the sperm enter the cytoplasm of the oocyte. Once the sperm penetrates the zona pellucida, a change in the properties of the zona pellucida called zona reaction occurs, making the zona pellucida impermeable to other sperms. The zona reaction is believed to result from the action of lysosomal enzymes released by cortical granules near the plasma membrane of the oocyte. The penetration of the oocyte by a sperm activates the secondary oocyte quickly completing the second meiotic division and forming a mature ovum and a second polar body. Third, following the decondensation of the maternal chromosomes, the nucleus of the mature oocyte becomes the female pronucleus. On the other hand, the nucleus of the sperm enlarges to form the male pronucleus, and the tail of the sperm degenerates. Then, both pronuclei approach the cellular center. As they are close enough to fuse into a single diploid aggregation of chromosomes, the cell becomes a zygote.

　　Significances of fertilization are as follows. First, fertilization restores the normal diploid number of chromosomes in the zygote. The zygote is genetically unique because half of its chromosomes came from the mother and half from the father. The zygote contains a new combination of chromosomes that is different from that in the cells of either of the parents. Second, fertilization determines the sex of the embryo. The sex of the embryo is determined at fertilization by the kind of sperm that fertilizes the oocyte. Fertilization by a 23, X sperm produces a 46, XX zygote, which develops into a female, while fertilization by a 23, Y sperm produces a 46, XY zygote, which develops into a male. Third, fertilization causes metabolic activation of the oocyte and initiates cleavage of the zygote to start the embryonic development.

2　Formation of Blastocyst and Implantation

2.1　Cleavage and Formation of Blastocyst

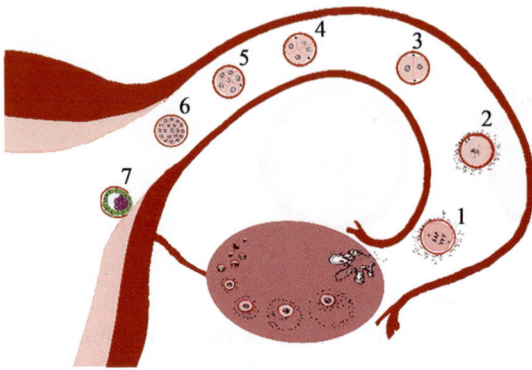

1. Ovulation; 2. Fertilization and beginning of cleavage; 3. Two-cell stage; 4. Four-cell stage; 5. Eight-cell stage; 6. Morula; 7. Blastocyst

Figure 21 - 2　Schematic summary of the ovulation, fertilization, cleavage and formation of the blastocyst

The zygote keeps moving from the uterine tube toward the uterus and starts to divide (Figure 21 - 2). The several mitotic divisions of the zygote at the beginning are called cleavage because the daughter cells are created by cleaving the parent cell in half. These daughter cells are also called blastomeres. At day 3 after fertilization, cleavage divisions produce 12 - 16 blastomeres to form a solid ball of cells, which is called morula. The embryo keeps moving towards the uterine cavity during these divisions. At day 4 - 5, morula enters the uterine cavity, and the cleavage keeps going on. When the blastomere number reaches about 100, a cavity forms within the morula, transforming the embryo into a blastocyst. The cells in the blastocyst can be divided into two groups. The cells on the interior form inner cell mass, which will form all the components of the embryo. The cells of a layer in the outer wall become trophoblast, which will form the extraembryonic tissues (Figure 21 - 3). The blastocyst enters the uterine cavity, and the zona pellucida surrounding the blastocyst starts to degenerate.

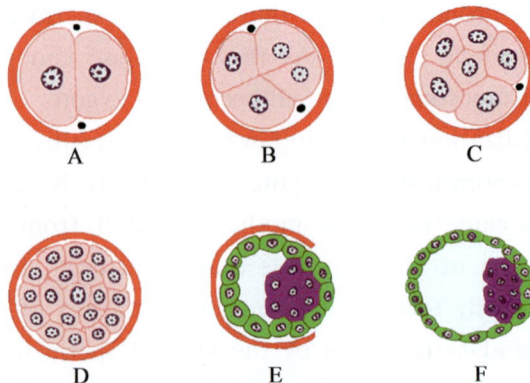

Figure 21 - 3　Drawings showing the cleavage and formation of the blastocyst
A. Two-cell stage; B. Four-cell stage; C. Eight-cell stage; D. Morula;
E. Early blastocyst with zona pellucida; F. Blastocytst

2.2 Implantation

Implantation is the process that the blastocyst embeds itself within the uterine endometrium. It begins on day 5 – 6 after fertilization. After the blastocyst hatches out, the polar trophoblast overlying the inner cell mass contacts with the endometrial lining of the uterus and secrets proteolytic enzymes to invade the endometrium, creating a wound in the uterine mucosa (Figure 21 – 4, Figure 21 – 5). By the day 11 – 12, the trophoblast has been almost completely embedded within the endometrium, and the uterine epithelium grows back over the embryo, thus healing the wound (Figure 21 – 5).

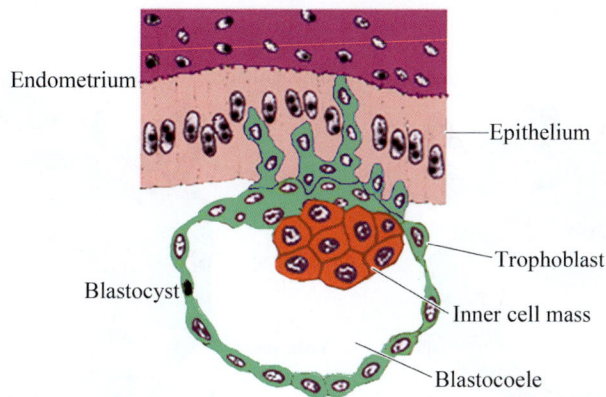

Figure 21 – 4 **Drawing showing a blastocyst invading the endometrium**

Because of the presence of an embryo, striking changes take place in uterine endometrium of the secretory phase, such as more blood supply, more gland secretion, being thicker, and enlarged stromal cells with more glycogen and lipid droplets. These changes of endometrium are called decidua reactions, and the stromal cells are called decidua cells. The endometrium is thus termed decidua. Based on the relationship with the embryo, the decidua is divided into 3 parts: decidua basalis, decidua capsularis and decidua parietalis (Figure 21 – 6). The decidua basalis is deeply behind the embryo; the decidua capsularis covers the part of the embryo in the uterine cavity; the rest of the decidua is the decidua parietalis.

Implantation is based on the secretory phase of endometrium. The disappearance of the zona pellucida and timely entry of the blastocyst into the uterine cavity are necessary conditions for implantation. If maternal endocrine disorders cause periodic changes in the endometrium that are not synchronized with the development of the blastocyst, and if there is inflammation or foreign matter in the endometrium, the implantation can be hindered.

Implantation of blastocysts usually occurs in the uterine endometrium in the body or fundus of the uterus, more often on the posterior uterine wall. In some cases, implantation occurs near the uterine cervix, resulting in placenta previa. Implantation sometimes occurs outside the uterus, such as the ovary, uterine tube and mesentery, which results in ectopic

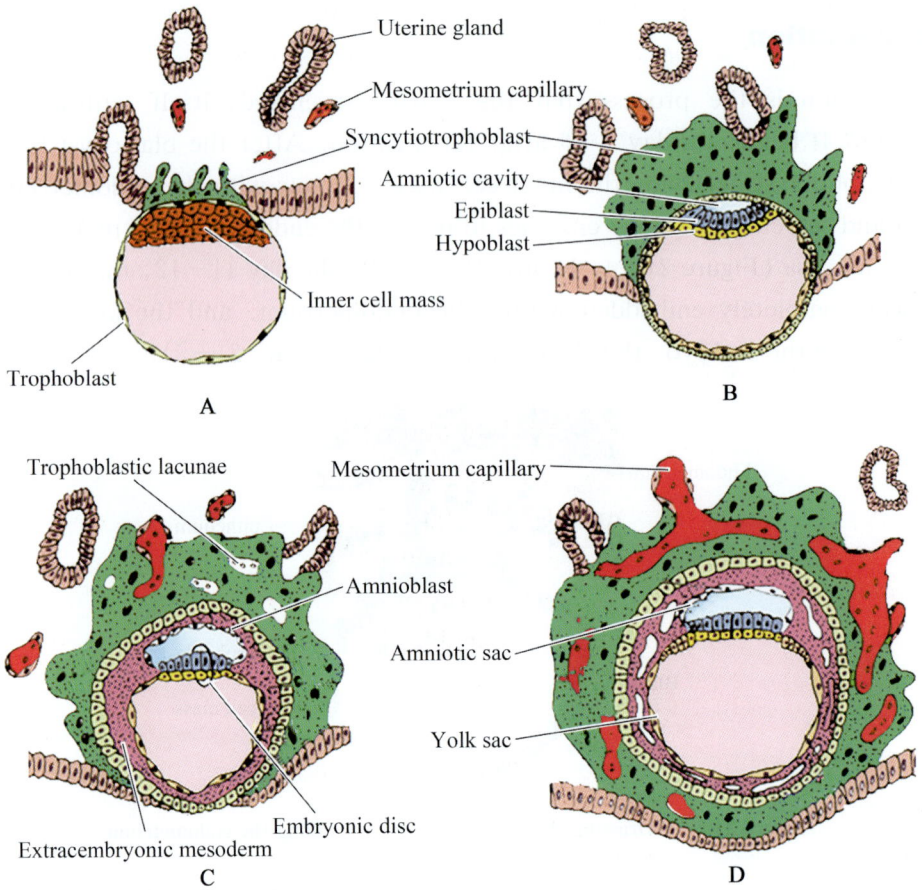

Figure 21-5   Drawings showing the implantation of a blastocyst
A. Day 7; B. Day 8; C. Day 9; D. Day 12

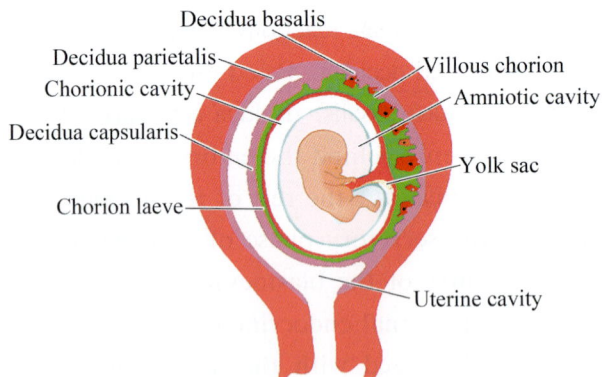

Figure 21-6   Drawing showing the relationship between the embryo and decidua

pregnancies.

During the implantation, the trophoblast cells proliferate and are subdivided into two distinct layers. The inner layer is composed of simple cuboidal cells, which is called cytotrophoblast. The outer layer is a single cell fused by some trophoblast cells, which is called syncytiotrophoblast. Soon irregular lacunae appear within the expanding syncytiotrophoblast, and maternal blood then fills them (Figure 21 – 5).

3 Formation of Germ Layers

As implantation of the blastocyst progresses, cells in the inner cell mass proliferate and differentiate to form circular plates of cells called germ layers. Adjacent germ layers closely adhere to each other, forming an elliptical cell disc, known as germ disk.

3.1 Formation of Bilaminar Germ Disk

In the 2-week human embryo, proliferation of the inner cell mass results in the formation of a circular bilaminar germ disk, consisting of two germ layers: the epiblast consisting of simple columnar cells and the hypoblast consisting of simple cuboidal cells. The two layers are closely attached and separated by a basement membrane. By the end of week 2, the bilaminar germ disk has been formed. Meanwhile, a cavity appears on the side of the upper embryonic layer near the trophoblast, called amniotic cavity, which is filled with amniotic fluid. The amniotic cavity wall is composed of a layer of flat amnioblasts that extend along the edge of the epiblast. The amnioblasts and the remaining epiblast form a sac called amniotic sac. Epiblast forms the base of the amniotic sac, while hypoblast grows and extends ventrally to form another sac called yolk sac (Figure 21 – 5).

As the formation of epiblast and hypoblast, some stellate cells and extracellular matrix appear in the blastocyst cavity between the cytotrophoblast and the yolk sac or amniotic sac, to form the extraembryonic mesoderm. Then a cavity appears between the cells in the extraembryonic mesoderm, and gradually increases, forming a large cavity in the extraembryonic mesoderm, called extraembryonic coelom. With the enlargement of the extraembryonic coelom, there is only a small amount of extraembryonic mesoderm called body stalk connecting the germ disk and cytotrophoblast, which develops into the main component of the umbilical cord in the future (Figure 21 – 5).

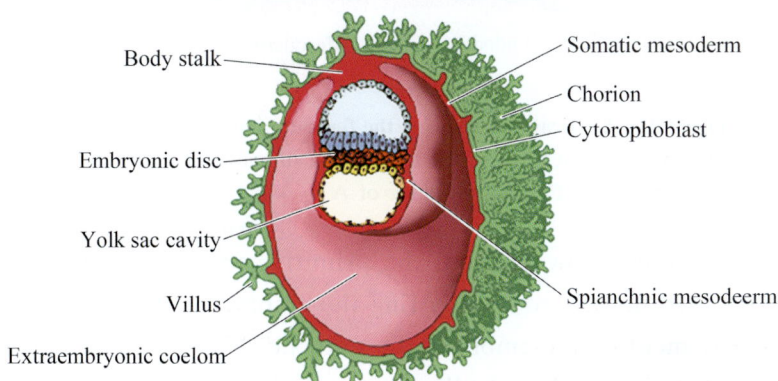

Figure 21 – 7　Drawing of a human embryo in early week 3

3.2 Formation of Trilaminar Germ Disk

At the beginning of week 3, a thickening of the epiblast appears in the middle line of the dorsal bilaminar germ disk, called primitive streak, indicating the caudal part of the embryo. The prominent cranial end of the primitive streak forms the primitive node. Concurrently, a narrow groove called primitive groove develops in the primitive streak, which is continuous with a small depression in the primitive node called primitive pit. The primitive groove and primitive pit result from the invagination of epiblast cells, which leave their deep surface and form a new layer termed mesoderm. Other cells from the epiblast displace the hypoblast, forming the endoderm in the roof of the yolk sac. The cells remaining in the epiblast form the ectoderm (Figure 21 – 8). By the end of week 3, a trilaminar germ disk has been developed, and all the cells in the three layers are derived from the epiblast.

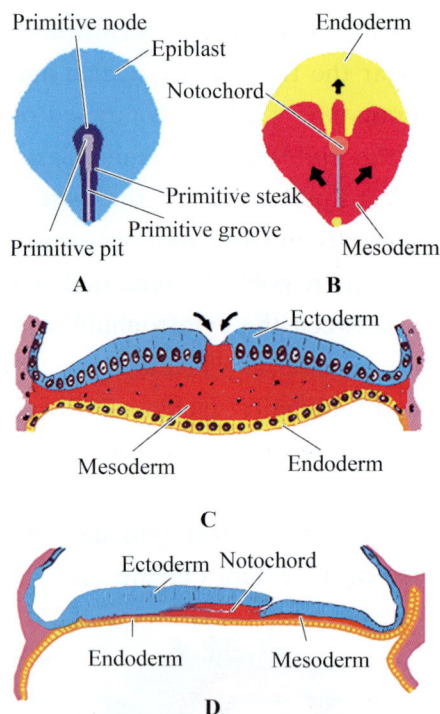

Figure 21 – 8　Drawings showing the formation of three germ layers
A. Surface plane of embryonic disc at day 16; B. Formation of mesoderm and notochord. The epiblast is removed; C. Transverse plane of A; D. Sagittal plane of A

Some mesoderm cells, growing from the primitive pit toward the cranial direction, form a cell chord called notochord, supporting the embryo in the early stage (Figure 21 – 8). With the development of the embryo, the notochord grows and extends cranially and caudally, and the primitive cord gradually shortens and finally disappears. If the primitive cord cells remain, they will differentiate and proliferate into a teratoma containing various tissues in the sacral region in the future. In the trilaminar germ disk, there are two small areas without mesoderm on the cranial side of the notochord and on the caudal side of the primitive streak, where the ectoderm and endoderm are close to each other and present a membrane, which are called oropharyngeal membrane and cloacal membrane, respectively.

4　Differentiation of Trilaminar Germ Layers and Formation of Embryonic Body

4.1　Differentiation of Trilaminar Germ Layers

During week 4 – 8, the trilaminar germ layers gradually differentiate into the primordia of various organs of the embryo.

4.1.1　Differentiation of Ectoderm

The notochord induces the ectodermal thickening of the dorsal midline in a plate shape, which is called neuronal plate. This part of the ectoderm is called neural ectoderm, and the rest ectoderm is called surface ectoderm. The neural plate grows with the growth of the notochord and sinks to the notochord to form a neural groove. The edges on both sides of the groove are raised and called nerve folds. The neuronal folds on both sides first approach each other, then fuse in the middle of the neuronal groove, and progress to both ends of the head and tail. Finally, two openings are formed at both ends, which are called anterior neural foramen and posterior neural foramen, respectively. The nerve foramens are closed in week 4, making the neuronal groove completely form the neuronal tube (Figure 21 – 9). At the same time, the cells at the lateral edge of the neuronal plate enter the dorsal side of the neuronal tube and soon migrate out of the tube wall to form two longitudinal cell cords located at the dorsal side of the neuronal tube, called neuronal crest (Figure 21 – 10). The neural tube is the primordium of the central nervous system, which will differentiate into the brain and spinal cord, retina, neurohypophysis, pineal gland and so on. The neural crest is the primordium of the peripheral nervous system, which will differentiate into brain ganglion, spinal ganglion, autonomic ganglion and peripheral nerve. Some neural crest cells migrate into the adrenal primordium and differentiate into chromaffin cells. Some neural crest cells migrate into the skin epidermis to form melanocytes. Some neural crest cells in the head are also involved in the formation of craniofacial bone and connective tissue. The surface ectoderm will differentiate into the epidermis of the skin and its accessory organs, enamel, corneal epithelium, lens, inner eardrum labyrinth, adenohypophysis, salivary gland, oral cavity, nasal cavity, and the epithelium of the lower segment of the anal canal.

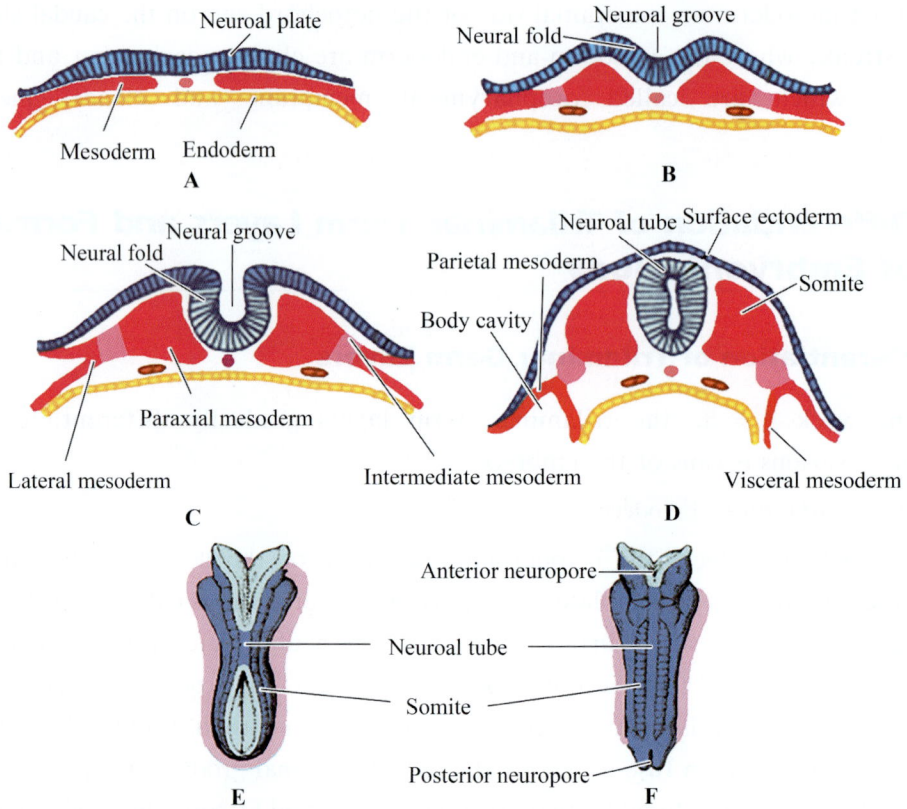

Figure 21 – 9   Drawings showing the formation of the neural tube and the early differentiation of mesoderm

A. Day 17; B. Day 19; C. Day 20; D. Day 21; E. Day 22; F. Day 23

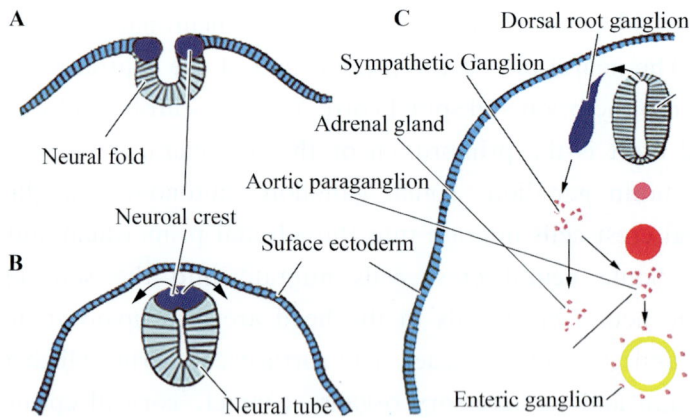

Figure 21 – 10   Drawings showing the formation of the neural crest and its migration

A. Formation of the neuronal crest; B. Neural crest cells starting to migrate after closure of neural tube; C. Different structures differentiated by the neuronal crest

4.1.2   Differentiation of Mesoderm

Mesoderm is usually first differentiated into mesenchymal and then into connective tissue, muscle tissue and blood vessels. Mesoderm cells on both sides of the notochord proliferate rapidly, forming paraxial mesoderm, intermediate mesoderm and lateral mesoderm from inside to outside (Figure 21 - 9). Paraxial mesoderm first forms segmental massive cell clusters, called somites, which are produced successively from the neck to the tail and paired left and right. In week 5, all somites are produced, a total of 42 - 44 pairs. Somites are mainly differentiated into the skin dermis, skeletal muscle and axial bone of the back. Most of the notochord degenerates and disappears, while the other parts form the nucleus pulposus in the intervertebral disk of the spine. Intermediate mesoderm differentiates into the main organs of the urinary system and the reproductive system. A small cavity is first formed in the lateral mesoderm and then fused into a large one, called intraembryonic body cavity, which is connected with the extraembryonic body cavity (Figure 21 - 11). So the lateral mesoderm is divided into two layers. The mesoderm of the body wall is connected with the ectoderm and mainly differentiates into skin, dermis,

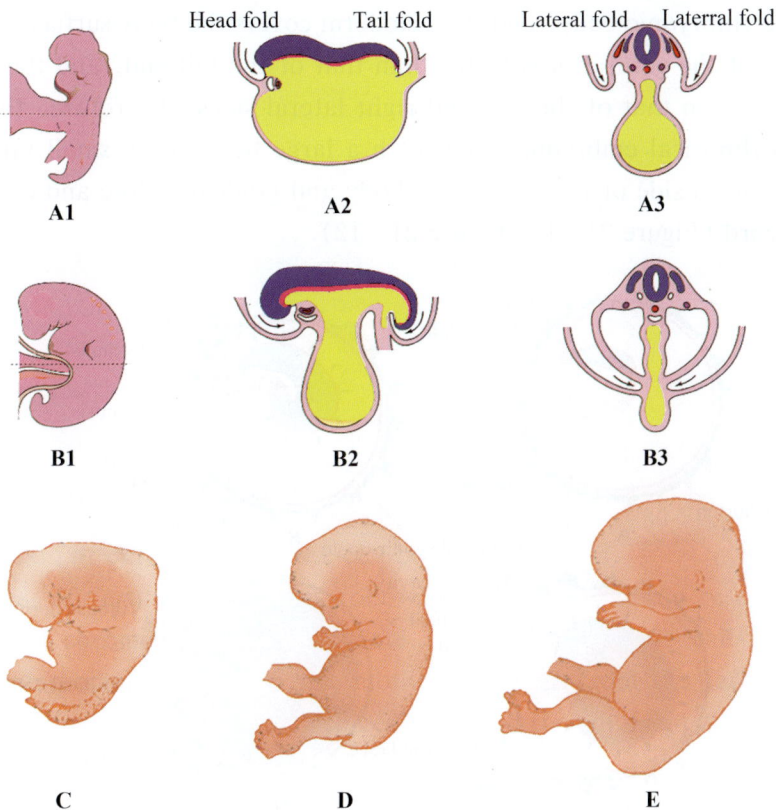

Figure 21 - 11   Drawings showing the development of the embryonic body
A. Day 23; B. Day 28; C. Day 48; D. Day 52; E. Day 56;
A1 and B1. Lateral view; A2 and B2. Sagittal plane; A3 and B3. Transverse plane

skeletal muscle, bone, and blood vessels of the chest, abdomen and limbs; the visceral wall mesoderm is connected with the endoderm and mainly differentiates into muscle tissue, blood vessels, connective tissue, and mesothelium of the digestive system and the respiratory system.

4.1.3 Differentiation of Endoderm

The endoderm forms the primitive gut, which will differentiate into the epithelial tissues of the digestive tube, digestive gland, respiratory tract, and lung below the throat, as well as the epithelial tissues of the middle ear, thyroid gland, parathyroid gland, thymus, bladder, and other organs.

4.2 Formation of Embryonic Body

With the differentiation of the three germ layers, the edge of the germ disk is folded to the ventral side to form head fold, tail fold, and lateral folds, respectively, so that the flat germ disk gradually becomes a cylindrical embryonic body. Because of the growth of neural tubes and somites, the central axis of the germ disk bulges to the dorsal side. The growth rate of the ectoderm is faster than that of the endoderm, so that the endoderm is involved in the embryonic body, and the ectoderm covers the body surface. The growth of the cranial end of the germ disk is faster than that of the tail end, and the growth of the tail end is faster than that of the left and right lateral sides. Therefore, the germ disk is folded into a cylindrical embryonic body with a large head and a small tail. The edge is folded to the ventral side of the embryonic body and gradually close and converge to form the umbilical cord (Figure 21 - 11, Figure 21 - 12).

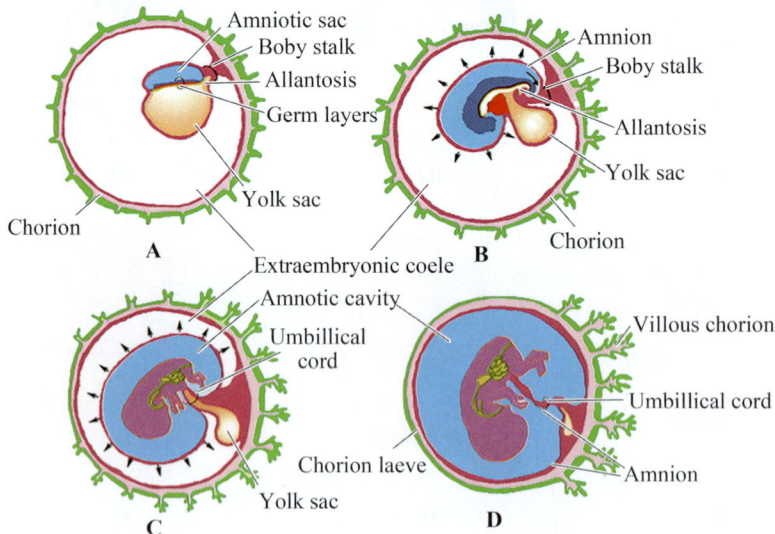

Figure 21 - 12 Drawings showing the development of the fetal membrane
A. Week 3; B. Week 5; C. Week 10; D. Week 20

At this time, the embryonic body protrudes into the amniotic cavity and grows in the amniotic fluid. The body stalk and yolk sac are combined on the ventral side of the embryonic body, wrapped with amnion to form umbilical cord. The ectoderm envelops the body surface. The endoderm folds into the embryo to form a primitive digestive tube, the middle part of which is connected with the yolk sac. The oropharyngeal membrane and cloacal membrane are transferred to the head and ventral side of the embryonic body respectively to seal the embryonic body. By the end of week 8, the embryo has eyes, ears, nose and limbs, showing a human shape (Figure 21 – 11).

5　Fetal Membrane and Placenta

The fetal membrane and placenta are accessory structures that play a role in protection, nourishment, breath, and excretion. Some of them have endocrine functions. After the fetus is delivered, the fetal membrane and placenta detach from the uterine wall and discharge out. They are also called afterbirth.

5.1　Fetal Membrane

The fetal membrane includes the chorion, amnion, yolk sac, allantois, and umbilical cord (Figure 21 – 12).

5.1.1　Chorion

Chorion consists of chorionic plate and various stem villi and villi. The chorionic plate consists of the trophoblast and extraembryonic mesoderm lining its inner surface. After implantation, the trophoblast has differentiated into syncytiotrophoblast and cytotrophoblast, and then the cells of cytotrophoblast proliferate and enter the syncytiotrophoblast to form villous processes. The villus at the end of week 2 is only composed of the outer syncytiotrophoblast and the inner cytotrophoblast, called primary stem villus. In week 3, the extraembryonic mesoderm gradually extends into the stem villus, and thus the primary stem villus is renamed the secondary stem villus. After that, the mesenchymal from the extraembryonic mesoderm in the stem villus differentiates into connective tissue and blood vessels, and the tertiary stem villus is formed. Among the stem villi, trophoblast lacunae develop into intervillous spaces, where maternal blood from the uterine spiral artery presents (Figure 21 – 13). The stem villus branches again to form many fine villi. At the same time, the cytotrophoblast cells at the end of the villus stem proliferate, penetrate out of the syncytiotrophoblast to the decidua, expand outward along the decidua, and connect with each other to form a layer of cytotrophoblast shell so that the chorion is firmly connected with the uterine decidua (Figure 21 – 14).

In the early stage of the embryo, the villi on the whole chorionic surface are evenly distributed. After that, due to the decrease of blood supply on the decidual side, the villi gradually degenerate and disappear, forming a chorion laeve (also called smooth chorion)

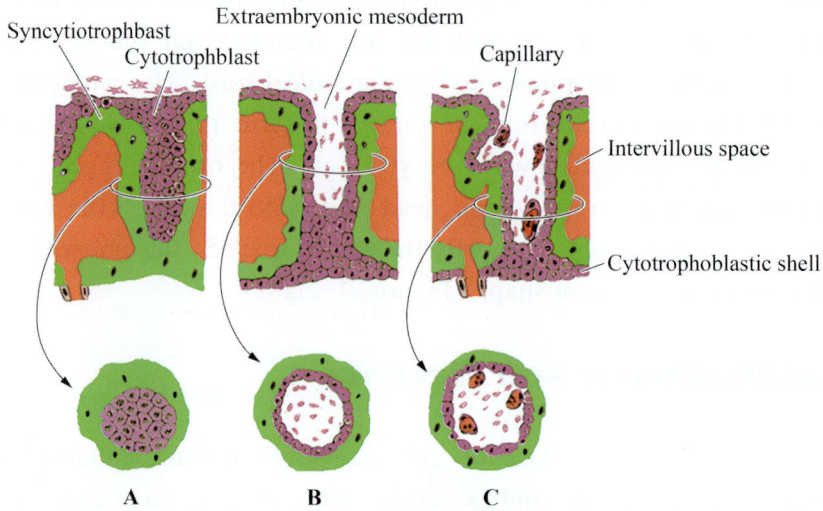

Figure 21 – 13 Drawings showing the development of the stem villus
A. The primary stem villus; B. The secondary stem villus; C. The tertiary stem villus

on the surface. While the blood supply on the basal decidual side is sufficient, the villi branch and grow repeatedly to form a villous chorion (Figure 21 – 12). The blood vessels in the chorion are connected with the blood vessels in the embryo through the umbilical cord. Since then, with the development of the fetus and the continuous expansion of the amniotic cavity, amnion, chorion leave, and decidua capsularis further protrude into the uterine cavity. The decidua capsularis contacts and then fuses with the decidua parietalis, thereby obliterating the uterine cavity gradually. Next, due to the reduced blood supply, the ducidua capsularis degenerates and disappears. Then the amnion and decidua parietalis fuse with each other (Figure 21 – 14).

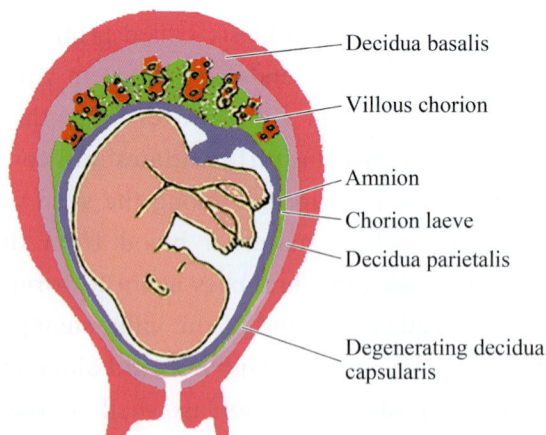

Figure 21 – 14 Drawing of the chorion and decidua in the late fetal period

The chorion provides nutrition and oxygen for early embryonic development, and the villous chorion forms a part of the placenta. Abnormal development of chorion endangers embryonic development. If the connective tissue in the villi is highly edema and the blood vessels disappear, the villi show hydatomorphic, which is called hydatidiform mole. Choriocarcinoma, a kind of malignant tumor, also endangers maternal health.

5.1.2   Amnion

Amnion is a translucent membrane composed of amniotic epithelium and few tissues of extraembryonic mesoderm (Figure 21 - 12). The amniotic cavity is filled with amniotic fluid, and the embryo grows and breeds in amniotic fluid. Amnion is initially attached to the edge of the embryonic disc. With the formation of the embryonic body, the expansion of the amniotic cavity, and the projection of the embryonic body into the amniotic cavity, the amnion wraps on the surface of the body stalk on the ventral side of the embryo to form the primitive umbilical cord. The enlargement of the amniotic cavity gradually makes the amnion close to the chorion, and the extraembryonic body cavity disappears. Amniotic fluid is weakly alkaline and contains exfoliated epithelial cells and some fetal metabolites. Amniotic fluid is mainly produced by continuous secretion of amnion, and is continuously absorbed by the amnion. From the medium term of pregnancy to the delivery, the fetus swallows the amniotic fluid, and the urine and feces enters amniotic fluid. Amnion and amniotic fluid play an important protective role in embryonic development. For example, embryos can move freely in the amniotic fluid, which is conducive to the normal development of skeletal muscles and prevents local adhesion, compression and vibration of embryos. During the delivery, amniotic fluid can also dilate the cervix and flush the birth canal. As the embryo grows up, the amniotic fluid also increases correspondingly, about 1 000 - 1 500 ml at delivery. Oligohydramnios (less than 500 ml) is prone to adhesion between amnion and fetus, affecting normal fetal development. Excessive amniotic fluid (more than 2 000 ml) can also affect normal fetal development. Abnormal amniotic fluid content is also related to some congenital malformations. For example, fetal absence of kidney or urethral atresia can cause oligohydramnios; fetal gastrointestinal atresia or incomplete neural tube closure can cause excessive amniotic fluid. Puncture and extraction of amniotic fluid, cell chromosome examination, or determination of the content of some substances in amniotic fluid can early diagnose some congenital abnormalities.

5.1.3   Yolk Sac

Yolk sac is located on the ventral side of the primitive gut (Figure 21 - 12). The yolk sac of a bird embryo is well developed, and a large amount of yolk is stored there to provide nutrition for embryonic development. There is not yolk in the yolk sac of human embryo. Yolk sac is a reflection of the germline genesis and evolution recapitulation. After the yolk sac of human embryo is wrapped into the umbilical cord, the yolk stalk connects with the primitive gut is closed in week 6, then the yolk sac gradually degenerates. Human hematopoietic stem cells and primordial germ cells come from the extraembryonic mesoderm and endoderm of the yolk sac respectively.

5.1.4 Allantois

Allantois is a blind tube extending from the tail of the yolk sac to the body stalk (Figure 21 - 12). With the formation of the embryonic body, it opens on the ventral side of the tail of the primitive gut; that is, it is connected with the future bladder. The median umbilical ligament from bladder to umbilicus is formed after allantoic atresia. The extraembryonic mesoderm on its wall forms allantoic arteries and allantoic veins, and then develops into umbilical arteries and umbilical veins.

5.1.5 Umbilical Cord

The umbilical cord is a cord-like structure connecting the umbilical part of the embryo and the placenta (Figure 21 - 12). It is covered with amnion and contains mucinous connective tissue differentiated by body stalk. In addition to the atretic yolk sac and allantois, there are also the umbilical arteries and umbilical vein in the connective tissue. The umbilical vessels connect embryonic vessels and placental villous vessels. There are two umbilical arteries that transport embryonic blood to the placental villi, in which the embryonic blood in the villi capillaries exchanges materials with the mother blood in the villi space. There is only one umbilical vein, which sends the blood collected by placental villi back to the embryo.

At birth, the umbilical cord is 40 to 60 cm long and 1.5 to 2 cm in diameter. If being too short, it is easy to cause premature separation of placenta and excessive bleeding when the fetus is delivered; if being too long, it is easy to wrap around the fetal limbs or neck, which may cause local dysplasia and even fetal asphyxia.

5.2 Placenta

5.2.1 Structure of Placenta

The placenta is a disc-shaped structure composed of fetal villous chorion and maternal decidua basalis (Figure 21 - 15). The placenta of a full-term fetus weighs about 500 g, with a diameter of 15 to 20 cm. It is thick in the center and thin around, with an average thickness of about 2.5 cm. The fetal surface of the placenta is smooth and covered with amnion. The umbilical cord is attached to the center or slightly deviated. Radial umbilical

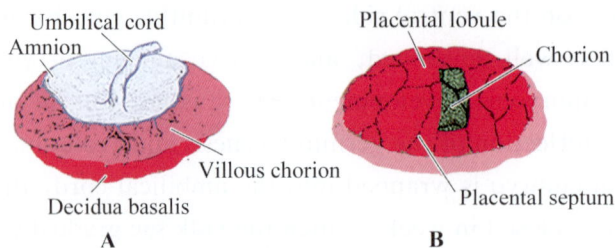

Figure 21 - 15 Drawings of a full-term placenta
A. Fetal side; B. Maternal side

vessel branches can be seen through the amnion. The maternal surface of the placenta is the rough stripped decidua basalis in which there are 15 to 30 placental lobules separated by shallow grooves.

On the vertical section of the placenta, the connective tissue of the chorion below the amnion and the branches of umbilical blood vessels are seen. The chorion emits about 40 to 60 stem villi, and each stem villi emits many villi. The end of the stem villus is fixed on the decidua basalis with the cytotrophoblast shell. The branches of umbilical vessels enter the villi along the stem villus to form capillaries. A short septum composed of basal decidua extends into the villous space, called placental septum. The placental septum divides the stem villi into the placental lobules, and each lobule contains 1 to 4 stem villi. The uterine spiral artery and uterine vein open in the villous space, so the villous space is filled with maternal blood, and the villi are immersed in maternal blood.

5.2.2   Blood Circulation of Placenta and Placental Membrane

There are two sets of maternal and fetal blood circulation in the placenta. Their blood circulates in their respective closed pipes, which are not mixed with each other but can exchange substances. Maternal arterial blood flows into the villous space from the uterine spiral artery. After material exchange with the fetal blood of the capillaries in the villus, it flows back into the mother from the uterine vein. The fetal venous blood flows into the villous capillaries through the umbilical artery and its branches. After material exchange with the maternal blood in the villous space, it becomes arterial blood and flows back to the fetus through the umbilical vein (Figure 21 - 16).

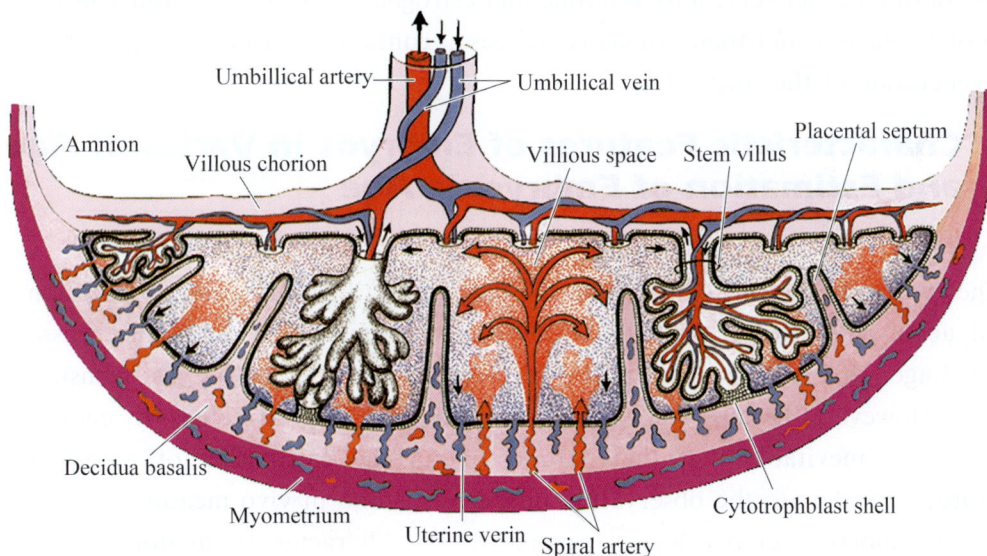

Figure 21 - 16   Drawing showing the placenta structure and blood circulation

The structure through which fetal blood and maternal blood exchange substances in the placenta is called placental membrane or placental barrier. The early placental membrane consists of syncytiotrophoblast, cytotrophoblast and its basement membrane, a thin layer of villous connective tissue, capillary endothelium and its basement membrane. In the later stage of development, because the cytotrophoblast disappears in many parts and the syncytiotrophoblast is only a thin layer of cytoplasm in some parts, the placental membrane becomes thinner, and there is only villous capillary endothelium, the thin syncytiotrophoblast, and their basement membrane between fetal blood and maternal blood, which is more conducive to the material exchange.

5.2.3 Functions of Placenta

Material exchange is the main function of the placenta. The fetus obtains nutrition and O_2 from the mother's blood through the placenta and discharges metabolites and CO_2. Therefore, the placenta has the function equivalent to the small intestine, lung and kidney after birth. Because some drugs, viruses and hormones can affect the fetus through the placental membrane, pregnant women should be careful with their medication and infections.

The syncytiotrophoblast of the placenta can secrete the following hormones, which play an important role in maintaining pregnancy. Human chorionic gonadotropin (HCG), similar to luteinizing hormone, can promote the growth and development of the corpus luteum to maintain pregnancy. It begins to secrete in week 2 of pregnancy, reaches the peak in week 8, and then decreases gradually. Human placental lactogen can promote the growth and development of the maternal mammary gland and the development of the fetus. It begins to be secreted in the second month of pregnancy and reaches its peak in the eighth month until delivery. Progesterone and estrogen begin to be secreted in the fourth month of pregnancy and then gradually increase, continuing to maintain pregnancy after the degeneration of the corpus luteum.

6 Characteristic Features of Embryos in Varies of Age and Estimation of Embryonic Age

The embryonic age calculated from the date of fertilization is the fertilization age, a total of about 38 weeks to delivery. Clinically, the embryonic age is often assessed by menstrual age, that is, it is about 40 weeks from the first day of the last menstruation to delivery. However, because the menstrual cycle is often affected by environmental changes, it is inevitable that there are errors in the calculation of embryonic age. Therefore, according to the observation in specimens and in vivo measurement of a large number of embryos, embryologists summarize the characteristic features and average lengths of embryos in each week, which can be used as the basis for estimating the embryonic age (Table 21-1, 21-2). The estimation of embryonic age is mainly based on the development of the germ disk, somite, face, limbs, skin, hair, and external genitalia, with reference to length and weight. There are three measurement standards for length.

The greatest length (GL) is mostly used to measure embryos of 1 − 3 weeks; crown-rump length (CRL), also known as sitting height, is used to measure embryos in and after week 4; crown-heel length (CHL), also called standing height, is used to measure the fetuses (Figure 21 − 17).

Table 21 − 1   Somite, length and characteristic features in varies of age during the preembryonic and embryonic Periods

Age (week)	Length (mm)	Somites (pairs)	Characteristic Features
1		0	blastocyst forming and implantating
2	0.2 − 0.4(GL)	0	appearance of bilaminar germ disk
3	0.5 − 1.5(GL)	1 − 4	trilaminar germ disk; primitive streak; neural groove; notochord
4	1.5 − 5(CRL)	4 − 29	embryonic folds; neural tube forming; optic vesicles and optic placodes forming; appearance of branchial arch 1,2,3
5	5 − 8(CRL)	30 − 44	branchial arch 4 occurring; hind-limb buds; optic vesicles; lens placodes and paddle-shaped forelimbs; C-shaped embryo
6	8 − 13(CRL)		Digital rays in hand or foot plates; prominent brain vesicle; external auricle forming; umbilical herniation developing
7	13 − 21(CRL)		pigmentation of retina; digital rays separating; nipples and eyelids formed; upper lip formed; obvious umbilical herniation
8	21 − 35(CRL)		long limbs with bent elbows or knees; free fingers and toes; more human-like face; umbilical herniation presenting

Table 21 − 2   Length, weight and characteristic features in varies of age during the fetal period

Age (week)	Length (CRL, mm)	Weight (g)	Characteristic Features
9	50	8	eyelids closed; umbilical herniation disappearing
10	61	14	fingernails developing
12	87	45	sex identifiable; eyes and ears lie close to definitive position
14	120	110	toenails developing; lower limbs well developing
16	140	200	ears erecting
18	160	320	appearance of vernix caseosa
20	190	460	appearance of lanugo hair
22	210	630	skin reddish and wrinkled
24	230	820	fingernail well developed; fetal body emaciated
26	250	1 000	eyebrows occurring; eyelids opening
28	270	1 300	eyelids well opened; head hair occurring
30	280	1 700	toenails well developed; testis beginning to descend
32	300	2 100	smooth and radish skin; body well-rounded contour
36	340	2 900	chubby body; lanugo disappearing; vernix caseosa covering
38	360	3 400	testes in scrotum; fingernails over top of fingers

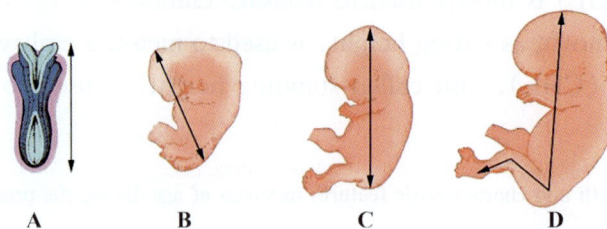

Figure 21 - 17   Drawings of methods used to measure the length of embryos
A. Great length (GL); B. and C. Crown-rump length (CRL); D. Crown-heel length (CHL)

7   Twins, Multiples and Conjoined Twins

7.1   Twins

The incidence of twins accounts for about 1% of newborns. There are two types of twins: dizygotic twins and monozygotic twins.

7.1.1   Dizygotic Twins

Dizygotic twins develop from two zygotes and may be of the same sex or different sexes. For the same reason, they are not more alike genetically than brothers or sisters born at different times. The only thing they have in common is that they are at the same age.

7.1.2   Monozygotic Twins

Monozygotic twins result from the fertilization of one oocyte and develop from one zygote, so they are of the same sex, genetically identical, and very similar in physical appearance. The reasons for monozygotic twins are as follows: ①One oocyte develops into two blastocysts and then develops into a complete embryo with his or her own amniotic cavity and placenta, respectively. ②There are two inner cell masses in each blastocyst, each of which develops into an embryo with his or her own amniotic cavity and a shared placenta. ③There are two primitive streaks and notochords in one germ disk, inducing the formation of two neural tubes and then developing into two embryos who are located in the same amniotic cavity and share a placenta.

7.2   Multiples

More than two newborns delivered at one time are called multiples. The causes of multiple births can be monozygotic, polyzygotic, or mixed. Mixed multiple births are more often seen. The incidence of multiple births is very low.

7.3   Conjoined Twins

In monozygotic twins, when two primitive streaks appear in one germ disk and then two embryos are developed, respectively, if the two primitive streaks are too close, local connection occurs during embryonic body formation, resulting in conjoined twins. Conjoined twins can be divided into symmetrical and asymmetric types. Symmetrical type refers to two embryos of the same size, which can be divided into cephalic conjoined bodies, thoracoabdominal conjoined bodies, hip conjoined bodies, etc. Asymmetric type refers to two embryos in different sizes, and the smaller one often develops incompletely, forming parasitic fetus or fetus in fetus.

(Yue Haiyuan)

第二十一章　胚胎发生总论

人类胚胎发育包括胚前期、胚期和胎期，持续约 266 天。在胚前期和胚期，受精卵发育为初具人形的胎儿，因此它们是胚胎发育的关键时期。本章主要叙述胚胎发生的总体过程以及胚体和母体的关系。

第一节　生殖配子和受精

一、生殖配子

人类生殖配子包括精子和卵子，均为单倍体细胞。配子由前体生殖细胞产生。与精子相比，卵子体积巨大，且几乎静止不动，而精子较小且具有很强的运动能力。在性染色体构成上，精子中的半数含 Y 染色体(23，Y)，半数含 X 染色体(23，X)，而卵子只含 X 染色体(23，X)。

二、受精

受精是由精子和卵子结合产生受精卵的过程(图 21-1)。受精部位通常在输卵管的壶腹部。卵母细胞通常在排卵后 12~24 h 内受精，否则很快退化。精子在子宫或输卵管中需要清除其头部表面的一层糖蛋白和精液蛋白才能获得使卵子受精的能力，这个过程叫作获能。精子在女性生殖管道内的受精能力一般可维持 24 h。

受精是一系列连续的过程。首先，大量获能的精子通过顶体释放顶体酶，溶解放射冠等卵泡细胞，这样部分精子可直接与透明带接触。接触到透明带的第一个精子与透明带上的精子受体结合，进一步释放顶体酶溶蚀透明带，形成一条孔道。精子释放顶体酶溶蚀放射冠和透明带的过程也称顶体反应。然后，精子的细胞膜和次级卵母细胞的细胞膜发生融合，精子的头部和尾部进入卵母细胞的细胞质。一旦有精子穿透透明带，卵母细胞胞质内的皮质颗粒释放溶酶体酶，使透明带的性质发生改变，精子受体失活，使其他精子不能再穿越透明带，这一过程称

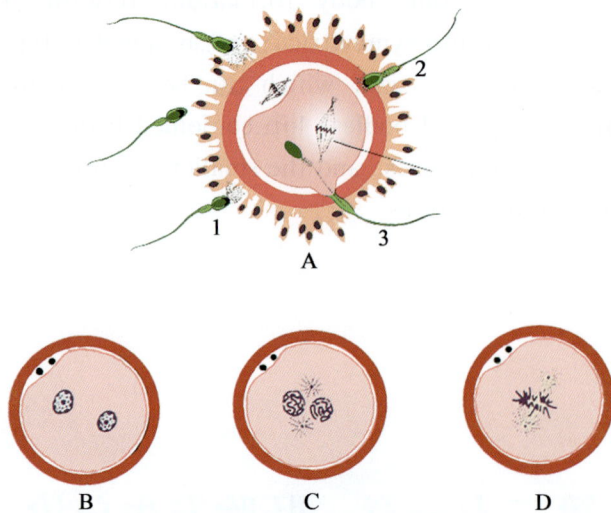

图 21 - 1　受精过程示意图

A：1—解离卵泡细胞；2—穿越透明带；3—精子入卵；B.次级卵母
细胞完成第二次减数分裂；C.原核形成；D.原核融合

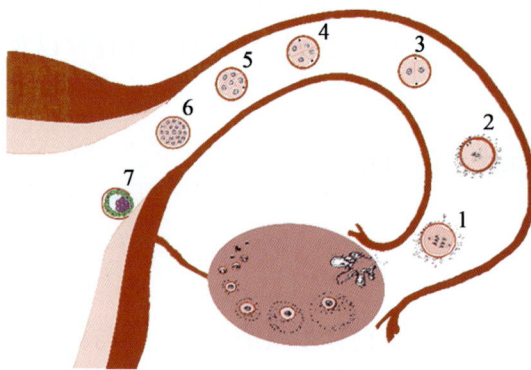

1—排卵；2—受精与卵裂；3—2 细胞期；4—4 细胞
期；5—8 细胞期；6—桑椹胚；7—胚泡

图 21 - 2　排卵、受精与卵裂过程模式图

透明带反应。此时，次级卵母细胞很快完成第二次减数分裂，形成卵细胞并排出第二极体。接下来，卵细胞的核和精子的核膨大分别形成雌原核和雄原核，精子的尾部退化。最后，雌原核、雄原核靠近并发生融合，形成二倍体的受精卵(图 21 - 2、图 21 - 3)。

受精的意义在于：①恢复受精卵的二倍体核型。受精卵在遗传上是独特的，因为它的染色体一半来自母亲，一半来自父亲。受精卵包含了一个新的染色体组合，与双亲的染色体组合不同。②决定胚胎的性别。胚胎的性别由使卵母细胞受精的精子种类决定。含 X 染色体的精子受精产生 46,XX 受精卵，发育为女性；而含 Y 染色体的精子受精产生 46,XY 受精卵，发育为男性。③激活卵母细胞的代谢并启动受精卵的分裂，胚胎发育开始。

第二节　胚泡形成和植入

一、卵裂和胚泡形成

受精卵形成后就向子宫腔移动，并开始细胞分裂。由于子代细胞是由母细胞分裂成两半而产生的，其细胞体积变小。这些子代细胞称卵裂球，这种特殊的有丝分裂称卵裂。受精后第 3 天，卵裂产生 12～16 个卵裂球，形成一个实心的胚，称桑椹胚，并到达子宫与输卵管交界的子宫腔侧。卵裂继续进行,细胞之间出现许多小腔隙,后逐渐融合成一个大腔。第 4~5 天,当卵裂球的数目达到 100 个左右时,出现一囊泡状结构,称胚泡。胚泡壁为单层细胞,称滋养层,将发育成胚外组织,主要是胎盘,支持胚胎的发育;胚泡的中心为胚泡腔,内含液体;胚泡腔内一侧的一团细胞称内细胞群,将发育成胚体。胚泡进入子宫腔后,透明带开始退化(图 21 - 2、图 21 - 3)。

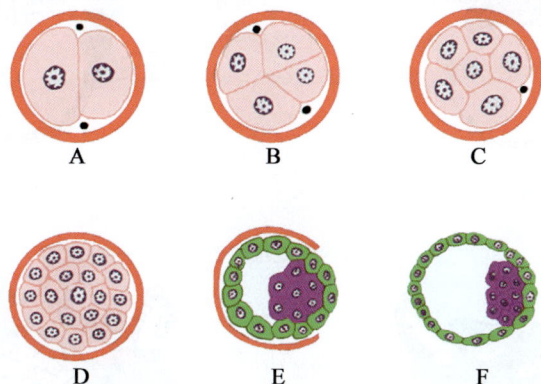

图 21 - 3 卵裂与胚泡形成模式图
A.2 细胞期;B.4 细胞期;C.8 细胞期;D.桑椹胚;E.早期胚泡;F.胚泡

二、植入

植入,也称着床,是胚泡埋入子宫内膜的过程,开始于受精后第 5~6 天。胚泡形成后,其内细胞团一侧的滋养层(极端滋养层)与子宫内膜相接触。随后,滋养层细胞开始增生,并分泌蛋白酶侵蚀子宫内膜,形成缺口,胚泡逐渐被子宫内膜包埋。到第 11~12 天,胚泡完全嵌入子宫内膜,子宫内膜上皮在胚泡外侧增生修复,使缺口愈合,植入完成(图 21 - 4,图 21 - 5)。

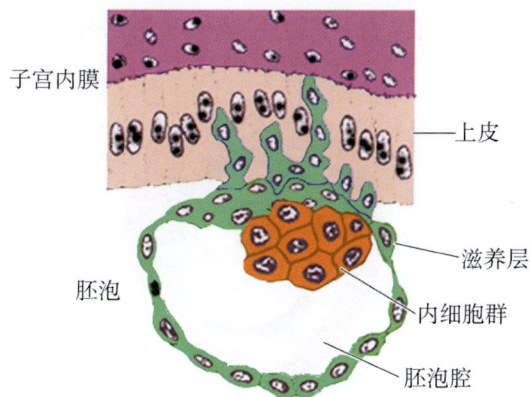

图 21 - 4 植入早期模式图

植入时的子宫内膜处于分泌期,植入后子宫血供增多、腺体分泌旺盛、内膜增厚、基质细胞肥大,富含糖原和脂滴。这些变化称为蜕膜反应,此时的子宫内膜称蜕膜,基质细胞称蜕膜细胞。根据蜕膜与胚的位置关系,将蜕膜分为三部分:基蜕膜、包蜕膜和壁蜕膜。基蜕膜位于胚

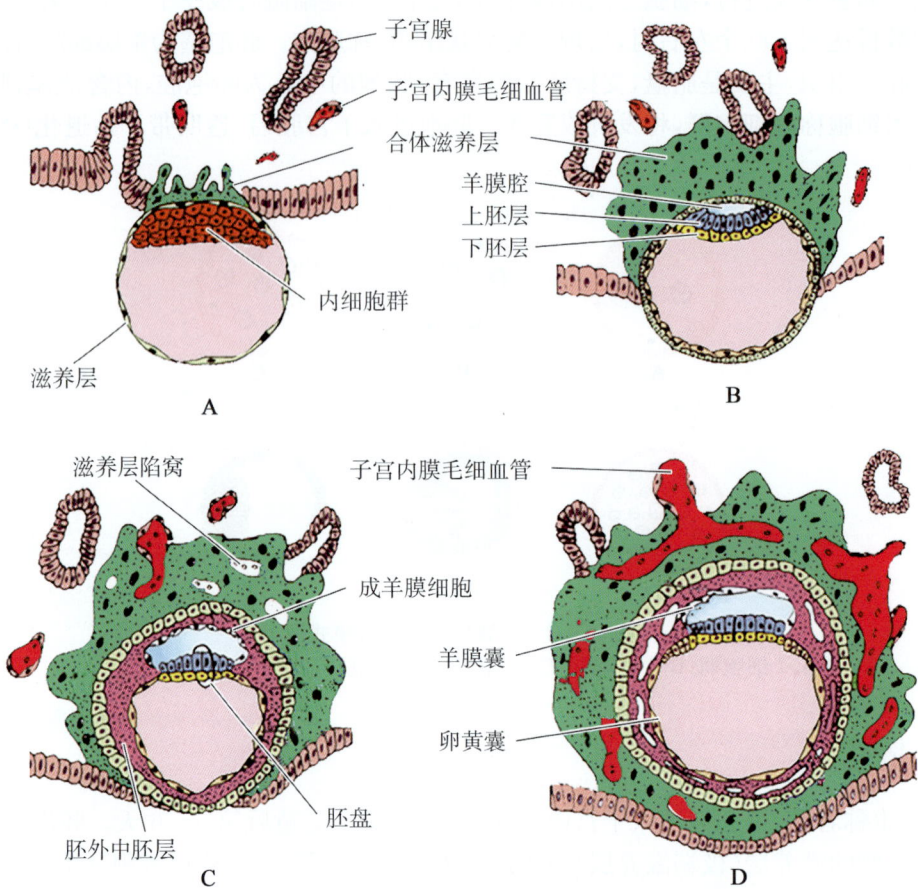

图 21-5　胚泡植入子宫内膜模式图
A. 第 7 天；B. 第 8 天；C. 第 9 天；D. 第 12 天

的深面，包蜕膜覆盖在胚的子宫腔侧，壁蜕膜为蜕膜的其余部分(图 21-6)。

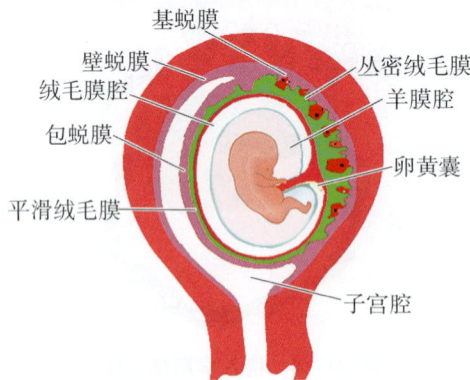

图 21-6　胚胎与子宫蜕膜的关系示意图

　　植入是以子宫内膜保持在分泌期为基础的，透明带消失和胚泡适时进入宫腔是植入的必要条件。若母体内分泌紊乱导致子宫内膜周期性变化与胚泡的发育不同步，或子宫内膜存在炎症或异物,均可阻碍胚泡的植入。

胚泡的植入通常发生在子宫体部和底部,多见于后壁。若植入发生在子宫以外部位,如卵巢、输卵管和肠系膜等,则称异位妊娠。若植入发生在近子宫颈处,会形成前置胎盘。

在植入过程中,滋养层细胞分化增殖为两层。内层为单层立方细胞,称细胞滋养层;外层细胞互相融合,细胞界线消失,称合体滋养层。随着滋养层的增厚,合体滋养层中出现一些不规则的腔隙,称滋养层陷窝,不久母体的血液流入并填充这些陷窝。

第三节　胚层的形成

胚泡植入的同时,内细胞群也不断增殖和分化,形成板层状结构,称胚层。相邻胚层紧密相贴形成椭圆形的细胞盘,称胚盘。

一、二胚层胚盘及相关结构的形成

在人胚发育第2周,内细胞群不断增殖形成胚层。靠近胚泡腔的是单层立方细胞,称下胚层;靠近极端滋养层的是单层柱状细胞,称上胚层。两个胚层紧密相贴,中间以基膜相隔。至第2周末,二胚层胚盘形成。同时,在上胚层靠近滋养层的一侧出现一个腔,称羊膜腔,其内充满液体,称羊水。羊膜腔壁由一层扁平的成羊膜细胞组成,与上胚层的边缘相延续,上胚层的其余部分共同包裹羊膜腔形成的囊状结构称羊膜囊。上胚层则形成羊膜囊的底。同时,下胚层细胞向腹侧生长延伸,形成由单层上皮细胞围成的另一个囊,称卵黄囊(图21-5)。

在上、下胚层形成的同时,胚泡腔中出现一些星状细胞和细胞外基质,填充在细胞滋养层和卵黄囊、羊膜囊之间,形成胚外中胚层。然后胚外中胚层细胞间出现腔隙,并逐渐增大,在胚外中胚层内形成一个大腔,称胚外体腔。随着胚外体腔的增大,二胚层胚盘和细胞滋养层之间仅由少量胚外中胚层连接,这部分胚外中胚层称体蒂,将发育成脐带的主要成分(图21-5、图21-7)。

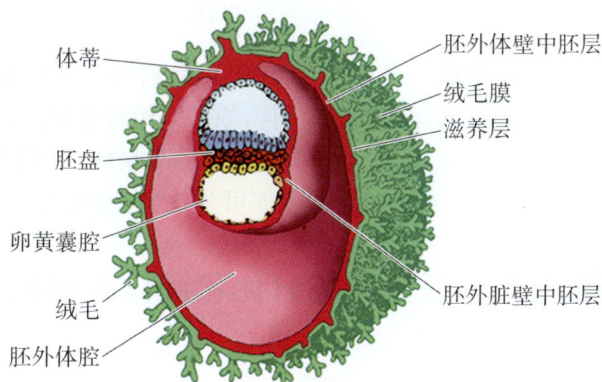

图21-7　第3周初胚的立体模式图

二、三胚层胚盘及相关结构的形成

第3周初,在二胚层胚盘背侧正中线出现一纵行的细胞柱,称原条。出现原条的一端成为胚的尾端。原条的头端膨大形成原节。继而在原条的中线出现浅沟，原结的中心出现浅凹，分别称原沟与原凹。原沟深部的胚层细胞不断增殖，在上、下胚层之间向周围迁移。其中一部分在上、下胚层之间形成一个新的夹层，称中胚层；另一部分进入下胚层并取代了下胚层，形成一新的细胞层，称内胚层。这时原上胚层则改称为外胚层，因此三个胚层均来自上胚层。到第 3 周末，三胚层胚盘建立（图 21 - 7、图 21 - 8）。

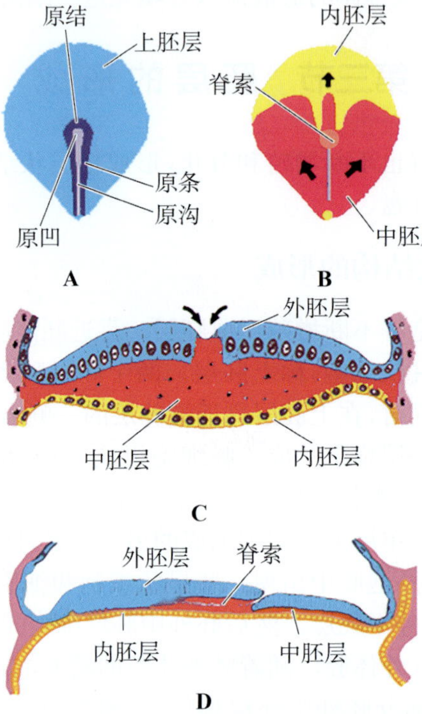

图 21 - 8 三胚层形成示意图

A.第 16 天胚盘表面观；B.原条和脊索形成（上胚层被去除，箭头示细胞迁移方向）；C.通过原条的胚盘横切面；D.胚盘中轴纵切面

从原凹向头端生长的细胞，形成一条中胚层细胞索，称脊索。脊索在胚胎早期起一定的支架作用。随着胚体的发育，脊索向头、尾端生长、延伸，原条则相对缩短。在脊索的头侧和原条的尾侧，各有一个没有中胚层的小区，此处外、内胚层紧贴，呈薄膜状，分别称口咽膜和泄殖腔膜。原条最终消失，如果原条细胞残留，未来在人体骶部可分化、增殖成由多种组织构成的畸胎瘤。

第四节 三胚层的分化和胚体的形成

一、三胚层的分化

在人胚第 4～8 周，三个胚层逐渐分化成胚体各种器官的原基。

1. 外胚层的分化

脊索诱导其背侧中线的外胚层增厚呈板状，称神经板。构成神经板的这部分外胚层，也称神经外胚层，其余的外胚层称表面外胚层。神经板随着脊索的生长而增长，并向脊索方向凹陷,形成神经沟,沟的两侧边缘隆起称神经褶。两侧神经褶首先在神经沟中段靠拢、融合,并向头尾两端进展,最后在两端各形成一开口,分别称前神经孔和后神经孔。神经孔在第4周闭合,使神经沟完全闭合形成神经管,同时神经板外侧缘的细胞随之进入神经管的背侧,并很快从管壁上迁移出来,形成位于神经管背外侧的两条纵行细胞索,称神经嵴(图21-9、图21-10)。

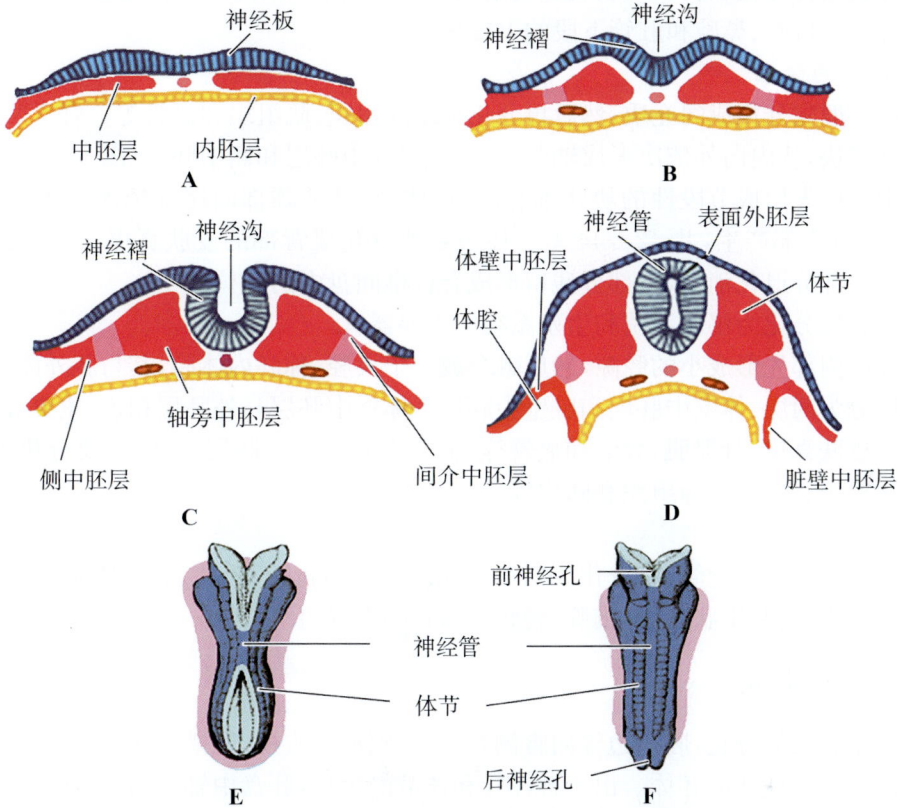

图 21-9 神经管形成与中胚层早期分化模式图
A.第17天;B.第19天;C.第20天;D.第21天;E.第22天;F.第23天

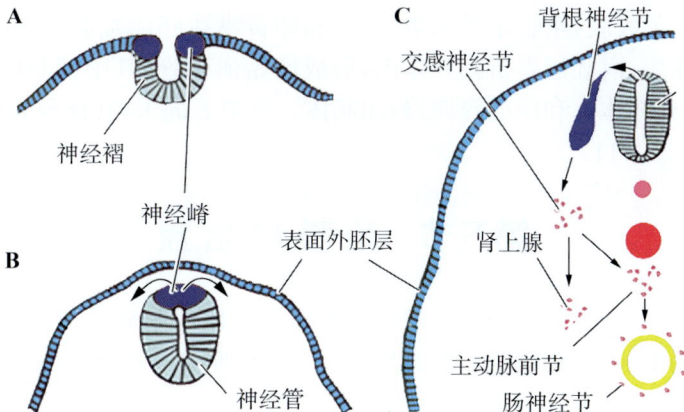

图 21-10 神经嵴的发生与细胞迁移模式图
A.神经嵴形成;B.神经嵴细胞开始迁移;C.神经嵴细胞分化为不同结构

神经管是中枢神经系统的原基,将分化为脑和脊髓、视网膜、神经垂体、松果体等。神经嵴是周围神经系统的原基,将分化为脑神经节、脊神经节、自主神经节和周围神经;部分神经嵴细胞迁入肾上腺原基,分化为嗜铬细胞;部分神经嵴细胞迁入皮肤表皮形成黑素细胞;头端的部分神经嵴细胞还参与颅面部骨骼和结缔组织的形成。

表面外胚层将分化成皮肤的表皮及其附属器官、牙釉质、角膜上皮、晶状体、内耳膜迷路、腺垂体、唾液腺、口腔、鼻腔和肛管下段的上皮等。

2. 中胚层的分化

中胚层一般先分化成间充质,然后再分化成结缔组织、肌组织和血管等。脊索两侧的中胚层细胞增殖较快,从内向外依次形成轴旁中胚层、间介中胚层和侧中胚层(图 21-9)。

轴旁中胚层先形成节段性的块状细胞团,称体节,其从颈部向尾部依次产生,左右成对。第 5 周时,体节全部产生,共 42～44 对。体节主要分化成背部的皮肤真皮、骨骼肌和中轴骨骼。脊索的大部分退化消失,少部分残留形成脊柱椎间盘内的髓核。

间介中胚层分化为泌尿系统和生殖系统的主要器官。

侧中胚层内部先形成小的腔隙,然后融合成一个大腔,称胚内体腔,其与胚外体腔相通,于是侧中胚层分为两层:体壁中胚层和脏壁中胚层。体壁中胚层与外胚层相连,主要分化为胸腹部和四肢的皮肤真皮、骨骼肌、骨骼和血管等;脏壁中胚层与内胚层相连,主要分化为消化、呼吸系统的肌组织、血管、结缔组织和间皮等。

3. 内胚层的分化

内胚层形成原始消化管,将分化成咽喉及其以下的消化管、消化腺、呼吸道和肺的上皮组织,以及中耳、甲状腺、甲状旁腺、胸腺、膀胱等器官的上皮组织。

二、胚体的形成

随着三个胚层的分化,胚盘边缘向腹侧卷折,分别形成头褶、尾褶和左右侧褶,使原本扁平的胚盘逐渐变成圆柱状的胚体。由于神经管和体节的生长,胚盘中轴部向背侧隆起,而外胚层的生长速度又快于内胚层,这样使得内胚层被卷入胚体内部,外胚层则覆盖于体表。胚盘头端的生长速度快于尾端,而尾端生长又快于左右侧向生长,因此胚盘卷折成头大尾小的圆柱形胚体,其边缘卷折到胚体腹侧,并逐渐靠拢、会聚形成脐部(图 21-11)。

此时,胚体凸入羊膜腔,生长于羊水中;体蒂和卵黄囊在胚体腹侧合并,外包羊膜,形成脐带;外胚层包裹于体表;内胚层卷折到胚体内,形成原始消化管,其中部与卵黄囊相通;口咽膜和泄殖腔膜分别转到胚体头和尾的腹侧,封闭胚体。至第 8 周末,胚体外表已可见眼、耳、鼻和四肢,初具人形(图 21-11)。

第五节 胎膜和胎盘

胎膜和胎盘是对胚胎起保护、营养、呼吸和排泄等作用的附属结构,有的还具有内分泌功能,但不参与胚体的形成,总称衣胞。胎儿娩出后,胎膜、胎盘与母体子宫分离,一并排出。

一、胎膜

胎膜包括绒毛膜、羊膜、卵黄囊、尿囊和脐带(图 21-12)。

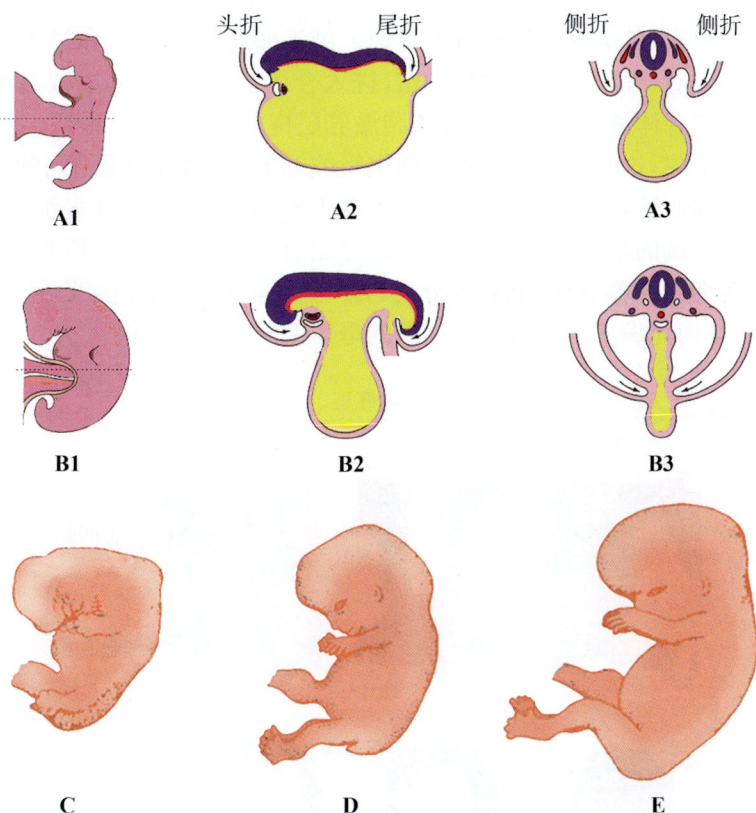

图 21-11　胚体形成示意图

A.第 23 天；B.第 28 天；C.第 48 天；D.第 52 天；E.第 56 天；A1、B1、C、D 和 E 为侧面观；A2 和 B2 为矢状面；A3 和 B3 为横切面

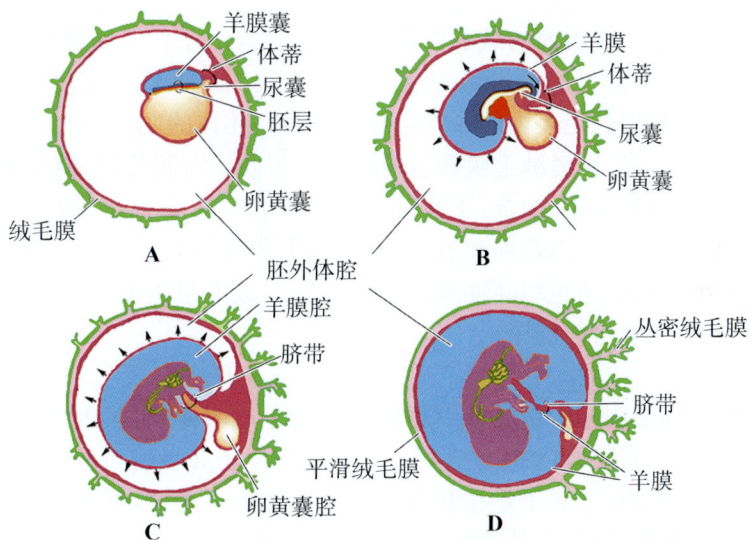

图 21-12　胎膜演变示意图

A.第 3 周；B.第 5 周；C.第 10 周；D.第 20 周

1. 绒毛膜

绒毛膜由绒毛膜板、各级绒毛干和绒毛组成。绒毛膜板由滋养层和衬于其内面的胚外中胚层组成。植入完成后,细胞滋养层细胞增殖,进入合体滋养层内,形成绒毛状突起。第2周末的绒毛仅由外表的合体滋养层和内部的细胞滋养层构成,称初级绒毛干。第3周时,胚外中胚层逐渐长入绒毛干内,这时初级绒毛干改称次级绒毛干。此后,绒毛干内的胚外中胚层间充质分化为结缔组织和血管,三级绒毛干形成。绒毛干发出分支,形成许多细小的绒毛(图21-13)。同时,绒毛干末端的细胞滋养层细胞增殖,穿出合体滋养层,直至蜕膜,并沿蜕膜向外扩展,彼此连接,形成细胞滋养层壳,牢固连接绒毛膜与子宫蜕膜。滋养层陷窝演变为绒毛间隙,位于绒毛干之间,其内充满从子宫螺旋动脉来的母体血液。

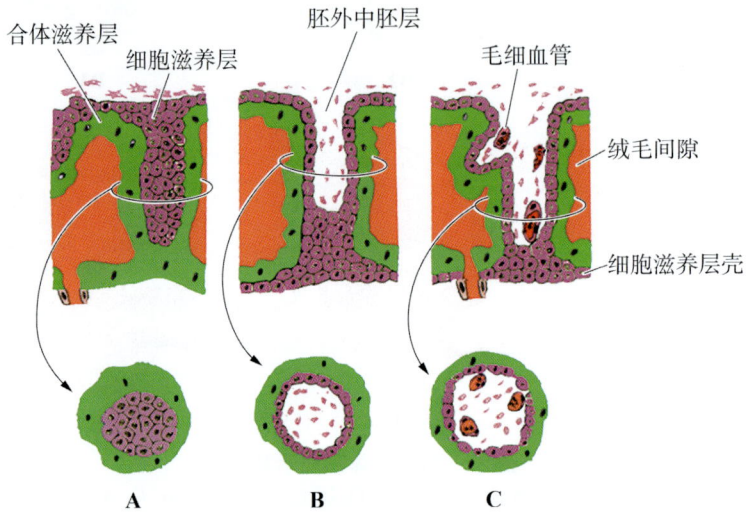

图21-13 绒毛干的分化发育模式图
A.初级绒毛干;B.次级绒毛干;C.三级绒毛干

在胚胎早期,整个绒毛膜表面的绒毛均匀分布。之后,由于包蜕膜侧的血供减少,绒毛逐渐退化、消失,形成表面无绒毛的平滑绒毛膜。而基蜕膜侧血液供应充足,绒毛反复分支、生长,形成丛密绒毛膜。丛密绒毛膜内的血管通过脐带与胚体内的血管连通。此后,随着胚胎的发育及羊膜腔的扩大,羊膜、平滑绒毛膜和包蜕膜进一步向子宫腔凸起,随后包蜕膜退化,最终羊膜、平滑绒毛膜与壁蜕膜靠近、融合,子宫腔消失(图21-12、图21-14)。

绒毛膜为早期胚胎发育提供营养和氧气,丛密绒毛膜参与组成胎盘。绒毛膜发育异常会危害胚胎发育。如绒毛内结缔组织高度水肿,血管消失,绒毛呈水泡状,称葡萄胎。绒毛膜癌是一种高度恶性肿瘤,危及母体健康。

2. 羊膜

羊膜是由单层羊膜细胞和少量胚外中胚层组成的半透明薄膜,膜内无血管。羊膜腔内充满羊水,胚胎在羊水中生长发育(图21-12)。羊膜最初位于胚盘的边缘,随着胚体形成、羊膜腔扩大,胚体凸入羊膜腔内,羊膜于是在胚胎腹侧包裹在体蒂表面,形成原始脐带。羊膜腔的扩大逐渐使羊膜与绒毛膜相贴,胚外体腔逐渐消失。羊水主要由羊膜不断分泌产生,又不断地被羊膜吸收,呈弱碱性,含有脱落的上皮细胞。妊娠中期以后,胎儿开始吞饮羊水,其泌尿系统

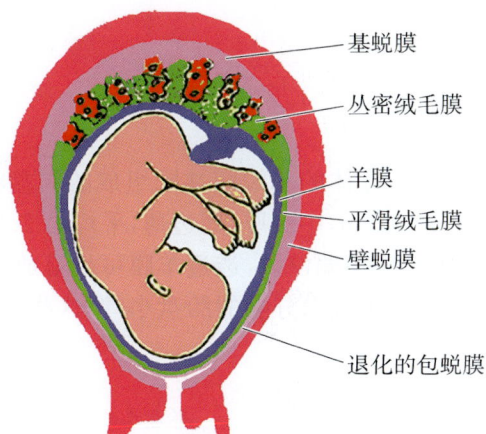

图 21-14　胎儿后期胎膜、蜕膜与胎盘模式图

基蜕膜
丛密绒毛膜
羊膜
平滑绒毛膜
壁蜕膜
退化的包蜕膜

和消化系统的排泄物也进入羊水。羊膜和羊水在胚胎发育中起重要的保护作用。羊水能缓冲外力的压迫与震荡，使胚胎在羊水中可较自由地活动，有利于骨骼肌的正常发育，并防止局部组织粘连。分娩时，羊水还具有扩张宫颈、冲洗产道的作用。随着胚胎的长大，羊水也相应增多，足月时有 1 000～1 500 ml。羊水过少（500 ml 以下），易发生羊膜与胎儿粘连，影响胎儿正常发育；羊水过多（2 000 ml 以上），也可影响胎儿正常发育。某些先天性畸形会使羊水含量异常，如胎儿无肾或尿道闭锁可致羊水过少；胎儿消化道闭锁或神经管封闭不全可致羊水过多。穿刺抽取羊水，进行染色体检查或测定其内某些物质的含量，有助于早期诊断某些先天性异常。

3. 卵黄囊

卵黄囊位于原始消化管腹侧（图 21-12）。卵生动物如鸟类的卵黄囊内贮有大量卵黄，为胚胎发育提供营养。人胚胎的卵黄囊内没有卵黄，它的出现也是种系发生和进化的重演。人胚胎卵黄囊被包入脐带后，与原始消化管相连的狭窄部分称卵黄蒂，其于第 6 周闭锁，卵黄囊也逐渐退化。人类的造血干细胞和原始生殖细胞分别来自卵黄囊的胚外中胚层和内胚层。

4. 尿囊

尿囊是从卵黄囊尾侧向体蒂内伸出的一个盲管，随着胚体的形成而开口于原始消化管尾段的腹侧，即与后来的膀胱通连（图 21-12）。尿囊先演化为脐尿管，然后闭锁形成脐中韧带，其壁上的胚外中胚层内形成尿囊动脉和尿囊静脉，这些血管以后演变为脐带内的脐动脉和脐静脉。

5. 脐带

脐带是连接胚胎脐部与胎盘的条索状结构（图 21-12、图 21-15）。脐带外被羊膜，内含由体蒂分化的黏液性结缔组织。结缔组织内除有闭锁的卵黄蒂和尿囊遗迹外，还有脐动脉和脐静脉。脐血管的一端与胚胎血管相连，另一端与胎盘绒毛血管续连。脐动脉有两条，负责将胚胎血液运送至胎盘绒毛内，在此与绒毛间隙内的母体血液进行物质交换。脐静脉仅有一条，负责将胎盘绒毛汇集的血液送回胚胎。胎儿出生时，脐带长 40～60 cm，粗 1.5～2 cm。脐带过短，胎儿娩出时易引起胎盘过早剥离，造成出血过多；脐带过长，易缠绕胎儿肢体或颈部，可致局部发育不良,甚至造成胎儿窒息死亡。

二、胎盘

(一) 胎盘的结构

胎盘是由胎儿的丛密绒毛膜与母体的基蜕膜共同组成的圆盘状结构(图 21-15)。足月胎儿的胎盘重约 500 g,直径 15~20 cm,中央厚,周边薄,平均厚 2.5 cm。胎盘的胎儿面光滑,表面有羊膜覆盖,脐带附着于中央或稍偏位置,透过羊膜可见呈放射状走行的脐血管的分支。胎盘的母体面粗糙,可见 15~30 个由浅沟分隔的胎盘小叶,这些小叶为从母体剥离出来的基蜕膜。

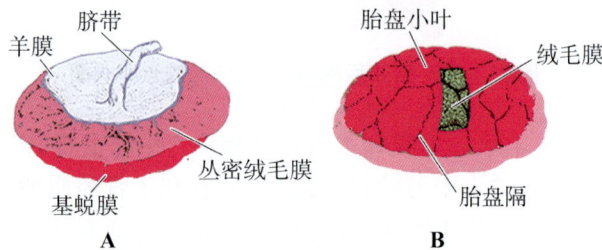

图 21-15 胎盘仿真图
A.羊膜面观;B.子宫蜕膜面观

在胎盘垂直切面上,可见羊膜下方脐血管的分支走行于其绒毛膜的结缔组织中。绒毛膜板发出 40~60 根绒毛干,其末端以细胞滋养层壳固着于母体基蜕膜上,绒毛干又发出许多细小绒毛。脐血管的分支沿绒毛干进入绒毛内,形成毛细血管。绒毛干之间为绒毛间隙,由基蜕膜构成的短隔伸入其间,称胎盘隔。胎盘隔将绒毛干分隔到各个胎盘小叶内,每个小叶含 1~4 根绒毛干。子宫螺旋动脉与子宫静脉开口于绒毛间隙,因此绒毛间隙内充满母体血液,绒毛浸在母血中。

(二) 胎盘的血液循环和胎盘膜

胎盘内有母体和胎儿两套血液循环系统,两者的血液在各自的封闭通道内循环,互不相混,但可进行物质交换(图 21-16)。母体动脉血从子宫螺旋动脉流入绒毛间隙,在此与绒毛内毛细血管的胎儿血进行物质交换后,再由子宫静脉回流入母体。胎儿的静脉血经脐动脉及其分支流入绒毛毛细血管,与绒毛间隙内的母体血进行物质交换后,成为动脉血,再经脐静脉回流到胎儿体内。

胎儿血与母体血在胎盘内进行物质交换所通过的结构,称胎盘膜或胎盘屏障。早期胎盘膜由合体滋养层、细胞滋养层和基膜、薄层绒毛结缔组织及毛细血管内皮和基膜组成。发育后期,细胞滋养层大部分消失且一些合体滋养层细胞仅剩一薄层胞质,此时的胎盘膜变得很薄,仅由绒毛毛细血管内皮和薄层合体滋养层及两者的基膜组成,这一变化更有利于母体和胎儿之间的物质交换。

(三) 胎盘的功能

1. 物质交换

进行物质交换是胎盘的主要功能,胎儿通过胎盘从母血中获得营养和 O_2,排出代谢产物

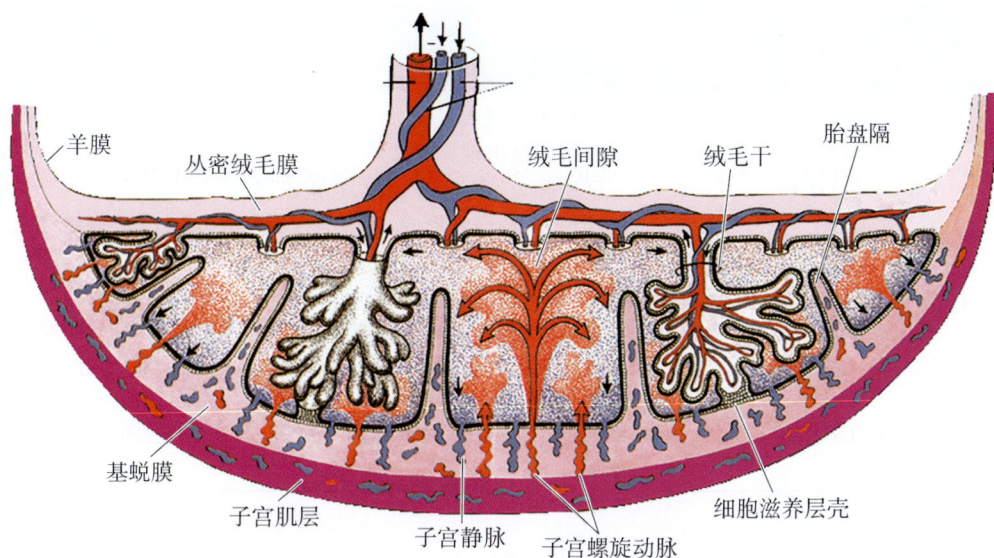

图 21 - 16　胎盘的结构与血液循环模式图

箭头示血流方向；红色示富含营养和 O_2 的血；蓝色示含代谢废物和 CO_2 的血

和 CO_2。因此胎盘具有相当于成体小肠、肺和肾的功能。某些病毒、药物和激素可以透过胎盘膜影响胎儿发育，故孕妇需避免感染并谨慎用药。

2. 内分泌功能

胎盘的合体滋养层可分泌数种激素，对维持妊娠起重要作用。这些激素主要有：①绒毛膜促性腺激素，其作用和黄体生成素类似，能促进母体黄体的生长发育以维持妊娠。其在妊娠第2周开始分泌，第8周达高峰，以后逐渐下降。②绒毛膜促乳腺生长激素，能促使母体乳腺生长发育，也可促进胎儿的发育。其分泌始于妊娠第2月，第8月达高峰，并直到分娩。③孕激素和雌激素，于妊娠第4月开始分泌，以后逐渐增多。当母体的黄体退化后，这两种激素起着继续维持妊娠的作用。

第六节　胚胎各期外形特征和胚胎龄的推算

从受精之日起计算的胚胎龄为受精龄，至分娩共约38周。临床上又常以月经龄表示胚胎龄，即从孕妇末次月经的第1天算起，至分娩共约40周。但由于妇女的月经周期常受环境变化的影响，故胚胎龄的推算难免有误差。因此，胚胎学者根据大量胚胎标本的观察和活体测量，总结归纳出各期胚胎的外形特征和平均长度，以此作为推算胚胎龄的依据。胚胎龄的推算主要根据胚盘、体节、颜面、四肢、皮肤、毛发、外生殖器等的发育状况，并参照长度和体重（表21-1、表21-2）。长度的测量标准有三种。最长值（great length，GL），多用于测量1～3周的胚胎；顶臀长（crown-rump length，CRL），又称坐高，用于测量第4周及以后的胚胎；顶跟长（crown-heel length，CHL），又称站高，用于测量胎儿（图21-17）。

表 21-1　胚胎的长度、体节和外形特征

胚龄（周）	长度（mm）	体节（对数）	外形特征
1		0	胚泡形成与植入
2	0.2~0.4(GL)	0	二胚层胚盘出现
3	0.5~1.5(GL)	1~4	三胚层胚盘、原条、神经沟、脊索出现
4	1.5~5(CRL)	4~29	胚褶形成,神经管形成,视泡与视板形成,第1、2、3对鳃弓出现
5	5~8(CRL)	30~44	第4对鳃弓出现,后肢芽形成,视泡与晶状体板出现,桨状前肢形成,胚胎呈"C"形
6	8~13(CRL)		手足板出现指(趾)线,脑泡显著,外耳郭形成,脐疝开始发育
7	13~21(CRL)		视网膜色素沉着,指(趾)线分离,乳头与眼睑形成,上唇形成,脐疝明显
8	21~35(CRL)		四肢增长且肘、膝关节弯曲,指(趾)分离独立,面部更具人形,脐疝显现

GL,最长值;CRL,顶臀长

表 21-2　胎儿的长度、重量和外形特征

胚龄（周）	长度（CRL,mm）	重量（g）	外形特征
9	50	8	眼睑闭合,脐疝消失
10	61	14	指甲开始发育
12	87	45	性别可辨,眼和耳接近最终位置
14	120	110	趾甲开始发育,下肢发育良好
16	140	200	耳郭竖立
18	160	320	胎脂出现
20	190	460	胎毛出现
22	210	630	皮肤呈红色且有皱纹
24	230	820	指甲发育完好,胎儿身体消瘦
26	250	1000	眼睑完全睁开,头发开始生长
28	270	1300	眉毛出现,眼睑张开
30	280	1700	趾甲发育完好,睾丸开始下降
32	300	2100	皮肤光滑,身体轮廓圆润
36	340	2900	身体丰满,胎毛脱落,胎脂覆盖全身
38	360	3400	睾丸降入阴囊,指甲超过指尖

CRL,顶臀长

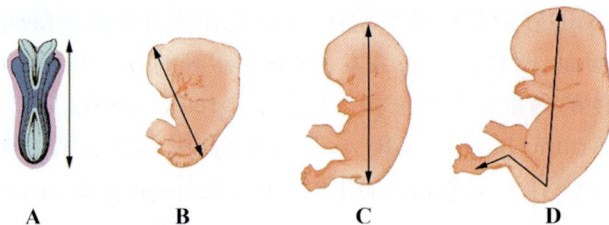

图 21-17　胚胎长度测量示意图
A.最长值(GL);B、C.顶臀长(CRL);D.顶跟长(CHL)

第七节　双胎、多胎和联胎

一、双胎

双胎又称孪生,双胎的发生率约占新生儿的1%。双胎有两种。

1. 双卵孪生

一次排出两个卵子分别受精后发育为双卵孪生,占双胎的大多数。他(她)们有各自的胎膜与胎盘,性别相同或不同,相貌和生理特性的差异如同一般兄弟姐妹,仅是同龄而已。

2. 单卵孪生

由一个受精卵发育为两个胚胎,故此种双胎儿的基因完全一样。他(她)们的性别一致,而且相貌和生理特征也极相似。单卵孪生的原因有:①受精卵发育成两个胚泡,然后分别发育为一个完整的胚,两个胚胎有各自的羊膜腔和胎盘。②一个胚泡内出现两个内细胞群,各发育为一个胚胎,两个胚胎有各自的羊膜腔,但共有一个胎盘。③胚盘上出现两个原条与脊索,诱导形成两个神经管,发育为两个胚胎,两个胚胎同位于一个羊膜腔内,也共有一个胎盘。

二、多胎

一次娩出两个以上新生儿为多胎。多胎的原因可以是单卵性、多卵性或混合性,常为混合性多胎。多胎发生率极低。

三、联体双胎

单卵孪生中,当一个胚盘出现两个原条并分别发育为两个胚胎时,若两原条靠得较近,胚体形成时发生局部联接,导致联体双胎。联体双胎有对称型和不对称型两类。对称型指两个胚胎大小相同,根据联结部位又可分为头联体、胸腹联体、臀联体等。不对称型指两个胚胎一大一小,小者常发育不全,形成寄生胎或胎中胎。

（岳海源）

Chapter 22

Development of the Face and Limbs

In a human embryo of 4 weeks, the blastoderm has folded into a cylindrical embryo. The anterior neural foramen gradually closes, and the head of the neural tube expands rapidly to form the brain vesicle, that is, the primordium of the brain. The mesenchyme on the ventral side of the brain vesicle proliferates locally, making a large circular bulge of the embryonic body, which is called frontonasal process. At the same time, the primitive heart on the caudal side of oropharyngeal membrane develops, grows, bulges, and finally forms the heart bulge (Figure 22 – 1).

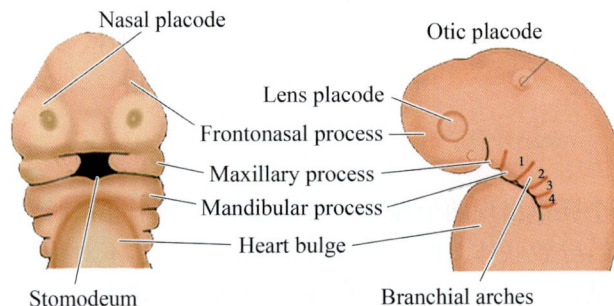

Figure 22 – 1   Drawings showing the human head of 4 weeks
A. Ventral view; B. Lateral view

1   Development of Branchial Apparatus

In week 4 – 5, with the emergence of frontonasal process and heart bulge, the mesenchymal hyperplasia in both sides of the head gradually forms 6 pairs of arcuate columnar protrusions called branchial arches, which are left-right and dorsoventrally symmetrical. The 5 pairs of strip depressions between adjacent branchial arches are branchial grooves. The first 4 pairs of branchial arches of human embryos are obvious. The pair 5 appear and then disappears soon. The pair 6 are very small and not obvious. At the same time, as the branchial arches develop, the endoderm in the lateral wall of the primitive pharynx bulges outward to form 5 pairs of saccular structures on the left and right, which are called pharyngeal pouches. They correspond to 5 pairs of branchial grooves, respectively (Figure 22 - 2). The branchial membranes exist between the grooves and pouches and are composed of ectoderm, mesoderm and endoderm as a lining.

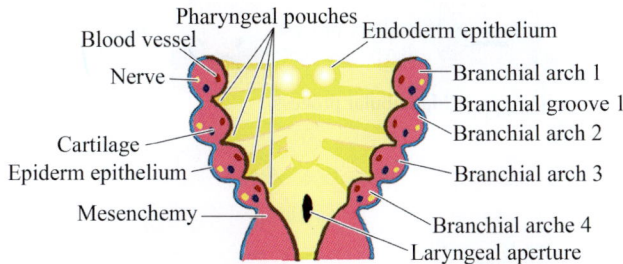

Figure 22 - 2   Drawing of the pharyngeal pouches and branchial arches

Branchial arches, branchial grooves, branchial membranes and pharyngeal pouches are collectively referred to as the branchial apparatus. The branchial apparatus of fish and amphibian embryos evolves into gills with respiratory function, whereas there is a short time existence in human embryo. The branchial arches will participate in the formation of the face and neck. The mesenchyme will differentiate into muscle tissue, cartilage and bone. The endoderm of pharyngeal pouches is the primordium of many important organs. The appearance of branchial apparatus in the early stage of a human embryo is not only a repetition of germline occurrence, but also one of the evidences for biological evolution and human origin.

2   Development of Face

After the appearance of the first pair of branchial arches, its ventral part rapidly bifurcates into upper and lower branches, called maxillary process and mandibular process, respectively. The left and right mandibular processes quickly fuse in the ventral midline, separating the oropharyngeal membrane from the heart bulge. At this time, if the embryo body is viewed from the front, its face is composed of the frontonasal process, left and right maxillary processes, fused left and right mandibular processes and a wide depression surrounded by these 5 bulges. This depression is called stomodeum, i.e., the primitive oral cavity (Figure 22 - 3). Its bottom is the oropharyngeal membrane, which separates the primitive oral cavity from the primitive pharynx. The oropharyngeal membrane ruptures around day 24, and the primitive oral cavity is then connected with the primitive pharynx.

The development of the face is closely related to the development of the nose. On both sides of the lower edge of the frontonasal process, local ectodermal tissue proliferates and thickens, forming a pair of nasal placodes on the left and right. Then, the center of the nasal placode is recessed to the deep to form a nasal pit, and its lower edge is connected with the stomodeum by a fine groove. The mesenchyme around the nasal pits proliferates and bulges. The bulge on the inner side of the nasal pit is called median nasal prominence,

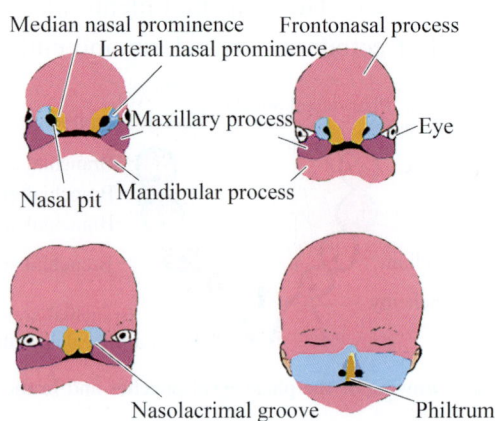

Figure 22 - 3 Schematic diagrams showing the development of face

while that on the outer side is called lateral nasal prominence. The upper parts of the early two bulges are continuous (Figure 22 - 3).

Face develops from both sides to the middle. In week 5, the left and right mandibular processes fuse with each other in the midline and develop into the mandible and lower lip. Then, the left and right maxillary processes also grow towards the midline. At the same time, the nasal pits on both sides are also close to each other, and the left and right median nasal processes gradually converge and migrate downward to fuse with the maxillary process. The medial nasal process will develop into the median part of the upper lip, including the philtrum, and the maxillary process will develop into the lateral part of the upper lip and the upper jaw. When the medial nasal process migrates downward, the lower median tissue of the frontal nasal process proliferates like a ridge, forming the bridge and tip of the nose, and the upper part develops into the forehead. The lateral nasal process is involved in the formation of the lateral nasal wall and nosewing. With the formation of external structures of the nose such as the bridge of the nose and the tip of the nose, the nasal pit originally opened in the front gradually turns downward to form the external nostril. The nasal pit expands to the deep to form the primitive nasal cavity. In the beginning, the primitive nasal cavity and the primitive oral cavity are separated by a very thin oronasal membrane. When the membrane was broken, the primitive nasal cavity is connected with the primitive oral cavity (Figure 22 - 4).

The opening of the original oral cavity is very wide in the beginning. With the convergence of the maxillary and mandibular processes on both sides to the midline and the formation of the upper and lower lips, the bifurcation of the ipsilateral maxillary and mandibular processes grows to the midline to form cheeks, so the oral fissure gradually becomes smaller. The development of the eye is initially in the ventrolateral part of the frontonasal process, and the 2 eyes are far apart. Later, with the rapid development of the brain, skull, maxilla and nose, the 2 eyes gradually approach the midline and stay in the same plane. The external auditory canal evolves from the first branchial groove, and the

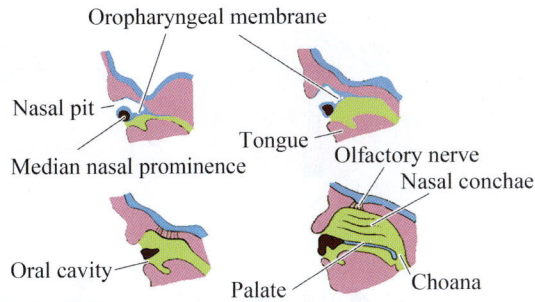

Figure 22 - 4   Drawings showing the development of nasal cavity

mesenchyme around the branchial groove proliferates to form the auricle. The outer ear stays at the low position in the beginning, but later it is pushed back and up with the development of the mandible and neck. By the end of the 8th week, the embryo resembles a human.

3   Development of Palate

The palate originates from the median palatine process and the lateral palatine process, which begins in week 5 and completes in week 12. After the fusion of the left and right medial nasal processes, a short protrusion, the median palatal process, will form a small part of the anterior palate. Then, the maxillary process extends to the left and right pair of flat processes growing in the primitive oral cavity, called lateral palatal process. At first, the lateral palatal process is obliquely downward on both sides of the tongue. Later, with the expansion of the oral cavity and the flattening and decline of the tongue, the left and right lateral palatal processes gradually grow horizontally above the tongue and fuse in the midline to form most of the palate. Its leading edge and median palatal process will converge and fuse, and there is a small hole at the intersection of the two, called incsive foramen. Later, the anterior palatal mesenchyme ossifies into the hard palate, and the posterior part becomes the soft palate. The tissue in the middle of the posterior edge of the soft palate proliferates and protrudes to the rear to form the uvula (Figure 22 - 5).

The formation of the palate separates the primitive oral cavity and the primitive nasal cavity again to become the permanent oral cavity and nasal cavity. The nasal cavity communicates with the pharynx at the posterior edge of the palate, which is called posterior nostril. With the development of the palate, the lower part of the frontonasal process not only forms the bridge and tip of the nose, but also grows a plate-shaped nasal septum into the primitive nasal cavity. It grows vertically downward and finally fuses with the palate in the midline, and the nasal cavity is immediately split into two. There are also 3 cristae folds on the lateral wall of the nasal cavity, forming the superior, middle, and inferior conchae turbinate, respectively (Figure 22 - 5).

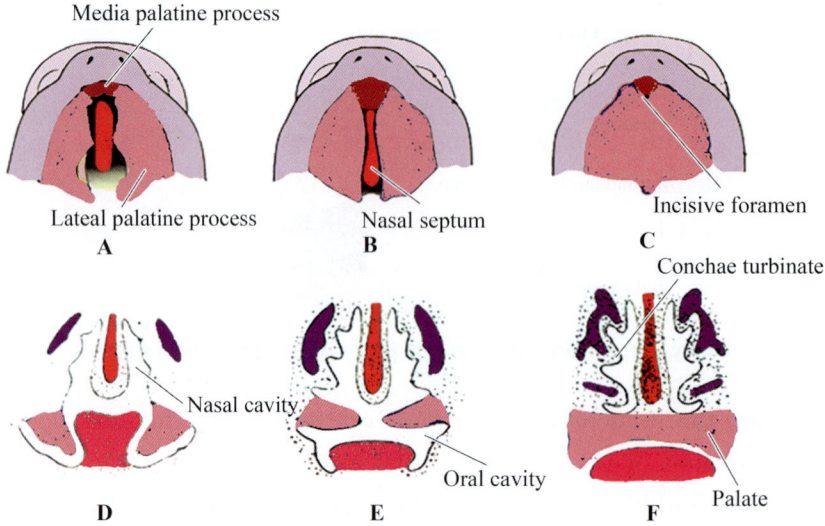

Figure 22 - 5   Drawings showing the development of palate and the split of the nasal cavity
A - C. Top view of the oral cavity; D - F. Coronal section of the head

4   Development of Tongue

At the end of the 4th week, the mesenchyme on the inner side of the left and right mandibular processes proliferates, forming a pair of lateral lingual swellings in the front and a tuberculum impar in the posterior midline in the primitive oral cavity. On the dorsal side of the tuberculum impar, the mesenchyme on the ventral part of the 2nd, 3rd and 4th branchial arch proliferates, forming copula and epiglottic copula. Both lateral lingual swellings converge and fuse with each other to form the most of the tongue body, and the tuberculum impar forms a small part of the tongue body in front of the foramen cecum. The copula develops into the root of the tongue. The tongue body and the root of the tongue fuse to form the lingual terminal sulcus, and its apex is the foramen cecum. Epiglottic copula develops into epiglottis (Figure 22 - 6).

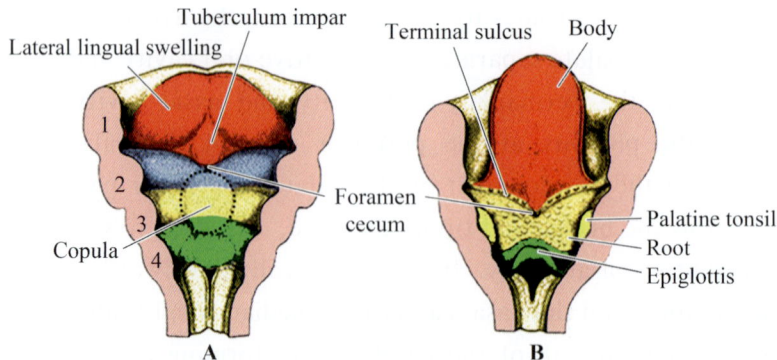

1 - 4 indictaing branchial arches
Figure 22 - 6   Drawing showing the development of tongue

5   Development of Neck

The neck is developed from the branchial arch 2 – 6 and the epicardial ridge. The left and right second branchial arches grow rapidly and fuse towards the midline, and grow to the cranial end to push the outer ear and the mandibular process to the side above; it extends caudally over the branchial arch 3 – 6 and covers their surfaces. The epicardial ridge is a crest like protuberance that grows from the mesenchymal hyperplasia at the upper edge of the heart bulge to the head of the embryo. After the fusion of the branchial arch 2 and epicardial ridge, the space among them and the 3 smaller branchial arches below are called cervical sinus. The cervical sinus closes and disappears soon. With the growth of branchial arches and the heart bulge, the elongation of the esophagus and trachea, and the decline of heart position, the neck gradually develops.

6   Development of Limbs

At the end of week 4, two pairs of small bulges appeared successively on the left and right lateral body walls of the embryo, called upper limb bud and lower limb bud, which are composed of deep proliferating mesoderm tissue and surface ectoderm. Limb buds gradually grow and become thicker, and 2 contraction rings appeared at the proximal and distal ends successively. Each limb bud is divided into 3 segments. The upper limb bud is divided into arm, forearm and hand, and the lower limb bud is divided into thigh, calf and foot. The mesenchyme of the middle axis of the limb first forms cartilage and then forms bone in the form of endochondral osteogenesis; the mesenchyme of the somite migrates into limb buds and differentiates into the skeletal muscles of limbs; the spinal nerve also grows into the limbs. At first, the hands and feet of the limbs are flat paddle-like. Then there are 4 longitudinal concave grooves at their distal end, and five fingers (toes) lines appear between the grooves. With the continuous apoptosis of cells between lines, fingers and toes are formed by the end of week 8.

7   Main Congenital Malformations

7.1 Cleft Lip

The cleft lip is the most common facial deformity, mostly caused by the non-fusion of the maxillary process and the ipsilateral medial nasal prominence. The cleft is located in the middle and outside of the philtrum. Cleft lip is mostly unilateral and bilateral. If the left and right medial nasal prominence is not fused or the mandibular prominence on both sides is not fused, it can lead to a median cleft lip of the upper lip or lower lip, respectively, while they are rare. If the middle defect is caused by the dysplasia of the medial nasal prominence, there will be a wide median cleft lip. Cleft lip may be accompanied by the alveolar cleft and cleft palate (Figure 22 - 7).

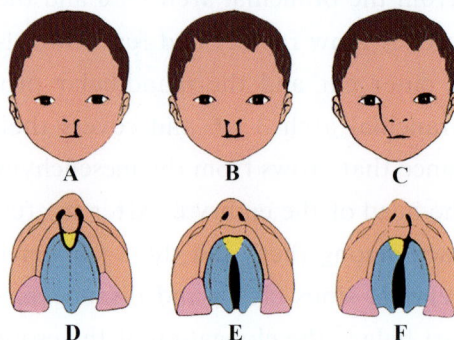

Figure 22 - 7   Drawings showing cleft lips and cleft palates
A. Unilateral cleft lip; B. Bilateral cleft lip; C. Oblique facial clef; D. Bilateral anterior cleft palate; E. Median cleft palate; F. Complete cleft palate

7.2   Cleft Palate

The cleft palate is also common with many phenotypes. The anterior cleft palate (unilateral or bilateral, often accompanied by cleft lip) is caused by the non-fusion of the median palatal process and lateral palatal process. The median cleft palate is caused by non-fusion of left and right lateral palatal process. If both of the anterior cleft palate and the median cleft palate occur, it is called complete cleft palate (Figure 22 - 7).

7.3   Oblique Facial Clefts

Oblique facial clefts are located between the inner canthus and the angle of mouth, caused by the non-fusion of the maxillary process and ipsilateral lateral nasal process (Figure 22 - 7).

7.4   Limb Deformities

Limb deformities have many phenotypes, which can occur in the upper, middle and lower segments of the limb. One phenotype is the limb absence, including transverse and longitudinal limb absence. The former type is the people without arms, hands, fingers, etc., while absence of the radial or ulnar side of the upper limb and the tibial or fibular side of the lower limb are found in the latter type. Another phenotype is the short limbs, such as seal-like hand or foot. The limb differentiation disorder is also one of the phenotypes including absence of a certain muscle or muscle group, joint dysplasia, bone deformity, bone fusion, polydactyly, syndactyly, clubfoot, etc.

(Yue Haiyuan)

第二十二章 颜面和四肢的发生

人胚第4周时,胚盘已向腹侧卷折成为圆柱状胚体。前神经孔逐渐闭合,神经管头端迅速膨大形成脑的原基,即脑泡。脑泡腹侧的间充质局部增生,使胚体头部外观呈较大的圆形隆起,称额鼻突。同时,口咽膜尾侧的原始心脏发育长大并隆起,称心隆起(图22-1)。

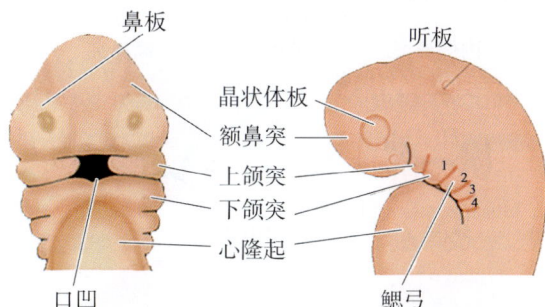

图 22-1 第4周人胚头部模式图
A.腹面观;B.侧面观

第一节 鳃器的发生

人胚第4~5周,伴随额鼻突与心隆起的出现,头部两侧的间充质增生,渐次形成左右对称、背腹方向的6对弓形柱状隆起,称鳃弓。相邻鳃弓之间的5对条形凹陷为鳃沟。人胚的前4对鳃弓明显,第5对出现不久即消失,第6对很小,不甚明显。在鳃弓发生的同时,原始咽侧壁内胚层向外膨出,形成左右5对囊状结构,称咽囊,它们分别与5对鳃沟相对应(图22-2)。咽囊顶壁内胚层与鳃沟底壁外胚层及二者之间的少量中胚层间充质构成鳃膜。

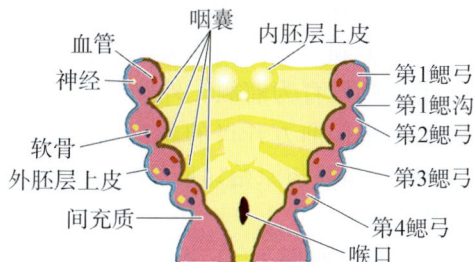

图 22-2 咽囊和鳃弓模式图

鳃弓、鳃沟、鳃膜与咽囊统称鳃器。鱼类和两栖类胚体的鳃器演化为具有呼吸功能的鳃等器官。人胚的鳃器存在时间短暂,鳃弓将参与颜面与颈的形成,其间充质分化为肌组织、软骨与骨;咽囊内胚层则是多种重要器官发生的原基。人胚早期鳃器的出现是重演种系发生的现象,也是生物进化与人类起源的佐证之一。

第二节　颜面的形成

第 1 鳃弓出现后,其腹侧份迅速分叉为上下两支,分别称为上颌突与下颌突。左右下颌突很快在腹侧中线融合,将口咽膜与心隆起隔开。此时正面观察胚体,其颜面是由额鼻突、左右上颌突、已融合的左右下颌突以及它们包围的一宽大凹陷构成的。这一凹陷称口凹(图 22 - 3)。口凹即原始口腔,其底是口咽膜,此膜将口腔与原始咽分隔开。口咽膜于第 24 天左右破裂,原始口腔便与原始咽相通。

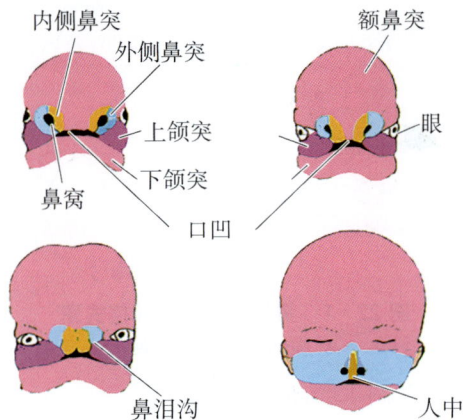

图 22 - 3　颜面形成过程示意图

颜面形成与鼻的发生密切相关。在额鼻突的下缘两侧,局部外胚层组织增生变厚,形成左右一对鼻板。继而鼻板中央向深部凹陷形成鼻窝,其下缘以一条细沟与口凹相通。鼻窝周缘部的间充质增生而隆起,鼻窝内侧的隆起称内侧鼻突,外侧的隆起称外侧鼻突,早期两个隆起的上部相连续(图 22 - 3)。

颜面的演化是从两侧向正中方向发展的。第 5 周,左右下颌突在中线融合,将发育形成下颌与下唇。随后,左右上颌突也向中线生长;同时,两侧的鼻窝亦彼此靠拢,左右内侧鼻突逐渐融合,并向下方迁移与上颌突愈合。内侧鼻突将发育形成包括人中在内的上唇正中部分,上颌突将发育形成上唇的外侧部分以及上颌。当内侧鼻突向下迁移时,额鼻突的下部正中组织呈嵴状增生,形成鼻梁和鼻尖,其上部则发育为前额。外侧鼻突参与组成鼻外侧壁与鼻翼。随着鼻梁、鼻尖等鼻外部结构的形成,原来向前方开口的鼻窝逐渐转向下方,形成外鼻孔。鼻窝向深部扩大形成原始鼻腔。起初,原始鼻腔与原始口腔之间隔以很薄的口鼻膜,该膜破裂后,原始鼻腔便与原始口腔相通(图 22 - 4)。

原始口腔的开口起初很宽大,随着两侧上、下颌隆起向中线会拢与上、下唇的形成,同侧上、下颌突的分叉处向中线方向生长形成颊,口裂因此逐渐变小。眼的发生最初是在额鼻隆起

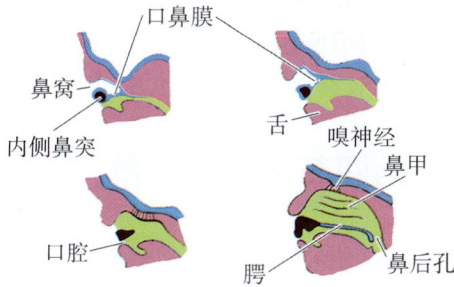

图 22 - 4　鼻腔形成示意图

的腹外侧,两眼相距较远。以后随着脑与颅的迅速增大以及上颌与鼻的形成,两眼逐渐向中线靠近,并处于同一平面。外耳道由第 1 鳃沟演变而成,鳃沟周围的间充质增生形成耳郭。外耳的位置原本很低,后来随着下颌与颈的发育而被推向后上方。至第 8 周末,胚胎初具人形。

第三节　腭 的 发 生

腭起源于正中腭突与外侧腭突两部分,从第 5 周开始发育,至第 12 周完成。

左右内侧鼻突融合后,向原始口腔内长出一个短小的突起,即正中腭突,它将演化为腭前部的一小部分。随后,左、右上颌突向原始口腔内长出左右一对扁平突起,即外侧腭突。外侧腭突起初位于舌的两侧斜向下方,之后随着口腔的扩大及舌变扁和位置下降,左右外侧腭突逐渐在舌的上方呈水平方向生长,并在中线愈合,形成腭的大部分。其前缘与正中腭突会拢愈合,两者正中交会处残留一小孔,即切齿孔。随后,腭前部间充质骨化为硬腭,后部则为软腭。软腭后缘正中部组织增生并向后方突出,形成悬雍垂(图 22 - 5)。

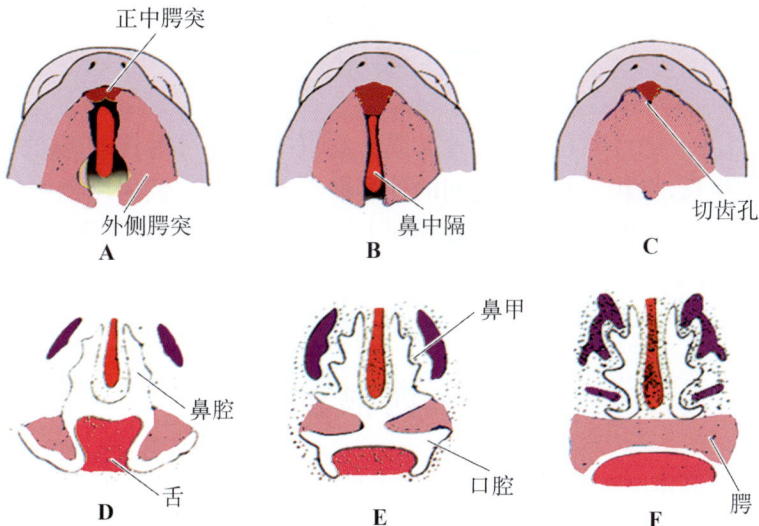

图 22 - 5　腭的发生及口腔与鼻腔的分隔示意图
A～C 为口腔顶部观;D～F 为头部冠状切面

腭的形成将原始口腔与原始鼻腔再次分隔为永久的口腔与鼻腔。鼻腔在腭的后缘与咽相通,该部位即为后鼻孔。伴随腭的形成,额鼻突的下部在形成鼻梁与鼻尖的同时,还向原始鼻腔内生长出板状的鼻中隔。鼻中隔向下垂直生长,最终与腭在中线愈合,鼻腔随即被一分为二。鼻腔外侧壁还生长出三个嵴状皱襞,分别形成上、中、下三个鼻甲(图22-5)。

第四节 舌 的 发 生

第4周末,左、右下颌突内侧面的间充质增生,在原始口腔内形成位于前方的左右一对侧舌膨大和位于后方中线处的一个奇结节。在奇结节的背侧,第2、3、4鳃弓腹侧份的间充质增生,形成联合突和会厌突。侧舌膨大左右融合形成舌体的大部分,奇结节则形成舌盲孔前方舌体的小部分。联合突发育为舌根,舌体和舌根融合形成舌界沟,其顶点为舌盲孔。会厌突发育为会厌(图22-6)。

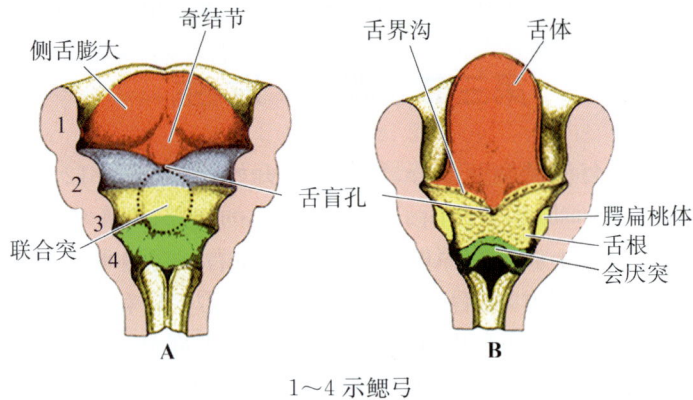

1~4 示鳃弓

图 22-6 舌的发生示意图

第五节 颈 的 发 生

颈是由第2、3、4、6鳃弓与心上嵴发育而成。左、右第2鳃弓生长迅速,它们向中线生长而愈合;它们向头端生长,将其与下颌突之间的外耳推向侧上方;它们向尾侧生长,越过第3、4、6鳃弓并覆盖在这些鳃弓表面。心上嵴是心隆起上缘的间充质增生向胚体头端生长出的嵴状隆起。当第2鳃弓与心上嵴愈合后,它们与下方3个较小鳃弓之间的间隙称颈窦。颈窦不久就闭锁、消失。随着鳃弓与心上嵴的生长、食管和气管的伸长及心脏位置的下降,颈逐渐形成。

第六节 四 肢 的 发 生

人胚第4周末,胚体左右外侧体壁上先后出现两对小隆起,即上肢芽与下肢芽,它们由深部的中胚层组织和表面外胚层组成。肢芽逐渐增长变粗,并先后出现近端和远端两个收缩环,将每一肢芽分为三段。上肢被分为上臂、前臂和手,下肢芽被分为大腿、小腿和足。肢体中轴的间充质先形成软骨,继而以软骨内成骨的方式形成骨;来自体节的间充质细胞迁移到肢芽,分化成肢体的骨骼肌;脊神经随后也长入肢体。肢体的手和足起初为扁平的桨板状,分别称手板和足板,之后其远端分别出现四条纵行凹沟,沟间出现 5 条指(趾)线,随着线间的细胞不断凋亡,至第 8 周末,手指和足趾形成。

第七节　常见畸形

一、唇裂

唇裂是最常见的一种颜面畸形,多因上颌突与同侧的内侧鼻突未愈合所致,裂沟位于人中外侧。唇裂多为单侧,也可见双侧者。如左、右内侧鼻突未愈合或两侧下颌突未愈合,可分别导致上唇或下唇的正中唇裂,但均较为少见。如内侧鼻突发育不良导致人中缺损,则出现宽大的正中唇裂。唇裂可伴有牙槽突裂和腭裂(图 22-7)。

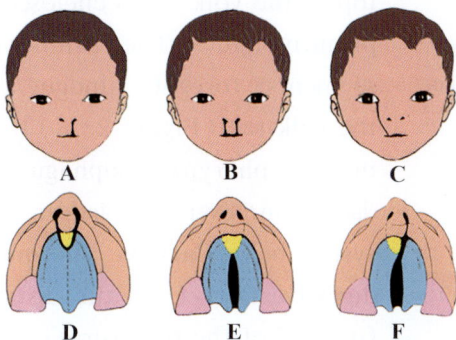

图 22-7　唇裂、腭裂与面斜裂仿真图
A.单侧唇裂;B.双侧唇裂;C.面斜裂;D.双侧前腭裂;E.正中腭裂;F.全腭裂

二、腭裂

腭裂也较常见,可有多种类型。因正中腭突与外侧腭突未愈合所致者称前腭裂(单侧或双侧,常伴发唇裂);因左、右外侧腭突未愈合所致者称正中腭裂;前腭裂和正中腭裂兼有者称全腭裂(图 22-7)。

三、面斜裂

面斜裂位于眼内眦与口角之间,因上颌突与同侧外侧鼻突未愈合所致(图 22-7)。

四、四肢畸形

四肢畸形种类众多,可发生在肢体的上、中、下各段。一类是肢体缺如,包括横向和纵向的肢体缺如。前者如无臂、无手、无指等,下肢亦然;后者如上肢桡侧或尺侧缺如,下肢胫侧或腓侧缺如。另一类是短肢,如海豹样手或足畸形。还有一类是肢体分化障碍,如某块肌或肌群缺如、关节发育不良、骨畸形、骨融合、多指(趾)、并指(趾)畸形、马蹄内翻足等。

(岳海源)

Chapter 23

Development of the Digestive and Respiratory Systems

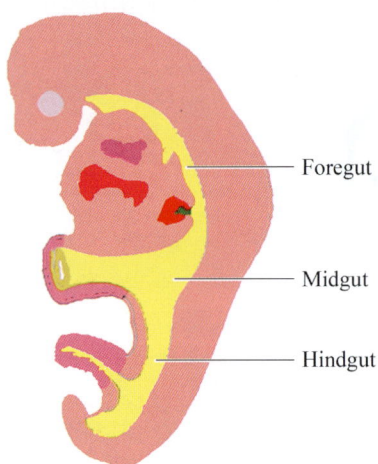

Figure 23 - 1   Drawing of the primitive gut

- Foregut
- Midgut
- Hindgut

In a human embryo of 3 - 4 weeks, with the development of blastocyst folding, the endoderm at the top of the yolk sac is enclosed in the embryo to form the primitive gut. The primitive gut is divided into 3 segments: foregut, hindgut and midgut connected with the yolk sac (Figure 23 - 1). The foregut differentiates into the pharynx, esophagus, stomach, proximal 2/3 of duodenum, liver, gallbladder, pancreas and the respiratory system below larynx. The midgut differentiates into the digestive tract from the distal 1/3 of duodenum to the first 2/3 of the transverse colon. The hindgut derivatives form the digestive tract from the distal 1/3 of the transverse colon to the upper part of anal canal. The mucosal epithelium, glandular epithelium and alveolar epithelium in these organs all derive from the endoderm, while the connective tissue, muscle tissue, vascular endothelium and mesothelium all derive from the mesoderm.

1   Development of Digestive System

1.1   Development of Primitive Pharynx and Pharyngeal Pouches

The primitive pharynx is an enlarged part of the cranial end of the foregut. It starts from the oropharyngeal membrane and ends at the beginning of the laryngotracheal diverticulum. It is funnel-shaped, wider in left and right, flatter in back and abdomen, thicker in cranial end, and thinner in caudal end. In week 4, the oropharyngeal membrane ruptures, and the primitive pharynx communicates with the outside world through the primitive oral cavity and primitive nasal cavity. There are 5 pairs of saccular processes on the lateral wall of the primitive pharynx, called pharyngeal pouches, which are opposite to the 5 pairs of the branchial grooves outside. With the development of the embryo, each pair of pharyngeal pouches has undergone important differentiation (Figure 23 – 2).

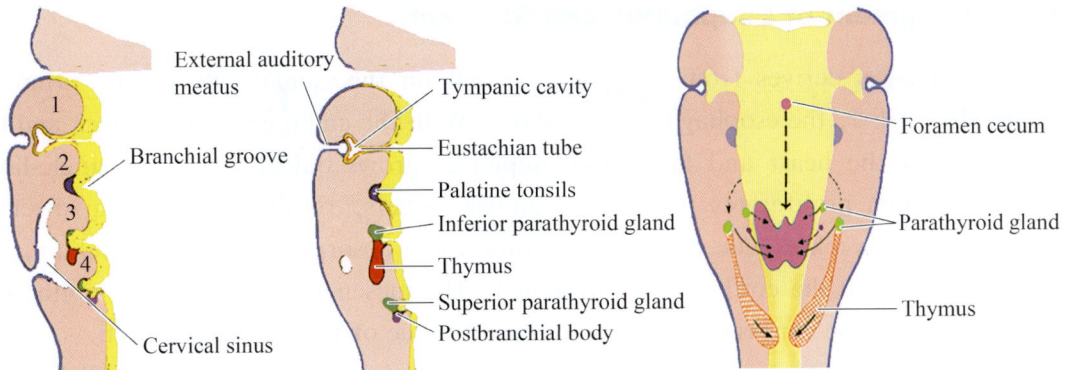

Figure 23 – 2　Drawings showing the derivatives of pharyngeal pouches and the development of thyroid

The lateral part of the first pair of pharyngeal pouches expands to form the middle ear tympanic cavity; the branchial membrane at the top of the pharyngeal pouch differentiates into the tympanic membrane; the outer side of the tympanic membrane is the external auditory canal formed by the first branchial groove, while the inner part elongates and evolves into the eustachian tube.

The second pair of pharyngeal pouches develop into palatine tonsils. Its surface epithelium derives from the endoderm, and the reticular tissue derives from the mesenchyme. Lymphocytes migrate and proliferate here.

The cells in the dorsal part of the 3rd pharyngeal pouches proliferate and move down to the dorsal side of the thyroid primordium to differentiate into the inferior parathyroid glands. The cells in the ventral part develop into thymus primordium.

The cells of the 4th pair of pharyngeal pouches proliferate and migrate to the upper dorsal side of the thyroid gland, which differentiate into the chief cells and form the superior parathyroid glands.

The 5th pair of pharyngeal pouches are very small and form a cell mass called postbranchial body. Some of its cells migrate into the thyroid primordium and differentiate into parafollicular cells. But some scholars believe that parafollicular cells derive from the neural crest cells.

1.2　Development of Thyroid Gland

At the beginning of week 4, the cells in the midline of the primitive pharyngeal wall proliferate and form a caudal blind tube, called thyroglossal duct, that is, the thyroid primordium. The thyroglossal duct extends down from the midline of the neck to the front of the future trachea, and the end expands to form left and right thyroid lateral lobes. In week 7, the upper segment of the thyroglossal duct degenerates and disappears (Figure 23 – 2). In week 11, follicles and colloids appear in the thyroid primordium, and the thyroid gland begins to secrete thyroid hormones at the beginning of week 13.

1.3 Development of Esophagus and Stomach

The esophagus derives from the primitive gut on the caudal side of the primitive pharynx. In week 4, the esophagus is very short. With the emergence of the neck and the development of the heart and lung, the esophagus grows quickly, and its single-layer surface epithelium proliferates to become multiple layers, resulting in the narrower or atretic lumen. In week 8, due to the degeneration and absorption of the epithelium, the lumen reappears and the epithelium is stratified. The mesenchyme around the epithelium differentiates into the connective tissue and muscle tissue of the esophageal wall.

In week 4 – 5, there is a fusiform dilation at the caudal end of the foregut, that is, the primordium of the stomach. In the beginning, the gastric primordium is close to the lower part of the primitive diaphragm, with a short dorsal mesangium and a long ventral mesangium. Then, with the elongation of the pharynx and esophagus, the stomach also moves to the caudal side, and its dorsal edge grows quickly to form the greater curvature of the stomach, while the ventral margin grows slowly to form the lesser curvature of the stomach. The cranial end of the greater curvature of the stomach bulges to form the gastric fundus. As the dorsal mesangium develops into the omental bursa protruding to the left, the greater curvature of the stomach turns from the back to the left, and the lesser curvature of the stomach turns from the ventral to the right, making the stomach rotate 90° clockwise to the right around the longitudinal axis of the embryo. Later, due to the enlargement of the liver, the cranial end of the stomach was pushed to the left. And, due to the fixation of the duodenum, the caudal end of the stomach is fixed to the posterior abdominal wall. As a result, the stomach turns from the original vertical orientation to the oblique orientation from upper left to lower right (Figure 23 – 3).

1.4 Development of Intestines

The intestine derives from the primitive gut below the stomach. The intestine is initially a straight tube parallel to the long axis of the embryo. The abdominal mesentery of the intestine degenerates and disappears very early, while the cranial dorsal mesentery fuses with the posterior abdominal wall and is fixed, and the rest extends with the development of the intestine tract. Because the growth rate of the intestine is much faster than that of the embryo, the intestinal tract forms a U-shaped bend protruding to the ventral side, which is called midgut loop. The top of the intestinal loop is connected with the yolk stalk, and the superior mesenteric artery runs along the central axis of the mesenteric loop, so the intestines are divided into 2 segments: the cephalic limb and the caudal limb (Figure 23 – 4).

In week 6, the intestinal loop grows rapidly, while the abdominal volume becames relatively small because of the development of the liver and mesonephros, resulting in the

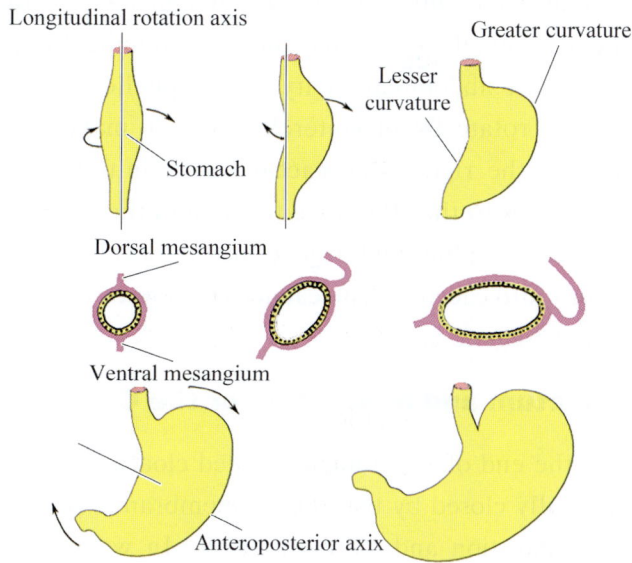

Figure 23 – 3   Drawings showing the development of stomach

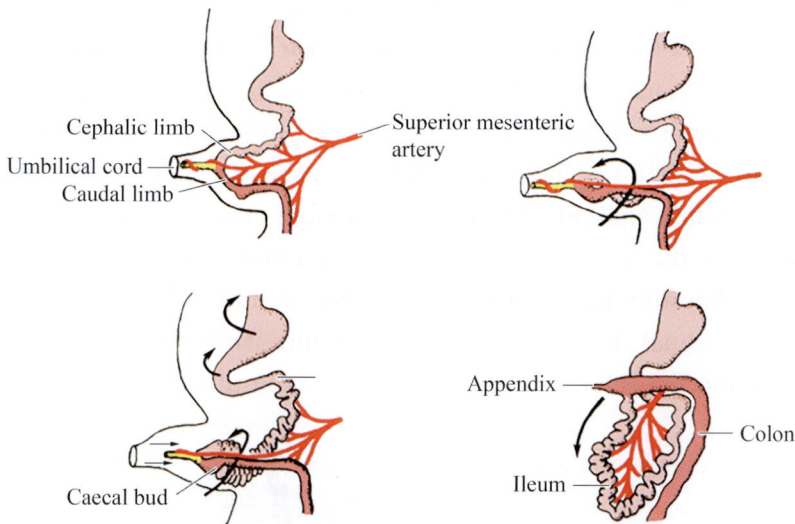

Figure 23 – 4   Drawings showing the rotation of intestinal loop

midgut loop entering the extraembryonic body cavity in the umbilical cord, that is, the umbilical coelom, forming a physiological umbilical hernia. The midgut loop continues to grow in the umbilical coelom, and rotates $90°$ counterclockwise with the superior mesenteric artery as the axis, resulting in the midgut loop turning from the sagittal direction to the horizontal direction, that is, the cephalic limb from the cranial position to the right, and the caudal limb from the caudal position to the left. There is a local dilatation in the caudal limb, namely the caecal bud, which is the primordium of caecum and appendix. In week 10, due to the atrophy of the mesonephros, the slow growth of the liver and the increase of the abdominal cavity, the midgut loop begins to return from the umbilical coelom to the abdominal cavity, and then the umbilical coelom is closed. When the midgut loop returns to the abdominal cavity, the cephalic limb goes first and the tail branch goes later, and they rotate 180° counterclockwise to make the cephalic limb to the left and the caudal limb to the right. The caecal bud is initially located in the position below the liver, then descends to the right iliac fossa, and the ascending colon forms. The distal part of the caecal bud atrophies and degenerates to develop into the appendix, while the proximal part develops into caecum. The caudal segment of the descending colon moves to the midline to form the sigmoid colon.

1.5 Formation of Rectum and Separation of the Cloaca

The enlargement at the end of the hindgut, called cloaca, is ventrally connected with the allantois and the caudally closed by the cloacal membrane. Rectum and anal canal are the products of cloacal separation and differentiation. In week 4 – 7, the mesenchymal between the initial part of allantois and the hindgut proliferates, forming a ridge protruding into the cloaca, which is called urorectal septum. This septum grows rapidly to the caudal and connects with the cloacal membrane, so the cloaca is divided into 2 compartments: one is the urogenital sinus for the formation of bladder and urethra; the other is the anorectal canal that differentiates into the rectum and upper anal canal. The cloacal membrane is also divided into 2 parts: the urogenital membrane and the anal membrane (Figure 23 – 5). The outer circumference of anal membrane is a shallow concave, which is called anal pit. The ectoderm of the anal pit is concave inward to form the lower segment of the anal canal. After anal membrane ruptures and is absorbed, the caudal end of the digestive tract connects with the outside. The epithelium of the upper segment of the anal canal derives from the endoderm, while the epithelium of the lower segment derives from the ectoderm. The border between them is named the dentate line.

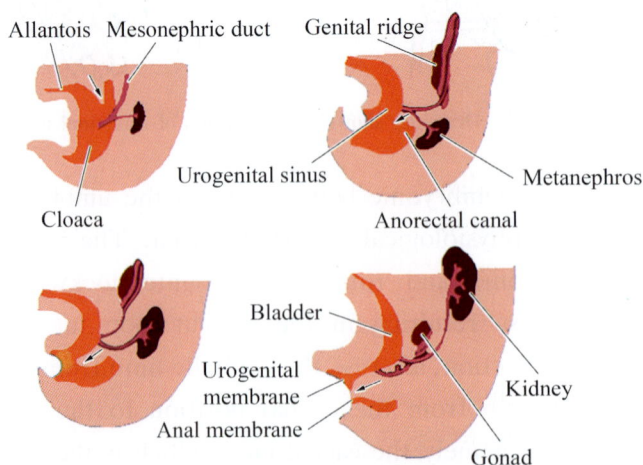

Figure 23 – 5   Drawings showing the separation of cloaca

1.6 Development of Liver and Gallbladder

In the beginning of the fourth week of the human embryo, the epithelium of the ventral wall at the end of the foregut proliferates and forms an outward protruding cystic process, called hepatic diverticulum, which is the primordium of the liver and gallbladder (Figure 23 - 6). The hepatic diverticulum rapidly enlarges and soon grows into the primitive diaphragm. Its end expands and divides into the cephalic limb and the caudal limb. The cephalic branches and grows rapidly. Its epithelial cells proliferate into many cell cords anastomosed, forming the hepatic cord. The hepatic cord is superimposed up and down to form the hepatic plate. The hepatic plate is arranged radially around the central vein to form hepatic lobules. The liver plate is initially composed of 2 - 3 layers of hepatocytes, and gradually becomes a single layer of hepatocytes in the later stage of the fetus. In the second month of embryo, bile canaliculi are formed between hepatocytes, and intrahepatic bile ducts are formed in the endoderm epithelium. The mesenchymal in the primitive diaphragm differentiates into the intrahepatic connective tissue and hepatic capsule.

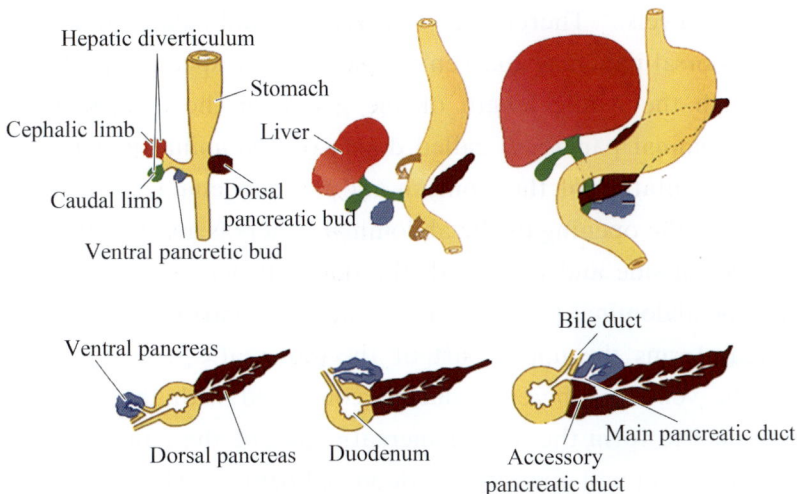

Figure 23 - 6   Drawings showing the development of the liver, gallbladder and pancreas

Embryonic liver is functionally active. In the 3rd month, hepatocytes begin to secrete bile. In week 6, hematopoietic stem cells migrate from the yolk sac wall into the liver and the liver begins to produce blood, mainly producing erythrocytes. After the 6th month, the hematopoietic tissue in the liver gradually decreases, and the liver basically stops hematopoietic before birth. Fetal liver began to synthesize and secrete a variety of plasma proteins. Before the 6th month, all fetal hepatocytes synthesize alpha fetoprotein. Then they gradually produce less and stop soon after birth.

The caudal limb develops into the gallbladder and cystic duct, and the root of the hepatic diverticulum develops into the common bile duct (Figure 23 - 6). Due to the excessive hyperplasia of the epithelium, the lumen of the cystic duct and common bile duct disappear. With the degeneration and absorption of intraluminal epithelial cells, the lumen reappears. Initially, the common bile duct opens in the ventral wall of the duodenum. With the transposition of the duodenum and the faster development of the right wall of duodenum than the left one, the opening of the common bile duct gradually moves to the dorsomedial side of the duodenum and opens in the duodenum together with the pancreatic duct.

1.7 Development of Pancreas

Pancreas derives from 2 primordia: the dorsal pancreatic bud and ventral pancreatic bud (Figure 23 - 6). At the end of week 4, the endoderm epithelium proliferates to form abdominal pancreatic buds in the ventral end of the foregut near the caudal edge of the hepatic diverticulum. The dorsal pancreatic bud is formed from the epithelial hyperplasia on the opposite side of the abdominal pancreatic bud, with a slightly higher position and a slightly larger volume. The epithelial cells of the 2 pancreatic buds proliferate and branch repeatedly, and acini are formed at the terminals. The branches connected with the acini form ducts at all levels. Therefore, the dorsal and abdominal pancreatic buds differentiated into dorsal pancreas and ventral pancreas, respectively. There is a common duct running through the whole length of the gland on the central axis of the dorsal pancreas or the abdominal pancreas, called dorsal or abdominal pancreatic duct. Due to the changes in the orientation of the stomach and the duodenum, and the unequal growth of the intestinal wall, the opening of the abdominal pancreas and the abdominal pancreatic duct turns to the dorsal side and fuses with the dorsal pancreas to form a single pancreas (Figure 23 - 6). The abdominal pancreas forms the lower part of the pancreatic head, and the dorsal pancreas forms the upper part of the pancreatic head, pancreatic body and pancreatic tail. The ventral pancreatic duct is connected with the distal segment of the dorsal pancreatic duct to form the main pancreatic duct of the pancreas, which converges with the common bile duct and opens to the duodenal papilla. The proximal segment of the dorsal pancreatic duct degenerates or forms an accessory pancreatic duct which opens in the duodenal accessory papilla.

During the differentiation of the pancreatic primordium, some epithelial cells separate from the cell cord to form isolated cell clusters, which differentiate into islands of pancreatic islets and begin to secrete hormones at the 5th month.

1.8 Main Congenital Malformations

1.8.1 Thyroglossal Duct Cyst

The thyroglossal duct is not completely closed or degenerated, forming a small cyst, which can move up and down with swallowing activity.

1.8.2 Digestive Tract Atresia or Stenosis

In the development of the digestive tract, epithelial cells in the wall once proliferate excessively, resulting in the atresia or stenosis of the lumen of a certain part of the digestive tract. Subsequently, as the hyperplastic cells die, the epithelium becomes thinner, and the narrowed or closed lumen returns to normal. If the hyperplastic epithelium does not die, it will form atresia or stenosis of a certain section of the digestive tract, commonly in the esophagus and duodenum.

1.8.3 Ileal Diverticulum

Also known as Meckel's diverticulum, it is a small cystic protrusion on the ileal wall $40-50$ cm away from the ileocecal part, with or without a fiber cord connected to the umbilicus at the top. This deformity is caused by incomplete degeneration of the yolk stalk. Most patients are asymptomatic, but abdominal pain and other diseases can occur during infection. It also occasionally causes the intestinal obstruction.

1.8.4 Congenital Umbilical Hernia

It is caused by the failure of umbilical coelom atresia. Although the umbilical cord is cut off at birth, a cavity is still left to communicate with the abdominal cavity. When the intra-abdominal pressure increases, the intestinal canal will bulge from the umbilicus and even cause incarcerated hernia.

1.8.5 Umbilical Fecal Fistula

Because the yolk stalk does not degenerate, there is a fistula between the intestine and the umbilicus. When the abdominal pressure increases, feces can overflow from the umbilicus through the fistula.

1.8.6 Congenital Megacolon

Also known as Hirschsprung's disease, it is more common in sigmoid colon. Because the neural crest cells fail to migrate to the intestinal wall, the parasympathetic ganglion cells in the wall are absent, so the intestinal wall contracted weakly, and the contents of the intestinal cavity could not be discharged well, expanding the intestinal canal.

1.8.7 Anal atresia

Also known as imperforate anus, it is caused by the absence of rupture of anal membrane or the failure of anal pit in communicating with the end of rectum.

1.8.8 Abnormal Transposition of Midgut Loop

When the midgut loop returns to the abdominal cavity from the umbilical coelom, it should rotate $180°$ counterclockwise. If there is no rotation, incomplete transposition, or reverse transposition, it will form a variety of ectopic digestive tracts, often accompanied by ectopic liver, spleen, pancreas, or even heart and lung.

2 Development of Respiratory System

2.1 Development of the Larynx, Trachea and Lung

Except that the nasal epithelium comes from the surface ectoderm, the epithelium of other parts of the respiratory system derives from the primitive gut endoderm.

In a human embryo of 4 weeks, a longitudinal shallow groove called laryngotracheal groove, appears in the middle line of the caudal bottom wall of the primitive pharynx. This groove gradually deepens and begins to gradually fuse from its ventral end to the cranial end, and finally forms a long blind sac, called laryngotracheal diverticulum, which is the primordium of the larynx, trachea, bronchus and lung (Figure 23 - 7). The laryngotracheal diverticulum is located on the ventral side of the esophagus. The mesenchymal septum between the two is called tracheoesophageal septum.

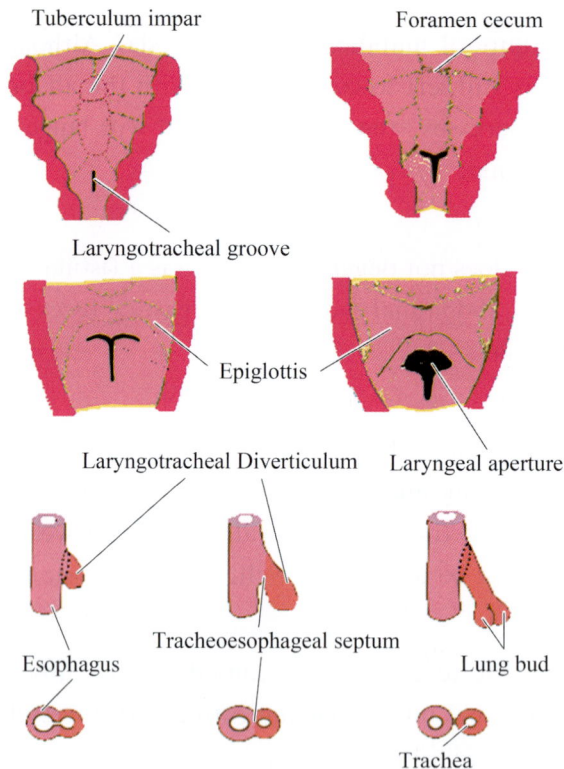

Figure 23 - 7　Drawings showing the development of the laryngotracheal diverticulum and esophagus

The upper part of the laryngotracheal diverticulum opening in the pharynx develops into the larynx, and the rest develops into the trachea. The end of the diverticulum is enlarged and divided into left and right branches, called lung buds, which are the primordium of bronchus and lung. The lung buds grow rapidly and form tree branches.

The left lung bud is divided into 2 branches while the right lung bud is divided into 3 branches, forming the lobar bronchi of the left lung and the right lung respectively. At the end of the second month, the lobar bronchi form segmental bronchi, with 8 – 9 branches in the left lung and 10 branches in the right lung. In the sixth month, the branches reach about the grade 17, and finally there are terminal bronchioles, respiratory bronchioles with gas exchange function, alveolar ducts and alveolar sacs (Figure 23 – 7, Figure 23 – 8). In the 7th month, the number of alveoli increases. In addition to type I cells, type II cells with secretory function appear in the alveolar epithelium, and began to secrete surfactant. At this time, the blood circulation in the lung is more perfect, and there are dense capillaries on the alveolar wall, so the premature fetus can have normal respiratory function at this time. The mesenchyme around the laryngotracheal diverticulum and lung buds differentiates into the connective tissue, cartilage and smooth muscle of larynx, trachea and bronchial wall at all levels.

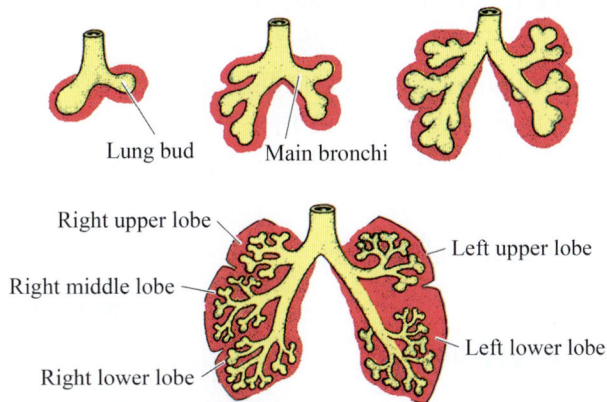

Lung bud   Main bronchi

Right upper lobe   Left upper lobe
Right middle lobe
Left lower lobe
Right lower lobe

Figure 23 – 8   Drawings showing the development of lung

2.2   Main Congenital Malformations

2.2.1   Tracheoesophageal Fistula

Due to the dysplasia of tracheoesophageal septum, the separation between trachea and esophagus is incomplete, and there is a fistula between them.

2.2.2   Hyaline Membrane Disease

Due to the poor differentiation of alveolar type II cells and the inability to secrete surfactant, resulting in the increase of alveolar surface tension, the alveolar cannot expand with respiratory movement after birth. Microscopic examination shows alveolar collapse, interstitial edema and a layer of plasma protein membrane on the surface of alveolar epithelium. The disease is mainly seen in preterm infants before week 28 of pregnancy.

(Yue Haiyuan)

第二十三章 消化系统和呼吸系统的发生

人胚第3～4周,随着胚盘卷折的发生,卵黄囊顶部的内胚层卷入胚体内,形成原始消化管。原始消化管从头端到尾端分为前肠、中肠和后肠三段,其中中肠和卵黄囊相连(图23-1)。前肠主要分化为咽、食管、胃、十二指肠上段、肝、胆囊、胰腺及喉以下的呼吸系统;中肠主要分化为从十二指肠中段至横结肠右2/3部的肠管;后肠主要分化为从横结肠左1/3至肛管上端的肠管。以上器官中的黏膜上皮、腺上皮和肺泡上皮均来自内胚层,而结缔组织、肌组织、血管内皮和外表面的间皮均来自中胚层。

第一节 消化系统的发生

一、原始咽的发生和咽囊的演变

原始咽为前肠头端的一个膨大部,从口咽膜起止于喉气管憩室起始部,呈左右宽、背腹扁、头端粗、尾端细的漏斗状。人胚第4周,口咽膜破裂,原始咽通过原始口腔和原始鼻腔和外界相通。在原始咽侧壁有5对囊状突起,称咽囊,分别与其外侧的5对鳃沟相对,随着胚胎的发育,各对咽囊也先后发生重要的分化和演变(图23-2)。

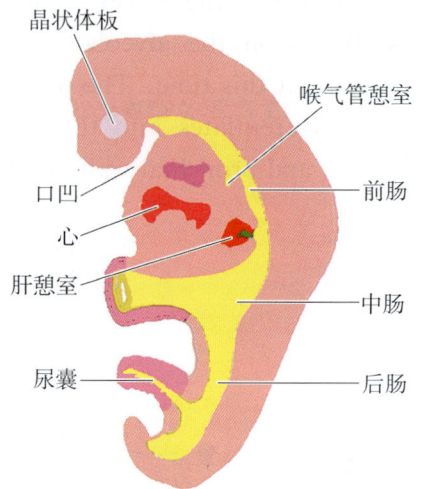

图 23-1 早期原始消化管示意图

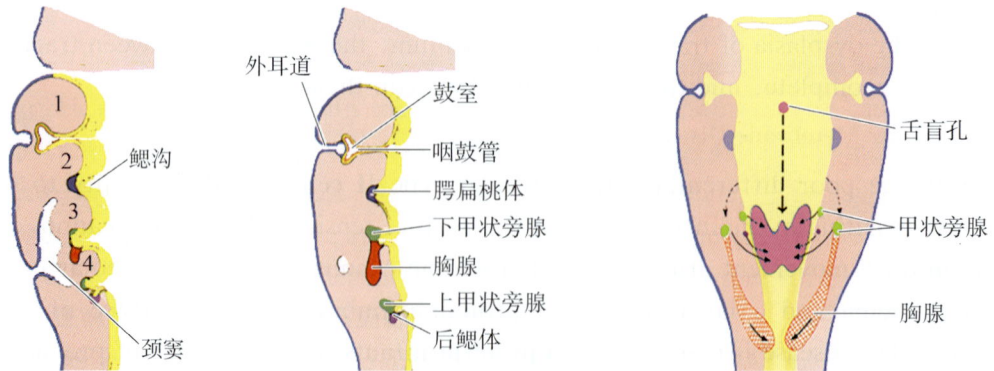

图 23-2 咽囊的演化及甲状腺的发生示意图

第1对咽囊的外侧份膨大,形成中耳鼓室,其顶部的鳃膜分化为鼓膜,鼓膜外侧为第一鳃沟形成的外耳道,而内侧份伸长,演化为咽鼓管。

第2对咽囊演化成腭扁桃体,其表面上皮来自内胚层,网状组织来自间充质,淋巴细胞迁移到此并大量增殖。

第3对咽囊的背侧份细胞增生并下移至甲状腺原基背侧,分化为下一对甲状旁腺;腹侧份细胞增生形成胸腺原基。

第4对咽囊的细胞增生并迁移至甲状腺背侧上方,形成上一对甲状旁腺,主要分化为主细胞。

第5对咽囊很小,形成一细胞团,称后鳃体,其部分细胞迁入甲状腺原基,分化为甲状腺滤泡旁细胞。也有学者认为,滤泡旁细胞来自神经嵴细胞。

二、甲状腺的发生

人胚第4周初,在原始咽底壁正中线处的细胞增生,形成一伸向尾侧的盲管,称甲状舌管,即甲状腺原基。此盲管沿颈部正中线下延伸至未来气管前方,末端向两侧膨大,形成左右两个甲状腺侧叶(图23-2)。第7周时,甲状舌管的上段退化消失。第11周时,甲状腺原基中出现滤泡并含有胶质,第13周初甲状腺开始出现分泌活动。

三、食管和胃的发生

食管由原始咽尾侧的一段原始消化管分化而来。人胚第4周时,食管很短。随着颈的出现和心、肺的发育,食管也迅速增长,其表面上皮增生,由单层变为复层,使管腔变窄,甚至闭锁。第8周,过度增生的上皮退化吸收,管腔重新出现,上皮仍保持为复层。上皮周围的间充质分化为食管壁的结缔组织和肌组织。

人胚第4~5周,前肠尾端出现一梭形膨大,即胃的原基。起初,胃原基紧靠原始横隔下方,其背系膜短,腹系膜长。之后,随着咽和食管的伸长,胃也向尾侧移动,其背侧缘生长迅速,形成胃大弯;腹侧缘生长缓慢,形成胃小弯。胃大弯的头端膨出,形成胃底。由于胃背系膜发育为突向左侧的网膜囊,致使胃大弯由背侧转向左侧,胃小弯由腹侧转向右侧,使胃沿胚体纵轴向右旋转90°。后由于肝的增大,胃的头端被推向左侧;由于十二指肠的固定,胃的尾端被固定于腹后壁上。结果,胃由原来的垂直方位变成了由左上至右下的斜行方位(图23-3)。

四、肠的发生

肠由胃以下的原始消化管分化而成。肠起初为一条与胚体长轴平行的直管。肠的腹系膜很早即全部退化消失,而头端背系膜与腹后壁融合而被固定,其余部分随着肠管的生长而增长。由于肠的增长速度远比胚体快,致使肠管形成一凸向腹侧的"U"形弯曲,称中肠袢。肠袢顶部与卵黄蒂通连,肠系膜上动脉走行于肠袢系膜的中轴部位。肠袢与卵黄蒂相连的头侧段为肠袢的头支,尾侧段为肠袢尾支。

第6周,肠袢生长迅速,加之肝和中肾的发育,腹腔容积相对变小,迫使肠袢进入脐带内的胚外体腔,即脐腔,形成生理性脐疝。肠袢在脐腔中继续增长,同时以肠系膜上动脉为轴心作逆时针方向旋转90°,致使肠袢由矢状方向转为水平方向,即头支从头侧至右侧,尾支从尾侧转至左侧。尾支出现一囊状突起,即盲肠突,为盲肠和阑尾的原基。第10周时,由于中肾萎缩、

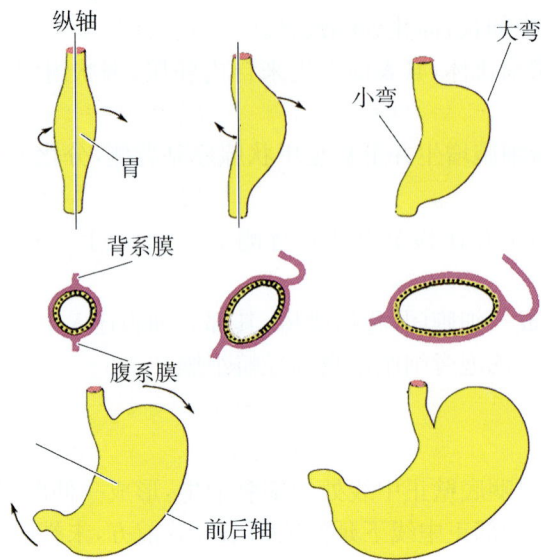

图 23-3 胃的发生示意图

肝生长减缓和腹腔的增大,肠袢开始从脐腔退回腹腔,脐腔随之闭锁。在肠袢退回腹腔时,头支在先,尾支在后,并且逆时针方向再旋转 180°,使头支转至左侧,尾支转至右侧。盲肠突初位于肝下,后下降至右髂窝,升结肠随之形成。盲肠突的远侧份萎缩退化,发育为阑尾,近侧份发育为盲肠。降结肠尾段移向中线,形成乙状结肠(图 23-4)。

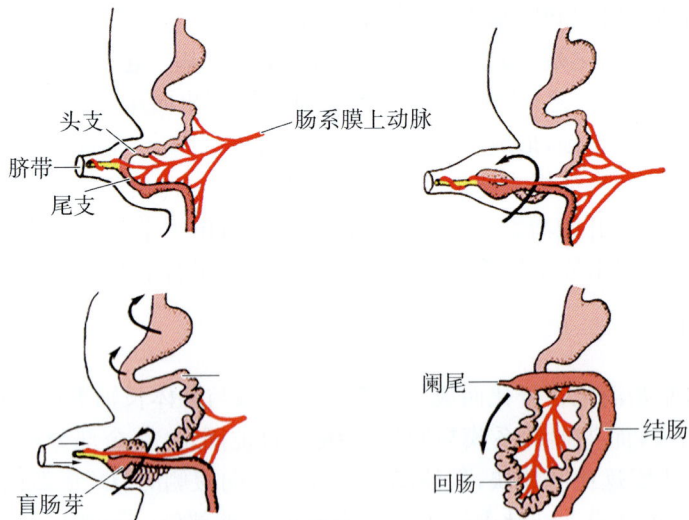

图 23-4 中肠袢的旋转示意图

五、直肠的发生与泄殖腔的分隔

后肠末端的膨大称泄殖腔,其腹侧与尿囊相连,尾端由泄殖腔膜封闭。直肠和肛管是泄殖腔分隔、分化的产物。人胚第4～7周,尿囊起始部分与后肠之间的间充质增生,形成一镰刀状隔膜突入泄殖腔内,称尿直肠隔。此隔迅速向尾端增长,并与泄殖腔膜相连,于是泄殖腔被分隔为背腹两份。腹侧份称尿生殖窦,主要分化为膀胱和尿道;背侧份为肛直肠管,分化为直肠和肛管上段。泄殖腔膜也被分为背腹两份,腹侧份称尿生殖窦膜,背侧份称肛膜(图23-5)。肛膜外周为一浅凹,称肛凹。肛凹的外胚层向内凹陷形成肛管下段。肛膜破裂被吸收后,消化管尾端与外界相通。肛管上段的上皮来自内胚层,下段的上皮来自外胚层,两者之间的分界线称齿状线。

六、肝和胆的发生

胚胎发育至第4周初,前肠末端腹侧壁的上皮增生,形成一个向外突出的囊状突起,称肝憩室,是肝与胆囊的原基(图23-6)。肝憩室迅速增大,很快长入原始横隔,其末端膨大,并分为头、尾两支。头支较大且生长迅速,其上皮细胞增殖,形成许多细胞索并分支吻合,即肝索。肝索上下叠加,形成肝板。肝板围绕中央静脉呈放射状排列,形成肝小叶。肝板最初由2～3层肝细胞组成,胎儿后期逐渐变为单层肝细胞。胚胎第2个月,肝细胞之间形成胆小管,内胚层上皮也相继形成肝内胆管。原始横隔中的间充质分化为肝内结缔组织和肝被膜。

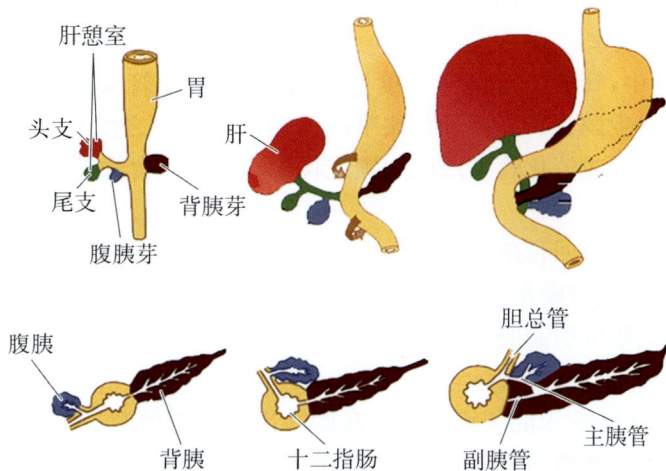

图23-6 肝、胆、胰的发生示意图

胚胎期肝的功能十分活跃。第3个月,肝细胞开始分泌胆汁。第6周时,造血干细胞从卵黄囊壁迁入肝,并开始造血,主要产生红细胞。第6个月后,肝造血逐渐减少,出生前肝基本停止造血。胎肝很早就开始合成和分泌白蛋白等多种血浆蛋白质。第6个月前,几乎所有的胎肝细胞都能合成甲胎蛋白,此后逐渐减少。出生后很快停止合成甲胎蛋白。

肝憩室的尾支发育为胆囊和胆囊管,肝憩室的根部则发育为胆总管(图23-6)。由于上皮的过度增生,胆囊管和胆总管的管腔曾一度消失。随着腔内上皮细胞的退化吸收,管腔重新出现。最初,胆总管开口于十二指肠的腹侧壁,随着十二指肠的转位及右侧壁的发育快于左侧壁,致使胆总管的开口逐渐移至十二指肠的背内侧,并与胰腺导管合并共同开口于十二指肠。

七、胰腺的发生

胰腺来源于两个原基,即背胰芽和腹胰芽(图 23-6)。胚胎第 4 周末,在前肠末端腹侧靠近肝憩室的尾缘,内胚层上皮增生,形成腹胰芽。背胰芽由腹胰芽对侧的上皮增生而成,位置稍高,体积略大。背、腹两个胰芽的上皮细胞不断增生并反复分支,其末端形成腺泡,与腺泡相连的各级分支形成各级导管,于是由背、腹两个胰芽分化成了背胰和腹胰。在背胰和腹胰的中轴线上均有一条贯穿腺体全长的总导管,分别称背胰管和腹胰管。由于胃和十二指肠方位的变化和肠壁的不均等生长,致使腹胰和腹胰管的开口转至背侧,并与背胰融合,形成一个单一的胰腺(图 23-6)。腹胰构成胰头的下份,背胰构成胰头上份、胰体和胰尾。腹胰管与背胰管远侧段通连,形成胰腺的主胰导管,它与胆总管汇合后共同开口于十二指肠乳头。背胰管的近侧段或退化或形成副胰导管,开口于十二指肠副乳头。

在胰腺原基的分化过程中,部分上皮细胞脱离细胞索,形成孤立存在的细胞团,由此分化为胰岛,并于第 5 个月开始分泌激素。

八、主要畸形

1. 甲状舌管囊肿

甲状舌管未完全闭锁、退化,形成小的囊肿,并可随吞咽活动而上下移动。

2. 消化管闭锁或狭窄

在消化管的发生中,管壁上皮细胞一度过度增生,使消化管某部的管腔闭锁或狭窄。随后,过度增生的细胞发生调亡,上皮变薄,狭窄或闭锁的管腔随之恢复正常。如果过度增生的上皮不发生调亡,就会形成消化管某段的闭锁或狭窄。常见于食管和十二指肠。

3. 回肠憩室

又称麦克尔憩室,是距回盲部 40~50 cm 处回肠壁上的一个小的囊状突起,有的在其顶端尚有一纤维索连于脐。这种畸形是由于卵黄蒂退化不全引起的。患者多无症状,但在感染时可出现腹痛等病症,偶尔可引起肠梗阻。

4. 先天性脐疝

先天性脐疝是由于脐腔未能闭锁所致。在胎儿出生脐带剪断后,脐部仍留有一腔与腹腔相通。当腹内压增高时,肠管便从脐部膨出,甚至造成嵌顿疝。

5. 脐粪瘘

由于卵黄蒂未退化,以致在肠与脐之间残存一瘘管,当腹压增高时,粪便可通过瘘管从脐部溢出。

6. 先天性巨结肠

又称 Hirschsprung 病,多见于乙状结肠。由于神经嵴细胞未能迁至该处肠壁中,致使肠壁内副交感神经节细胞缺如,肠壁收缩无力,肠腔内容物不能很好地排出,因而肠管扩大。

7. 肛门闭锁

又称不通肛,是由于肛膜未破裂或者肛凹未能与直肠末端相通引起。

8. 肠袢转位异常

当肠袢从脐腔退回腹腔时,应发生逆时针方向旋转 180°。如果未发生旋转,或转位不全,或反向转位,就会形成各种消化管异位,并且常常伴有肝、脾、胰,甚至心、肺的异位。

第二节　呼吸系统的发生

一、喉、气管和肺的发生

人胎第 4 周时,原始咽的尾端底壁正中出现一纵行浅沟,称喉气管沟。此沟逐渐加深,并从其尾端开始愈合,愈合过程向头端推移,最后形成一个长形盲囊,称气管憩室,是喉、气管、支气管和肺的原基(图 23 - 7)。喉气管憩室位于食管的腹侧,两者之间的间充质称为气管食管隔。

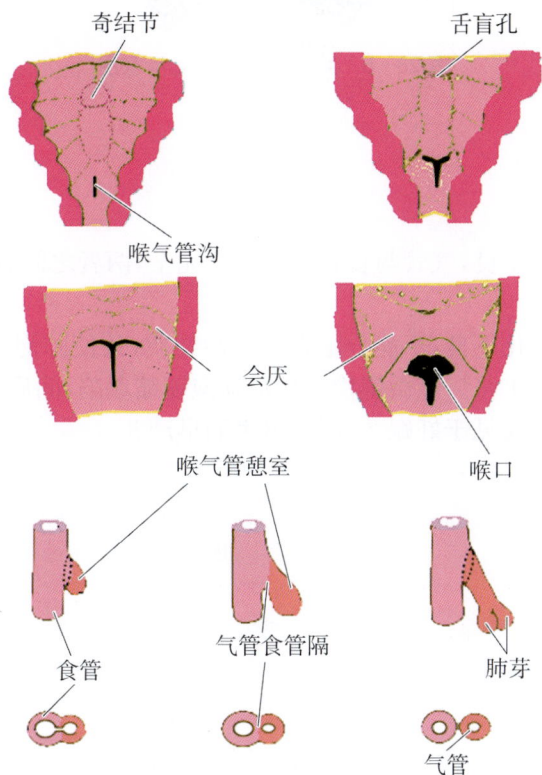

图 23 - 7　喉气管憩室的发生和演化示意图

喉气管憩室的上端开口于咽的部分发育为喉,其余部分发育为气管。憩室的末端膨大并分成左右两支,称肺芽,是支气管和肺的原基。肺芽迅速生长并成树状分支。左肺芽分为两支,右肺芽分为三支,分别形成左肺和右肺的肺叶支气管。至第 2 个月末,肺叶支气管分支形成肺段支气管,左肺 8~9 支,右肺 10 支。第 6 个月时,分支达 17 级左右,出现了呼吸性细支气管、肺泡管和肺泡囊(图 23 - 7,图 23 - 8)。至第 7 个月,肺泡数量增多,肺泡上皮除 Ⅰ 型肺泡细胞外,还出现了有分泌功能的 Ⅱ 型肺泡细胞,并开始分泌表面活性物质。此时,肺内血液循环完善,肺泡壁上有密集的毛细血管,故在此时早产的胎儿可进行正常的呼吸功能。喉气管憩室和肺芽周围的间充质分化为喉、气管和各级支气管壁的结缔组织、软骨、平滑肌,以及肺内间质中的结缔组织。

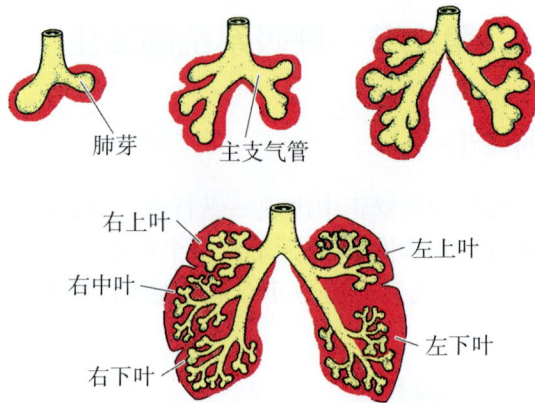

图 23-8 肺的发生和演化示意图

二、主要畸形

1. 气管食管瘘

由于气管食管隔发育不良,气管与食管的分隔不完全,两者之间有瘘管相连。

2. 透明膜病

由于Ⅱ型肺泡细胞分化不良,不能分泌表面活性物质,致使肺泡表面张力增大,胎儿出生后肺泡不能随呼吸运动而扩张。显微镜检查显示肺泡萎缩塌陷,间质水肿,肺泡上皮表面覆盖一层血浆蛋白膜。该病主要见于妊娠28周前出生的早产儿。

（岳海源）

Chapter 24

Development of the Urogenital System

The main organs of the urinary and reproductive systems originate from intermediate mesoderm. At the beginning of week 4 of the human embryo, the cranial intermediate mesoderm grows in segments called nephrotome, while the caudal part grows longitudinally in a strip shape called nephrogenic cord. At the end of week 4, the nephrotomes separate from the somites, and its volume increases continuously. It protrudes from the posterior wall of the embryo to the body cavity, forming a pair of left-right symmetrical longitudinal ridges on both sides of the dorsal aorta, called urogenital ridges. The urogenital ridge develops further, and a longitudinal groove appears in the middle, which divides the ridge into the inner and lateral parts. The lateral part called mesonephric ridge is long and thick, while the inner part called genital ridge is short and thin (Figure 24 - 1).

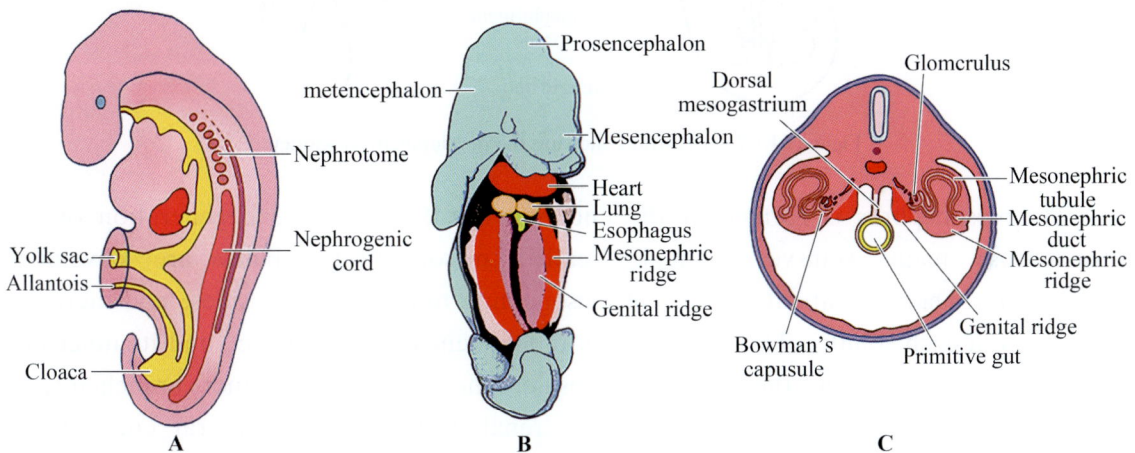

Figure 24 - 1　Drawings showing the development of the mesonephric ridge and genital ridge
A. Lateral view in the end of week 4; B. Ventral view in the end of week 4; C. Transverse pane in week 5

1　Development of Urinary System

1.1　Development of Kidney and Ureter

The development of the human embryonic kidney can be divided into 3 successive stages: pronephros, mesonephros and metanephros from the neck to the lumbosacral portion.

The pronephros is formed the earliest. At the beginning of week 4, it is located outside the 7 – 14th somites of the neck. The cranial nephrotome develops several transverse cell cords, then forms pronephric tubules whose inner ends open in the body cavity of the embryo. The lateral ends of the pronephric tubules extend to the tail, and connect each other to form a longitudinal pronephric duct. The pronephros includes the pronephric tubules and the pronephroic duct, which is not functionally significant in humans. The pronephric tubules totally degenerate at the end of week 4, but most of the pronephric duct remains and continues to extend to the tail to become the mesonephric duct (Figure 24 – 2).

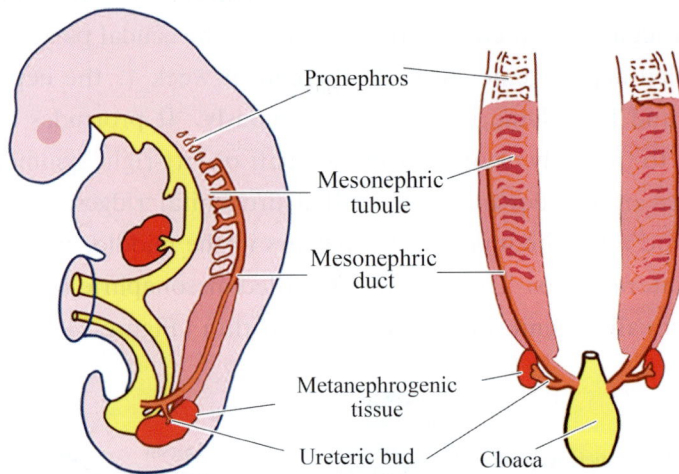

Figure 24 – 2　Drawings showing the development of kidney

The mesonephros is formed at the end of week 4. After the degeneration of the pronephros, many transverse tubules called mesonephric tubules are developed successively. There are about 80 pairs of mesonephric tubules on both sides, and there are 2 – 3 pairs in each somite. The mesonephric tubule bends in an S shape, and its inner end expands and is sunken into the Bowman's capsule. There are capillary knots branched from the dorsal aorta, which together form the renal corpuscle. The lateral ends of the mesonephric tubules coincide with the pronephric duct extending to the caudal end; then the pronephric duct is renamed mesonephric duct. The caudal end of the mesonephric duct leads into the cloaca (Figure 24 – 2). In humans, the mesonephros may have transient functional activity until the formation of metanephros. At the end of the second month, most of the mesonephros also degenerate, just leaving the mesonephric duct and a small part of the caudal mesonephric tubules.

The metanephros develops into an adult permanent kidney. At the beginning of week 5 of the human embryo, when the mesonephros is still developing, metanephros begins to form. After week 11 – 12, the metanephros begins to produce urine, and its function continues throughout the fetal period. The urine is discharged into the amniotic cavity and constitutes the main component of the amniotic fluid. Because the metabolites of the embryo are mainly excreted by the placenta, the excretion function of the kidney in the fetal period is very small. The posterior kidney originates from 2 different parts: the metanephrogenic tissue and the ureteric bud that both derive from the mesoderm.

The ureteric bud is a blind tube growing dorsolaterally near the cloaca at the end of the mesonephric duct. It extends to the dorsal and cranial sides of the embryo and grows into the mesoderm tissue at the caudal end of the mesonephic ridge. The ureteric bud repeatedly branches to more than 12 grades and gradually develops into the ureter, renal pelvis, renal calyces and collecting tubule. The collecting tubule develops T-shaped branches whose arcuate blind end induces the adjacent metanephrogenic tissue to differentiate into nephrons (Figure 24 – 3, 24 – 4).

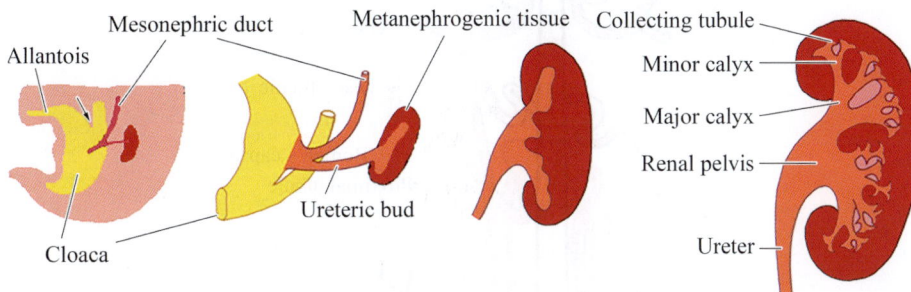

Figure 24 – 3   Drawings showing the development of metanephros

The metanephrogenic tissue is developed by the mesoderm at the caudal mesorenal ridge induced by the ureteric bud. The cells of the mesonephric duct are dense and cap-shaped around the end of the ureteric bud, which becomes the metanephric tissue. The peripheral part of the metanephrogenic tissue develops into the renal capsule, and the inner part forms multiple cell clusters that gradually differentiate into S-shaped tubules. One end of this tubule connects the blind end of arcuate collecting tubules, the other end expands and concaves to develop into the Bowman's capsule, forming renal corpuscles with the glomeruli extending into the capsule. The rest of these tubules gradually grows and differentiates into the segments of renal tubules, which form the nephron with renal corpuscles. A distal convoluted tubule connects an arcuate collecting tubule, and then their lumens are communicated. The juxtamedullary nephrons develop earlier. As the end of the collecting duct continues to grow and branches to the superficial cortex, the metanephrogenetic tissue is induced to form cortical nephrons (Figure 24 – 4).

In week 12, the posterior kidney begins to produce urine, which constitutes the main source of the amniotic fluid. Because the metanephros develops at the caudal side of the mesonephric ridge, the original position of the kidney is low. With the growth of the embryo abdomen, the extension of the ureter and the erection of the embryo body, the

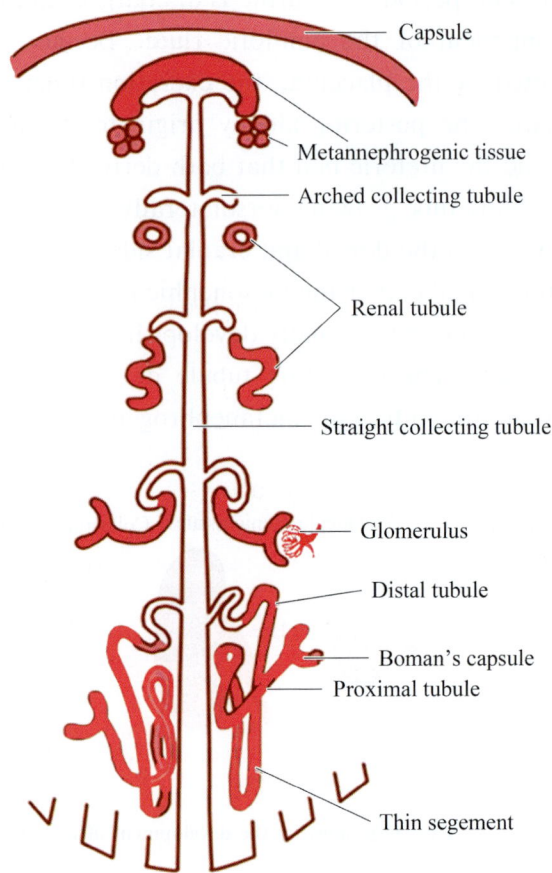

Figure 24 - 4　Drawing showing the development of the collecting tubule and nephron

kidney gradually rises to the waist, and rotates along the central axis of the embryo body, making the renal hilum turn from the ventral side to the inside.

1.2　Development of Bladder and Urethra

In week 4 - 7, the urorectal septum divides the cloaca into 2 parts: the dorsal primitive rectum and the ventral urogenital sinus. The urogenital sinus consists of 3 segments. The upper segment is large and develops into the bladder that will connect the allantois. Before birth, the allantois from the umbilical cord to the top of the bladder degenerates into a fibrous cord, which is named the middle umbilical ligament. The left and right mesonephric ducts are open to the bladder, respectively. With the expansion of the bladder, the mesonephric duct below the beginning of the ureter also expands and gradually merges into the bladder to become a part of its back wall. Therefore, the ureter and the middle renal duct are open in the bladder, respectively. The middle segment is quite narrow and tubular, forming most of the urethra in women and the prostatic and membranous urethra in men. Due to the migration of the kidney to the cephalic side and the continuous downward growth of the middle renal duct, the ureteral opening moves outward and upward, and the opening of the mesonephric duct moves downward to the urethra and prostate in men; in women, the site of access to the urethra will degenerate. The lower segment forms the corpus cavernosum of the urethra in men and expands into the vaginal vestibule in women.

1.3   Main Congenital Malformations

1.3.1   Polycystic Kidney

Because the collecting tubules and distal tubules are not connected, urine accumulates in the renal tubules, and many cysts in different sizes appear in the kidney, resulting in compression, atrophy of normal renal tissue, and renal dysfunction (Figure 23 – 7).

1.3.2   Ectopic Kidney

The kidneys are blocked in the rising process, so that the postnatal kidneys cannot reach the normal position and will be located in the pelvis usually.

1.3.3   Horseshoe Kidney

It is formed by the abnormal fusion of the lower ends of kidneys, resulting from the obstruction of the root of the inferior mesenteric artery when the kidney rises (Figure 23 – 7).

1.3.4   Double Ureter

It is caused by the premature branching of the ureteral bud. Various malformations can be induced because of the branches, such as incomplete renal ureteral branches, separating kidneys, and double ureters.

1.3.5   Urachal Fistula

The urachal tube between the top of the bladder and umbilicus is not closed, and urine can leak out of the umbilicus after birth.

1.3.6   Exstrophy Bladder

There is no mesenchymal between the urogenital sinus and the surface ectoderm. Therefore, there are no muscles covering the bladder in the anterior abdominal wall, resulting in the destruction of the thin epidermis, the anterior wall of the bladder, and the exposure of the bladder mucosa.

2   Development of Reproductive System

Although the sex of an embryo is genetically determined by the karyotype of sperm at the time of fertilization, the gonads do not show the morphological characteristics of sex until week 7 of the embryo. The gender of the external genitalia cannot be recognized until week 12. The reproductive system (including the gonad, reproductive ducts and external genitalia) can be divided into 2 stages: sexual indifferent stage and sexual different stage.

2.1 Development of Testes and Ovaries

The gonads originate from 3 different sources: the mesothelium on the genital ridge, the underlying mesenchyme, and the primordial germ cells.

2.1.1 Indifferent Stage

In week 5 of the human embryo, the mesothelium on the genital ridge proliferates to form many irregular cell cords, which are known as primary sex cords, extending into the mesenchyme. In week 4, many large round cells are derived from the endoderm near the root of allantois at the posterior wall of the yolk sac, which are called primordial germ cells (Figure 24 - 5, 24 - 6). In week 6, these cells successively migrate into the genital ridge through the dorsal mesentery. The migration will be completed within about 1 week, and the primordial germ cells enter the primary sex cords (Figure 24 - 5, 24 - 6). At this time, the gonads do not show sexual characteristics, hence are called indifferent gonads.

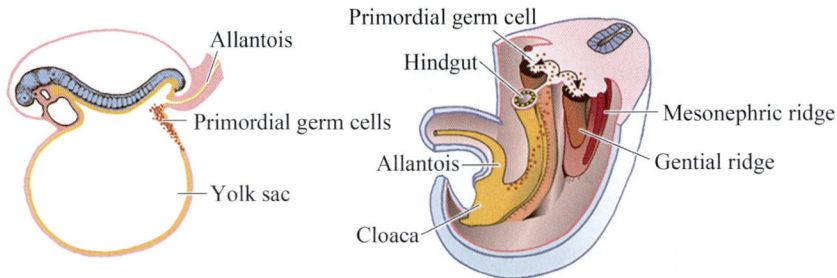

Figure 24 - 5   Drawings showing the migration of the primordial germ cells

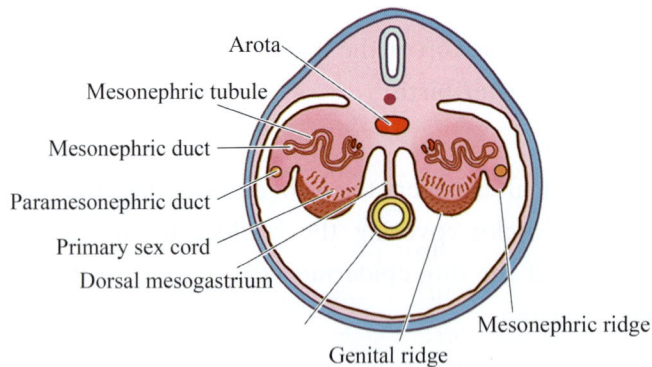

Figure 24 - 6   Drawing showing the development of indifferent gonads

2.1.2 Development of Testes

If the gender of the embryo is male, the primordial germ cells carry XY chromosomes. The sex determining region of the Y chromosome encodes a testis-determining factor, which determines the indifferent gonads to differentiate into testis. In a male embryo of 7 - 8 weeks, the primary sex cords separate from the surface mesothelium, keep proliferating toward the deep, and form many slender and curved testis cords that communicate with each other. The epithelium of the primary sex cords develops into Sertoli cells; the primordial germ cells differentiate into spermatogonia; the ends of testis cords communicate each other to form rete testis; the mesenchyme underlying the surface epithelium forms the tunica albuginea while that between testis cords differentiates into testicular interstitial cells (also called Leydig cells) (Figure 24 – 7). In adolescence, the testis cords develop into the seminiferous tubules.

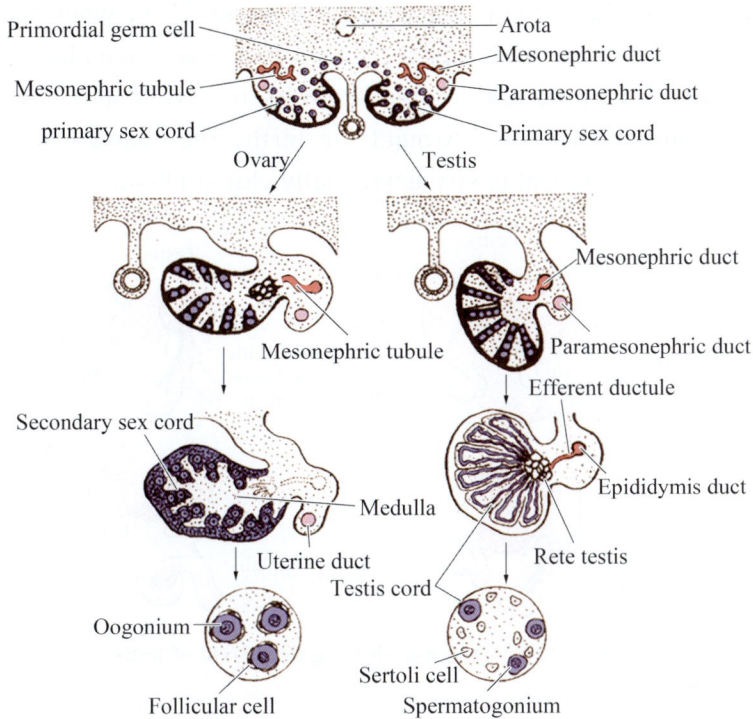

Figure 24 – 7   Drawings showing the development of the testis and ovary

2.1.3   Development of Ovaries

A female embryo carries XX chromosomes. Without a testis-determining factor, the indifferent gonads naturally differentiate into ovaries, which are formed later than testes. After week 10, the primary sex cords degenerate and are replaced by matrix and blood vessels, forming the ovarian medulla. Then, the surface mesothelium proliferates and extends into the mesenchyme again, forming the secondary sex cords (also called cortical cords). In week 16, the cortical cord breaks into many isolated cell clusters, forming the primordial follicles. In the center of the follicle there is an oogonium derived from the primordial germ cells, surrounded by a layer of small and flat follicular cells differentiated from the cortical cord cells. The mesenchyme underlying the surface epithelium forms tunica albuginea. In the embryonic stage, oogonia divide, proliferate, and differentiate into the primary oocytes (Figure 24 - 7). There are 700 - 2 000 thousand primordial follicles in the ovaries at birth.

2.1.4 Descent of Gonads

The gonads are initially located at the posterior abdominal wall. The gubernaculum connects the caudal end of the gonad and the labio-scrotal swelling. With the growth of the embryo, the gubernaculum is relatively shortened, resulting in the decline of gonads. In the third month, the testes continue to decline, and reach the inner opening of the inguinal canal, while the ovaries stay in the pelvic cavity. In month 7 - 8, when the testis descends through the inguinal canal, the peritoneum forms a processus vaginalis around the testis, entering the scrotum. The processus vaginalis covers the front and lateral sides of the testes, forming the tunica vaginalis. Around the birth, the channel between the tunica vaginalis cavity and the peritoneal cavity is gradually closed (Figure 24 - 8).

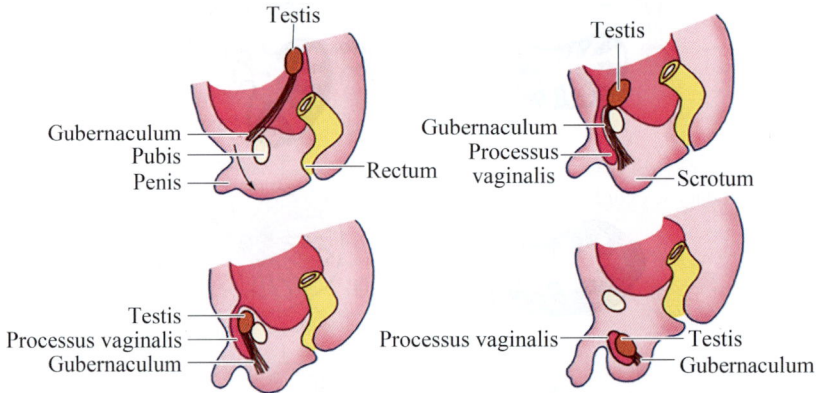

Figure 24 - 8 Drawings showing the descent of testis

2.2 Development of Genital Ducts

2.2.1 Indifferent Stage

In week 6, both male and female embryos have 2 sets of germ ducts, which are called mesonephric duct and paramesonephric duct (also known as Müller duct). The paramesonephric duct is formed by the invagination and convolution of the body cavity epithelium. Its upper segment is located outside and parallel the mesonephric duct; its middle segment bends inside, crosses the ventral surface of the mesonephric duct, and reaches the inside of the mesonephric duct; both of its lower segments combine in the midline; its upper end is a funnel-shaped opening in the abdominal cavity, its lower end is the blind end. It protrudes into the dorsal wall of the urogenital sinus and forms a bulge in the sinus cavity, which is called sinus tubercle (also known as Müller nodule). The mesonephric ducts open on both sides of the sinus tubercle (Figure 24 - 9).

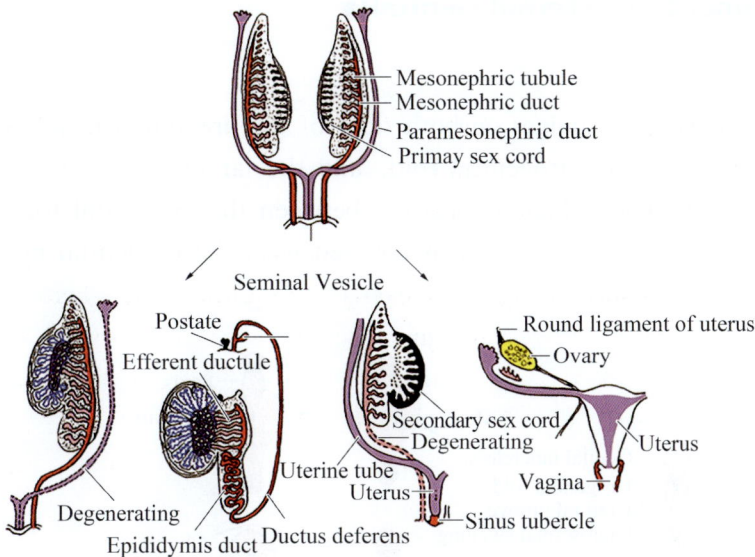

Figure 24 - 9   Drawing showing the development of the genital ducts

2.2.2   Development of Male Genital Ducts

Sertoli cells in testis secrete anti-paramesonephric duct hormone, which degenerates the paramesonephric ducts. Leydig cells secrete testosterone to induce the mesonephric duct to develop into the epididymal duct, vas deferens, seminal vesicle and ejaculatory duct (Figure 24 - 9).

2.2.3   Differentiation of Female Genital Ducts

Due to the lack of androgen, the mesonephric duct degenerates. Due to the lack of anti-Mullerian hormone, the paramesonephric duct continues to develop. Its upper and middle segments form oviducts; the upper opening forms the infundibulum of oviducts; the combined lower segments form the uterus. The sinus nodules continue to proliferate into a solid vaginal plate, in which the cells degenerate to form the vagina and the hymen (Figure 24 - 9, 24 - 10).

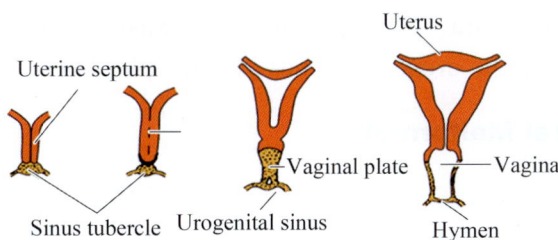

Figure 24 - 10   Drawings showing the development of the uterus and the vagina

2.3 Development of External Genitalia

2.3.1 Indifferent Stage

In week 5, there are 2 bulges on both sides of the urogenital membrane, the smaller one on the inner side is the urogenital fold, and the larger one on the outer side is the labioscrotal swelling. The volume depression between the urogenital folds is the urethral groove, and the bottom of the groove is covered with the urogenital membrane (Figure 24 - 11).

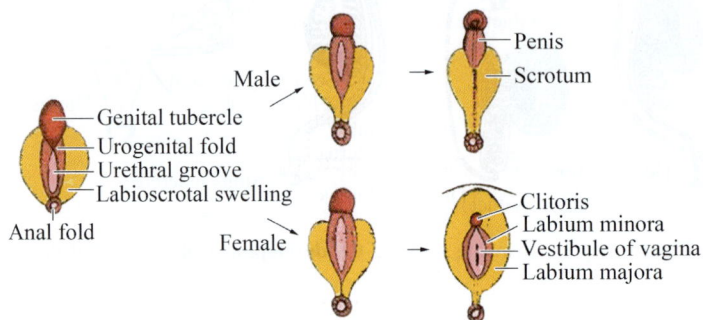

Figure 24 - 11   Drawings showing the development of external genitalia

2.3.2 Development of Male External Genitalia

Under the action of androgen, the genital tubercle elongates to form the penis; the urogenital folds on both sides merge together to form the corpus cavernosum of the urethra; both sides of the labio-scrotal swelling fuse at the midline to form the scrotum (Figure 24 - 11).

2.3.3 Development of Female External Genitalia

Due to the absence of androgen, the genital tubercle is slightly enlarged to form the clitoris. The urogenital folds on both sides are not combined to form labia minora. Both sides of the labio-scrotal swelling fuse in front of the clitoris to form the pubic caruncle, and the rear fuse to form the posterior commissure of the labia, while the most parts do not fuse to become the labia majora. The urethral sulcus expands and forms a vaginal vestibule with the lower segment of the urogenital sinus (Figure 24 - 11).

2.4 Main Congenital Malformations

2.4.1 Cryptorchidism

It is caused by the fact that the testis does not descend to the scrotum but stays in the abdominal cavity or groin. It is unilateral or bilateral. Because the temperature of the abdominal cavity is higher, bilateral cryptorchidism affects spermatogenesis, or even causes infertility.

2.4.2   Congenital Inguinal Hernia

It is more common in men. If the channel between the abdominal cavity and the sheath process is not closed, when the abdominal pressure increases, some intestinal loops can protrude into the sheath cavity.

2.4.3   Double Uterus

It is caused by the fact that both sides of the lower segment of the paramesonephric ducts do not fuse. It is often accompanied by the double vagina.

2.4.4   Vaginal Atresia

It is caused by the non-formation of the vaginal plate or no canal in the vaginal plate.

2.4.5   Hypospadias

It is due to the failure of the left and right urogenital folds to fuse, resulting in urethral openings on the ventral side of the penis.

2.4.6   Abnormal Sexual Differentiation

It leads to different degrees of gender deformity. The external genitalia of patients are often between men and women. According to different gonads, this malformation can be divided into 3 types: true hermaphroditism, male pseudohermaphroditism and female pseudohermaphroditism. The true hermaphroditism is very rare, in which the sex chromosome belongs to the chimeric type so that there are testis and ovary in the body at the same time. In male pseudohermaphroditism, there are testes in the body, but due to insufficient androgen secretion, the external genitalia look like a female. In the female pseudohermaphroditism, there are ovaries in the body, but the external genitalia look like a man due to the excessive androgen secretion.

2.4.7   Androgen Insensitivity Syndrome

Also known as testicular feminization syndrome. The patient has testis with the normal function for secreting androgen. However, due to the lack of androgen receptors, the reproductive duct and external genitalia fail to differentiate into the male. The anti-paramesonephric duct hormone produced by Sertoli cells inhibits the development of paramesonephric duct, so the oviducts and uterus fail to develop. The patient has female external genitalia and female secondary sexual characteristics.

(Yue Haiyuan)

第二十四章　泌尿系统和生殖系统的发生

泌尿系统和生殖系统的主要器官起源于间介中胚层。人胚第 4 周初,间介中胚层头端呈节段性生长,称生肾节,尾端呈纵行条索状生长,称生肾索。第 4 周末,生肾索与体节分离,体积不断增大,从胚体后壁突向体腔,在背主动脉两侧形成左右对称的一对纵行隆起,称尿生殖嵴。尿生殖嵴进一步发育,中部出现一条纵沟,将其分成内、外两部分。外侧部分较长而粗,为中肾嵴;内侧部分较短而细,为生殖腺嵴(图 24-1)。

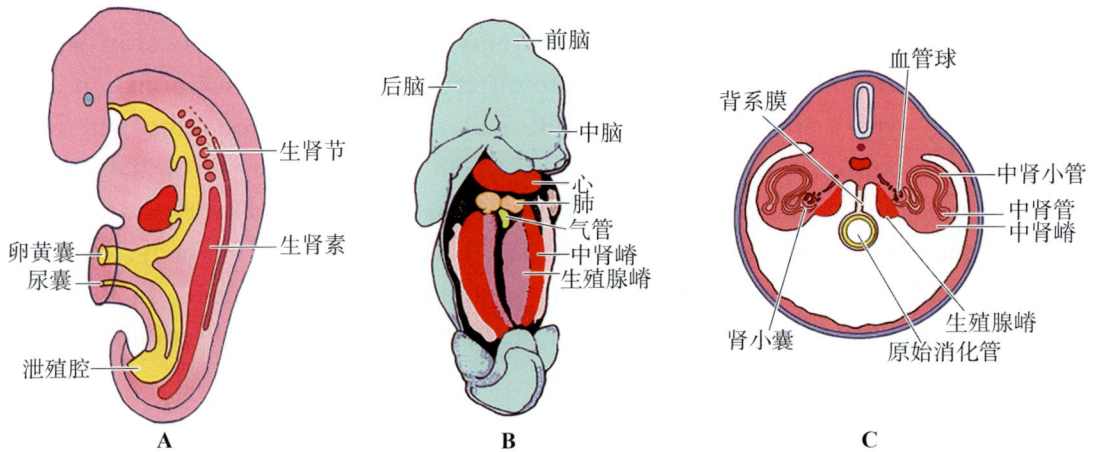

图 24-1　中肾嵴和生殖腺嵴的发生示意图
A.第 4 周末人胚内部侧面观;B.第 4 周末人胚内部腹面观;C.第 5 周人胚横断面

第一节　泌尿系统的发生

一、肾和输尿管的发生

人胚肾的发生可分为 3 个阶段,即从胚体颈部向腰骶部相继出现的前肾、中肾和后肾。

(一) 前肾

发生最早,人胚第 4 周初,位于颈部第 7～14 体节的外侧,生肾索的头端部分形成数条横行细胞索,称前肾小管,其内侧端开口于胚内体腔,外侧端均向尾部延伸,并互相连接成一条纵行的前肾管。前肾在人类无功能意义,于第 4 周末即退化,但前肾管的大部分保留,向尾部继续延伸,成为中肾管。

(二) 中肾

发生于第 4 周末。继前肾退化之后,在生肾索和中肾嵴内,相继产生许多横行小管,称中肾小管。两侧中肾小管共约 80 对,每个体节相应位置有 2~3 条。中肾小管呈"S"形弯曲,其内侧端膨大并凹陷成肾小囊,内有从背主动脉分支而来的毛细血管球,两者共同组成肾小体。中肾小管外侧端与向尾部延伸的前肾管相吻合,于是前肾管改称为中肾管,中肾管尾端通入泄殖腔(图 24-2)。在人类,中肾可能有短暂的功能活动,直至后肾形成。至第 2 个月末,中肾大部分退化,仅留下中肾管及尾端小部分中肾小管。

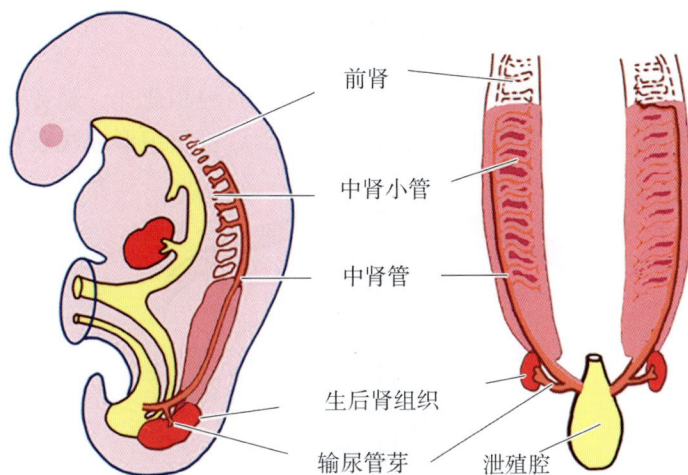

图 24-2　前肾、中肾和后肾的发生示意图

(三) 后肾

发育为成体的永久肾。人胚第 5 周初,当中肾仍在发育中,后肾即开始形成。第 11~12 周,后肾开始产生尿液,其功能持续于整个胎儿期。尿液排入羊膜腔,组成羊水的主要成分。由于胚胎的代谢产物主要由胎盘排泄,故胎儿期肾的排泄功能极微。后肾起源于生后肾组织和输尿管芽两个不同的部分,但均源于中胚层。

1. 输尿管芽

输尿管芽是中肾管末端近泄殖腔处向背外侧长出的一个盲管。它向胚体背、外侧方向延伸,长入中肾嵴尾端的中胚层组织中。输尿管芽反复分支达 12 级以上,逐渐演变为输尿管、肾盂、肾盏和集合管。输尿管芽的起始两级分支扩大合并为肾盂,第 3~4 级分支扩大为肾盏,其余的分支为集合管。集合管的末端呈"T"形分支,它的弓形盲端诱导邻近的生后肾组织分化为肾单位(图 24-3、图 24-4)。

2. 生后肾组织

生后肾组织是中肾嵴尾端的中胚层组织受输尿管芽的诱导而产生的。中肾嵴的细胞密集并呈帽状包围在输尿管芽的末端,形成生后肾组织。生后肾组织的外周部分演变为肾的被膜,内侧部分形成多个细胞团,附着于弓形集合管末端两侧。这些上皮细胞团逐渐分化成"S"形弯曲的肾小管,一端与弓形集合管的盲端相连,另一端膨大凹陷形成肾小囊,并与伸入囊内的毛细血管球组成肾小体。这些小管的其他部分逐渐增长,分化成肾小管各段,与肾小体共同组成

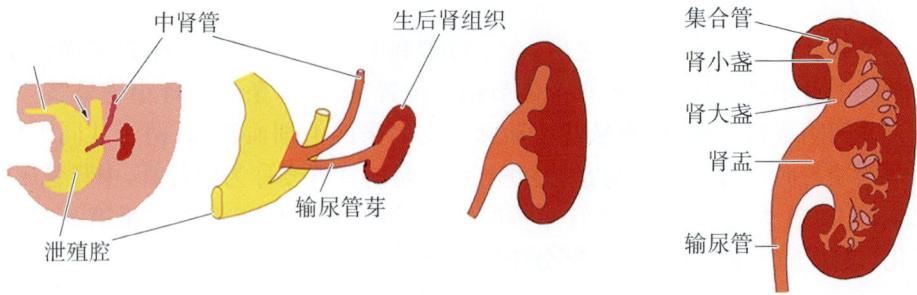

图 24-3　后肾的发生示意图

肾单位。每个远曲小管与一个弓形集合管相连接,继而内腔相通连。髓旁肾单位发生较早,随着集合管末端不断向皮质浅层生长并分支,陆续诱导生后肾组织形成浅表肾单位(图 24-4)。

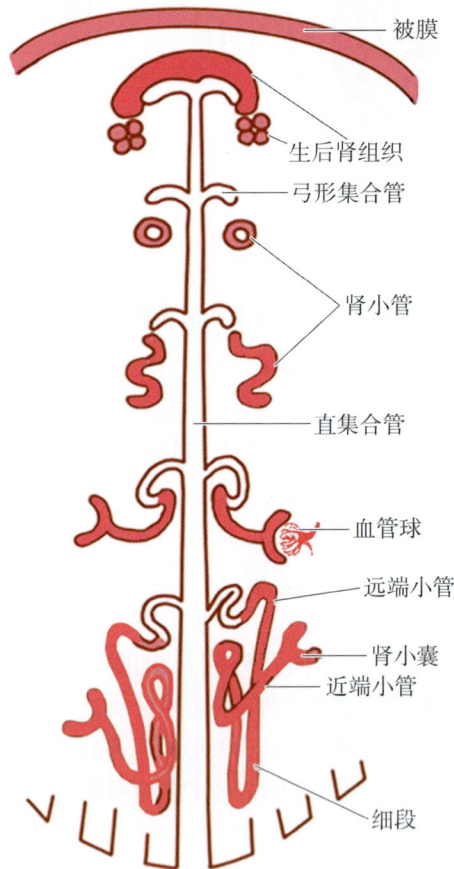

图 24-4　集合管与肾单位的发生示意图

人胚第 12 周左右,后肾开始产生尿液,构成羊水的主要来源。由于后肾发生于中肾嵴尾侧,故肾的原始位置较低。随着胚胎腹部生长、输尿管伸展和胚体的直立,肾逐渐上升至腰部,同时也沿胚体中轴旋转,使肾门从腹侧转向内侧。

二、膀胱和尿道的发生

在人胚第 4～7 周时，尿直肠隔将泄殖腔分隔为背侧的原始直肠和腹侧的尿生殖窦两个部分。尿生殖窦又分为三段：①上段较大，发育为膀胱，它的顶端与尿囊相接，在胎儿出生前从脐到膀胱顶的尿囊退化成纤维索，称脐中韧带。左、右中肾管分别开口于膀胱。随着膀胱的扩大，输尿管起始部以下的一段中肾管也扩大并渐并入膀胱，成为其背壁的一部分，于是输尿管与中肾管即分别开口于膀胱。②尿生殖窦的中段颇为狭窄，保持管状，在女性形成尿道大部分，在男性成为尿道的前列腺部和膜部。由于肾向头侧迁移及中肾管继续向下生长等因素的影响，使输尿管开口移向外上方，而中肾管的开口在男性下移至尿道前列腺部；在女性，其通入尿道的部位将退化。③下段在男性形成尿道海绵体部，女性则扩大成阴道前庭。

三、常见先天畸形

1. 多囊肾
由于集合管与远端小管未接通，使肾小管内尿液积聚，肾内出现许多大小不等的囊泡，致使正常肾组织受压而萎缩，造成肾功能障碍。

2. 异位肾
肾在上升过程中受阻，出生后肾未达到正常位置，常见位于盆腔内。

3. 马蹄肾
由于两肾的下端异常融合而形成一个马蹄形的大肾，其成因为肾上升时被肠系膜下动脉根部所阻而致。

4. 双输尿管
由于输尿管芽过早分支所致。按其分支的程度不同，可诱导出各种畸形，如分支不完全形成肾输尿管分支及分隔肾，若分支完全则成为双输尿管。

5. 脐尿瘘
由于膀胱顶端与脐之间的脐尿管未闭锁，出生后尿液可从脐部漏出。

6. 膀胱外翻
在尿生殖窦与表面外胚层之间没有间充质长入，因此在前腹壁无肌肉覆盖膀胱，致使薄的表皮和膀胱前壁破裂，膀胱黏膜外翻。

第二节　生殖系统的发生

一、睾丸和卵巢的发生

胚胎的遗传性别虽决定于受精时与卵子结合的精子核型，但直到胚胎第 7 周，生殖腺才开始有性别的形态学特征。在胚胎早期，男性和女性的生殖系统是相似的，称为生殖器官未分化期。胚胎的外生殖器则要到第 12 周才能辨认性别，因此，生殖系统（包括生殖腺、生殖管道及外生殖器）在发生中均可分为性未分化阶段和性分化阶段。

生殖腺来自体腔上皮、上皮深部的间充质及原始生殖细胞三个不同的部分。

(一) 未分化性腺的发生

人胚第 5 周时,左、右中肾嵴内侧的表面上皮下方间充质细胞增殖,形成一对纵行的生殖腺嵴。不久,生殖腺嵴的表面上皮向其下方的间充质生出许多不规则的细胞索,称初级性索。胚胎第 4 周时,位于卵黄囊后壁近尿囊处有许多源于内胚层的大的圆形细胞,称原始生殖细胞。它们于第 6 周经背侧肠系膜陆续向生殖腺嵴迁移,约在 1 周内迁移完成,原始生殖细胞进入初级性索内(图 24 - 5、图 24 - 6)。

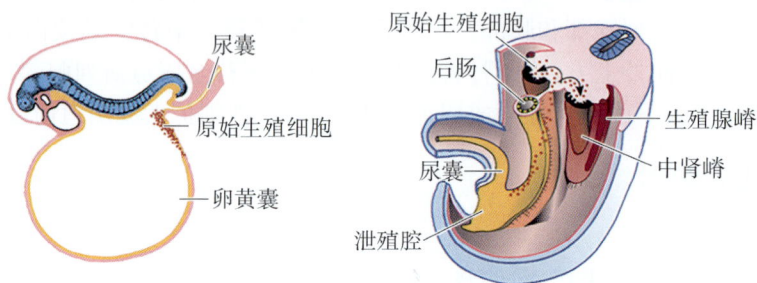

图 24 - 5 原始生殖细胞迁移示意图

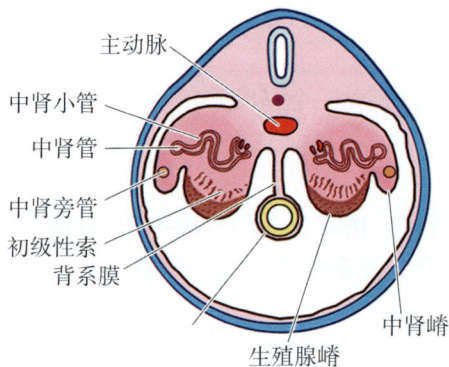

图 24 - 6 未分化性腺的发生示意图

(二) 睾丸的发生

若胚胎的性别为男性,其原始生殖细胞携带 XY 染色体,其中 Y 染色体上的性别决定区编码睾丸决定因子,使未分化性腺分化为睾丸。在人胚 7～8 周,初级性索与表面上皮分离,继续向深部增生,形成许多相互吻合的细长弯曲的睾丸索。初级性索上皮细胞发育成支持细胞,原始生殖细胞分化为精原细胞,睾丸索末端吻合成睾丸网,表面上皮深层的间充质形成白膜,睾丸索间的间充质分化为睾丸间质细胞(图 24 - 7)。在青春期,睾丸索演化为生精小管。

(三) 卵巢的发生

女性胚胎携带 XX 染色体,没有睾丸决定因子,未分化性腺自然分化为卵巢。卵巢的形成比睾丸晚。人胚第 10 周后,初级性索退化,被基质和血管取代,形成卵巢髓质。然后,表面上皮增生并再次延伸到间充质,形成次级性索(皮质索)。第 16 周,皮质索断裂成许多孤立的细胞团,形成原始卵泡。在卵泡的中心有一个由原始生殖细胞分化而来的卵原细胞,周围有一

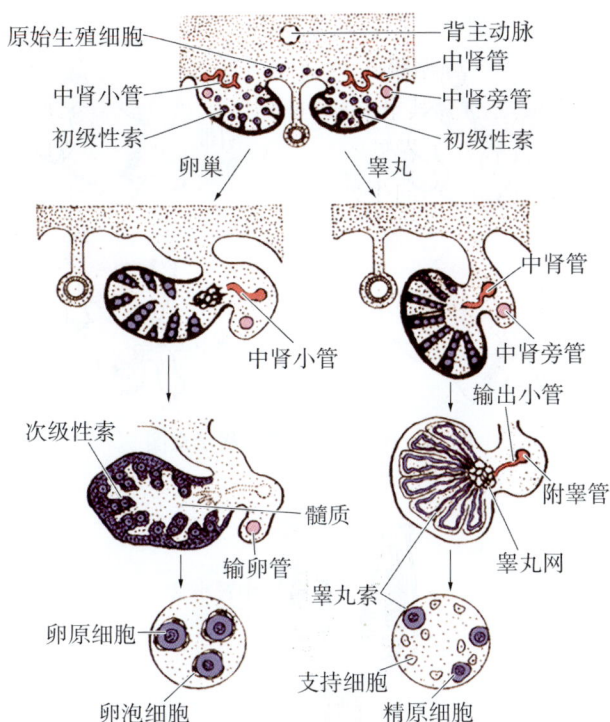

图 24-7 睾丸与卵巢的发生示意图

层由皮质索细胞分化而来的小而扁平的卵泡细胞。表面上皮深层的间充质形成白膜。在胚胎期,卵原细胞分裂、增殖并分化为初级卵母细胞(图 24-7)。出生时卵巢中有 70～200 万个初级卵泡。

(四)睾丸和卵巢的下降

生殖腺最初位于后腹壁,在其尾侧有一条由中胚层形成的索状结构,称引带,它的末端与阴唇阴囊隆起相连。随着胚体长大,引带相对缩短,导致生殖腺的下降。第 3 个月时,生殖腺已位于盆腔,卵巢即停留在骨盆缘下方,睾丸则继续下降,于第 7～8 个月时抵达阴囊。当睾丸下降通过腹股沟管时,腹膜形成鞘突包于睾丸的周围,随同睾丸进入阴囊,覆盖在睾丸的前面和侧面,成为鞘膜。然后,鞘膜腔与腹膜腔之间的通道逐渐封闭(图 24-8)。

二、生殖管道的发生与演化

(一)未分化期

人胚第 6 周时,男女两性胚胎都具有两套生殖管,即中肾管和中肾旁管(米勒管)。中肾旁管由体腔上皮内陷卷褶而成,上段位于中肾管的外侧,两者相互平行;中段弯向内侧,越过中肾管的腹面,到达中肾管的内侧;下段的左、右中肾旁管在中线合并。中肾旁管上端呈漏斗形开口于腹腔,下端是盲端,突入尿生殖窦的背侧壁,在窦腔内形成一隆起,称窦结节。中肾管开口于窦结节的两侧(图 24-9)。

(二)男性生殖管道的分化

在男性,由于 Y 染色体的存在,性腺分化为睾丸时,在人绒毛膜促性腺激素刺激下,睾丸

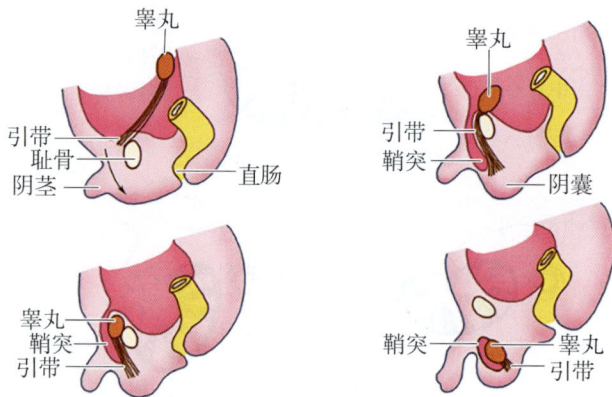

图 24-8　睾丸下降过程示意图

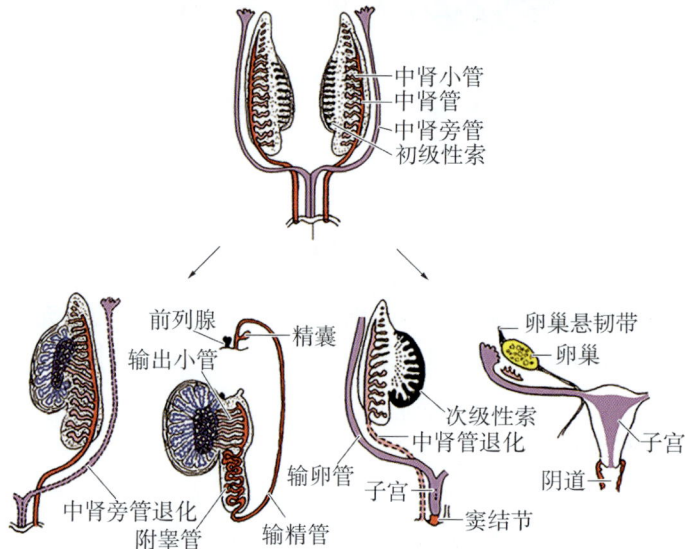

图 24-9　生殖管道的演变示意图

内间质细胞产生的雄激素刺激中肾管继续发育为附睾管、输精管、精囊和射精管；同时，睾丸内的支持细胞分泌抗中肾旁管激素抑制中肾旁管的发育，使其逐渐退化吸收，从而使生殖管道向男性分化(图 24-9)。

（三）女性生殖管道的分化

由于缺乏雄激素，中肾管退化。同时由于缺乏抗中肾旁管激素，中肾旁管继续发育。中肾旁管的上中段形成输卵管，上口形成输卵管漏斗部，合并的下段形成子宫。窦结节继续增殖成阴道板，然后阴道板中的细胞退化，阴道和处女膜形成(图 24-9、图 24-10)。

三、外生殖器的发生

（一）未分化期

第 5 周初，尿生殖膜的头侧形成一隆起，称生殖结节。尿生殖膜的两侧各有两条隆起，内

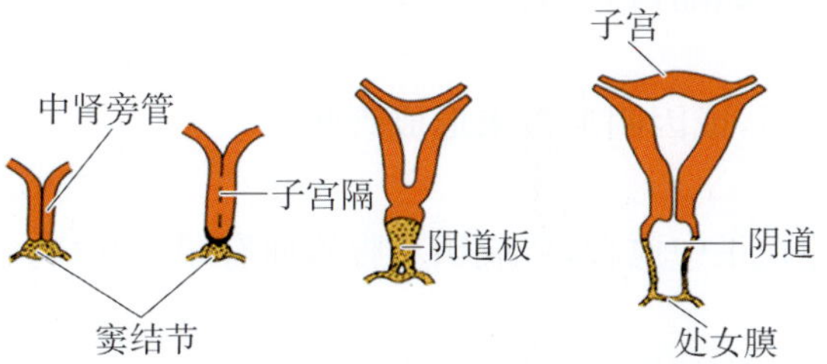

图 24 - 10　子宫与阴道的发生示意图

侧的较小，为尿生殖褶，外侧的较大，为阴唇阴囊隆起。尿生殖褶之间的凹陷为尿道沟，沟底覆有尿生殖膜。第 9 周时，尿生殖膜破裂（图 24 - 11）。

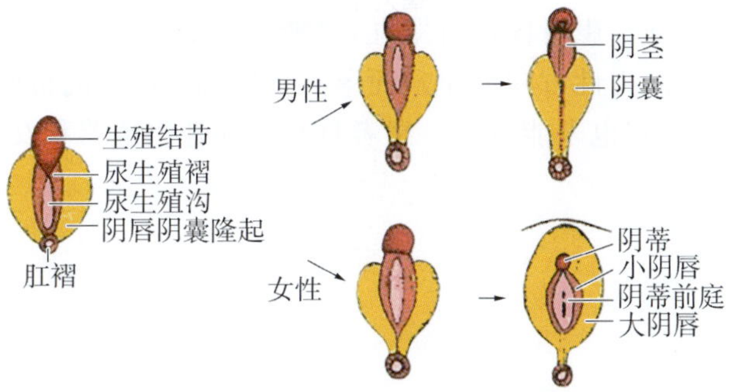

图 24 - 11　外生殖器的演变示意图

（二）男性外生殖器的发生

在雄激素的作用下，生殖结节伸长形成阴茎；两侧的尿生殖褶合并形成尿道海绵体部；左右阴唇阴囊隆起在中线处愈合成阴囊（图 24 - 11）。

（三）女性外生殖器的发生

女性因无雄激素的作用，外生殖器自然向女性分化。生殖结节略增大，形成阴蒂。两侧的尿生殖褶不合并，形成小阴唇。左右阴唇阴囊隆起发育成大阴唇，并在阴蒂前方愈合，形成阴阜；后方愈合形成阴唇后连合。尿道沟扩展，并与尿生殖窦下段共同形成阴道前庭（图 24 - 11）。

四、主要先天畸形

1. 隐睾

睾丸未下降至阴囊而停留在腹腔或腹股沟等处，称隐睾，可单侧或双侧。因腹腔温度高，隐睾会影响精子发生，双侧隐睾可造成不育。

2. 先天性腹股沟疝

多见于男性。因腹腔与鞘膜腔之间的通道没有闭合，当腹压增大时，部分肠管可突入鞘膜腔。

3. 双子宫

左右中肾旁管的下段未愈合所致。较常见的是中肾旁管下段的上半部未完全愈合，形成双角子宫。若同时伴有阴道纵隔,则为双子宫双阴道。

4. 阴道闭锁

因窦结节未形成阴道板,或因阴道板未形成管腔。

5. 尿道下裂

因左右尿生殖褶未能在正中愈合,造成阴茎腹侧面有尿道开口。

6. 两性畸形

性分化异常导致不同程度的性别畸形,患者的外生殖器常介于男女之间。根据生殖腺不同,此畸形分为三种:①真两性畸形,极为罕见,性染色体属嵌合型,体内同时有睾丸及卵巢。②男性假两性畸形,体内有睾丸,但由于雄激素分泌不足所致,外生殖器似女性;③女性假两性畸形,体内有卵巢,但由于雄激素分泌过多,外生殖器似男性。

7. 雄激素不敏感综合征

又称睾丸女性化综合征。患者体内有睾丸,也能分泌雄激素,但因细胞缺乏雄激素受体,生殖管道和外生殖器未能向男性方向分化。而睾丸支持细胞产生的抗中肾旁管激素抑制中肾旁管的发育,故输卵管与子宫也未能发育。患者具有女性外生殖器和女性第二性征。

(岳海源)

Chapter 25

Development of the Cardiovascular System

The cardiovascular system is the first major system to function in the embryo, which is derived mainly from mesoderm. Because of the rapid growth of human embryo, the cardiovascular system functions and the blood circulation starts in the end of the third week of embryonic development to acquire oxygen and nutrients and dispose waste products.

1 Establishment of Primordial Cardiovascular System

The primordial cardiovascular system is symmetrical on the left and right and composed of the cardiac tube, primordial arterial system and primordial venous system.

1.1 Extraembryonic Angiogenesis

In a human embryo of 3 weeks, the cells in the extraembryonic mesoderm of the yolk sac wall, somatic pedicle and chorion are successively concentrated into cords or clusters, which are called blood islands. Then gaps appear between the blood island cells. The surrounding cells of the blood island differentiate into the flat endothelial cells, and the central cells differentiate into free hematopoietic stem cells. The endothelial tube sprouts and extends outward, fusing with the endothelial tubes formed by the adjacent blood islands. An extraembryonic capillary network is gradually formed (Figure 25 – 1).

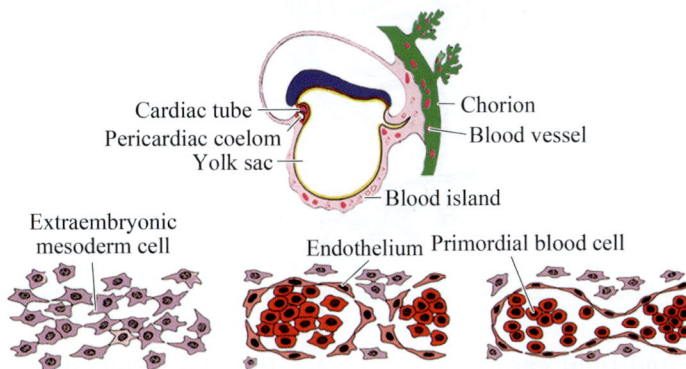

Figure 25 – 1　Drawings showing the formation of the blood islands and primitive blood vessels

1.2   Angiogenesis in Embryo

At day 18 – 20, there are gaps in the mesenchyme, and the surrounding cells differentiate into endothelial cells, forming intraembryonic capillaries. The adjacent vascular endothelium was connected by budding to form a primitive capillary network in the embryo. Then, the capillary network inside and outside the embryo is connected through the pedicle, and hematopoietic stem cells enter into the embryo, forming the early primitive vascular pathway.

At this time, the structure of blood vessels cannot be distinguished between arteries and veins, so they can only be named according to their attribution and the relationship with the heart. Lately, the mesenchymal cells around the vascular endothelium differentiate into smooth muscle fibers and connective tissue, forming tunica media and tunica adventitia of arteries and veins.

1.3   Early Blood Circulation of Embryo

At the end of the third week, a pair of cardiac tubes, a pair of abdominal aorta, a pair of dorsal aorta and the first pair of pharyngeal arch arteries connecting the ipsilateral abdominal aorta and dorsal aorta are formed. The dorsal aorta will be divided into several pairs of vitelline arteries in the wall of the yolk sac and a pair of umbilical arteries in the chorion through the pedicle. The yolk sac capillaries converge into a pair of vitelline veins, and the chorionic capillaries converge into an umbilical vein. The vitelline vein and umbilical vein transport blood back to the venous end of the cardiac tube, thus forming yolk sac circulation and umbilical circulation, respectively (Figure 25 – 2).

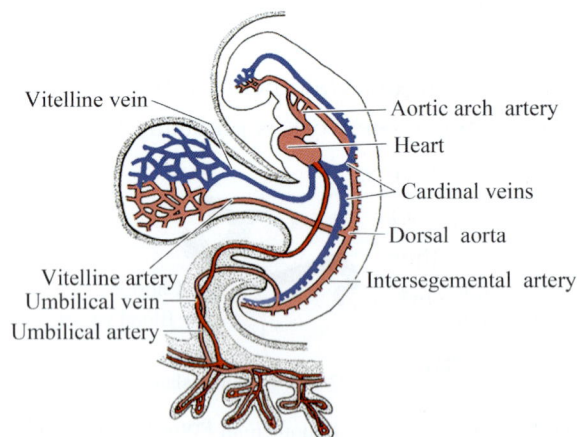

Figure 25 – 2   Drawing of the primitive cardiovascular system

When the left and right cardiac tubes merge, the two abdominal aortas fuse into the aortic sac, and the two dorsal aortas merge. The branches of the aortas transport blood along the way to each part of the embryonic body. At this time, a pair of anterior cardinal veins are formed at the front of the embryo body, and a pair of posterior cardinal veins are formed at the back of the embryo body, which confluence to the left and right common cardinal veins, respectively, and then connect to the venous end of the cardiac tube to form embryo body circulation.

2 Establishing of Heart

The mesoderm cells converge between the oropharyngeal membrane and the primordial diaphragm to form the cardiogenic area where the heart appears.

2.1 Development of Cardiac Tube

At day 19 – 19, there is a cavity in the cardiogenic area called pericardial coelom. The mesoderm cells on the ventral side of the pericardial coelom converge to form a pair of endothelial strands, and then the strands canalize to form two thin cardiac tubes. As the head fold occurs, both the pericardial coelom and cardiac tubes turn 180°. The pericardial coelom comes to lie ventral side while the cardiac tubes lie dorsal to the pericardial coelom (Figure 25 – 3). As the lateral fold occurs, the two tubes approach each other and fuse to form a single cardiac tube at day 22 or 23 (Figure 25 – 4).

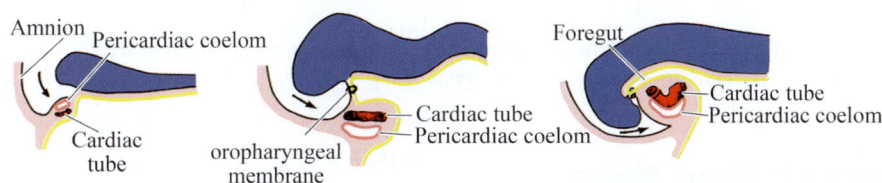

Figure 25 – 3 Drawings showing the position changes of the early heart in longitudinal section

As the heart elongates and bends, it gradually invaginates into the pericardial coelom. The heart is initially suspended from the dorsal wall by a mesentery, the dorsal mesocardium, but the central part of this mesentery soon degenerates, forming a communication, the transverse pericardial sinus, between the right and left sides of the pericardial coelom. The heart is then attached only at its cranial and caudal ends. Then pericardial coelom develops into pericardial cavity.

2.2 Formation of Heart Wall

When the cardiac tubes fuse, the endothelial tube becomes the internal endothelium. The myocardium and epicardium are derived from the myoepicardial mantle developed by the splanchnic mesoderm surrounding the cardiac tubes. The gelatinous connective tissue, known as cardiac jelly, lies between the endothelial tube and myocardium, developing into the connective tissue in the endocardium (Figure 25 – 4).

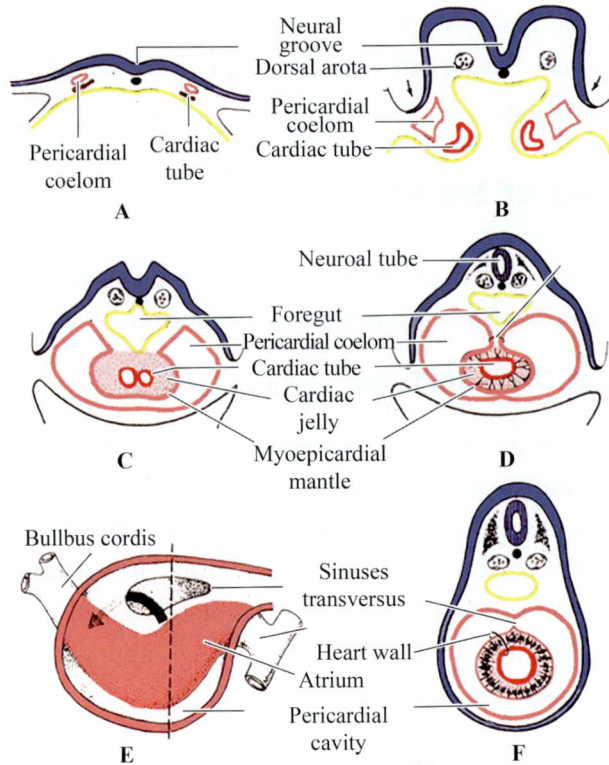

Figure 25 - 4 Drawings showing the early development of the heart
A. Day 19; B. Day 20; C. Day 21; D. Day 22; E. Day 28 in lateral view; F. Day 28

2.3 Changes in Heart Shape

The cardiac tube elongates and develops alternate dilations and constrictions: the bulbus cordis, ventricle, atrium, and sinus venosus (Figure 25 - 5). The distal part of the bulbus cordis is thinner and continuous cranially with the aortic sac, from which the arch arteries arise. The end of the sinus venosus is divided into left and right horns to receive the left and right umbilical, vitelline, and common cardinal veins from the chorion, umbilical vesicle, and embryo, respectively. The arterial and venous ends of the heart are fixed by the pharyngeal arches and diaphragm, respectively. The tubular heart undergoes a dextral (i. e., right-handed) loop approximately from day 23 to day 28, forming a U-shaped loop that results in a heart with the apex pointing to the left (Figure 25 - 5).

Subsequently, the atrium gradually moves away from the diaphragm and moves to the dorsal end of the ventricular head, slightly to the left. The sinus venosus also dissociates from the diaphragm and is located on the posterior and caudal sides of the atrium. At this point, the shape of the heart is in an S shape. The atrium is limited by the anterior cardiac bulb and the posterior esophagus, thus expanding to the left and right, resulting in swelling on both sides of the arterial trunk. The atrium expands and the atrioventricular sulcus

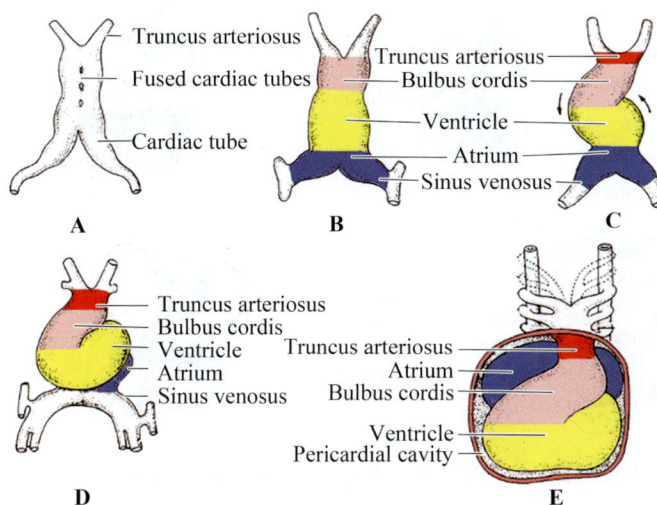

Figure 25 – 5   Drawings showing the establishment of the appearance of heart
A. Day 21; B. Day 22; C. Day 23; D. Day 24; E. Day 25

deepens, so that a narrow atrioventricular canal is formed. The proximal segment of the bulbus cordis is absorbed by the ventricle, becoming the right ventricle. The ventricle became the left ventricle. The interventricular sulcus appears on the surface between the left and right ventricles. At this point, the heart has taken on the shape of an adult one, but its interior has not yet been completely separated (Figure 25 – 5).

2.4   Partitioning of Heart

The shape of the heart is initially established at the beginning of the 5th week, but the internal separation of the heart is not complete at this time. The separation of all parts of the heart is carried out at the same time and completed at the end of the 7th week.

2.4.1   Partitioning of Atrioventricular Canal

At the 4th week, the endocardium of the dorsal and ventral sides of the atrioventricular canal proliferates to form the atrioventricular endocardial cushion. The atrioventricular canal will be divided into the left and right atrioventricular canals (Figure 25 – 6). The mesenchyme around the atrioventricular foramen proliferates and protrudes into the cavity to form an atrioventricular valve.

2.4.2   Partitioning of Primitive Atrium

When the endocardial cushions are forming, the septum primum, a thin crescent-shaped membrane, grows toward the fusing endocardial cushions from the roof of the primordial atrium. As this septum grows, a large opening, the foramen primum, is located between its crescentic free edge and the endocardial cushions. Before the foramen primum disappears, perforations appear in the central part of the septum primum, forming another opening in the septum primum, the foramen secundum. Concurrently, the free edge of the

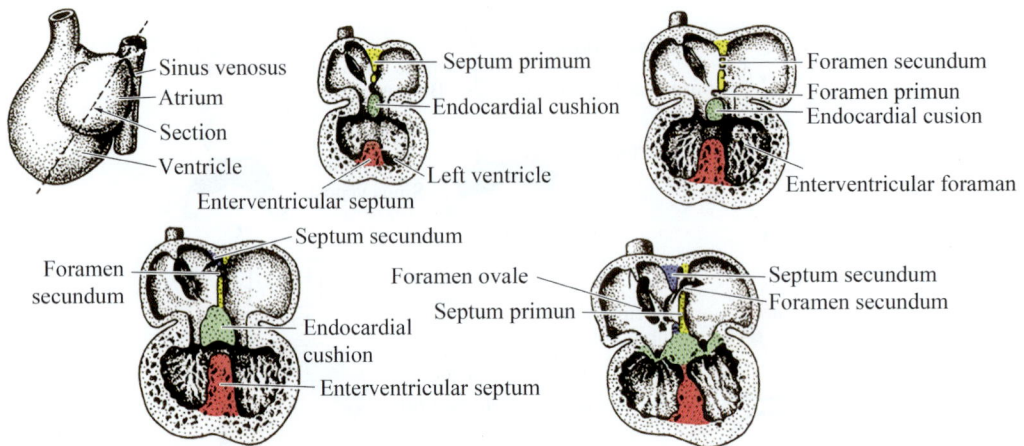

Figure 25 – 6 Drawings showing the partitioning of the heart

septum primum fuses with the left side of the fused endocardial cushions, obliterating the foramen primum. The septum secundum, a thick crescentic muscular fold, grows from the ventrocranial wall of the right atrium, immediately adjacent to the septum primum in the 5th week. It gradually overlaps the foramen secundum in the septum primum. The septum secundum forms an incomplete partition between the atria. Consequently, an oval foramen named foramen ovale forms. The cranial part of the septum primum, initially attached to the roof of the left atrium, gradually disappears. The remaining part of the septum primum, attached to the fused endocardial cushions, forms the flap-like valve of the foramen ovale. Before birth, the foramen ovale allows most of the oxygenated blood entering the right atrium to pass into the left atrium. This foramen prevents the passage of blood in the opposite direction because the septum primum closes against the relatively rigid septum secundum. After birth, the foramen ovale will be closed functionally because of the higher pressure in the left atrium. The valve of the foramen ovale fuses with the septum secundum, forming the fossa ovalis. So far, the atriums have been completely separated (Figure 25 – 6).

2.4.3 Partitioning of Primitive Ventricle

Division of the primordial ventricle is first indicated by a median ridge, the muscular interventricular septum. Until the 7th week, there is a crescent-shaped foramen between the free edge of the septum and the fused endocardial cushions, which permits communication between the right and left ventricles. The interventricular foramen usually closes by the end of the 7th week as the bulbar ridges fuse with the endocardial cushion. Closure of the interventricular foramen and formation of the membranous interventricular septum result from the fusion of tissues from 3 sources: the right bulbar ridge, the left bulbar ridge and the endocardial cushion. So far, the ventricles have been completely separated (Figure 25 – 6, Figure 25 – 7).

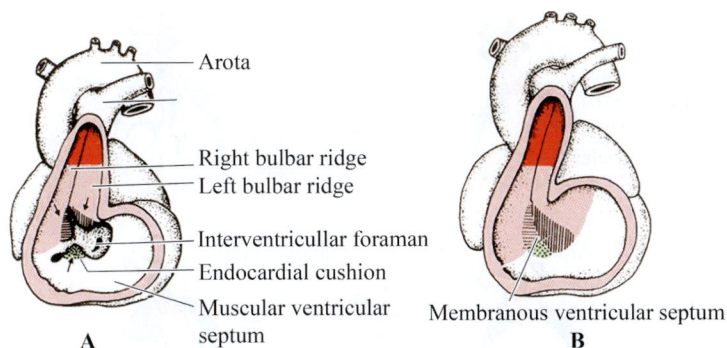

Figure 25 - 7 Drawings showing the formation of the interventricular septum
A. Week 5; B. Week 7

2.4.4 Changes of Sinus Venosus and Formation of Right and Left Atrium

The opening of the sinus venosus into the single primordial atrium, is initially located in the posterior wall of the primordial atrium. Its right and left horns are similar in size, which connect to the ipsilateral common cardinal vein, umbilical vein, and vitelline vein, respectively. As the right horn receives most of the blood, it enlarges, and the sinoatrial orifice moves to the right. The left horn is gradually shrinking, and its proximal part becomes the coronary sinus while the distal part becomes the root of the oblique vein of Marshall. At 7 - 8th week, the primordial atrium expands rapidly, and the right horn of the venous sinus is gradually absorbed into the right atrium, forming an adult right atrium proper. The primitive right atrium becomes the right auricle.

Meanwhile, due to the enlargement of the left atrium, the root and branches of the pulmonary veins gradually merge into the left atrium, so that 4 pulmonary veins open directly into the left atrium. The pulmonary veins and its left and right branches participate in the formation of the left atrial proper, and the primitive atrium becomes the left auricle.

2.4.5 Partitioning of Truncus Arteriosus and Bulbus Cordis

The truncus arteriosus is divided into 2 channels in a similar manner with that in the endocardial cushions. At the 5th week, the endocardial tissue of the truncus arteriosus and bulbus cordis is locally proliferated, forming a pair of bulbar ridges and a pair of truncus ridges. The ridges grow in the opposite direction, and merge in the middle line to form a spiral septum called aortico-pulmonary septum, which divides the truncus arteriosus and bulbus cordis into the aorta and pulmonary artery. The endocardial tissue in the beginning of the aorta and pulmonary artery proliferates into the lumen, forming three thin bulges, and gradually evolves into semilunar valves. After closure of the interventricular foramen, the pulmonary artery communicates with the right ventricle, and the aorta connects with the left ventricular (Figure 25 - 8).

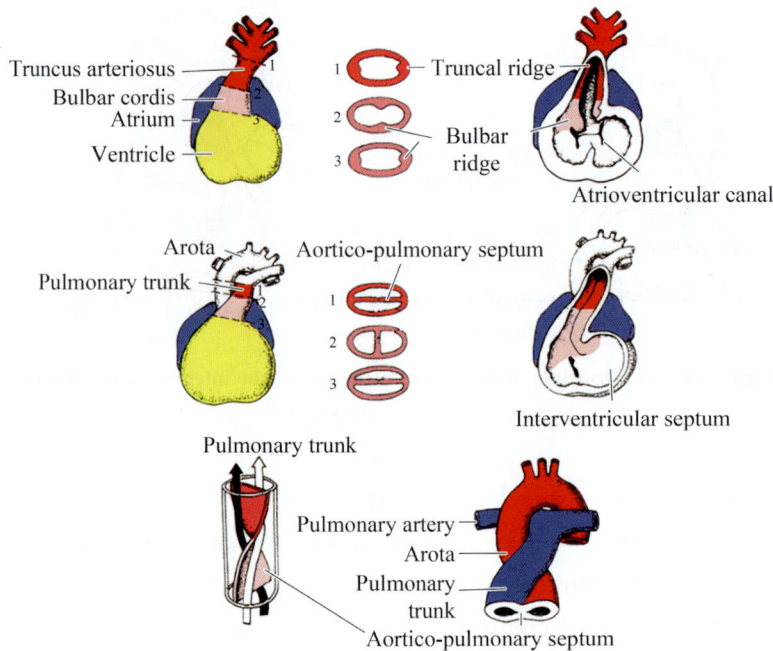

Figure 25 - 8 Drawing showing the partitioning of the truncus arteriosus and the bulbus cordis

3 Derivatives of Main Blood Vessels

The arcuate artery starts from the aortic sac, and there are 6 teams running in each pair of parotid arches from week 4 to week 6, connecting with the ipsilateral dorsal aorta. During week 6 - 8, the derivatives of the arcuate artery are as follows. The 1st and 2nd pair degenerate and disappear, but a segment of the dorsal aorta connected with them remains. The 3rd pair branches to form the left and right external carotid arteries. The proximal end and part of the aortic sac develop into the common carotid artery, and the distal segment and connected dorsal aorta form the internal carotid artery. The left 4th arch artery and the artery sac form the aortic arch. The right half of the arterial sac forms the brachiocephalic trunk. The left subclavian artery is formed by the 7th internode artery from the left dorsal aorta. The right subclavian artery is formed by the right 4th arch artery, the caudal dorsal aorta and the 7th internode artery. The dorsal aorta between the 3rd and 4th arch arteries atrophies and disappears. The 5th pair are of hypoplasia and then rapid degenerate. The proximal ends of the 6th pair form the base of the pulmonary artery, the left distal segment forms the ductus arteriosus, while the right distal ends degenerate. With the division of the arterial trunk, the pulmonary artery is connected with the pulmonary trunk.

The left and right vitelline veins, together with the vitelline pedicle, enter the embryo body and venous sinus through the original diaphragm. There are many anastomotic branches between the yolk sac and the original diaphragm. Following the formation of the liver, the original vitelline vein will be divided into 3 segments: a segment connected with the liver that will enter into to form the hepatic sinusoid; at the proximal end of the liver, the left branch disappears, and the right branch forms the proximal segment of the hepatic vein and inferior vena cava; at the distal end of the liver, an S-shaped blood vessel develops into the portal vein.

The branches of the umbilical vein enter liver and communicate with the hepatic sinuses. After that, the right umbilical vein degenerates completely. The left umbilical vein between the liver and the sinuses also degenerates and disappears. The umbilical to liver segment remains until birth. The small blood vessels passing through the liver expand to form the ductus venosus. One end of the ductus venosus is connected with the left umbilical vein, and the other end enters the inferior vena cava. Blood from the placenta enters the inferior vena cava and then enters the right corner of the venous sinus.

4   Fetal Blood Circulation and Changes in Neonatal Blood Circulation

4.1   Fetal Blood Circulation

Before birth, oxygenated blood from the placenta returns to the fetus through the umbilical vein. On approaching the liver, the main portion of this blood flows through the ductus venosus directly into the inferior vena cava. A small portion enters the liver sinusoids and mixes here with blood from the portal circulation. The blood in the inferior vena cava enters the right atrium. The entrance of the inferior vena cava directly faces the foramen ovale so that most blood streams enter the left atrium. A small portion remains in the right atrium, mixing with the blood from the superior vena cava. The blood stream from the left atrium enters the left ventricle and ascending aorta. The heart is supplied with well-oxygenated blood via the arch of the aorta and its 3 large branches. The poorly-oxygenated blood from the superior vena cava flows from the right ventricle into the pulmonary trunk. Because of the high resistance in the pulmonary vessels of the fetal, the main portion of blood passes directly through the ductus arteriosus in the descending aorta. The blood stream flows into the placenta through 2 umbilical arteries (Figure 25 - 9).

4.2   Changes in Neonatal Blood Circulation

After birth, placenta circulation stops and pulmonary circulation begins, leading to a series of changes in blood circulation—closure of the umbilical vessels, ductus arteriosus, ductus venosus and foramen ovale.

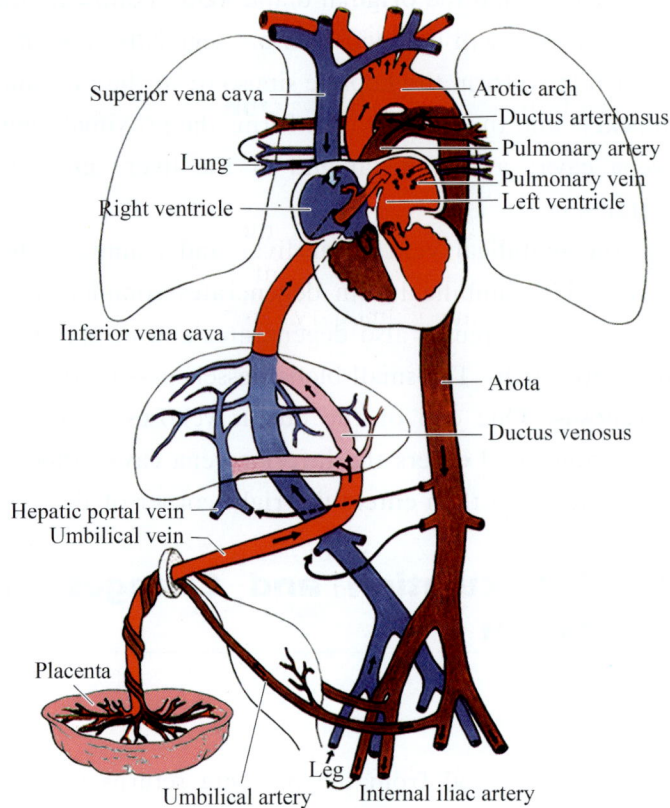

Figure 25 - 9   Drawing showing the fetal blood circulation

5   Main Congenital Malformations

5.1   Atrial Septal Defects

They are mainly caused by perforation of the foramen ovale valve, excessive absorption of the septum primum, hypoplasia of the septum secundum, hypoplasia of the endocardial cushion and oversized or abnormal position of the septum secundum.

5.2   Ventricular Septal Defects

They occur in the membranous or muscular ventricular septum. Membranous ventricular septal defects are most common, mainly due to the poor hyperplasia of the endocardial cushion, which cannot fuse with the bulbar ridges and muscular ventricular septum. Muscular ventricular septal defect happens rarely, mainly due to its over-absorption during development.

5.3   Patent Ductus Arteriosus

It is caused by the fact that the ductus arteriosus is too long or its external muscle fibers cannot contract after birth, resulting in the connection between the pulmonary artery and aorta, which is more common in women.

5.4 Anomalies of Aortopulmonary Septation

5.4.1 Aorta and Pulmonary Artery Dislocation

The main reason for the dislocation is that the aortico-pulmonary septum does not spiral, resulting in that the aorta is located in front of the pulmonary artery and sent out from the right ventricle, while the pulmonary artery trunk is sent out from the left ventricle.

5.4.2 Aorta stenosis or Pulmonary Artery stenosis

The main reason for the stenosis is that the aortico-pulmonary septum deviates to one side. If it is on the side of the pulmonary artery, it often leads to the coexistence of 4 defects: the pulmonary artery stenosis, overriding aorta, ventricular septal defect, and right ventricular hypertrophy, which is called tetralogy of Fallot.

(Yue Haiyuan)

第二十五章　心血管系统的发生

心血管系统是最早产生功能的系统,主要来源于中胚层。人胚早期以物质弥散方式进行代谢,由于胚体生长快速,大约在第 3 周末就开始血液循环,以获取更多的氧气和营养物质并排泄废物。

第一节　原始心血管系统的建立

原始心血管系统呈左、右对称,由心管、原始动脉系统和原始静脉系统组成。

一、胚外血管的发生

人胚第 3 周,卵黄囊壁的胚外中胚层、体蒂和绒毛膜等部位的细胞相继分化,形成细胞索或细胞团,称血岛。随后,血岛细胞间出现空隙,其周围的细胞分化成扁平的内皮细胞,而中央的细胞分化则成游离的造血干细胞。内皮管不断向外出芽延伸,并与相邻血岛形成的内皮管互相融合,逐渐形成胚外毛细血管网(图 25 - 1)。

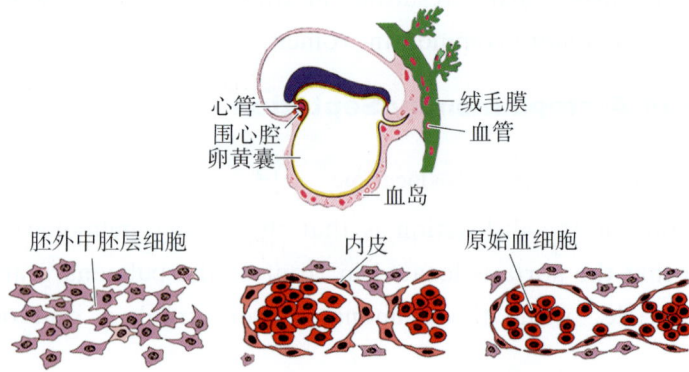

图 25-1　血岛和血管的形成示意图

二、胚内血管的发生

人胚第 18~20 天,体内各处间充质内出现空隙,其周围的细胞分化成内皮细胞,进而形成胚内毛细血管。相邻血管内皮以出芽方式连接,形成胚内原始毛细血管网。随后,胚体内、外的毛细血管网通过体蒂相通,造血干细胞进入胚体内,形成早期的原始血管通路。

此时的血管在结构上尚无法明确区分动脉和静脉,只能根据它们的归属及与心脏的关系进行命名。之后,血管内皮周围的间充质细胞分化成为平滑肌纤维和结缔组织,形成血管的中膜和外膜,进而演化成动脉或静脉。

三、胚体早期血液循环

人胚第 3 周末已形成一对心管,一对腹主动脉,一对背主动脉以及连接同侧腹主动脉和背主动脉的第 1 对弓动脉。背主动脉在卵黄囊壁分出若干对卵黄动脉,这些动脉经过体蒂在绒毛膜处分出一对脐动脉。卵黄囊的毛细血管汇合成一对卵黄静脉,而绒毛膜中的毛细血管则汇合成一条脐静脉。卵黄静脉和脐静脉分别输送血液回心管的静脉端,从而形成了卵黄囊循环和脐循环(图 25-2)。

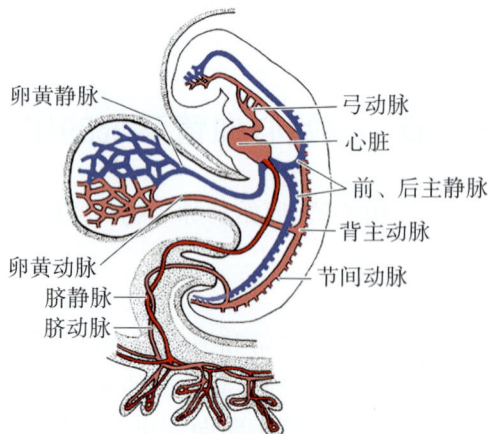

图 25-2　人胚早期血液循环示意图

当左、右心管合并时，两条腹主动脉融合成主动脉囊，两条背主动脉也合并，沿途的分支将血液输送至胚体的各个部分。此时，胚体的前部形成了一对前主静脉，后部形成一对后主静脉，它们分别汇流至左、右总主静脉，再连接心管的静脉端，形成胚体循环。

第二节　心脏的发生

在三胚层胚盘中，部分中胚层细胞在胚盘前缘口咽膜的头端和原始横膈的尾端之间汇聚形成生心区，心脏发生于此。

一、原始心脏的形成

（一）心管的形成

在人胚第 18～19 天，生心区出现腔隙，称围心腔。其腹侧的间充质细胞聚集成一对长条细胞索，称生心索。随后，生心索中央出现腔隙，形成左、右两个细的心管（图 25 - 3）。当胚胎发生卷折时，围心腔转至心管腹侧，两个心管相互靠近，并在第 22～23 天融合形成一个心管（图 25 - 4）。

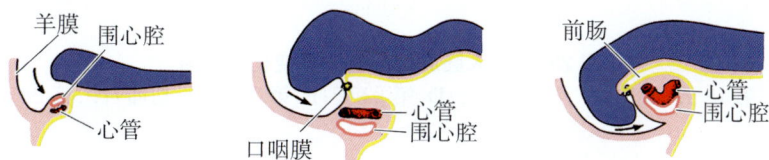

图 25 - 3　人胚原始心脏位置变化示意图（头端纵切面）

围心腔不断向心管的背侧扩大，使心管与前肠之间的间充质变窄，形成心背系膜。围心腔将心管悬连于背侧壁，随后其中央部逐渐退化消失，形成一个通道，称心包横窦。除了头、尾侧留有心背系膜外，心管其余部分完全游离于围心腔内。之后，围心腔发育为心包腔。

（二）心壁的形成

心管合并时，心管内皮成为心内膜的内皮。心管周围的间充质形成心肌外套层，之后分化成心肌膜和心外膜。位于心管内皮和心肌外套层之间的胶状结缔组织，称心胶质，它形成内皮下层的结缔组织（图 25 - 4）。

二、心脏外形的演变

随着心管的拉长以及交替扩张和收缩，形成 4 个膨大，依次为心球、心室、心房和静脉窦。心球的远侧较细，称动脉干，与主动脉囊相连，主动脉囊又与弓动脉相连。静脉窦末端分为左、右角，分别与卵黄静脉、脐静脉、和总主静脉相连。

由于心脏的动脉端和静脉端分别由腮弓和横膈固定，而心球和心室的生长速度远大于心包腔的扩展速度，因此管状心脏在大约第 23～28 天时经历右旋，形成一个“U”字形球室袢，此时心尖指向左侧（图 25 - 5）。

随后，心房逐渐离开原始横膈，位置逐渐移至心室头端的背侧，并稍偏左。静脉窦也从原始横膈内游离出来，位于心房的背面尾侧。此时的心脏外形呈“S”形。心房受前面的心球和后

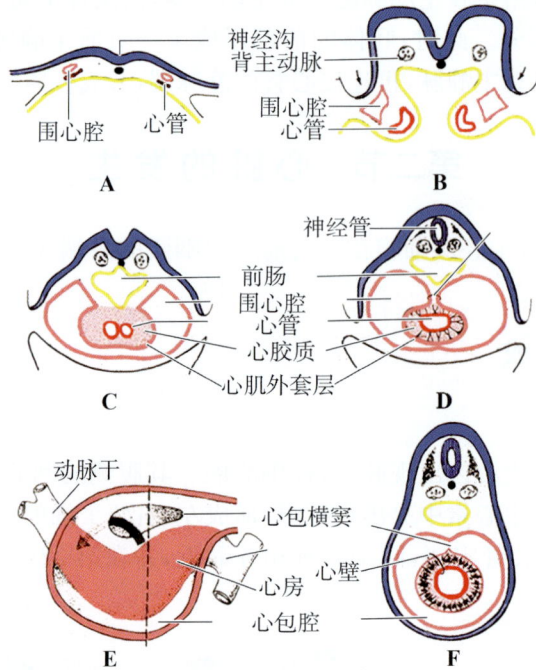

图 25‐4　人胚原始心脏位置变化示意图
A.第 19 天;B.第 20 天;C.第 21;D.第 22 天;E.第 28 天(纵切面);F.第 28 天

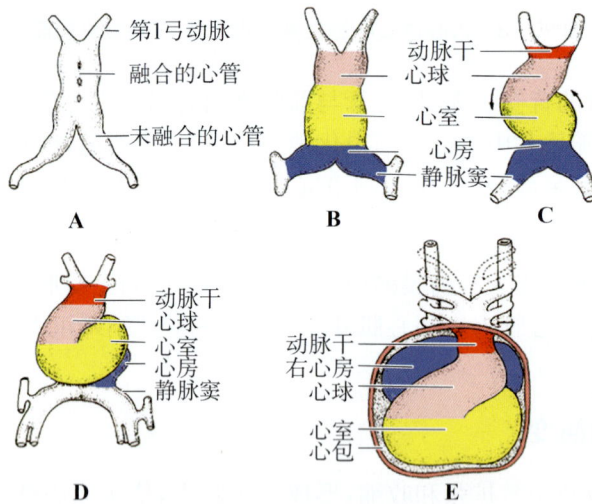

图 25‐5　心脏外形的演变示意图
A.21 天;B.22 天;C.23 天;D.24 天;E.25 天

面的食管限制,故向左、右方向扩展,结果便膨出于动脉干的两侧。心房扩大,房室沟加深,房室之间遂形成狭窄的房室管。心球近侧段被心室吸收,成为原始右心室。原来的心室成为原始左心室。左、右心室之间的表面出现室间沟。至此,心脏已初具成体心脏的外形,但内部仍未完全分隔(图 25‐5)。

三、心脏内部的分隔

心脏外形于第 5 周初初步建立,但此时心脏内部的分隔尚不完全。心脏各部的分隔同时进行,于第 7 周末完成。

(一) 房室管的分隔

心房和心室之间的房室沟逐渐加深,形成一狭窄的通道,称房室管。第 4 周,房室管背侧和腹侧心内膜增生形成心内膜垫。心内膜垫向中央生长并融合,将房室管分为左、右房室管(图 25-6)。围绕房室孔的间充质向腔内增生、隆起,形成房室瓣。

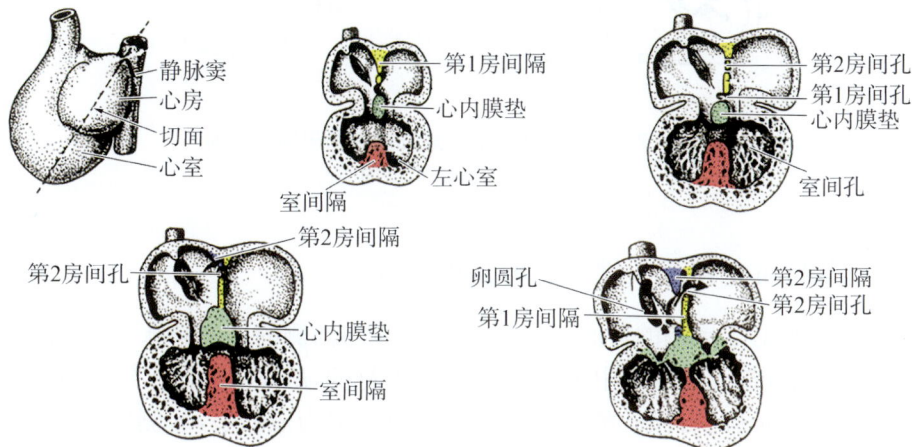

图 25-6 心脏内部的分隔示意图

(二) 心房的分隔

第 4 周,心房头端背侧壁的正中线处发生一个薄的半月形薄膜,称第一房间隔。第一房间隔向心内膜垫方向生长,其游离缘与心内膜垫之间暂时留有一个孔,称第一房间孔。随着第一房间隔的继续生长,其上部中央变薄,出现若干小孔,并逐渐融合成一大孔,称第二房间孔。然后,心内膜垫向上生长并与第一房间隔融合,封闭第一房间孔。

第 5 周末,在第一房间隔的右侧,从心房的头端腹侧再生长出一较厚的新月形隔,称第二房间隔。此隔逐渐向心内膜垫方向生长,覆盖第二房间孔。当其前后缘与心内膜垫接触时下方留有一孔,称卵圆孔。卵圆孔的位置比第二房间孔稍低,两孔交错重叠。第一房间隔在左侧下方覆盖卵圆孔。此时,第一房间隔相当于瓣膜,称卵圆孔瓣。出生前,由于肺循环不行使功能,左心房压力低于右心房,右心房的血液可经卵圆孔流入左心房,反之则不能。出生后肺循环开始,左心房压力增大,致使两个隔靠近并发生融合,卵圆孔关闭,一个完整的房间隔形成,至此左、右心房完全分隔(图 25-6)。

(三) 心室的分隔

第 4 周末,心尖处心室底壁组织向上增生形成,一半月形的肌性隔膜,称室间隔肌部。此隔向心内膜垫方向生长,直到第 7 周,在其自由边缘和心内膜垫之间有一个新月形的孔,称室间孔。第 7 周末,由于左、右心球嵴彼此对向生长、融合并向下延伸,分别与室间隔肌部的前缘和后缘融合,关闭了室间孔上部的大部分。同时,心内膜垫的间充质增生,室间隔肌部上缘向上生长与心球嵴愈合,形成室间隔膜部。至此,左右室间孔封闭,心室完全分隔(图 25-6、图 25-7)。

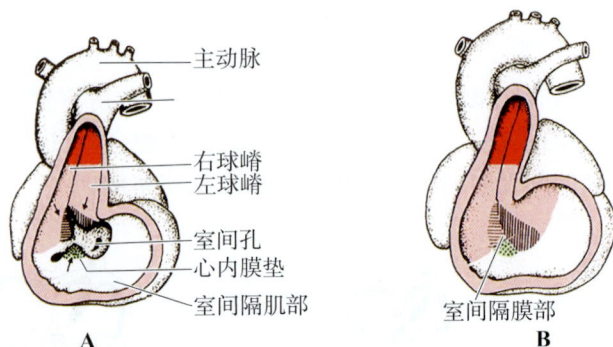

图 25-7　室间隔膜部的形成及室间孔闭锁示意图
A.第 5 天;B.第 7 周

四、静脉窦的演变和永久性左右心房的生成

静脉窦位于原始心房尾端的背面,窦的左右角分别与同侧的总主静脉、脐静脉和卵黄静脉相连。起初,静脉窦开口于心房的中央部,两个角是对称的,后来因血液多经右角回流心脏,右角逐渐扩大,窦房口逐渐向右移。窦左角逐渐萎缩,近侧成为冠状窦,远侧成为左心房斜静脉的根部。第 7~8 周,原始心房扩展很快,静脉窦右角被逐渐吸收并入右心房,形成永久性的右心房固有部。原始右心房则变为右心耳。同时,由于原始左心房的扩大,逐渐把原始肺静脉的根部及其左右属支逐渐并入左心房,形成永久性左心房固有部,原始的左心房则成为左心耳。

五、心球与动脉干的分隔

心球与动脉干以类似于心内膜垫的方式被分隔成两个通道。第 5 周,心球与动脉干的内膜组织局部增生,形成一对心球嵴和动脉干嵴。相应的嵴向对侧生长,在中线融合,形成螺旋状走行的隔,称主动脉肺动脉隔,将心球与动脉干分割成相互缠绕的主动脉和肺动脉。主动脉和肺动脉起始处的心内膜组织向腔内增生,各形成三个薄片状隆起,逐渐演变为半月瓣。室间孔封闭后,肺动脉干与右心室相通,主动脉与左心室相通(图 25-8)。

第三节　主要血管的演变

一、弓动脉的发生和演变

弓动脉起至主动脉囊,第 4~6 周相继产生 6 对,分别走行于各对腮弓内,与同侧的背主动脉相连。第 6~8 周弓动脉的演变如下:

第 1、2 对弓动脉基本退化消失,但与其相连的一段背主动脉保留。

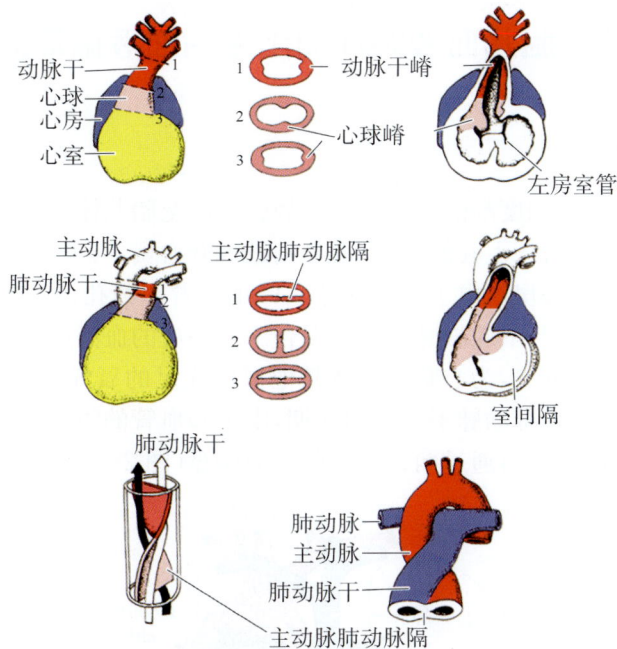

图 25-8　心球及动脉干的分隔示意图

第3对弓动脉左、右各发出一个分支,形成左、右颈外动脉。以颈外动脉的起始为界,近侧端及部分主动脉囊发育成颈总动脉,远侧段及其相连的背主动脉共同形成颈内动脉。

左侧第4弓动脉与动脉囊共同形成主动脉弓,动脉囊右半形成头臂干,左侧背主动脉发出的第7节间动脉形成左锁骨下动脉;右侧第4弓动脉与其相连的尾侧背主动脉和右侧第7节间动脉共同形成右锁骨下动脉。第3对和第4对弓动脉之间的背主动脉萎缩消失。

第5对动脉弓发育不全并很快退化。

第6对动脉弓近侧端形成肺动脉的基部,左侧远侧段形成动脉导管,右侧远侧端退化。随着动脉干的分割,肺动脉与肺动脉干相连。

二、卵黄静脉的演变

左、右卵黄静脉与卵黄蒂一同进入胚体,经过原始横膈注入静脉窦。在卵黄囊与原始横膈之间,左、右卵黄静脉形成众多吻合支。肝形成后,原来的卵黄静脉被分化为三段:与肝相连的一段进入肝内形成肝血窦;出肝后的近心段,左侧支消失,右侧支形成肝静脉和下腔静脉的近心段;出肝后的远心段,形成一段"S"形的血管,最终发育成门静脉。

三、脐静脉的演变

脐静脉的分支进入肝并与肝血窦相通。随后,右脐静脉完全退化,左脐静脉在肝与静脉窦之间的一段也退化消失,而脐至肝的一段则保留至出生,穿行于肝内的小血管扩大,形成一条静脉导管。静脉导管一端连接左脐静脉,另一端连接下腔静脉,负责将从胎盘回流的血液导入下腔静脉,再流入静脉窦右角。

第四节 胎儿血液循环和出生后血液循环的变化

一、胎儿血液循环

出生前,胎盘中血氧饱和度高的血液通过脐静脉回流至胎儿体内。当血液接近肝脏时,其大部分通过静脉导管直接流入下腔静脉,小部分则进入肝血窦,与来自门静脉的血液混合。下腔静脉的血液随后进入右心房。由于下腔静脉入口正对着卵圆孔,其血流的大部分进入左心房,只有小部分留在右心房与上腔静脉的血液混合。左心房的血液进入左心室和升主动脉,再通过主动脉弓及其三个大分支,为心脏和身体其他提供充足的氧气。来自上腔静脉的血氧饱和度低的血液经右心室流入肺动脉干。在胎儿期,由于肺血管的阻力高,大部分血液通过动脉导管直接进入降主动脉,然后再通过两条脐动脉流向胎盘(图 25 - 9)。

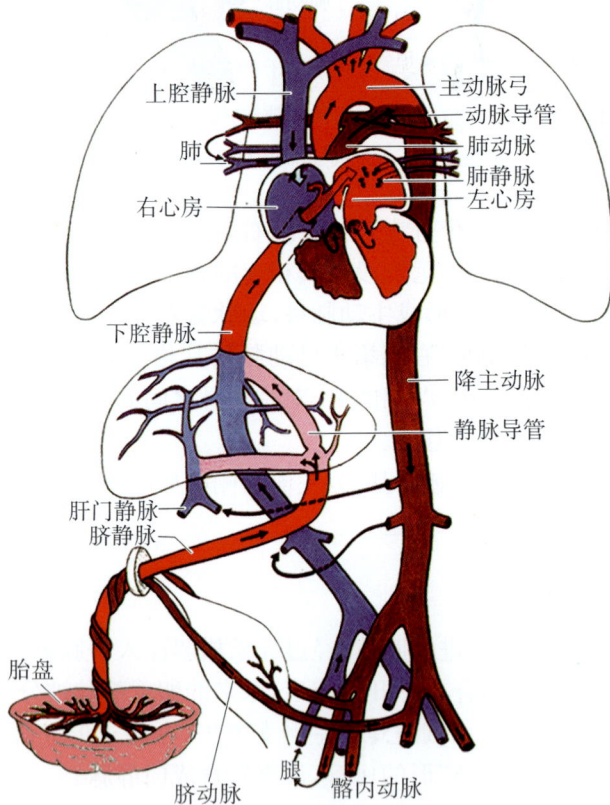

图 25 - 9 胎儿血液循环示意图

二、出生后血液循环的变化

胎儿出生后,胎盘循环停止,肺循环开始,导致一系列的血液循环变化:脐血管闭合、动脉导管闭合、静脉导管闭合及卵圆孔闭合。

第五节　主要先天性畸形

一、房间隔缺损

其产生的原因包括卵圆孔瓣穿孔、第一房间隔吸收过度、第二房间隔发育不全、心内膜垫发育不全以及第二房间孔过大或者位置异常。

二、室间隔缺损

室间隔膜部缺损最为常见，其主要原因是心内膜垫增生不良，导致其无法和心球嵴及室间隔肌部正常愈合。而室间隔肌部缺损则较为少见，主要是由于其在形成过程中被过度吸收。

三、动脉导管未闭

其主要原因是动脉导管过长或在出生后其肌纤维无法收缩，从而导致肺动脉和主动脉之间保持相通。此畸形在女性中较为多见。

四、动脉干和心球分隔异常

1. 主动脉和肺动脉错位

主要原因为主动脉肺动脉隔不呈螺旋状走行，导致主动脉位于肺动脉前面，由右心室发出，而肺动脉干则由左心室发出。

2. 主动脉或肺动脉狭窄

主要原因为主动脉肺动脉隔偏于一侧。如果偏于肺动脉一侧，常造成肺动脉狭窄、主动脉骑跨、室间隔缺损和右心室肥大四个缺陷共存，称为法洛四联症。

（岳海源）

Chapter 26

Development of the Nervous System, Eyes and Ears

1 Development of Nervous System

The nervous system originates from the neuroectoderm and is differentiated from the neural tube and neural crest.

1.1 Early Differentiation of Neural Tube and Neural Crest

At the beginning of the 3rd week of the human embryo, under the influence of the nearby notochord, part of the neuroectoderm forms the neural tube (Figure 21 – 9). The cephalic portion of the neural tube expands to form the brain, while the caudal portion is relatively thin and differentiates into the spinal cord. During the formation of the neural tube, some neuroectodermal cells at the edge of the neural fold dissociate, forming 2 cell cords parallel to the neural tube, located on the dorsal lateral side of the neural tube, called the neural crest (Figure 21 – 10). The neural crest differentiates into ganglia and glial cells of the peripheral nervous system, chromaffin cells of the adrenal medulla, melanocytes, etc.

The epithelium in the neural tube is a pseudostratified columnar structure, known as neuroepithelium, with a thicker basement membrane called external limiting membrane. There is also a layer of membrane on the inner surface of the neural tube, called internal limiting membrane. Neuroepithelial cells continuously divide and proliferate, and some of them migrate to the periphery of the neuroepithelium, becoming neuroblasts and glioblasts to form a new layer of cells, called mantle layer. The original neuroepithelium stops differentiating and becomes a layer of cubic or short columnar cells called ependymal layer. The spherical neuroblast in the mantle layer is called apolar neuroblast, and then it owns 2 processes, called bipolar neuroblast. One process grows towards the periphery of the mantle layer, extending into a new structure called marginal layer (Figure 26 – 1). The other faces the neural tube lumen, and subsequently degenerates and disappears, while the process extending towards the marginal layer rapidly grows, forming the primitive axon. At this time, the neuroblast is called unipolar neuroblast, subsequently forming several short processes from its soma to form primitive dendrites, thus becoming the multipolar neuroblast (Figure 26 – 1, 26 – 2).

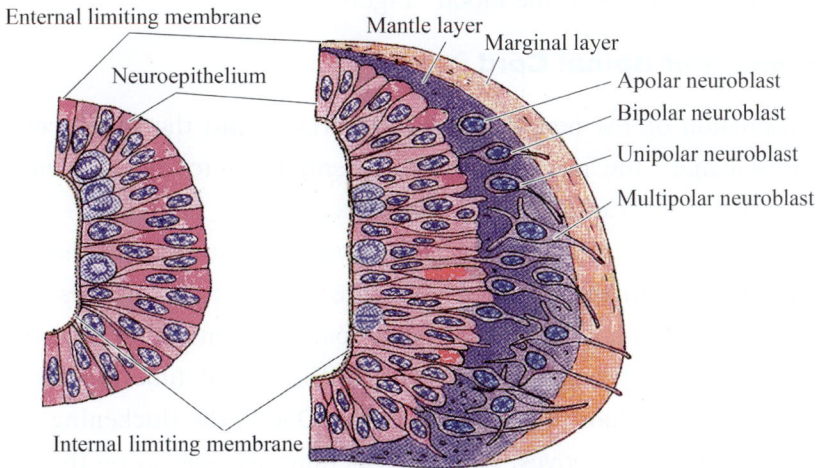

Figure 26 – 1   Drawings showing the early differentiation of neuroepithelium

The number of initially generated neurons is much higher than the number remaining later, and those neurons failing to establish a connection with the target cells die within a certain period of time. The survival and development of nerve cells are mainly regulated by neurotrophic factors produced by target cells, such as nerve growth factor, fibroblast growth factor, epidermal growth factor, insulin-like growth factor, etc.

The development of glial cells occurs later. Glioblasts first differentiate into the precursor cells of various types of glial cells, namely astroblasts and oligodendroblasts. Then, astroblasts differentiate into protoplasmic and fibrous astrocytes, while oligodendroblasts differentiate into oligodendrocytes (Figure 26 – 2), with some cells entering the marginal layer. The development of microglia occurs relatively late and

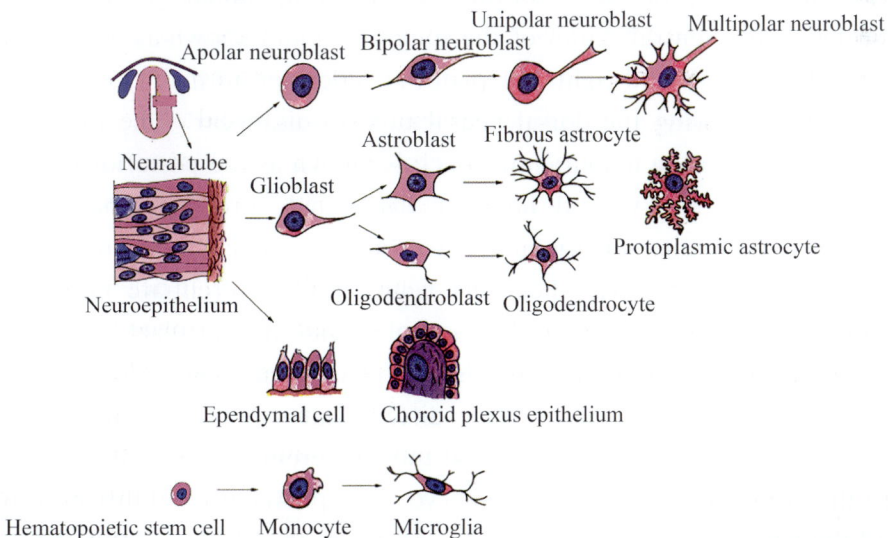

Figure 26 – 2   Schematic diagrams showing the differentiation of neuroepithelium and derivation of microglia

originates from the monocytes in the blood (Figure 26 - 2).

1.2　Development of Spinal Cord

The caudal portion of the neural tube differentiates into the spinal cord. The lumen forms the central canal; the mantle layer differentiates into the gray matter; and the marginal layer differentiates into the white matter.

The walls on both sides of the neural tube rapidly thicken due to the proliferation of neuroblasts and glioblasts in the mantle layer. The ventral part thickens to form the left basal plate and right basal plate, while the dorsal part thickens to form the right alar plate and left alar plate. The top and bottom walls of the neural tube are thin and narrow, forming a roof plate and a floor plate, respectively. Due to the thickening of the basal and alar plates, two longitudinal grooves, called sulcus limitans, appear on the inner surface of the neural tube (Figure 26 - 3).

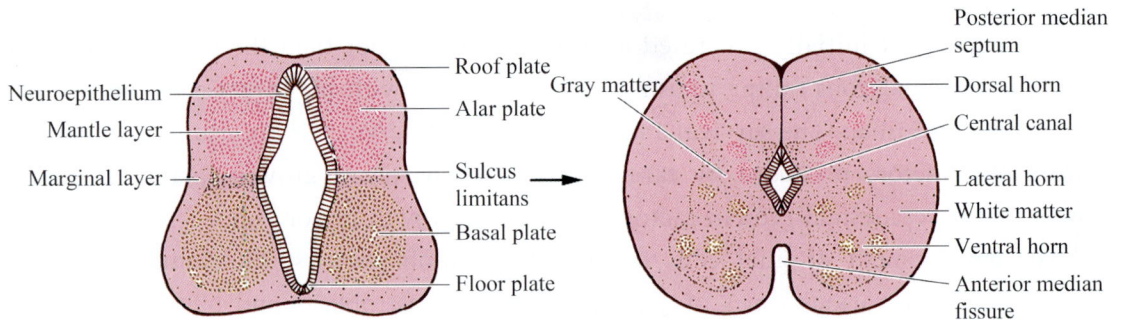

Figure 26 - 3　Drawings showing the development of the spinal cord

Due to the increase of neuroblasts and glioblasts, the left and right basal plates protrude towards the ventral side, forming a deep longitudinal groove between them, which is located in the ventral center of the spinal cord and known as the anterior median fissure. Similarly, the left and right alar plates also develop to mainly extend inward and fuse at the midline, causing the dorsal neural tube to disappear. The fusion of the alar plates at the midline forms a diaphragm, which is known as the posterior median septum. The basal plate forms the ventral horn of the spinal cord gray matter, where the neuroblasts differentiate into somatic motor neurons. The alar plate forms the dorsal horn of the spinal cord gray matter, where the neuroblasts differentiate into interneurons. Several neuroblasts aggregate between the basal plate and the alar plate, forming the spinal lateral horn, and they differentiate into visceral efferent neurons (Figure 26 - 3). Thus far, the caudal portion of the neural tube differentiates into the spinal cord, and the surrounding mesenchymal tissue of the neural tube differentiates into the meninges.

Before the 3rd month of the human embryo, the spinal cord and the spine are equal in length, and the lower end of the spinal cord can reach the coccyx. After the 3rd month, due to the faster growth of the spine when compared to the spinal cord, it gradually extends beyond the spinal cord to the tail end, and the position of the spinal cord is relatively upward. Before birth, the lower end of the spinal cord is at the level of the 3rd lumbar vertebra, and only connected to the coccyx with the filum terminale. Due to the fact that the spinal nerves distributed in each segment are formed in the early embryonic stage and penetrate through the intervertebral foramen of the corresponding segment, when the position of the spinal cord is relatively upward, the spinal nerve roots below the cervical segment of the spinal cord become more and more inclined towards the caudal side. The spinal nerve roots extend to the lumbar, sacral, and caudal segments, and then descend vertically within the spinal canal, together with the filum terminale, to form the cauda equina (Figure 26 – 4).

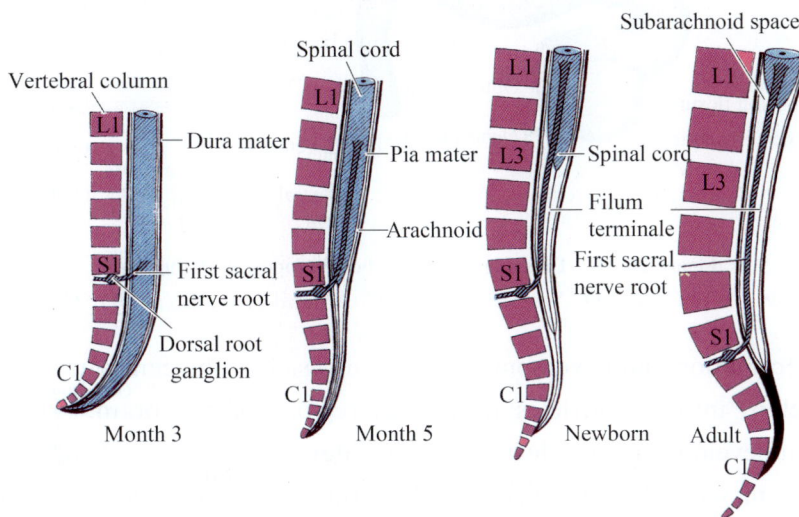

Figure 26 – 4   Drawings showing the relationship between the development of the spinal cord and the vertebral column

1.3 Development of Brain

The brain originates from the cephalic portion of the neural tube.

1.3.1   Formation and Development of Brain Vesicles

At the end of the 4th week of the human embryo, the anterior end of the neural tube forms 3 primary vesicles: the prosencephalon, mesencephalon, and rhombencephalon. By the 5th week, the prosencephalon expands to both sides, forming 2 telencephalons on the left and right, which later form 2 cerebral hemispheres, while the tail of the prosencephalon forms a diencephalon. The changes in the mesencephalon are not significant, which will form the midbrain. The rhombencephalon divides into the cephalic metencephalon and the caudal myelencephalon, thus forming 5 secondary vesicles. The cephalic mesencephalon forms the pons and cerebellum, while the caudal myelencephalon forms the medulla oblongata (Figure 26 – 5).

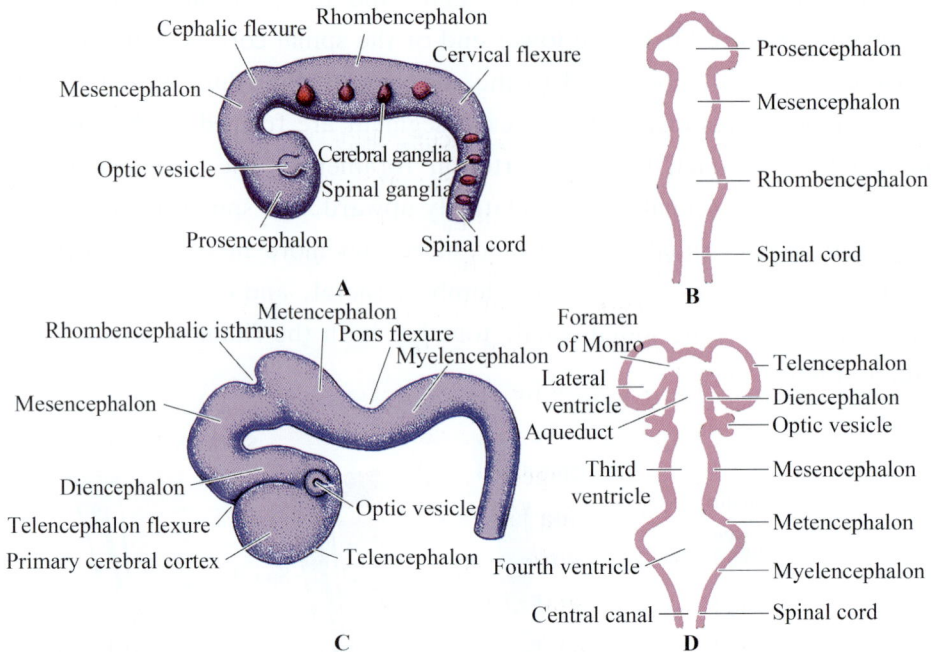

Figure 26 - 5   Drawings showing the development of the brain

A. and B. Week 4; C. and D. Week 6; A. and C. Lateral view; B. and D. Coronal section

With the formation and development of brain vesicles, the central canal of the neural tube also develops into 4 ventricles in various regions of the brain. The canal in the prosencephalon develops into the left and right lateral ventricles and the third ventricle; the canal in the mesencephalon is very small, forming a narrow mesencephalic aqueduct; the canal in the rhombencephalon develops into the broad fourth ventricle (Figure 26 - 5).

The brain region bends and several flexures develop meanwhile. The cervical flexure and cephalic flexure appear first. The former is located between the brain and spinal cord, while the latter is located in the midbrain. Afterwards, two more flexures appear at the pons and telencephalon, known as pons flexure and telencephalon flexure respectively (Figure 26 - 5).

The development of the brain wall is similar to that of the spinal cord, where the neuroectodermal cells on the lateral wall of the neural tube proliferate and migrate laterally, and then differentiate into neuroblasts and glioblasts, forming a mantle layer. Due to the thickening of the mantle layer, the lateral wall is divided into the basal plate and alar plate. The telencephalon and diencephalon mostly form an alar plate, with very small basal plates. Most cells of the layers in the telencephalon migrate to the outer surface, forming the cerebral cortex; a small number of cells aggregate into clusters, forming neural nuclei. The mantle layer cells in the mesencephalon, metencephalon and myelencephalon aggregate into cell clusters or columns, forming various neural nuclei. The neural nuclei in the alar plate are mostly sensory relay nuclei, while those in the basal plate are mostly motor nuclei.

1.3.2   Development of Cerebral Cortex

The organization of the cerebral cortex is formed by the migration and differentiation of neuroblasts in the mantle layer of the telencephalons. The phylogenetic development of the cerebral cortex can be divided into 3 stages: archicortex, paleocortex and neocortex. The hippocampus and dentate gyrus are the earliest formed cortical structures, equivalent to the archicortex. At the 7th week of the human embryo, a large number of neuroblasts gather and differentiate on the outer side of the striatum, forming the pyriform cortex that is equivalent to the paleocortex. Soon after the formation of the paleocortex, neuroepithelial cells divide, proliferate, and migrate to the surface in batches and differentiate into neurons, forming the neocortex, which is the latest and largest part of the cerebral cortex. Due to the staged generation and migration of neuroblasts, the neurons in the cortex are arranged in a layered manner. The earlier the cells are generated and migrated, the deeper their positions are. At the time of birth, the neocortex has formed 6 layers. The archicortex and paleocortex have no certain regularity in layers. Some areas of them have few obvious layers, and some of the others show 3 layers.

1.3.3   Development of Cerebellar Cortex

The cerebellar cortex originates from the rhombic lip in the dorsal part of the metencephalon alar plates. The fusion of the left and right rhombic lips in the midline forms the cerebellar plate, which is the primordium of the cerebellum. At the 12th week of the embryo, two lateral parts of the cerebellar plate expand and form the cerebellar hemisphere, while the middle part becomes thinner and forms the vermis. Then, the nodulus is separated from the vermis, and the flocculus is separated from the cerebellar hemisphere respectively by a transverse fissure (Figure 26 – 6). The flocculonodular lobe is composed of the flocculus and nodulus, which is the earliest part of the cerebellar lineage.

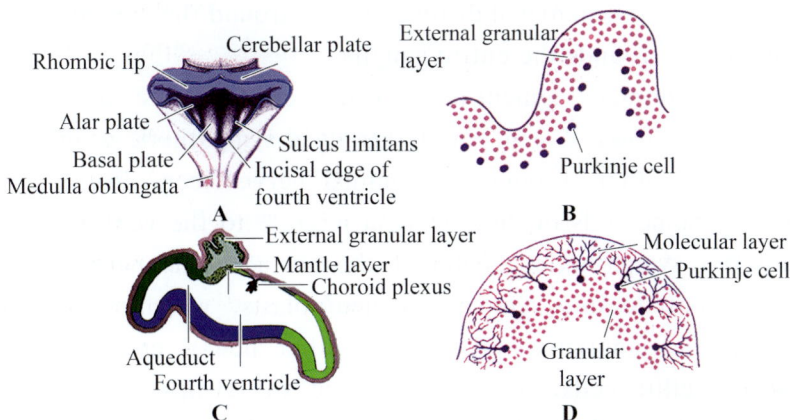

Figure 26 – 6   Drawings showing the development of the cerebellum
A. Dorsal view of the mesencephalon and rhombencephalon in week 8 when the top of the fourth ventricle is removed; B. Cerebellar cortex in fetus; C. Sagittal section of A; D Cerebellar cortex after birth

It is also known as the archicerebellum and still maintains contacts with the vestibular system.

At first, the cerebellar plate was composed of the neuroepithelium, the mantle layer, and the marginal layer. Then the neuroepithelial cells proliferate and migrate to the outer surface of the cerebellar plate through the mantle, forming an external granular layer. This layer of cells still maintains the ability to divide and proliferate, forming a proliferative zone on the surface of the cerebellum, which rapidly expands and produces wrinkles, forming cerebellar lobes. By the 6th month, the external granular layer cells begin to differentiate into different cell types. Some of them migrate inward and then differentiate into granular cells, which are located deep in the Purkinje cell layer to form the internal granular layer. The neuroblasts in the outer mantle layer differentiate into Purkinje cells and Golgi cells, forming the Purkinje cell layer, while those in the inner layer aggregate into clusters and differentiate into nuclei in the cerebellar white matter. The cells in the external granular layer become fewer due to the emigration, and they will differentiate into basket cells and astrocytes, forming the molecular layer of the cerebellar cortex. The internal granular layer is then renamed the granular layer (Figure 26 - 6).

1.4　Development of Ganglia and Peripheral Nerves

1.4.1　Development of Ganglia

Neural crest cells migrate and divide into cell clusters on the dorsal and lateral sides of the neural tube, differentiating into cerebral and spinal ganglia. These ganglia belong to the sensory ganglia. Neural crest cells first develop into neuroblasts and satellite cells, and then neuroblasts differentiate into sensory neurons. Neuroblasts first produce 2 processes to form bipolar neurons. Due to uneven growth on sides of the cell body, the starting parts of the 2 processes gradually converge and eventually merge, resulting in bipolar neurons becoming pseudo unipolar neurons. Satellite cells are a type of glial cell that surrounds the neuronal cell body. The mesenchymal differentiation around the ganglia forms a capsule of connective tissue that surrounds the entire ganglia.

Some cells in the thoracic segment of the neural crest migrate to the dorsal outer part of the aorta, forming 2 rows of segmentally arranged sympathetic ganglia. These ganglia are connected to each other through longitudinal nerve fibers, forming 2 longitudinal sympathetic trunks. Some cells in these ganglia migrate to the ventral side of the aorta, forming the anterior sympathetic ganglia of the aorta. Some neural crest cells in the ganglion first differentiate into sympathetic neuroblasts, which then differentiate into multipolar sympathetic ganglion neurons. The other neural crest cells in the ganglia differentiate into satellite cells. The periphery of the sympathetic ganglia also has a connective tissue membrane derived from mesenchymal differentiation.

The origin of the parasympathetic ganglia is still controversial. Some people believe that the neurons in the parasympathetic ganglia originate from the neural tubules, while others believe that they originate from the neuroblasts in the cerebral ganglia.

1.4.2   Development of Peripheral Nerves

The peripheral nerve is composed of sensory nerve fibers and motor nerve fibers. The nerve fiber is composed of neural processes and Schwann cells. The processes in sensory nerve fibers are the peripheral processes of sensory ganglion neurons; the processes in the somatic motor nerve fibers are axons of motor neurons in the brainstem and anterior horn of the spinal cord gray matter; the processes in the preganglionic fibers of the visceral motor nerves are axons of neurons in the lateral horn of the spinal cord gray matter and brainstem visceral motor nuclei; the processes in the postganglionic fibers are axons of ganglion neurons in the autonomic nervous system.

Schwann cells are differentiated neural crest cells that proliferate and migrate synchronously with the developing axons or peripheral processes. The Schwann cells are concave at the junction with the processes, forming a deep groove where axons are embedded. A flattened mesangium will be formed between the Schwann cells and the axon. In the myelinated nerve fibers, the mesentery continuously grows and surrounds the axon, forming a myelin sheath surrounded by multiple layers of cell membranes around the axon. In unmyelinated nerve fibers, a Schwann cell adheres to multiple axons and forms multiple deep grooves that wrap around the axons, forming a flat mesangium without a myelin sheath.

1.5   Development of Pituitary Gland

The pituitary gland develops from 2 sources: Rathke's pouch and the neurohypophyseal bud. Rathke's pouch eventually forms the adenohypophysis, while the neurohypophyseal bud forms the neurohypophysis (Figure 26 – 7).

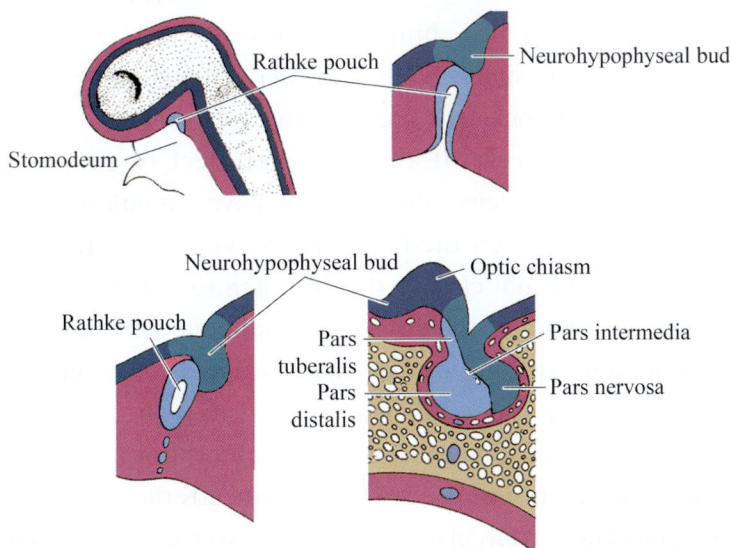

Figure 26 – 7   Drawings showing the development of pituitary gland

At the 4th week of embryonic development, the epithelium of the ectoderm at the top of the oral cavity descends towards the dorsal side, forming a sac-like protrusion called Rathke's pouch. Later, the basal neuroectoderm of the diencephalon protrudes towards the ventral side, forming a funnel-shaped protrusion called neurohypophyseal bud. Rathke's pouch and the neurohypophyseal bud gradually grow and approach each other. At the end of the 2nd month, the root of Rathke's pouch degenerates and disappears, and its distal end adheres to the neurohypophyseal bud. The distal expansion of the neurohypophysis bud forms the neurohypophysis. Its starting part becomes thinner, forming the infundibular stem. Afterwards, the anterior wall of Rathke's pouch rapidly enlarges, forming the pars distalis. A nodular protrusion grows upwards from the pars distalis of the pituitary gland and surrounds the infundibular stem, forming the pars tuberalis. The posterior wall of Rathke's pouch grows slowly, forming the pars intermedia (Figure 26 – 7). Most of the cavity disappears, leaving only a small fissure. Multiple types of glandular cells differentiate from the pituitary gland, while the neurohypophysis is mainly composed of nerve fibers and glial cells.

1.6 Development of Pineal Gland

At the 7th week of the human embryo, the caudal part of the diencephalon roof protrudes dorsally to form a sac-like protrusion that is the primordium of the pineal gland. The cells in the sac wall proliferate, the cavity disappears, and substantially a pineal like organ called pineal gland forms. The neuroepithelium differentiates into pinealocytes and glial cells.

1.7 Main Congenital Malformations

The neural tube defect is caused by the incomplete closure of the neural tube, mainly manifested as abnormalities in the brain and spinal cord, often accompanied by abnormalities in the skull and spine. Under normal circumstances, the neural groove (including anterior neural foramen and posterior neural foramen) should be completely closed by the end of the 4th week. If the inducing effect of the notochord is lost or affected by environmental teratogens, the neural groove cannot be properly closed into neural tubes. If the nerve groove on the head side is closed, the anencephaly will form, and if that on the caudal side is not closed, the myeloschisis will form. The anencephaly is often accompanied by hypoplasia of the cranial parietal bone, known as exencephaly. The myeloschisis is often accompanied by corresponding segments of spinal bifida.

The cause of hydrocephalus is developmental disorders of the ventricular system and an imbalance between cerebrospinal fluid generation and absorption. The stenosis or occlusion of the mesencephalic aqueduct or interventricular foramen is the most common. Due to the inability of cerebrospinal fluid to circulate normally, a large amount of fluid accumulates in the ventricles (internal hydrocephalus) or subarachnoid space (external hydrocephalus).

Its clinical symptom mainly includes enlargement of the brain, thinning of the skull, and widening of the cranial sutures.

2   Development of Eyes

2.1   Development of Eyeball

At the 4th week of the human embryo, two optic vesicles protrude on both sides of the prosencephalon. The distal end of the optic vesicle expands and is close to the surface ectoderm, forming a double layered cup-shaped structure called optic cup. The proximal end of the optic vesicle becomes thinner, known as the optic stalk, which is connected to the diencephalon which differentiates from the prosencephalon. Meanwhile, the surface ectoderm thickens under the induction of optic vesicle development, forming lens placodes. Subsequently, the placode recesses into the optic cup, gradually detaches from the surface ectoderm, and finally develops into lens vesicles (Figure 26 – 8). Mesenchyme is distributed between the optic cup and the lens vesicle, around the optic cup, and between the optic cup and the surface ectoderm. Various parts of the eye are formed by the further development of the optic cup and stalk, lens vesicles, and the surrounding mesenchyme.

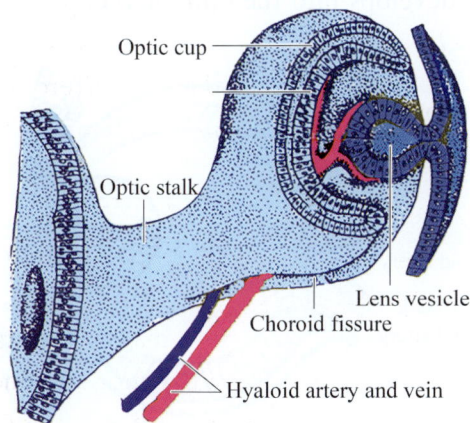

Figure 26 – 8   Drawing showing the optic cup and the lens in week 5

2.2   Development of Retina and Optic Nerve

The optic cup is composed of 2 layers with an intervening space. The outer layer becomes much thinner and differentiates into retinal pigment epithelium, while the inner layer thickens and has a structure similar to the walls of brain vesicles, which later differentiates into rod cells, cone cells, bipolar cells, and ganglion cells. The space between the 2 layers narrows and eventually disappears, so the 2 layers directly adhere to each other, forming the optic part of the retina. At the edge of the optic cup opening, the inner epithelium does not thicken and adheres to the differentiated pigment epithelium of the outer layer, extending in the mesenchymal space between the lens vesicle and the cornea, forming the epithelium of the ciliary body and iris. The inner layer epithelium of the ciliary body differentiates into non-pigmented epithelium, while the inner layer epithelium of the iris differentiates into pigmented epithelium. The outer layer of the pigment epithelium of the iris also differentiates into the sphincter pupillae and dilator pupillae.

In the 5th-week embryo, the optic cup and stalk are concave inward, forming a longitudinal groove called choroid fissure. The choroidal fissure contains mesenchymal and hyaloid arteries and veins, providing nutrients for the development of the vitreous and lens. The hyaloid artery also branches out to nourish the retina. The choroidal fissure is closed at the 7th week of a human embryo. The hyaloid artery and vein pass through a segment of the vitreous and degenerate, leaving a residue called hyaloid canal, while the proximal segments become the central artery and vein of the retina (Figure 26 - 9). The optic stalk is connected to the optic cup, and is also divided into 2 layers with a space between the layers. As the retina develops and differentiates, the axons of ganglion cells gather towards the inner layer of the optic stalk. The inner layer of the optic stalk gradually thickens and fuses with the outer layer, and the space between the 2 layers disappears. The optic stalk develops into the optic nerve.

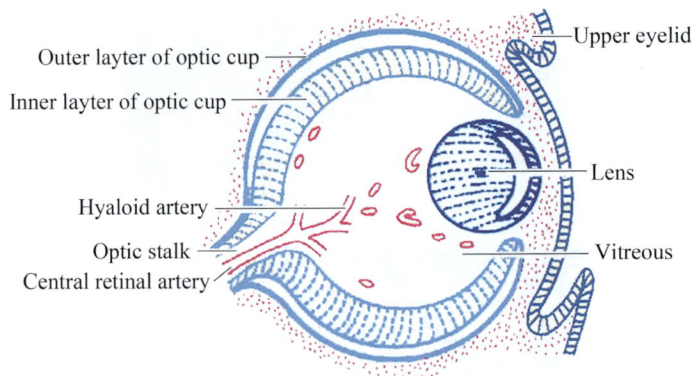

Figure 26 - 9　Drawing showing the eyeball and the eyelid in week 7

2.3　Development of Lens, Cornea and Eye chamber

The lens is formed from the lens vesicle. Initially, the lens vesicle is composed of a single layer of epithelium and a cavity (Figure 26 - 8). The anterior wall cells are cubic and differentiate into lens epithelium; the posterior wall cells are tall and columnar, gradually elongating towards the anterior wall to form primary lens fibers. The cavity gradually shrinks and disappears (Figure 26 - 9). Afterwards, the epithelial cells in the equatorial region of the lens continuously proliferate and grow, forming secondary lens fibers. The original primary lens fibers and their nuclei gradually degenerate to form the lens nucleus. New secondary lens fibers are added layer by layer around the lens nucleus, and the lens and nucleus gradually increase in size. This process lasts for a lifetime, but the rate of growth slows down with age, so the lens nucleus can be distinguished into embryonic nucleus, fetal nucleus, infant nucleus, and adult nucleus.

Under the development of the lens vesicle, the corresponding surface ectoderm differentiates into corneal epithelium. A cavity called anterior chamber, appears in the space between the lens vesicle and the corneal epithelium. The mesenchymal cells behind the corneal epithelium differentiate into the remaining layers of the cornea. The mesenchymal layer in front of the lens forms a membrane. Its thick periphery later forms the iris stroma, while the thin central part closes the opening of the optic cup, known as the pupillary membrane. After the formation of the iris and ciliary body, the posterior chamber is formed between the iris, ciliary body and lens. Before birth, the pupillary membrane is absorbed and disappears, and the anterior and posterior chambers are connected through the pupil (Figure 26 – 9).

2.4   Development of Vascular Membrane and Sclera

The mesenchyme around the optic cup divides into 2 layers. The inner layer is rich in blood vessels and pigment cells, which differentiate into the vascular membrane of the eyeball wall. The majority of the vascular membrane attached to the outside of the retina is called choroid membrane, while the part attached to the edge of the optic cup differentiates into the main body of the iris stroma and ciliary body. The outer layer is relatively dense and differentiated into the sclera. The choroid membrane and sclera are respectively connected to the pia mater and dura mater around the optic nerve respectively (Figure 26 – 9).

2.5   Development of Eyelid and Lacrimal Gland

At the 7th week of the human embryo, the surface ectoderm adjacent to the corneal epithelium in front of the eyeball forms 2 folds, namely the upper and lower eyelids. The surface ectoderm that folds back to the inner surface of the eyelids differentiates into a layered columnar conjunctival epithelium, which continues with the corneal epithelium. The surface ectoderm outside the eyelids differentiates into the epidermis. The mesenchyme within the folds differentiates into other structures of the eyelids. At the 10th week, the edges of the upper and lower eyelids merge with each other, and do not reopen until the 7th or 8th month.

The lacrimal gland is formed by the sinking of the surface ectodermal epithelium. The development of the lacrimal gland is relatively late, and it takes 6 weeks after birth to start secreting tears.

2.6 Main Congenital Malformations

2.6.1 Coloboma of Iridis

If the choroid fissure is not completely closed at the iris, it will cause a defect of the iris, resulting in a keyhole pupil called coloboma of iridis. Severe cases of this deformity can extend to the ciliary body, retina and optic nerve, often accompanied by other abnormalities in the eye.

2.6.2 Persistent Pupillary Membrane

If the pupillary membrane is not fully absorbed before birth, resulting in the remaining connective tissue network remaining in front of the lens. It is called persistent pupillary membrane (Figure 26 - 4), which can be gradually absorbed with the age after birth. It can be surgically removed if damaging vision.

2.6.3 Congenital Cataract

It is caused by the opacity of the lens before birth, which is often hereditary and can also be caused by early pregnancy infection with the rubella virus.

2.6.4 Congenital Glaucoma

It is characterized by abnormal or absent development of the scleral venous sinus, which obstructs aqueous drainage, increases intraocular pressure, causes eyeball enlargement, and ultimately may lead to retinal damage and blindness. Genetic mutations or early maternal infection with the rubella virus are the main causes.

2.6.5 Cyclopia, Microphthalmia and Anophthalmia

If both sides of the optic vesicles merge in the midline, it will result in cyclopia. If the development of optic vesicles is obstructed or do not occur, it will result in microphthalmia and anophthalmia respectively.

3　Development of Ears

3.1　Development of the Inner Ear

At the 4th week of the human embryo, the superficial ectoderm on either side of the neural plate becomes thickened, which is the start of the otic placode. The placode invaginates downward into the mesenchymal, forming the otic pit. Then the pit finally closes off from the ectoderm to form a sac called otic vesicle (Figure 26 - 10). At the beginning, the otic vesicle is pear-shaped and then extends dorsoventrally, dividing it into the dorsal vestibular sac and the ventral cochlear sac. It also develops a small tubular extension on the inner side of its dorsal end, which is known as the endolymphatic duct. The vestibular sac forms the epithelium of 3 semicircular ducts and the utricle while the cochlear sac forms the epithelium of the saccule and membranous cochlear canal. In this way, the otic vesicle and its surrounding mesenchymal tissue develop into an inner ear membranous labyrinth (Figure 26 – 11). At the 3rd month of human embryo, the mesenchymal tissue surrounding the membranous labyrinth differentiates into a cartilage sac. Around the 5th month, the cartilage sac ossifies into an osseous labyrinth. So, the membranous labyrinth is completely trapped within the osseous labyrinth, separated only by a narrow outer lymphatic space.

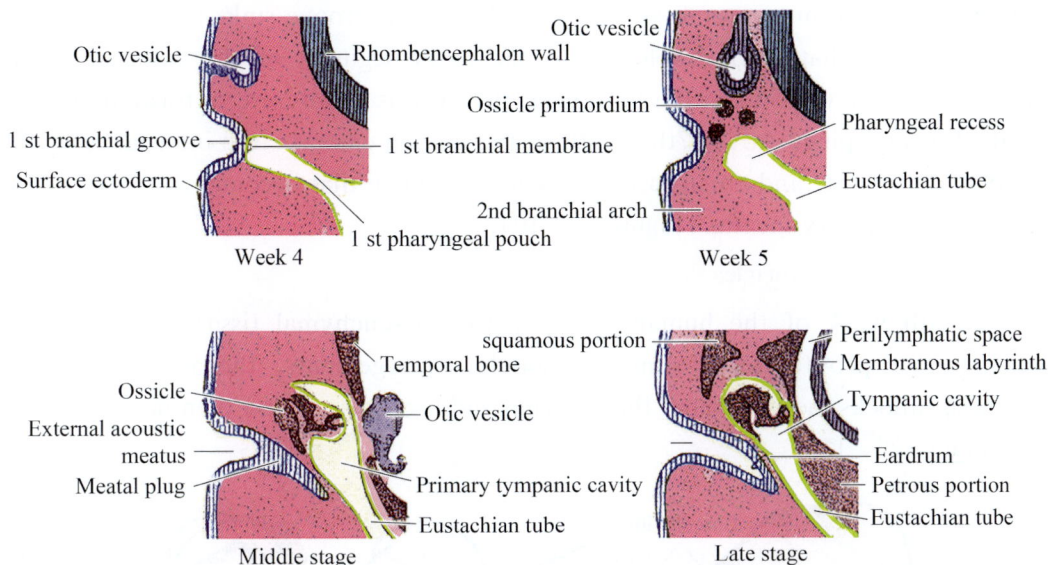

Figure 26 – 10　Drawing showing the development of ear

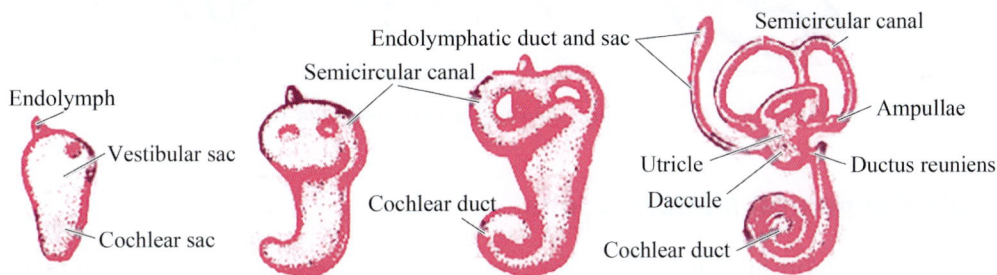

Figure 26 – 11　Drawing showing the development of the otic vesicle from week 5 to week 8

3.2　Development of the Middle Ear

At the 9th week of human embryo, the first pharyngeal pouch expands dorsolaterally. The distal blind end expands into the tympanic cavity, and the proximal end narrows to form the eustachian tube. The inner layer of the tympanic cavity is adjacent to the outer layer of the first branchial groove, forming the inner and outer epithelium of the tympanic membrane, respectively. The mesenchymal tissue between the 2 layers forms the connective tissue of the tympanic membrane. The mesenchymal tissue around the tympanic cavity differentiates into 3 auditory ossicles, which gradually protrude into the tympanic cavity (Figure 26 - 10).

3.3 Development of the External Ear

3.3.1 Development of Auditory Meatuses

The external auditory meatus develops from the first branchial groove. At the end of the 2nd month of the human embryo, the first branchial groove sinks inward, forming a funnel-shaped duct that later develops into the outer segment of the external auditory meatus. The outer layer cells at the bottom of the meatus proliferate to form an epithelial plate called meatal plug. At the 7th month of the human embryo, the internal cells of the meatal plug degenerate and are absorbed, forming a lumen that becomes the inner segment of the external auditory meatus (Figure 26 - 10).

3.3.2 Development of Auricles

At the 6th week of the human embryo, the mesenchymal tissue around the first branchial groove proliferates, forming 6 nodular enlargements, the auricular hillocks. Later, these hillocks merge around the external auditory meatus and then develop into the auricle (Figure 26 - 12).

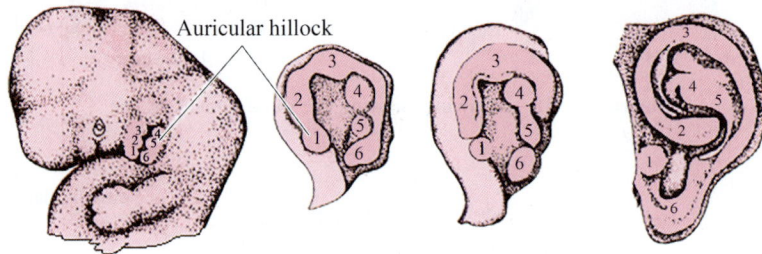

Figure 26 - 12   Drawings showing the development of the auricle

3.4 Main Congenital Malformations

The most common malformations are congenital deafness and auricular deformities. Abnormalities in the development of the inner, middle, and outer ears can all lead to congenital deafness, such as external auditory canal atresia, atresia of the middle ear and tympanic cavity, stiffness of the ossicular chain caused by the ossicle abnormality and abnormal development of internal ear osseous labyrinth or membrane labyrinth. The congenital deafness is mostly caused by genetic factors, but some are caused by the teratogens such as early pregnancy infection with rubella virus, strong noise in late pregnancy.

(Yue Haiyuan)

第二十六章　神经系统、眼和耳的发生

第一节　神经系统的发生

神经系统起源于神经外胚层，由神经管和神经嵴分化而成。

一、神经管和神经嵴的发生和早期分化

人胚第3周初，在脊索的诱导下，部分神经外胚层形成神经管（图21-9）。神经管的前段膨大，发育为脑；后段较细，发育为脊髓。

在神经管的形成过程中，神经褶边缘的一些神经外胚层细胞游离出来，形成左右两条与神经管平行的细胞索，位于神经管的背外侧，称神经嵴（图21-10）。神经嵴分化为周围神经系统、肾上腺髓质细胞、黑素细胞等。

神经管上皮为假复层柱状上皮，称神经上皮。上皮外包的基膜较厚，称外界膜；神经管内表面也有一层膜，称内界膜。神经上皮细胞不断分裂增殖，部分细胞迁至神经上皮的外周，分化为成神经细胞和成神经胶质细胞。于是，在神经上皮的外周由成神经细胞和成神经胶质细胞构成一层新的细胞层，称套层。原来的神经上皮则停止分化，变成一层立方形或矮柱状细胞，称室管膜层。套层的成神经细胞起初为圆球形，无突起，称无极成神经细胞；然后向套层外周和神经管腔方向各长出1个突起，称双极成神经细胞。成神经细胞朝向套层外周的突起扩展形成一层新的结构，称边缘层（图26-1）。随后，双极成神经细胞朝向神经管腔的突起退化

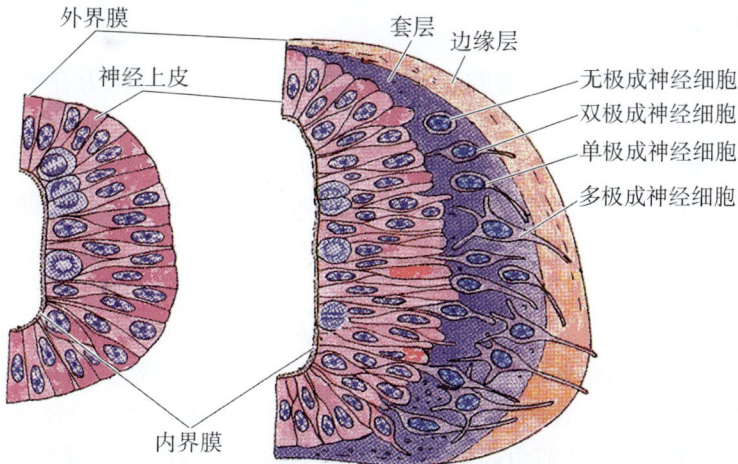

图26-1　神经管上皮的早期分化模式图

消失,而伸向边缘层的突起迅速增长,形成原始轴突。此时的成神经细胞称单极成神经细胞,然后其内侧端又形成若干短突起,成为原始树突,于是成为多极成神经细胞(图26-1、图26-2)。

在神经细胞的发生过程中,最初生成的细胞数目远比以后存留的数目多,那些未能与靶细胞建立连接的神经细胞都在一定时间内死亡。神经细胞的存活及其突起的发生主要受靶细胞产生的神经营养因子的调控,如神经生长因子、成纤维细胞生长因子、表皮生长因子、类胰岛素生长因子等。

胶质细胞的发生晚于神经元。成胶质细胞首先分化为各类胶质细胞的前体细胞,即成星形胶质细胞和成少突胶质细胞。然后,成星形胶质细胞分化为原浆性和纤维性星形胶质细胞,成少突胶质细胞分化为少突胶质细胞并有部分细胞进入边缘层。小胶质细胞的发生较晚,来源于血液中的单核细胞(图26-2)。

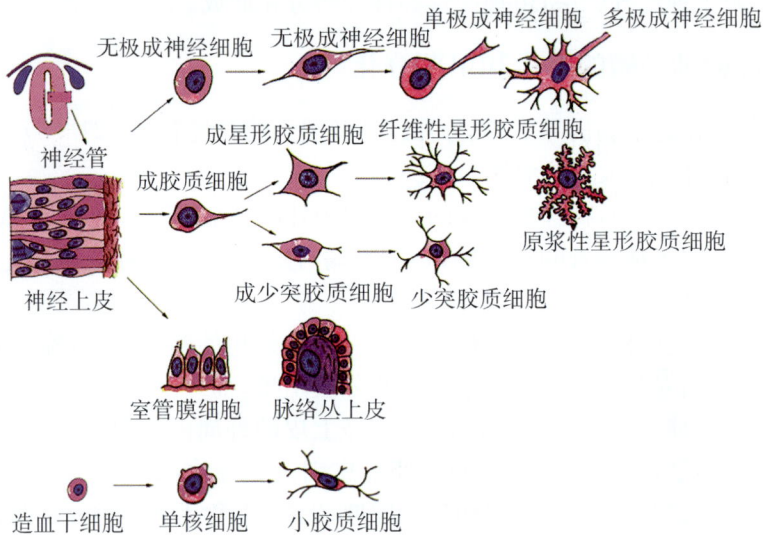

图26-2　神经上皮细胞的分化与小胶质细胞起源模式图

二、脊髓的发生

神经管的下段发育为脊髓,其管腔演化为脊髓中央管,套层分化为脊髓的灰质,边缘层分化为白质。

神经管的两侧壁由于套层中成神经细胞和成胶质细胞的增生而迅速增厚,腹侧部增厚形成左右两个基板,背侧部增厚形成左右两个翼板。神经管的顶壁和底壁都薄而窄,分别形成顶板和底板。由于基板和翼板的增厚,在神经管的内表面出现了左右两条纵沟,称界沟(图26-3)。

随着成神经细胞和成胶质细胞的增多,左右两基板向腹侧突出,致使在两者之间形成了一条纵行的深沟,位于脊髓的腹侧正中,称前正中裂。同样,左右两翼板也增大,但主要是向内侧推移并在中线愈合,导致神经管的背侧份消失。左右两翼板在中线的融合处形成一隔膜,称后正中隔。基板形成脊髓灰质的前角,其中的成神经细胞分化为躯体运动神经元。翼板形成脊髓灰质后角,其中的神经细胞分化为中间神经元。若干成神经细胞聚集于基板和翼板之间,形成脊髓侧角,其内的成神经细胞分化为内脏传出神经元(图 26-3)。神经管周围的间充质分化成脊膜。

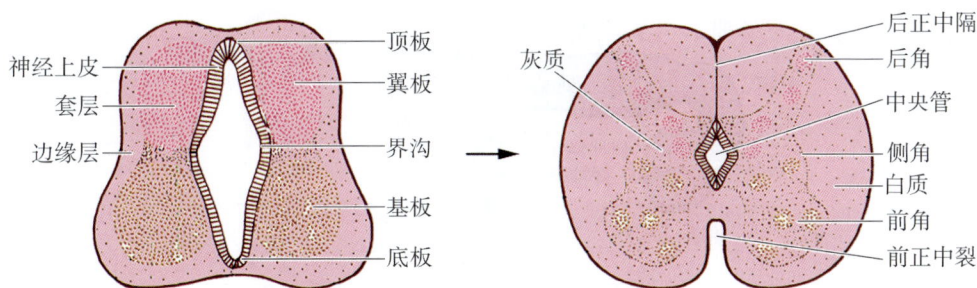

图 26-3 脊髓的发生示意图

胚胎第 3 个月之前,脊髓与脊柱等长,其下端可达脊柱的尾骨。第 3 个月后,由于脊柱增长比脊髓快,脊柱逐渐超越脊髓向尾端延伸,脊髓的位置相对上移。至出生前,脊髓下端与第 3 腰椎平齐,仅以终丝与尾骨相连。由于节段分布的脊神经均在胚胎早期形成,并从相应节段的椎间孔穿出,当脊髓位置相对上移后,脊髓颈段以下的脊神经根便越来越斜向尾侧,至腰、骶和尾段的脊神经根则在椎管内垂直下行,与终丝共同组成马尾(图 26-4)。

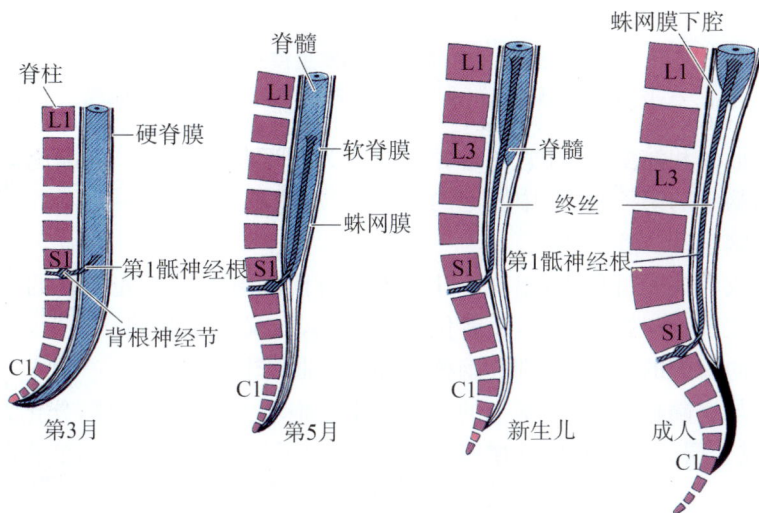

图 26-4 脊髓发育与脊柱的关系示意图

三、脑的发生

脑起源于神经管的头段。

(一) 脑泡的形成和演变

胚胎第 4 周末,神经管头段形成三个膨大,即初级脑泡,由前向后分别为前脑泡、中脑泡和菱脑泡。至第 5 周时,前脑泡的头端向两侧膨大,形成左右两个端脑,而菱脑泡演则变为头侧的后脑和尾侧的末脑。至此,形成了 5 个次级脑泡。随后,端脑演变为大脑两半球,前脑泡的尾端则形成间脑；中脑泡变化不大，演变为中脑；后脑演变为脑桥和小脑；末脑演变为延髓（图 26-5）。

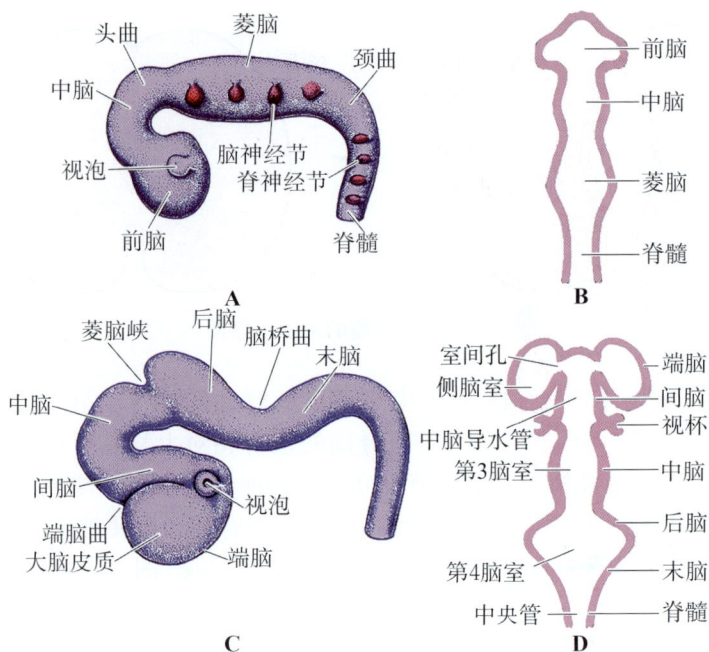

图 26-5 脑的各部发生模式图
A、B.第 4 周；C、D.第 6 周；A、C.侧面观；B、D.冠状切面观

随着脑泡的形成和演变，神经管的管腔也演变为各部位的脑室。前脑泡的腔演变为左右两个侧脑室和间脑中的第三脑室；中脑泡的腔很小，形成狭窄的中脑导水管；菱脑泡的腔则演变为宽大的第四脑室（图 26-5）。

在脑泡的形成和演变过程中，出现了几个不同方向的弯曲。首先出现的是凸向背侧的颈曲和头曲。前者位于脑与脊髓之间，后者位于中脑部，故又称中脑曲。之后，在脑桥和端脑处又出现了两个凸向腹侧的弯曲，分别称脑桥曲和端脑曲（图 26-5）。

脑壁的演化与脊髓相似，其侧壁上的神经上皮细胞增生并向侧迁移，分化为成神经细胞和成胶质细胞，形成套层。由于套层的增厚，侧壁被分成了翼板和基板。端脑和间脑的侧壁大部分形成翼板，基板较小。端脑套层中的大部分细胞都迁至外表面，形成大脑皮质；少部分细胞聚集成团，形成神经核。中脑、后脑和末脑中的套层细胞多聚集成细胞团或细胞柱，形成各种神经核。翼板中的神经核多为感觉中继核，基板中的神经核多为运动核。

（二）大脑皮质的发生

大脑皮质由端脑套层内的成神经细胞迁移和分化而来。大脑皮质的种系发生分三个阶段，即最早出现的古皮质，继之出现的旧皮质和最晚出现的新皮质。海马和齿状回是最早出现的皮质结构，相当于古皮质。胚胎第 7 周时，在纹状体的外侧，大量成神经细胞聚集并分化，形成梨状皮质，相当于旧皮质。旧皮质出现后不久，神经上皮细胞分裂增殖，分批分期地迁至表层并分化为神经元，形成了新皮质，这是大脑皮质中出现最晚、面积最大的部分。由于成神经细胞分批分期地产生和迁移，皮质中的神经元呈层状排列。越早产生和迁移的细胞，其位置越深。胎儿出生时,新皮质已形成6层结构。古皮质和旧皮质的分层无一定规律性,有的分层不明显,有的分为3层。

(三)小脑皮质的发生

小脑起源于后脑翼板背侧部的菱唇。左右两菱唇在中线融合,形成小脑板,这就是小脑的原基(图26-6)。胚胎第12周时,小脑板的两外侧部膨大,形成小脑半球;板的中部变细,形成小脑蚓。之后,横裂将小结和绒球分布从小脑蚓和小脑半球分出。由小结和绒球组成的绒球小结叶是小脑种系发生中最早出现的部分,故称原小脑,仍然保持着与前庭系统的联系。

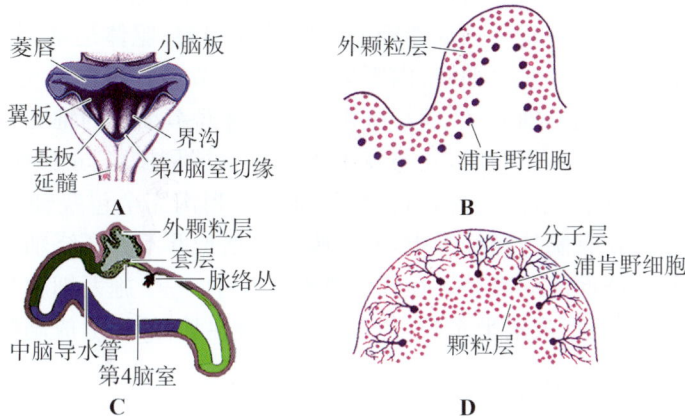

图26-6 小脑的发生模式图
A.第8周第4脑室顶切除后中脑和菱脑背面观;B.胚胎期小脑皮质;C.A的矢状切面;D.出生后小脑皮质

起初,小脑板由神经上皮、套层和边缘层组成。然后,神经上皮细胞增殖并通过套层迁至小脑板的外表面,形成了外颗粒层,此层细胞仍然保持分裂增殖的能力,在小脑表面形成一个细胞增殖区,使小脑表面迅速扩大并产生皱褶,形成小脑叶片。至第6个月,外颗粒层细胞开始分化出不同的细胞类型,部分细胞向内迁移,分化为颗粒细胞,位居浦肯野细胞层深面,构成内颗粒层。套层的外层成神经细胞分化为浦肯野细胞和高尔基细胞,构成浦肯野细胞层;内层的成神经细胞则聚集成团,分化为小脑白质中的核团。外颗粒层的细胞因大量迁出而数量减少,分化为篮状细胞和星形细胞,形成了小脑皮质的分子层。原来的内颗粒层则改称颗粒层(图26-6)。

四、神经节和周围神经的发生

(一)神经节的发生

神经节起源于神经嵴。神经嵴细胞向两侧迁移,分列于神经管的背外侧并聚集成细胞团,分化为脑神经节和脊神经节。这些神经节均属感觉神经节。神经嵴细胞首先分化为成神经细胞和卫星细胞,再由成神经细胞分化为感觉神经元。成神经细胞最先长出两个突起,成为双极神经元。由于细胞体各面的不均等生长,使两个突起的起始部逐渐靠拢,最后合二为一,于是双极神经元变成假单极神经元。卫星细胞是一种神经胶质细胞,包绕在神经元胞体的周围。神经节周围的间充质分化为结缔组织的被膜,包绕整个神经节。

位于胸段的神经嵴,有部分细胞迁至背主动脉的背外侧,形成两列节段性排列的神经节,即交感神经节。这些神经节通过纵行的神经纤维彼此相连,形成两条纵行的交感链。节内的部分细胞迁至主动脉腹侧,形成主动脉前交感神经节。节中的部分神经嵴细胞首先分化为交感成神经细胞,再由此分化为多极的交感神经节细胞。节中的另一部分则神经嵴细胞分化为卫星细胞。交感神经节的外周也有由间充质分化来的结缔组织被膜。

副交感神经节的起源问题尚有争议。有人认为副交感神经节中的神经细胞来自中枢神经系统的原基,即神经管,也有人认为来源于脑神经节中的成神经细胞。

(二) 周围神经的发生

周围神经由感觉神经纤维和运动神经纤维构成。这些神经纤维由神经元的突起和施万细胞构成。感觉神经纤维中的突起是感觉神经节细胞的周围突;躯体运动神经纤维中的突起是脑干及脊髓灰质前角运动神经元的轴突;内脏运动神经的节前纤维中的突起是脊髓灰质侧角和脑干内脏运动核中神经元的轴突,节后纤维则是植物神经节细胞的轴突。

施万细胞由神经嵴细胞分化而成,并与发生中的轴突或周围突同步增殖和迁移。施万细胞与突起相贴处凹陷,形成一条深沟,沟内包埋着轴突。当沟完全包绕轴突时,施万细胞与轴突间形成一扁的系膜。在有髓神经纤维中,此系膜不断增长并不断环绕轴突,于是在轴突外周形成了由多层细胞膜环绕而成的髓鞘。在无髓神经纤维中,一个施万细胞与多条轴突相贴,并形成多条深沟包绕轴突,也形成扁平系膜,但系膜不环绕生长,故不形成髓鞘。

五、垂体和松果体的发生

(一) 垂体的发生

垂体是由两个截然不同的原基共同发育而成的。腺垂体来自拉特克囊,神经垂体来自神经垂体芽(图 26-7)。

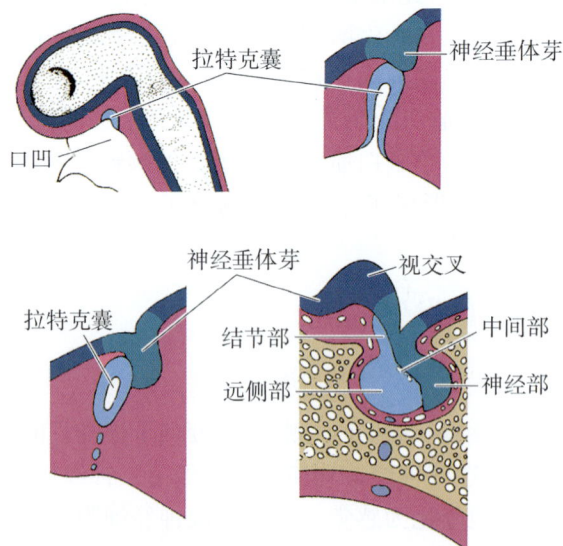

图 26-7　垂体的发生模式图

胚胎发育至第 4 周时,口凹顶的外胚层上皮向背侧下陷,形成一囊状突起,称拉特克囊。稍后,间脑的底部神经外胚层向腹侧突出,形成一漏斗状突起,称神经垂体芽。拉特克囊和神经垂体芽逐渐增长并相互接近。至第2月末，拉特克囊的根部退化消失，其远端长大并与神经垂体芽相贴。神经垂体芽的远端膨大，形成神经垂体；其起始部变细，形成漏斗柄。之后，囊的前壁迅速增大，形成垂体远侧部。从垂体远侧部向上长出一结节状突起并包绕漏斗柄，形成垂体的结节部。拉特克囊的后壁生长缓慢，形成垂体的中间部。拉特克囊腔大部消失，只残留一小的裂隙。腺垂体中分化出多种腺细胞，神经垂体则主要由神经纤维和神经胶质细胞构成。

（二）松果体的发生

胚胎第7周，间脑顶部向背侧突出，形成一囊状突起，即松果体原基。囊壁细胞增生，囊腔消失，形成一实质性松果样器官，即松果体。其中的松果体细胞和神经胶质细胞均由神经上皮分化而来。

六、神经系统的常见畸形

1. 神经管缺陷

这是由神经管闭合不全所引起的一类先天畸形，主要表现是脑和脊髓的异常，并常伴有颅骨和脊柱的异常。正常情况下，胚胎第4周末，神经沟（包括两端的神经孔）应完全闭合。如果失去了脊索的诱导作用或受到环境致畸因子的影响，神经沟就不能正常闭合为神经管。如果头侧的神经沟未闭，就会形成无脑畸形；如果尾侧的神经沟未闭，就会形成脊髓裂。无脑畸形常伴有颅顶骨发育不全，称露脑；脊髓裂常伴有相应节段的脊柱裂。

2. 脑积水

脑积水是一种比较多见的先天畸形，多由脑室系统发育障碍、脑脊液生成和吸收失去平衡所致，其中以中脑导水管和室间孔狭窄或闭锁最为常见。由于脑脊液不能正常流通循环，致使阻塞处以上的脑室或蛛网膜下腔中积存大量液体，前者称脑内脑积水，后者称脑外脑积水。其临床特征主要是颅脑增大，颅骨变薄，颅缝变宽。

第二节　眼 的 发 生

一、眼球的发生

胚胎第4周，前脑两侧突出左、右两个视泡。视泡远端膨大，贴近表面外胚层，并凹陷形成双层杯状结构，称视杯。视泡近端变细，称视柄，与前脑分化成的间脑相连。与此同时，表面外胚层在视泡的诱导下增厚，形成晶状体板。随后晶状体板凹陷入视杯内，渐与表面外胚层脱离，发育成晶状体泡（图26-8）。在视杯内与晶状体泡之间、视杯周围及其与表面外胚层之间充填有间充质。眼的各部分就是由视杯与视柄、晶状体泡及它们周围的间充质进一步发育形成的。

（一）视网膜和视神经的发生

视杯分为内、外两层。外层分化为视网膜色素上皮层；内层增厚，其结构与脑泡壁类似，分化形成视杆细胞、视锥细胞、双极细胞和节细胞等。两层之间的视泡腔变窄，最后消失，于是两层直接相贴，构成视网膜视部。在视杯口边缘部，内层上皮不增厚，与外层分化的色素上皮相

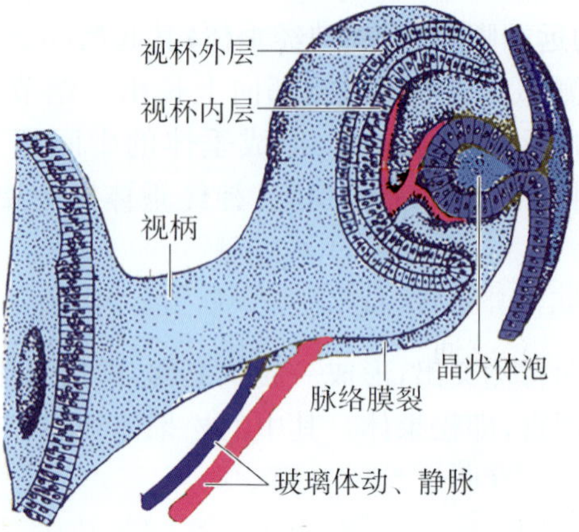

图 26-8 视杯与晶状体的发生模式图(第 5 周)

贴,并在晶状体泡与角膜之间的间充质内延伸,形成睫状体与虹膜的上皮。睫状体内层上皮分化为非色素上皮,虹膜内层上皮分化为色素上皮。虹膜的外层色素上皮层还分化出虹膜中的瞳孔括约肌和瞳孔开大肌。

胚胎第 5 周,视杯及视柄下方向内凹陷,形成一条纵沟,称脉络膜裂。脉络膜裂内含间充质和玻璃体动、静脉,为玻璃体和晶状体的发育提供营养。玻璃体动脉还发出分支营养视网膜。脉络膜裂于胚胎第 7 周封闭。玻璃体动、静脉穿经玻璃体的一段退化,并遗留一残迹称玻璃体管,而近段则成为视网膜中央动、静脉(图 26-9)。视柄与视杯相连,也分内、外两层,两层之间夹一腔隙。随着视网膜的发育分化,节细胞的轴突向视柄内层聚集,视柄内层逐渐增厚,并与外层融合,两层之间的腔隙消失。视柄最终演变为视神经。

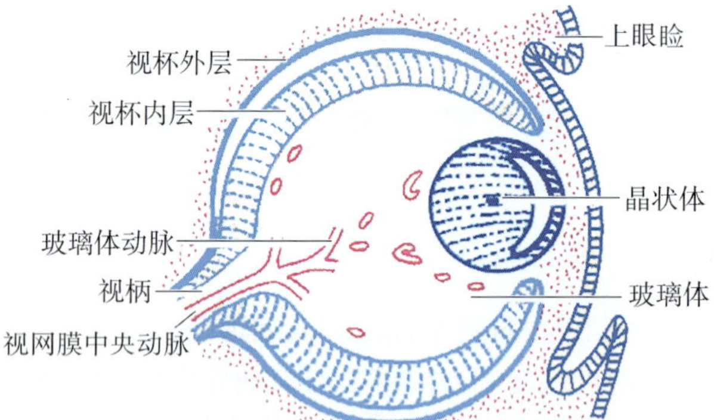

图 26-9 眼球与眼睑的发生模式图(第 7 周)

(二) 晶状体、角膜和眼房的发生

晶状体由晶状体泡演变而成(图 26-8、图 26-9)。最初,晶状体泡由单层上皮组成。前壁细胞呈立方形,分化为晶状体上皮;后壁细胞呈高柱状,并逐渐向前壁方向伸长,形成初级晶状体纤维。泡腔逐渐缩小,直至消失,晶状体变为实体的结构。此后,晶状体赤道区的上皮细胞不断增生、变长,形成次级晶状体纤维。原有的初级晶状体纤维及其胞核逐渐退化,形成晶状体核。新的次级晶状体纤维逐层添加到晶状体核的周围，晶状体及晶状体核逐渐增大。此过程持续终身，但随年龄的增长速度减慢，故晶状体核可区分为胚核、胎核、婴儿核及成人核等。

在晶状体泡的诱导下，与其相对的表面外胚层分化为角膜上皮。在晶状体泡与角膜上皮之间充填的间充质内出现一个腔，即前房。角膜上皮后面的间充质分化为角膜的其余各层。晶状体前面的间充质形成一层膜，周边部较厚，以后形成虹膜的基质；中央部较薄，封闭视杯口，称为瞳孔膜。虹膜与睫状体形成后，虹膜、睫状体与晶状体之间形成后房。出生前瞳孔膜被吸收而消失，前、后房经瞳孔相连通。

（三）血管膜和巩膜的发生

视杯周围的间充质分为内、外两层。内层富含血管和色素细胞，分化成眼球壁的血管膜。血管膜的大部分贴在视网膜外面，即为脉络膜；少部分贴在视杯口边缘的则分化为虹膜基质和睫状体的主体。外层较致密，分化为巩膜。脉络膜与巩膜分别与视神经周围的软脑膜和硬脑膜相连续。

二、眼睑和泪腺的发生

胚胎第7周时，眼球前方与角膜上皮毗邻的表面外胚层形成上、下两个皱褶，分别发育为上、下眼睑。反折到眼睑内面的表面外胚层分化为复层柱状的结膜上皮，与角膜上皮相延续。眼睑外面的表面外胚层则分化为表皮。皱褶内的间充质则分化为眼睑的其他结构。第10周时，上、下眼睑的边缘互相融合，至第7或第8个月时才重新张开。

泪腺的发育较晚，由表面外胚层上皮下陷而形成，出生后6周才具有分泌泪液的功能。

三、眼的常见畸形

1. 虹膜缺损
若脉络膜裂在虹膜处未完全闭合，造成虹膜下方缺损，致使圆形的瞳孔呈钥匙孔样，称虹膜缺损。此种畸形严重者可延伸到睫状体，视网膜和视神经，并常伴有眼的其他异常。

2. 瞳孔膜存留
若覆盖在晶状体前面的瞳孔膜在出生前吸收不完全，致使在晶状体前方保留着残存的结缔组织网，称瞳孔膜存留。出生后可随年龄增长而逐渐吸收。若残存的瞳孔膜影响视力，可手术剔除。

3. 先天性白内障
出生前晶状体不透明，多为遗传性，也可由于妊娠早期感染风疹病毒而引起。

4. 先天性青光眼
巩膜静脉窦发育异常或缺失，致使房水回流受阻，眼压增高，最终可导致视网膜损伤而失明。基因突变或母亲妊娠早期感染风疹病毒是产生此畸形的主要原因。

5. 独眼、小眼和无眼畸形
如果两侧视泡在中线合并，则产生独眼畸形；如果视泡发育受阻或视泡未发生，则分别产生小眼和无眼畸形。

第三节 耳的发生

一、内耳的发生

胚胎第 4 周,神经板上的表面外胚层变厚,形成听板。随后听板向下内陷到间充质中,形成听窝。听窝最终从外胚层分离,形成一个囊,即听泡(图 26 - 10)。听泡初为梨形,以后向背腹方向延伸增大,分为背侧的前庭囊和腹侧的耳蜗囊,并在背端内侧长出一小囊管,为内淋巴管。前庭囊形成三个半规管和椭圆囊的上皮;耳蜗囊形成球囊和膜蜗管的上皮。听泡及其周围的间充质演变为内耳膜迷路(图 26 - 11)。胚胎第 3 个月时,膜迷路周围的间充质分化成一个软骨囊,包绕膜迷路。约在胚胎第 5 个月时,软骨囊骨化成骨迷路。于是膜迷路就完全被套在骨迷路内,两者间仅隔以狭窄的外淋巴间隙。

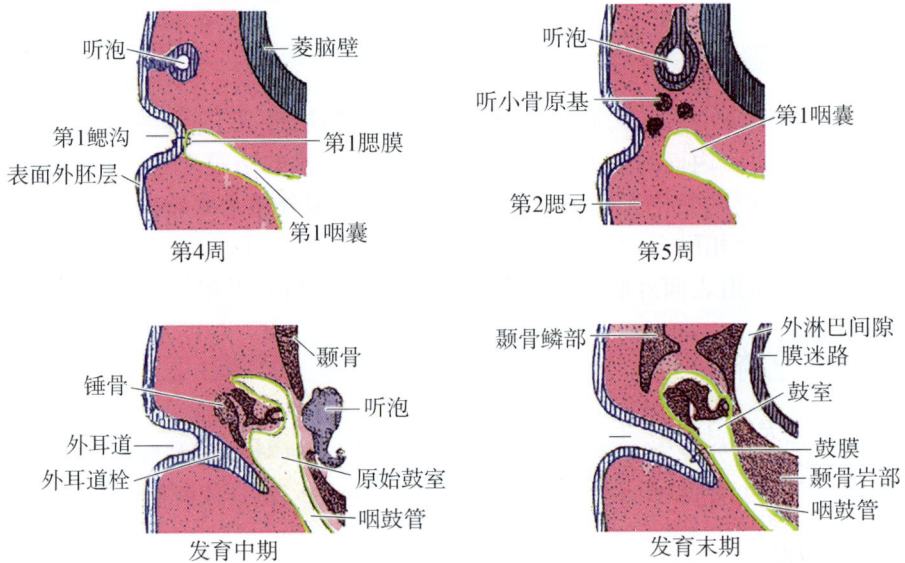

图 26 - 10 耳的发生模式图

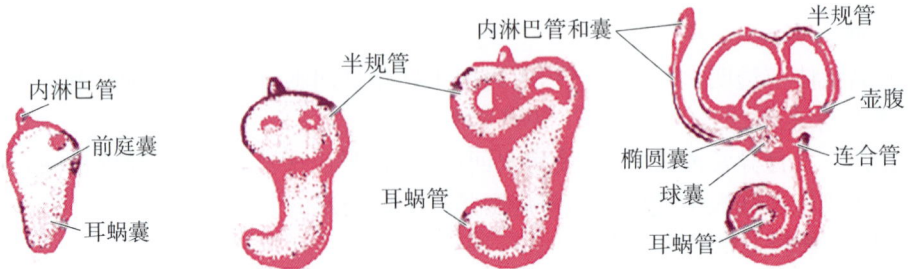

图 26 - 11 听泡的发育模式图(第 5~8 周)

二、中耳的发生

胚胎第9周时,第1咽囊向背外侧扩伸,远侧盲端膨大成鼓室,近端细窄形成咽鼓管。鼓室内胚层与第1鳃沟底的外胚层相贴,分别形成鼓膜内、外上皮,两者之间的间充质形成鼓膜的结缔组织。鼓室周围的间充质分化成三块听小骨,听小骨渐突入鼓室内(图26-10)。

三、外耳的发生

外耳道由第1鳃沟演变形成。胚胎第2个月末,第1鳃沟向内深陷,形成漏斗状管道,以后演变成外耳道外侧段。管道的底部外胚层细胞增生成一上皮细胞板,称外耳道栓。胚胎第7个月时,外耳道栓内部细胞退化吸收,形成管腔,成为外耳道的内侧段(图26-10)。

胚胎第6周时,第1鳃沟周围的间充质增生,形成6个结节状隆起,称耳丘。后来这些耳丘围绕外耳道口合并,演变成耳郭(图26-12)。

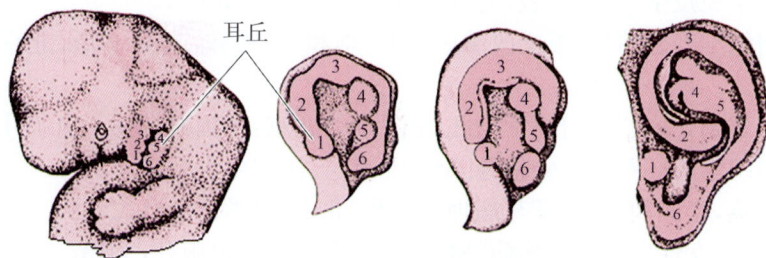

图26-12　耳郭的发生模式图

四、耳的常见畸形

最常见的是先天性耳聋和耳郭畸形。内、中、外耳的发育异常均可导致先天性耳聋,如外耳道闭锁、中耳鼓室闭锁、听小骨发生异常造成的听骨链僵直、内耳骨迷路或膜迷路发育异常等。先天性耳聋大多是遗传因素引起,但有些是由于环境致畸因子的作用如妊娠早期感染风疹病毒、妊娠后期强噪声等。

（岳海源）

参考文献

［１］ 李继承,邵淑娟.组织学与胚胎学［M］.10 版.北京:人民卫生出版社,2024.

［２］ 陈罡,余水长,祝辉.组织学与胚胎学［M］.4 版.北京:科学出版社,2023.

［３］ 周德山,张雷,张宏权.组织学与胚胎学［M］.5 版.北京:北京大学医学出版社,2023.

［４］ 曹雪涛.医学免疫学［M］.8 版.北京:人民卫生出版社,2024.

［５］ 梅舍尔.组织学与胚胎学:英文改编版［M］.李和,陈活彝,改编.2 版.北京:科学出版社,
2021.

［６］ 吴春云,李娟娟,马太芳.组织学与胚胎学［M］.北京:中国科学技术出版社,2020.

［７］ 李继承.组织学与胚胎学实验指导［M］.北京:人民卫生出版社,2018.

［８］ 贾筱琴,郑英,李国利.组织学与病理学［M］.北京:科学出版社,2018.

［９］ 李旭,徐丛剑.女性生殖系统疾病［M］.北京:人民卫生出版社,2015.

［10］ 李和,黄辰.生殖系统［M］.北京:人民卫生出版社,2015.

［11］ 李和,李继承.组织学与胚胎学［M］.北京:人民卫生出版社,2015.

［12］ 吴春云,林荣安.Histology practical handbook［M］.北京:科学出版社,2014.

［13］ 成令忠,钟翠平,蔡文琴.现代组织学［M］.上海:上海科学技术文献出版社,2003.

［14］ Ovalle WK, Nahirney PC. Netter's essential histology: with correlated histopathology
［M］. 3rd ed. Amsterdam: Elsevier, 2020.

［15］ Lowe JS, Anderson PG, Anderson SI. Stevens & Lowe's human histology［M］. 5th
ed. Philadelphia: Elsevier, 2019.

［16］ Mescher AL. Junqueira's basic histology: text & atlas［M］. 16th ed. New York:
McGraw-Hill Medical, 2021.

［17］ Gartener LP, Hiatt JL. Color Atlas and Text of Histology［M］. 7th ed.
Philadelphia: Wolters Kluwer, 2018.

［18］ Dudek RW. High-yield histopathology［M］. 2nd ed. Baltimore: Lippincott Williams
& Wilkins, 2013.

［19］ Pawlina W. Histology: A text and atlas with correlated cell and molecular biology
［M］. 7th ed. Philadelphia: Wolters Kluwer, 2016.

［20］ Gartener LP, Hiatt JL. Color textbook of histology［M］. 3rd ed. Amsterdam:
Elsevier, 2007.

［21］ Ge T, Yuan L, Xu L, et al. Coiled-coil domain containing 159 is required for
spermatid head and tail assembly in mice［J］. Biol Reprod, 2024,110(5):877 − 894.

［22］ Du L, Chen W, Cheng Z, et al. Novel Gene Regulation in Normal and Abnormal Spermatogenesis [J]. Cells, 2021,10(3):666.

［23］ Neto FT, Bach PV, Najari BB, et al. Spermatogenesis in humans and its affecting factors [J]. Semin Cell Dev Biol, 2016,59:10 - 26.

［24］ Reynolds SD, Giangreco A, Power JH, et al. Neuroepithelial bodies of pulmonary airways serve as a reservoir of progenitor cells capable of epithelial regeneration [J]. Am J Pathol, 2000,156(1):269 - 278.

［25］ McDaniel ML, Kwon G, Hill JR, et al. Cytokines and nitric oxide in islet inflammation and diabetes [J]. Proc Soc Exp Biol Med, 1996,211(1):24 - 32.